Surgery
REVIEW

THIRD EDITION

Surgery
REVIEW

THIRD EDITION

MARTIN A. MAKARY, MD, MPH, FACS

Associate Professor of Surgery, Health Policy and Management
Johns Hopkins University School of Medicine
Director, Johns Hopkins Pancreas Islet Transplantation Center
Director, Surgical Quality and Safety, Johns Hopkins Hospital
Baltimore, Maryland

MICHOL A. COOPER, MD, PHD

General Surgery Resident
Department of Surgery, Johns Hopkins University School
  of Medicine
Baltimore, Maryland

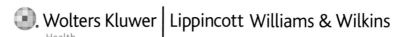

Wolters Kluwer | Lippincott Williams & Wilkins
Health

Philadelphia • Baltimore • New York • London
Buenos Aires • Hong Kong • Sydney • Tokyo

Acquisitions Editor: Keith Donnellan
Product Manager: Brendan Huffman
Vendor Manager: Bridgett Dougherty
Senior Manufacturing Manager: Beth Welsh
Design Coordinator: Stephen Druding
Production Service: Integra Software Services Pvt. Ltd.

Library of Congress Cataloging-in-Publication Data
Surgery review.
  Surgery review / [edited by] Martin A. Makary, Michol A. Cooper. — Third edition.
      p. ; cm.
  Preceded by General surgery review / [edited by] Martin A. Makary. 2nd ed. c2008.
  Includes index.
  ISBN 978-1-4511-8405-1
  I. Makary, Martin A., editor of compilation.   II. Cooper, Michol A., editor of compilation.   III. Title.
  [DNLM: 1. Surgical Procedures, Operative—Examination Questions.   2. Clinical Medicine—methods—Examination Questions.   3. Diagnostic Techniques and Procedures—Examination Questions.   4. Signs and Symptoms—Examination Questions. WO 18.2]
  RD37.2
  617.0076—dc23
                                                                                              2013028380

Care has been taken to confirm the accuracy of the information presented and to describe generally accepted practices. However, the authors, editors, and publisher are not responsible for errors or omissions or for any consequences from application of the information in this book and make no warranty, expressed or implied, with respect to the currency, completeness, or accuracy of the contents of the publication. Application of the information in a particular situation remains the professional responsibility of the practitioner.

The authors, editors, and publisher have exerted every effort to ensure that drug selection and dosage set forth in this text are in accordance with current recommendations and practice at the time of publication. However, in view of ongoing research, changes in government regulations, and the constant flow of information relating to drug therapy and drug reactions, the reader is urged to check the package insert for each drug for any change in indications and dosage and for added warnings and precautions. This is particularly important when the recommended agent is a new or infrequently employed drug.

Some drugs and medical devices presented in the publication have Food and Drug Administration (FDA) clearance for limited use in restricted research settings. It is the responsibility of the health care provider to ascertain the FDA status of each drug or device planned for use in their clinical practice.

To purchase additional copies of this book, call our customer service department at (800) 638-3030 or fax orders to (301) 223-2320. International customers should call (301) 223-2300.

Visit Lippincott Williams & Wilkins on the Internet at: LWW.com. Lippincott Williams & Wilkins customer service representatives are available from 8:30 am to 6:00 pm, EST.

10   9   8   7   6   5   4   3   2   1

To the Halsted residents of the Johns Hopkins Hospital, whose enthusiasm for learning has advanced the great heritage of surgical education.

Nita Ahuja, MD
Associate Professor of Surgery, Oncology, and Urology
Johns Hopkins University School of Medicine
Chief of the Section of GI Oncology, Breast,
    Melanoma and Endocrine Tumors
Director, Soft Tissue Sarcomas and
    Director, Peritoneal Surface Malignancies Program
Baltimore, Maryland

Adesola Akinkuotu, MD
Assistant Resident
Department of Surgery
Johns Hopkins Hospital
Baltimore, Maryland

Dean J. Arnaoutakis, MD
Assistant Resident, Department of Surgery
Johns Hopkins Hospital
Baltimore, Maryland

J.W. Awori Hayanga, MD, MPH
Cardiothoracic Transplant Fellow
University of Pittsburgh Medical Center
Pittsburgh, Pennsylvania

David Axelrod, MD, MBA
Assistant Professor of Surgery
Dartmouth University School of Medicine
Manchester, New Hampshire

Talia B. Baker, MD
Associate Professor of Surgery
Northwestern University School of Medicine
Director, Living Donor Liver Transplant Program
Comprehensive Transplant Center
Chicago, Illinois

Adrian Barbul, MD, FACS
Vice-Chair
Department of Surgery
Surgical Director, Operating Rooms
Washington Hospital Center
Washington, DC

Jennifer L. Bennett, BA
Department of Medicine
Johns Hopkins University School of Medicine
Baltimore, Maryland

Denis D. Bensard, MD
Professor of Surgery
University of Colorado School of Medicine
Chief of Pediatric Surgery
Denver Health Medical Center
Denver, Colorado

George Berberian, MD
Cardiothoracic Surgeon
Southeast Health
Cape Girardeau, Missouri

Danielle A. Bischof, MD, FRCSC
Surgical Oncology Fellow
Department of Surgery
Johns Hopkins University
Baltimore, Maryland

Debashish Bose, MD, PhD
Assistant Professor of Surgery
University of Central Florida College of Medicine
Director, The Pancreas Center
MD Anderson Cancer Center Orlando
Orlando, Florida

Karen E. Boyle, MD, FACS
Clinical Instructor of Urology
George Washington University School of
    Medicine
Washington, DC

Caroline Chebli, MD
Kennedy-White Orthopaedic Center
Sarasota, Florida

Joseph E. Chebli, MD, FACS
Staff Surgeon
Overlake Metabolic and Bariatric Surgery
Bellevue, Washington

Herbert Chen, MD, FACS
Chairman, Division of General Surgery
Layton F. Rikkers M.D. Chair in Surgical
    Leadership
Professor of Surgery
Vice-Chair of Research Department of Surgery
University of Wisconsin
Madison, Wisconsin

Albert Chi, MD
Assistant Professor of Surgery
Division of Acute Care Surgery
Johns Hopkins Hospital
Baltimore, Maryland

Alan P.B. Dackiw, MD, PhD
Assistant Professor of Surgery
Johns Hopkins University School of Medicine
Baltimore, Maryland

Estefania de la Paz Nicolau, MD, MPH
Johns Hopkins Bloomberg School of Public
    Health
Baltimore, Maryland

Nestor F. Esnaola, MD, MPH, MBA
Attending Surgeon, Fox Chase Cancer Center
Chief, Division of Surgical Oncology
    and Vice Chair of Clinical and Academic
    Affairs
Department of Surgery
Temple University School of Medicine
Philadelphia, Pennsylvania

Carole Fakhry, MD, MPH
Assistant Professor of Otolaryngology
Head and Neck Surgery
Johns Hopkins University School of
    Medicine
Baltimore, Maryland

Samir M. Fakhry, MD, FACS
Charles F. Crews Professor and Chief,
    Physician Leader, Surgical Acute and
    Critical Care Surgery
Department of Surgery
Medical University of South Carolina
Charleston, South Carolina

Robert J. Feezor, MD, FACS
Assistant Professor of Vascular Surgery
    and Endovascular Therapy
Department of Surgery
University of Florida
Gainesville, Florida

Jordan E. Fishman, MD, MPH
Surgical House Officer
Department of Surgery
New Jersey Medical School,
    Rutgers University
Newark, New Jersey

Lee A. Fleisher, MD, FACC
Robert Dunning Dripps
Professor and Chair, Department of Anesthesiology
    and Critical Care
Professor of Medicine
Perelman School of Medicine
University of Pennsylvania Health System
Philadelphia, Pennsylvania

Gary L. Gallia, MD, PhD
Assistant Professor of Neurosurgery, Otolaryngology
Head and Neck Surgery, and Oncology
Department of Neurosurgery
Johns Hopkins University School of Medicine
Director, Neurosurgery Skull Base Center
Baltimore, Maryland

Ruchi Garg, MD
Associate Clinical Professor
Department of Ob/Gyn
George Washington University
Medical Director, Minimally Invasive Gynecologic
    Surgery Division and Fellowship
INOVA Fairfax Hospital
Gynecologic Oncologist
Mid-Atlantic Pelvic Surgery Associates
Annandale, Virgiania

Ana L. Gleisner, MD
Department of Surgery
Johns Hopkins University School of Medicine
Baltimore, Maryland

Bradley J. Goldstein, MD, PhD
Assistant Professor, Otolaryngology
Investigator, Interdisciplinary Stem Cell Institute
Miller School of Medicine
University of Miami
Miami, Florida

Jeffrey M. Hardacre, MD, FACS
Section Head, Pancreatic Surgery
University Hospitals Seidman Cancer Center
Associate Professor of Surgery
Case Western Reserve University School of Medicine
Cleveland, Ohio

Richard J. Hendrickson, MD, FACS, FAAP
Associate Professor of Surgery
University of Missouri-Kansas City School of
    Medicine
Director, Small Intestinal Rehabilitation
Children's Mercy Hospital and Clinics
Kansas City, Missouri

Michael G. House, MD
Assistant Professor
Department of Surgery
Indiana University
School of Medicine
Indianapolis, Indiana

Lisa Jacobs, MD
Assistant Professor of Surgery
Division of Surgical Oncology
Johns Hopkins University School of Medicine
Baltimore, Maryland

Matthew L. Kashima, MD, MPH
Assistant Professor of Otolaryngology
Chair, Department of Otolaryngology
Head and Neck Surgery
Baltimore, Maryland

Edmund S. Kassis, MD
Assistant Professor Surgery
Division of Thoracic Surgery
The Ohio State University Medical Center
Columbus, Ohio

Lisa M. Kodadek, MD
Resident in General Surgery
Johns Hopkins Hospital
Baltimore, Maryland

Jeremy D. Kukafka, MD
Assistant Professor of Clinical Anesthesiology
    and Critical Care Cardiovascular Thoracic
    Anesthesia
Perelman School of Medicine
University of Pennsylvania Health System
Philadelphia, Pennsylvania

Sandhya Lagoo-Deenadayalan, MD
Assistant Professor of Surgery
Duke University School of Medicine
Durham, North Carolina

Joshua L. Levine, MD
Division of Plastic Surgery
Memorial Sloan-Kettering Cancer Center
New York, New York

Anne O. Lidor, MD, MPH
Associate Professor of Surgery
Johns Hopkins University School of Medicine
Surgical Clerkship and Curriculum Director
Director, Minimally Invasive Surgery Fellowship
Baltimore, Maryland

Nicole E. Lopez, MD
Department of Surgery
University of California, San Diego
San Diego, California

Ying Wei Lum, MD
Assistant Professor
Division of Vascular Surgery and Endovascular
    Therapy
Johns Hopkins University School of Medicine
Baltimore, Maryland
Section Director for Anatomy
Perdana University Graduate School of Medicine
Serdang, Malaysia

Heather G. Lyu, BA
Johns Hopkins University School of Medicine
Baltimore, Maryland

Thomas H. Magnuson, MD
Associate Professor of Surgery
Johns Hopkins University School of Medicine
Chair, Department of Surgery
Johns Hopkins
Bayview Medical Center
Baltimore, Maryland

Martin A. Makary, MD, MPH
Associate Professor of Surgery
Health Policy and Management
Johns Hopkins University School of Medicine
Director, Johns Hopkins Pancreas Islet
    Transplantation Center
Director, Surgical Quality and Safety
Johns Hopkins Hospital
Baltimore, Maryland

Michael R. Marohn, DO
Associate Professor of Surgery
Johns Hopkins University School of Medicine
Baltimore, Maryland

Justin B. Maxhimer, MD
Division of Plastic and Reconstructive Surgery
UCLA Medical Center
Los Angeles, California

Robert A. Meguid, MD, MPH
Assistant Professor of Surgery
Section of General Thoracic Surgery
Division of Cardiothoracic Surgery
Department of Surgery
University of Colorado School of Medicine
Aurora, Colorado

Genevieve Melton-Meaux, MA, MD, FACS, FASCRS
Associate Professor, Department of Surgery
Core Faculty, Institute for Health Informatics
University of Minnesota
Chief Medical Information Officer
University of Minnesota Physicians/University of Minnesota Medical Center
Minneapolis, Minnesota

Nicholas F. Montanaro, BSN
Department of General Surgery
University of Michigan Health Systems
University of Michigan School of Medicine
Ann Arbor, Michigan

Eric K. Nakakura, MD, PhD
Assistant Professor of Surgery
University of California, San Francisco
San Francisco, California

Peter R. Nelson, MD, MS
Associate Professor of Surgery and Molecular Pharmacology and Physiology
Morsani College of Medicine
University of South Florida
James A. Haley VA Medical Center
Tampa, Florida

Kathryn O'Keefe, MD
Cardiothoracic Surgery Fellow
The Ohio State University
Columbus, Ohio

Catherine Pesce, MD
Resident, Department of Surgery
Johns Hopkins University School of Medicine
Baltimore, Maryland

P. Pravin Reddy, MD
Midtown Aesthetic and Reconstructive Surgery
Atlanta, Georgia

Peter J. Pronovost, MD, PhD
Professor of Anesthesiology and Critical Care
Departments of Anesthesia, Surgery and Health Policy & Management
Johns Hopkins University School of Medicine
Baltimore, Maryland

Sashank K. Reddy, MD, PhD
Resident in Plastic and Reconstructive Surgery
Johns Hopkins Hospital
Baltimore, Maryland

Srinevas K. Reddy, MD
Department of Surgery
Duke University School of Medicine
Durham, North Carolina

Richard J. Redett, MD
Associate Professor and Program Director, Johns Hopkins/University of Maryland Plastic Surgery Residency
Department of Plastic Surgery
Johns Hopkins University School of Medicine
Baltimore, Maryland

Joseph J. Ricotta II, MD, MS, FACS
Chair, Department of Vascular Surgery and Endovascular Surgery
Director, Heart and Vascular Institute
Northside Hospital
Atlanta, Georgia

Joseph V. Sakran, MD, MPH
Assistant Professor of Surgery
Director, Global Health & Disaster Preparedness
Medical University of South Carolina
Charleston, South Carolina

J.R. Salameh, MD, FACS
Clinical Associate Professor of Surgery
Georgetown University School of Medicine
Chairman, Department of Surgery
Virginia Hospital Center
Director, Center for Bariatric Surgery
Arlington, Virginia

Diane A. Schwartz, MD
Trauma, Acute Care Surgery, and Surgical Critical Care
Johns Hopkins University School of Medicine
Bayview
Baltimore, Maryland

Steven J. Schwartz, MD
Associate Professor of Surgery
University of Maryland School of Medicine
Director, Critical Care Medicine
Baltimore Washington Medical Center
Clinical Assistant Professor of Anesthesia and Adult Critical Care
Johns Hopkins University School of Medicine
Baltimore, Maryland

Molly Sebastian, MD
Fellow in Laparoscopic Surgery
Johns Hopkins University School of Medicine
Baltimore, Maryland

Jason K. Sicklick, MD
Assistant Professor of Surgery
Division of Surgical Oncology
Moores UCSD Cancer Center
University of California, San Diego
UC San Diego Health System
San Diego, California

Vijay A. Singh, MD
Cardiovascular and Thoracic Surgery
Southside Hospital/Long Island Jewish Medical
    Hospital
Director, Thoracic Surgery Huntington Hospital
Assistant Professor, Hofstra North Shore-Long
    Island Jewish School of Medicine
Bay shore, New York

Sunil Singhal, MD
Assistant Professor of Surgery
Department of Surgery
University of Pennsylvania School of Medicine
Philadelphia, Pennsylvania

Rebecca S. Sippel, MD, FACS
Associate Professor of Surgery
Chief of Endocrine Surgery
University of Wisconsin School of Medicine and
    Public Health
Madison, Wisconsin

Kimberley Eden Steele, MD
Assistant Professor of Surgery and
    Assistant Director of Surgical Clerkship
Johns Hopkins Bayview Medical Center
Baltimore, Maryland

Dora Syin, MD
Assistant Professor of Anesthesiology and Critical
    Care Medicine
Johns Hopkins University School of Medicine
Baltimore, Maryland

Vicente Valero III, MD
Halsted Resident
Department of Surgery
Johns Hopkins University School of
    Medicine
Baltimore, Maryland

Jon D. Vogel, MD
Associate Staff Surgeon
Department of Colorectal Surgery
The Cleveland Clinic
Cleveland, Ohio

Elizabeth C. Wick, MD
Assistant Professor of Surgery and
    Oncology
Johns Hopkins University School of
    Medicine
Baltimore, Maryland

Christopher L. Wolfgang, MD, PhD
Department of Surgery
Johns Hopkins University School of
    Medicine
Baltimore, Maryland

Tinsay A. Woreta, MD, MPH
Assistant Professor of Medicine
Division of Gastroenterology and Hepatology
Johns Hopkins University
Baltimore, Maryland

Kashif A. Zuberi, MD, MRCSI
Fellow in Minimally Invasive Surgery
General and Gastrointestinal Surgery
Johns Hopkins University School of
    Medicine
Baltimore, Maryland

The third edition of *Surgery Review*, as the first two editions, will find an expanding audience of surgeons in search of a concise publication with which to review the broad field of general surgery. The book is presented in outline form and each topic is preceded by a case presentation of a set of clinical circumstances. These clinical scenarios are then reviewed with a series of high-yield facts and sentences, in a Socratic fashion, that lends itself to a rapid review of the topic. Each case presentation is followed by a treatment regimen that represents current standard of care. The text basically covers general and GI surgery, but the surgical specialties are also included, as well as a section on anesthesia, trauma, and critical care. There is also a short section on basic science that should be familiar to the general surgeon as well as a section on ethics.

The book is relatively short and is easy to hold and manage, unlike the ponderous large surgical texts that in years past were used by medical students, trainees, and practicing surgeons. This book certainly is not a substitute for those large texts, but should be used by someone who has basic knowledge of general surgery and would like a rapid review. If one is researching a topic, disease, or operative procedure, one of the standard texts is essential. The trainee or surgeon who is looking to review a topic, about which they are already well versed, will find this book particularly useful.

Dr. Makary is an outstanding, well-trained general surgeon, whose career happens to be in an academic institution. He is a very busy surgeon however, and has recruited a large number of busy, active surgeons to participate in this text. The book has clearly found its niche, and this is the third edition of what will probably be many, many more. It is well written, well illustrated, and highly readable. It is an excellent contribution to the series of surgical texts currently available.

John L. Cameron, MD
The Alfred Blalock Distinguished Service Professor
Johns Hopkins University School of Medicine

Dear Colleague,

Many surgical texts are burdened with controversial teaching points, which can cloud the teaching of surgical fundamentals. While the frontier of surgical science is the livelihood of academia, many students and surgeons studying for recertification exams have insisted that they want to focus on the accepted standard of care, not what is controversial. To this end, we crafted clinical scenarios that mandate a surgical decision and highlight the standard of care. Our emphasis on the Socratic method and high-yield facts is designed to provide an easy-to-read text with a classic yet innovative method of learning and retention. The case-based questions present information in a practical way and the italicized pearls indicate "take-home" points. The book is designed to be versatile, serving as both a quick review and a companion to other major texts.

We are especially proud to present this book as the collected work of over 70 outstanding teachers. Each one was invited to contribute because they have received teaching awards or have a strong track record of excellence in teaching. They are "in-tune" with basic learning objectives and have expertise in their specialty area. The third edition also represents the incorporation of hundreds of suggestions by readers who provided feedback on the publisher's website. We also added several dedicated chapters to topics traditionally over-represented on exams.

In the spirit of community, we welcome any suggestions you may have to improve this book for future editions. We hope that this text will be an opportunity for you to solidify fundamental principles across the great field of surgery and that it may ultimately benefit your command of all areas of surgery as they apply to your patients.

Martin A. Makary, MD, MPH
Department of Surgery
Johns Hopkins University School of Medicine

Michol Cooper, MD, PhD
Department of Surgery
Johns Hopkins University School of Medicine

CONTENTS

1 | Neurosurgery

Gary L. Gallia

A 40-year-old male is brought to the emergency department by ambulance after a motor vehicle accident. On examination, he opens his eyes in response to voice, is confused, and follows commands. What is his Glasgow Coma Scale (GCS) score?

This patient's GCS = Eye³Verbal⁴Motor⁶ = 13.

Glasgow Coma Scale

- Assesses level of consciousness
- Appropriate for ≧4 years of age
- Range of scores: 3 to 15 (extubated); 3T to 11T (intubated)
- Coma is defined as a GCS ≦ 8

Points	Best eye opening	Best verbal response[a]	Best motor response
6	—	—	Obeys commands
5	—	Oriented	Localizes pain
4	Spontaneous	Confused	Withdraws to pain
3	To voice	Inappropriate	Flexor (decorticate)
2	To pain	Incomprehensible	Extensor (decerebrate)
1	None	None	None

[a]In an intubated patient, 1T is assigned for verbal response (if the patient in the above example was intubated, his GCS = E³V¹ᵀM⁶ = 10T)

A 60-year-old woman is struck by a motor vehicle and is brought to the emergency department by ambulance. On examination, her GCS is 6. The patient has no systemic injuries. A head CT scan demonstrates diffuse cerebral edema. What is the next step in the management of this patient?

Placement of an intracranial pressure (ICP) monitor.

Indications for Intracranial Pressure Monitoring

- GCS ≤ 8 after resuscitation and an abnormal head CT scan
- GCS ≤ 8 and a normal head CT scan but with ≥2 risk factors for intracranial hypertension, including age >40 years, SBP < 90 mmHg, and motor posturing
- Multi-system trauma with an altered level of consciousness where therapies for other injuries may have deleterious effects on ICP (i.e., high positive end-expiratory pressure, need for large volumes, etc.)

Intracranial Pressure Monitoring

- Options include intraventricular catheters (IVCs), subarachnoid bolts, intraparenchymal monitors, and subdural and epidural catheters
- A major contraindication to ICP monitor placement is coagulopathy
- Normal ICP in adults is 10 to 15 mmHg
- Ketamine increases ICP and should be avoided in patients with head injury

Brain edema is greatest 2 to 3 days following a head injury.

Cerebral Blood Flow and Cerebral Perfusion Pressure

- Normal cerebral blood flow (CBF) is 50 to 55 mL per 100 g/min
- Impaired neural function occurs with CBF < 23 mL per 100 g/min
- Ischemic penumbra (cells can be functionally salvaged with return of blood flow) occurs at 8 to 23 mL per 100 g/min.
- Irreversible damage occurs at CBF < 8 mL per 100 g/min
- CBF is difficult to quantitate and is measured with a specialized equipment
- CBF depends on cerebral perfusion pressure (CPP) which is related to ICP by the following equation
    - CPP = MAP (mean arterial pressure) − ICP
    - Normal CPP in adults is >50 mmHg

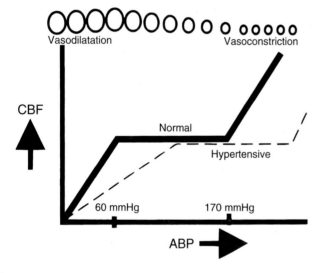

Cerebral perfusion pressure (CPP). Below 60 mmHg and above 170 mmHg, autoregulation of CPP breaks down. (With permission from O'Leary JP, Tabuenca A, eds. *Physiologic Basis of Surgery.* 4th ed. Philadelphia, PA: Wolters Kluwer Health/Lippincott Williams & Wilkins; 2007.)

Goals of Therapy for Intracranial Hypertension

- ICP < 20 mmHg
- CPP ≥ 60 mmHg

Intracranial Hypertension
- May see Cushing triad of hypertension, bradycardia, and respiratory irregularity
- Medical management includes elevation of the patient's head, sedation/paralysis, cerebrospinal fluid (CSF) drainage (when IVC utilized), osmotic therapy including mannitol and furosemide, hyperventilation (do not use prophylactically), barbiturate therapy, and hypothermia
- There is no role for steroids in head trauma
- The end result of uncontrolled intracranial hypertension is herniation

A unilaterally dilating pupil is the earliest sign of uncal herniation.

A 24-year-old man is brought to the emergency department following a motor vehicle crash with a GCS of 9. The patient's head CT demonstrates a 1-cm epidural hematoma (EDH). What is the next step in the management of this patient?

Emergent surgical evacuation is indicated for an EDH in a patient with compromised mental status.

Epidural Hematoma
- Collection of blood between skull and dura
- Usually associated with a skull fracture
- Source of bleeding is usually arterial (middle meningeal artery)
- Classic presentation is a brief post-traumatic loss of consciousness, followed by a several hour "lucid interval" (observed in only one-third of cases), then subsequent obtundation, contralateral hemiparesis, ipsilateral pupillary dilation, coma, and death
- Hyperdense biconvex (lenticular) shape on head CT scan

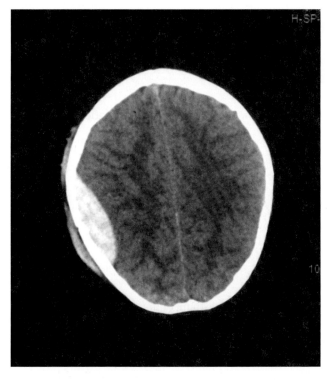
Epidural hematoma.

- Treatment is prompt surgical evacuation in most cases
- A small (<1 cm) EDH in an asymptomatic patient may resolve spontaneously and not require evacuation

The most common cause of an EDH is injury to the middle meningeal artery.

What is the usual source of bleeding in a subdural hematoma (SDH)?

Tearing of bridging cortical veins.

Subdural Hematoma

- Accumulation of blood between dura and underlying brain
- Usually due to torn bridging cortical veins
- Crescent shape on head CT scan

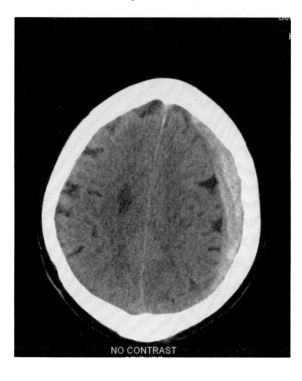

Subdural hematoma.

- With time, these lesions undergo clot lysis, organization, and neomembrane formation
- Density of the lesion changes with time:

Category	Density on CT scan	Time frame
Acute	Hyperdense	1–3 d
Subacute	Isodense	4 d to 3 wk
Chronic	Hypodense	>3 wk

- Mortality for acute SDH is greater than for an EDH
- Treatment is surgical evacuation for symptomatic SDH greater than 1 cm (at its thickest point)

A 20-year-old man is ejected during a high-speed motor vehicle crash. On arrival, he is hemodynamically stable with a GCS of 5T. His initial head CT is significant for a small left parietal traumatic subarachnoid hemorrhage (SAH). His neurologic examination and repeat head CT scan the following day remain unchanged. What is the most likely diagnosis?

Diffuse axonal injury.

Diffuse Axonal Injury

- Most common traumatic brain injury
- Axonal shearing injury
- Induced by sudden acceleration/deceleration or rotational forces
- Responsible for severely impaired neurologic function in patients without gross parenchymal contusions or hematomas
- Initial head CT scans are often normal
- Most common finding on MRI is multifocal hyperintense foci on T2-weighted images
- Punctate hemorrhages occur at the gray-white matter interface, corpus callosum, upper brainstem and superior cerebellar peduncle
- Histology reveals axonal swelling, disruption of axons and retraction balls (swollen proximal ends of severed axons)

Cerebral Contusion

- Second most common traumatic brain injury
- Induced by the brain striking an osseous ridge (or less frequently a dural fold) and occurs when differential acceleration/deceleration forces are applied to the head
- Common locations are the temporal lobes (50%), frontal lobes (30%), and parasagittal/convexity
- Initial head CT scan findings include patchy, ill-defined, low-density lesions that may be mixed with hyperdense foci of hemorrhage
- Serial CT scans may show more and/or larger lesions and delayed hemorrhages

---

A 40-year-old female is brought to the emergency department with an initial GCS of 15. On examination, she has bilateral periorbital ecchymoses and a small amount of clear fluid dripping from her nose. Her head CT scan demonstrates a basilar skull fracture. What is the initial management of this patient?

Conservative management (surgery is not indicated).

Basilar Skull Fracture

- Presents with CSF otorrhea or rhinorrhea, hemotympanum, postauricular ecchymoses (Battle's sign), periorbital ecchymoses (raccoon's eyes), and cranial nerve injuries
- Nasogastric tube placement is contraindicated in trauma patients with suspected basilar skull fractures
- Most do not require further treatment

Cerebrospinal Fluid Fistula

- Trauma is the most common cause (other causes include post-procedure and spontaneous)
- Occurs in about 2% of patients with head injury
- 70% occur with 48 hours of injury and 98% are clinically evident by 3 months
- Complications include meningitis (25%) and pneumocephalus (25%)
- Diagnosis of traumatic CSF fistula
  - Fluid is clear
  - Target sign
    - Performed when a CSF leak is suspected but fluid is blood tinged
    - Fluid is placed on a piece of filter paper or absorbent cloth

- If CSF is present, a "halo sign" will form as the CSF content of the fluid migrates farther out
  - The final product looks like a bull's eye with the thicker blood or mucus in the center and the lighter-colored CSF migrating beyond the inner ring
- Presence of beta-2 transferrin, a substance only found in CSF, perilymph, and vitreous humor of the eye
- Neuroimaging techniques, including fine-cut CT with coronal and axial images, contrast or radionuclide cisternography and nasal endoscopy, can be helpful in diagnosis
- Treatment of traumatic CSF fistula
  - 70% resolve within 7 days with conservative treatment (head-up in bed, bowel regimen to avoid straining, avoidance of maneuvers that increase ICP such as nose blowing, coughing, sneezing)
  - For persistent leaks, lumbar puncture (LP) or lumbar drainage may be beneficial
  - Surgical repair is rarely necessary

A 6-year-old child is brought to the emergency department after a fall from his bike with transient loss of consciousness. On examination, he is awake, interactive, and appropriate. A head CT scan demonstrates a 3-cm linear nondisplaced skull fracture in the right parietal region; there is no underlying brain abnormality. Does this fracture need operative fixation?

Operative fixation is not indicated in this case.

Criteria for Surgery for a Depressed Skull Fracture

- Depth of depressed fracture > width of surrounding bone (closed depressed skull fractures in a neurologically intact patient overlying a dural sinus may be managed conservatively)
- Open fracture

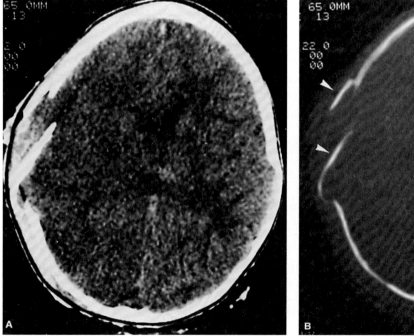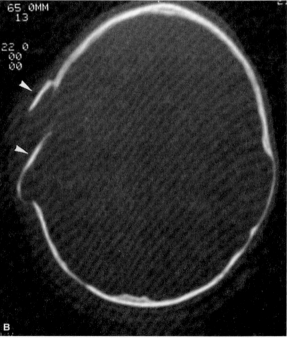

Depressed skull fracture. (With permission from Mulholland MW, Lillemoe KD, Doherty GM, Maier RV, Upchurch GR, eds. *Greenfield's Surgery.* 4th ed. Philadelphia, PA: Lippincott Williams & Wilkins; 2005.)

- Fracture associated with a significant underlying intracranial hematoma that requires evacuation
- Fracture over cosmetic areas

A mother brings her 15-month-old daughter to the emergency department because of lethargy. The mother states the infant accidentally fell off a 5-foot-tall changing table onto the floor. On examination, the child has numerous bruises. Ophthalmologic examination reveals retinal hemorrhages. Skull X-rays demonstrate a linear skull fracture and a small chronic SDH. What is the most likely diagnosis?

Child abuse should be suspected.

Cranial Findings Associated with Child Abuse
- Retinal hemorrhages
- Bilateral chronic SDHs
- Multiple skull fractures

A patient develops hyponatremia while on the floor and is found to have syndrome of inappropriate antidiuretic hormone secretion (SIADH). His neurologic examination is unchanged. What is the first step in management?

The mainstay of treatment for SIADH is fluid restriction.

Syndrome of Inappropriate Antidiuretic Hormone Secretion
- Release of antidiuretic hormone (ADH) in the absence of physiologic stimuli
- Etiologies
  - Intracranial processes (stroke, hemorrhage, trauma, tumors, SAH, post craniotomy, infection)
  - Tumors (small cell carcinoma of the lung, carcinoma of the pancreas and duodenum)
  - Drugs (chlorpropamide, carbamazepine, vincristine, vinblastine)
  - Infectious pulmonary diseases (tuberculosis, pneumonia)
  - Idiopathic
- Symptoms are secondary to hyponatremia (confusion, lethargy, nausea, vomiting, restlessness, irritability, seizure, and coma)
- Patients are usually euvolemic, but may be hypervolemic (pitting edema is almost always absent)
- Diagnosis
  - Hyponatremia
  - Low serum osmolality
  - High urine sodium
  - Normal renal, adrenal, and thyroid functions
  - No signs of dehydration or fluid overload
  - Water load test if diagnosis unclear
- Treatment
  - Mild/asymptomatic SIADH: Fluid restriction
  - Severe or symptomatic SIADH: Fluid restriction, hypertonic saline, furosemide
  - Chronic SIADH: Fluid restriction, demeclocycline (tetracycline antibiotic that partially antagonizes the effects of ADH on renal tubules), furosemide

Cerebral Salt Wasting

- Renal loss of sodium as a result of intracranial disease (especially SAH), causing hyponatremia and a decrease in extracellular fluid volume
- Laboratory values may be identical with SIADH and cerebral salt wasting (CSW)
- Difference between SIADH and CSW is volume status (patients with CSW are hypovolemic)
- Treatment is volume replacement and positive salt balance

Central pontine myelinolysis may result from excessively rapid correction of hyponatremia.

Central or Neurogenic Diabetes Insipidus

- Due to decreased release of ADH (in contrast to nephrogenic diabetes insipidus which is due to renal resistance to normal or supranormal levels of ADH)
- Caused by neoplastic or infiltrative lesions of the hypothalamus or pituitary, pituitary surgery, and severe head injuries
- Symptoms include polyuria, polydypsia, and excessive thirst
- Diagnosis is based on:
    - Hypernatremia
    - High urine output (>250 cc/hour)
    - Low urine specific gravity
    - Water deprivation test if diagnosis is unclear
- Treatment is vasopressin

A 70-year-old man is brought to the emergency department following a fall in which he struck his forehead. On physical examination, he has a large forehead laceration. Neurologic examination is significant for bilateral weakness in the upper extremities greater than the lower extremities, decreased sensation over the shoulders and arms and urinary retention. Cervical spine X-rays demonstrate no fracture or subluxation. What is the most likely diagnosis?

Acute central cervical spinal cord injury.

Types of Spinal Cord Injury

- Complete: No preservation of any motor or sensory function below the level of injury
- Incomplete: Any residual motor or sensory function below the level of injury
    - Acute central cervical spinal cord injury
    - Anterior cord syndrome
    - Brown-Séquard syndrome

Acute Central Cervical Spinal Cord Injury (Central Cord Syndrome)

- Most common type of incomplete spinal cord injury
- Typically follows a hyperextension injury in an older patient with pre-existing cervical spine stenosis
- Findings include: Weakness of upper extremities > lower extremities, varying degrees of sensory loss below the level of injury, and bladder dysfunction (usually urinary retention)
    - Often affects fine motor movement of the hands
- Surgical decompression is often performed on a non-urgent basis

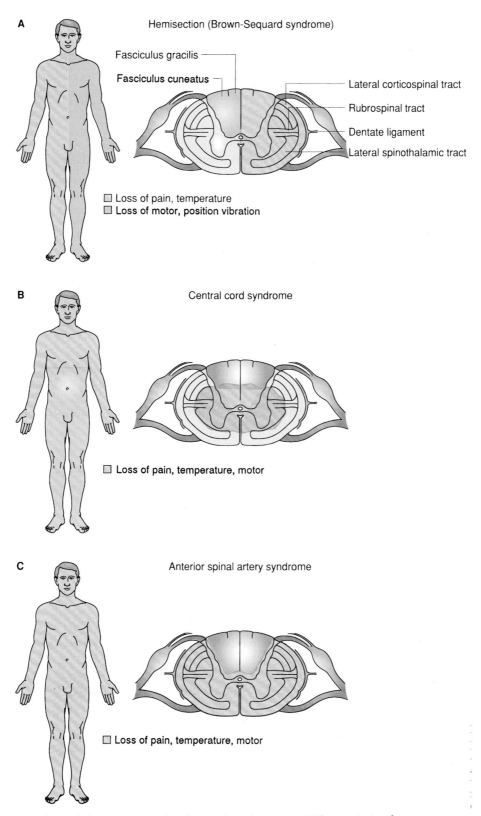

A   Hemisection (Brown-Sequard syndrome)

Fasciculus gracilis

Fasciculus cuneatus

Lateral corticospinal tract

Rubrospinal tract

Dentate ligament

Lateral spinothalamic tract

☐ Loss of pain, temperature
☐ **Loss of motor, position vibration**

B   Central cord syndrome

☐ Loss of pain, temperature, motor

C   Anterior spinal artery syndrome

☐ Loss of pain, temperature, motor

Neurologic defects associated with spinal cord injuries. (With permission from Mulholland MW, Lillemoe KD, Doherty GM, Maier RV, Upchurch GR, eds. *Greenfield's Surgery*. 4th ed. Philadelphia, PA: Lippincott Williams & Wilkins; 2005.)

> A patient who is paraplegic following trauma has preservation of touch, position, and vibration sense below the level of the lesion. What is the most likely reason for this finding?

Anterior cord syndrome.

Anterior Cord Syndrome

- Also known as anterior spinal artery syndrome
- Occurs with hyperflexion injuries and is due to compression or injury to the anterior spinal artery
- Characterized by motor paralysis (due to corticospinal tract lesion), dissociated sensory loss below lesion with loss of pain and temperature sensation (due to spinothalamic tract lesion), and intact proprioception and vibration sense (intact posterior column function)
- Poorest prognosis of incomplete spinal cord injuries

The pathway for nociceptive stimuli is the contralateral spinothalamic tract.

Brown-Séquard Syndrome

- Hemisection of the spinal cord
- Typically results from penetrating trauma
- Characterized by:
  - Ipsilateral motor paralysis (due to corticospinal tract lesion)
  - Ipsilateral loss of proprioception and vibratory sense (due to posterior column lesion)
  - Contralateral loss of pain and temperature sensation (due to spinothalamic tract lesion)
- Best prognosis of incomplete spinal cord injuries

> A 27-year-old male with a complete cervical spinal cord injury at T3 remains hypotensive and bradycardic following adequate intravascular resuscitation and a normal hematocrit. What is the next most appropriate treatment?

Dopamine.

Neurogenic and Spinal Shock

- Neurogenic shock: Hypotension and bradycardia resulting from interruption of sympathetic nervous system pathways within the spinal cord
- Spinal shock: Transient loss of all neurologic function below the level of injury leading to flaccid paralysis and areflexia lasting a varying amount of time followed by hypertonia, exaggerated reflexes, and spasticity

Blood Pressure Management after Acute Spinal Cord Injury

- Hypotension (SBP < 90 mmHg) should be avoided if possible or corrected as soon as possible after an acute spinal cord injury
- Maintenance of MAP at 85 to 90 mmHg for the first 7 days after acute spinal cord injury is recommended to improve spinal cord perfusion
- Pressors are recommended once volume resuscitation is completed
- Dopamine is the agent of choice

> Should a patient who presents 9 hours after an incomplete spinal cord injury due to non-penetrating trauma be treated with methylprednisolone?

Steroids are only indicated within 8 hours of a spinal cord injury secondary to blunt trauma.

Steroids in Spinal Cord Injury

- Although there is insufficient evidence to support treatment standards and guidelines, treatment with methylprednisolone is recommended as an option in the treatment of patients with acute spinal cord injuries
- Beneficial effects are seen for complete and incomplete spinal cord injuries when administered within 8 hours of injury
- Administration
  - Loading dose: 30 mg/kg IV over 15 minutes
  - 45-minute pause
  - Maintenance infusion: 5.4 mg/kg/hour continuous infusion
- Duration of maintenance infusion
  - If therapy is initiated <3 hours after injury, infusion is continued for 23 hours
  - If therapy is initiated between 3 and 8 hours, infusion continues for 47 hours

---

A 38-year-old unbelted driver involved in a motor vehicle accident is brought to the emergency room in a hard neck collar. His injuries include a left open tibial fracture. His admission GCS is 15. He has full strength in his upper extremities bilaterally and right lower extremity. His left lower extremity movement is limited secondary to pain. His head CT scan shows no acute intracranial pathology. His lateral cervical spine X-ray demonstrates no fracture or subluxation down to C7. What is the next step in the neurosurgical management of this patient?

Continue neck immobilization until evaluation of the cervical spine is complete.

Radiographic Assessment of the Cervical Spine in Trauma Patients

- Radiographic assessment of the cervical spine is not recommended in trauma patients who are awake, alert, and not intoxicated, who are without neck pain or tenderness, and who do not have significant associated injuries that are distracting to them
- Trauma patients who are symptomatic (neck pain, cervical spine tenderness, signs or symptoms of neurologic deficit) and those who cannot be assessed (unconscious, uncooperative, intoxicated, or have associated traumatic injuries that distract from assessment) require radiographic evaluation of the cervical spine before cervical spine immobilization can be discontinued
- The craniocervical junction must be adequately visualized down through and including C7-T1 junction
- A CT of the neck is the diagnostic gold standard

Discontinuation of Cervical Spine Immobilization

- Cervical spine immobilization in awake patients with neck pain or tenderness and normal cervical spine X-rays (including supplemental CT if necessary) can be discontinued after either:
  - Normal and adequate CT of the neck or
  - A normal MRI obtained within 48 hours of injury
- Cervical spine immobilization in obtunded patients with normal cervical spine X-rays (including supplemental CT if necessary) can be discontinued after:
  - Dynamic flexion/extension studies under fluoroscopic guidance, or
  - A normal MRI obtained within 48 hours of injury or
  - At the discretion of the treating physician

Atlas (C1) Fractures

- A "Jefferson fracture" is a burst fracture through the C1 ring
- Caused by an *axial load*
- Rarely have neurologic deficits if isolated (due to large canal and tendency for fragments to be forced outward)

Jefferson Fracture

C1 (Atlas)

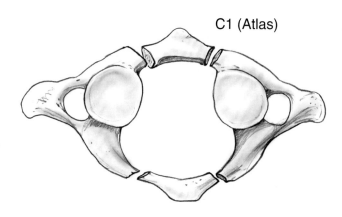

Caused by axial load

- Rule of Spence: On AP or open-mouth odontoid views, if the sum of the excursion of C1 lateral masses over C2 lateral masses >7 mm, the transverse atlantal ligament is probably disrupted
- If the transverse atlantal ligament is intact (<7 mm), the fracture can be treated with external cervical immobilization with rigid collar, a sternal-occipital-mandibular immobilizer (SOMI) brace, or halo orthosis
- If the transverse atlantal ligament is disrupted (>7 mm), halo orthosis and surgical stabilization and fusion is recommended

Axis (C2) Fractures

- **Odontoid Fracture**
- Most common traumatic axis fracture
- Neurologic deficits are uncommon
- Patients usually complain of occipital or high cervical pain
- Type I odontoid fracture
  - Involves avulsion of the distal odontoid process
  - Uncommon
  - Usually treated with cervical immobilization
- Type II odontoid fracture
  - Fracture through the base of the dens at the junction with the axis body
  - Most common odontoid fracture
  - Treatment options include halo immobilization and surgical fixation
- Type III odontoid fracture
  - Fracture through the odontoid that extends through the C2 body
  - Usually treated with cervical collar or halo immobilization
- Types I–III may be managed initially with external cervical immobilization

C2 Odontoid Fracture Classification

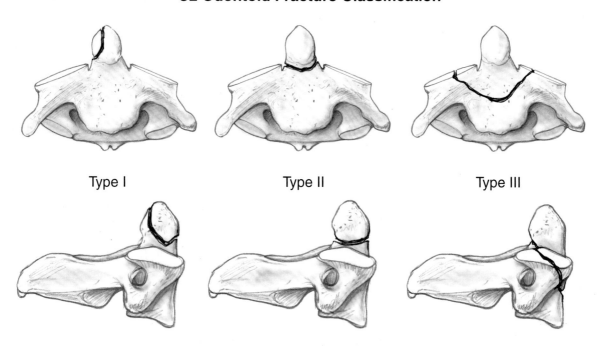

Type I   Type II   Type III

- Surgical fixation should be considered for Types II and III in cases of dens displacement ≥5 mm, comminution of the odontoid fracture, and/or inability to achieve or maintain fracture alignment with external immobilization

Hangman Fracture

- AKA traumatic spondylolisthesis of the axis
- Bilateral fractures through the pars interarticularis of C2
- Caused by a *hyperextension injury*

Hangman's Fracture

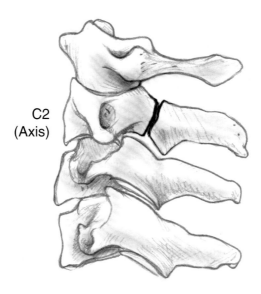

C2
(Axis)

Caused by hyperextension injury

- Most are neurologically intact
- Most can be treated with external immobilization
- Surgical stabilization is indicated in cases of severe angulation, disruption of the C2 to C3 disk space or inability to establish or maintain fracture alignment with external immobilization

Subaxial Fractures and Dislocations

- Include compression fractures, burst fractures, teardrop fractures, unilateral and bilateral locked facets, and clay shoveler fracture

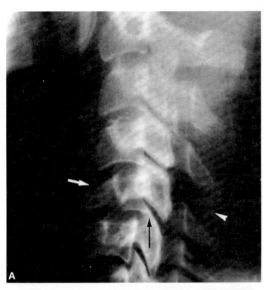

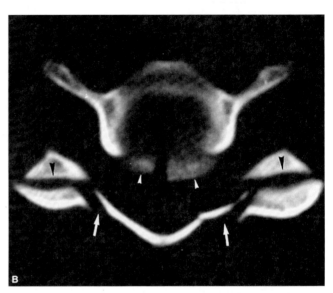

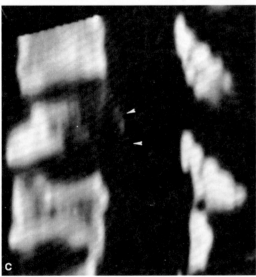

Vertebral compression fracture. (With permission from Mulholland MW, Lillemoe KD, Doherty GM, Maier RV, Upchurch GR, eds. *Greenfield's Surgery*. 4th ed. Philadelphia, PA: Lippincott Williams & Wilkins; 2005.)

Clay Shoveler Fracture

- Classically used to describe avulsion of the C7 spinous process, however, often used to describe fracture of any cervical spinous process
- Usually due to direct blow to the spinous process or flexion injury
- Stable fractures

A 38-year-old female presents to the emergency department with complaints of severe low back pain following a fall from a horse. She is neurologically intact and is found to have a T12 compression fracture with minimal loss of anterior vertebral body height and kyphotic angulation. What is the next step in management?

External immobilization.

The Three Functional Columns of the Thoracolumbar Spine

- Anterior column: Anterior half of the vertebral body and disk, anterior longitudinal ligament and anterior annulus fibrosis
- Middle column: Posterior half of the vertebral body and disk, posterior longitudinal ligament and posterior annulus fibrosis
- Posterior column: Posterior bony arch and posterior ligaments (supraspinous, interspinous, joint capsule, and ligamentum flavum)

Vertebral Compression Fracture

- Failure of anterior column; wedging of vertebral body anteriorly
- Middle column is intact
- Posterior column may or may not be damaged by distraction forces
- Usually no neurologic deficit
- Usually stable injury
- Treatment: Typically with external immobilization
- Surgical intervention is indicated if there is significant loss of anterior vertebral body height or kyphotic angulation (often associated with ligamentous incompetency of posterior elements)

Burst Fracture

- Results from a pure axial load
- Failure of anterior and middle columns
- Occurs mainly at thoracolumbar junction
- Findings include comminution of vertebral body, increase in interpedicular distance, retropulsion of fractured posterior vertebral body into the canal, and loss of posterior vertebral body height
- Neurologic deficits are present in 50%
- Treatment options include external bracing and surgical intervention depending on presence of neurologic symptoms, degree of spinal canal compromise, amount of kyphotic deformity, and loss of vertebral body height

Seat Belt Type Fracture

- Failure of middle and posterior columns
- Results from a flexion vector acting around an anteriorly placed axis of rotation
- Associated with the use of seat belts where the lower spine is fixed against the seat and the upper spine pivots around an axis anterior to the spine
- Usually no neurologic deficit
- Treatment usually external bracing

Fracture–Dislocation

- Failure of all three columns under compression, tension, rotation, shear, or extension
- Unstable
- Most patients have neurologic deficits
- Most require surgical treatment

A 45-year-old man presents with the sudden onset of low back pain radiating down both legs and urinary incontinence. On physical examination, he has a right-sided foot drop, decreased perineal sensation, and loss of Achilles reflexes bilaterally. What is the most likely diagnosis? What is the next step in management?

Cauda equina syndrome. This patient should undergo an MRI urgently.

Cauda Equina Syndrome

- Injury to nerve roots arising from the conus medullaris
- Can be seen with herniated disk, tumor, trauma, spinal EDH
- Patients present with sphincter disturbances, saddle anesthesia, asymmetric motor weakness, low back pain or sciatica, areflexia
- Diagnostic test of choice: MRI (if no contraindications)
- Treatment: Urgent decompression

What is the most common cause of SAH?

Trauma.

Subarachnoid Hemorrhage

- Trauma is the most common cause
- The most common cause of non-traumatic SAH is ruptured intracranial aneurysm (75%)
- Other causes of spontaneous SAH include cerebral arteriovenous malformations, vasculitides, benign perimesencephalic SAH, blood disorders, neoplasms, drugs
- 7% to 10% are idiopathic

A 52-year-old woman is brought to the emergency department complaining of the worst headache of her life. On neurologic examination, she is awake but confused and has a left-sided third nerve palsy. What is the most likely diagnosis?

A ruptured intracranial aneurysm.

Aneurysmal Subarachnoid Hemorrhage

- Clinical features: Hallmark is the sudden onset of severe headache ("worst headache of my life")
- Other features include nausea, vomiting, loss of consciousness, meningismus, focal neurologic deficits, seizures, ocular hemorrhage, lethargy, somnolence, and coma
- Workup for suspected SAH
  - Unenhanced head CT
  - LP if head CT normal

Cerebral Aneurysm

- Risk of bleeding: 1% to 2% per year
- Most common locations: Anterior communicating artery
- Most frequent presentation: SAH
- Gold standard diagnostic test: four-vessel cerebral angiogram
- Treatment: open (craniotomy) and endovascular options

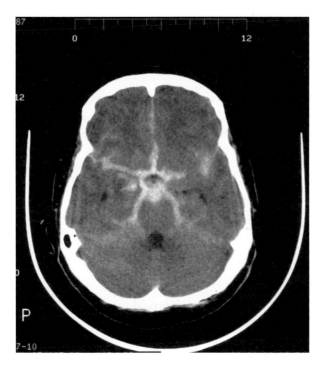

Subarachnoid hemorrhage.

Major Complications of Aneurysmal Subarachnoid Hemorrhage

- Re-bleeding
    - Peak risk within 24 hours after SAH
    - 50% re-bleed within 6 months
    - There is a 15–20% risk of re-bleeding with the first 2 weeks and 50% within 6 months

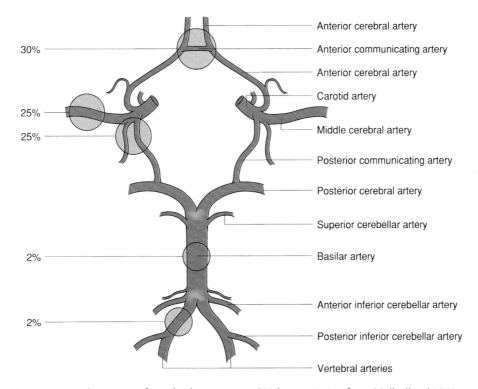

Most common locations of cerebral aneurysms. (With permission from Mulholland MW, Lillemoe KD, Doherty GM, Maier RV, Upchurch GR, eds. *Greenfield's Surgery*. 4th ed. Philadelphia, PA: Lippincott Williams & Wilkins; 2005.)

- Cerebral vasospasm
  - Occurs 3 to 12 days after hemorrhage
  - Symptoms range in severity from mild reversible neurologic deficit to severe permanent deficits secondary to infarction
  - The best predictor for the development of vasospasm is the amount of blood on CT scan
  - Treatment: Prophylactic administration of calcium channel antagonists (nimodipine), triple H therapy (hypervolemic, hypertensive, hemodilutional therapy), percutaneous transluminal balloon angioplasty, and intra-arterial papaverine
- Hydrocephalus
- Cerebral edema
- Seizures

Traumatic Aneurysm

- Rare
- Can be secondary to penetrating or nonpenetrating trauma
- With nonpenetrating trauma, these typically occur on peripheral intracranial vessels such as the distal anterior cerebral artery or at the skull base involving the petrous cavernous or supraclinoid internal carotid artery
- The most common presentation is delayed intracranial hemorrhage

Mycotic Aneurysm

- Technically denotes an aneurysm of fungal origin, but used in reference to all aneurysms of infectious origin
- Most common site: Thoracic aorta
- Most common intracranial site: Distal middle cerebral artery branches
- More than 80% of patients with infectious aneurysms have underlying endocarditis; 2% of patients with endocarditis are diagnosed with infectious aneurysms
- The most common organism is *Streptococcus*

Fusiform Aneurysm

- Also known as an atherosclerotic aneurysm
- Usually occurs in older patients
- Vertebrobasilar system commonly affected
- May thrombose, causing brainstem infarction

A 32-year-old woman is brought to the emergency department after developing a severe headache. A head CT demonstrates a left parietal intraparenchymal hematoma. What is the most likely diagnosis?

Arteriovenous malformation.

Arteriovenous Malformation

- Abnormal collection of blood vessels in which blood flows directly from enlarged feeding arteries to dilated draining veins without an intervening capillary bed or brain parenchyma
- Peak presentation is at age 20 to 40 years
- The most common presentation is hemorrhage (50%)
- The risk of hemorrhage is 2% to 4% per year

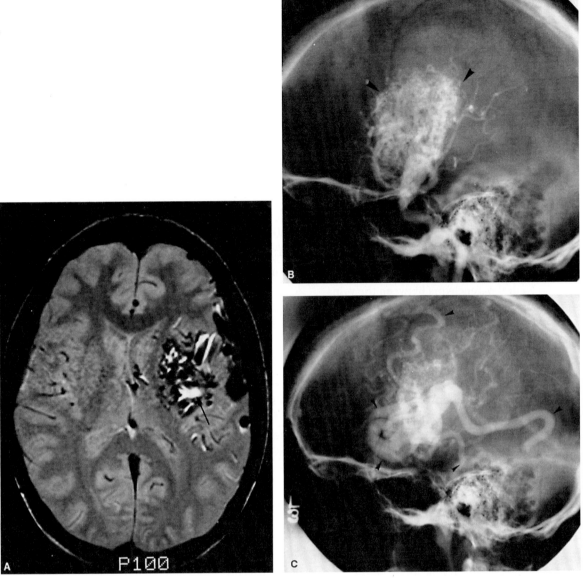

Large cerebral AVM. (With permission from Mulholland MW, Lillemoe KD, Doherty GM, Maier RV, Upchurch GR, eds. *Greenfield's Surgery*. 4th ed. Philadelphia, PA: Lippincott Williams & Wilkins; 2005.)

Cavernous Malformation

- Also known as cavernous hemangioma, cavernoma, cavernous angioma
- Well-circumscribed, endothelial-lined, sinusoidal vascular channels located within the brain but lacking intervening neural parenchyma
- Common presenting symptoms are seizure, focal neurologic deficit, and headache
- Peak presentation at age 20 to 40 years
- Angiographically occult
- MRI demonstrates a "popcorn-like" lesion with well-delineated reticulated core of mixed signal intensities representing hemorrhage in different stages of evolution

Capillary Telangiectasia

- Nest of dilated capillaries with interposed normal brain

- Usually located in pons, spinal cord, and cerebellum
- Most often found incidentally at autopsy
- MRI demonstrates black spots on T2-weighted images

A 23-year-old female presents for evaluation of chronic headaches. A contrast-enhanced head CT demonstrates a prominent left parietal vein. An angiogram demonstrates a wedge-shaped collection of dilated veins converging into an enlarged transcortical vein. What is the next step in management?

A venous angioma is treated with conservative management.

Venous Angioma

- Also known as a developmental venous anomaly
- The most common intracranial vascular malformation
- Tufts of dilated anomalous veins that converge in an enlarged transcortical draining vein
- Neural parenchyma between the veins
- Classic angiographic appearance of a "caput medusae"
- Usually clinically asymptomatic
- Rarely require surgical treatment

A 35-year-old female presents with complaints of neck pain radiating into her right upper extremity with paresthesias and numbness of her forearm and thumb. Neurologic examination reveals mild weakness of the right biceps and a decreased right biceps tendon reflex. What is the most likely diagnosis?

Right C6 radiculopathy due to a herniated right C5 to C6 disk. C5 to C6 is the most common location of a cervical disk herniation.

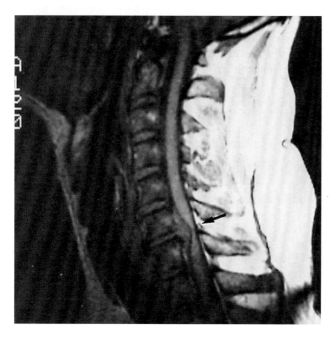

Cervical disk herniation. (With permission from Mulholland MW, Lillemoe KD, Doherty GM, Maier RV, Upchurch GR, eds. *Greenfield's Surgery*. 4th ed. Philadelphia, PA: Lippincott Williams & Wilkins; 2005.)

Cervical Disk Herniation

- There are eight cervical nerve roots (C1 to C8) but only seven cervical vertebrae
- Cervical roots exit above the pedicle of their like-numbered vertebra (i.e., the C5 nerve root exits between C4 and C5)
- Clinical presentation: Neck pain, radiculopathy (pain, weakness, sensory changes, and/or reflex changes associated with a particular nerve root)
- Over 90% will improve with conservative treatment
- Surgery is indicated for patients with progressive motor deficit and intractable pain

Cervical Disk Herniation Physical Examination Findings

	C4–C5	C5–C6	C6–C7	C7–C8
% of cervical disk herniations	2	19	69	10
Compressed root	C5	C6	C7	C8
Motor weakness	Deltoid	Biceps, brachioradialis	Triceps	Hand intrinsics
Paresthesia and hypesthesia	Shoulder	Upper arm, radial forearm, thumb	Second and third fingers	Ulnar forearm, fourth and fifth fingers
Reflex diminished		Biceps	Triceps	Finger jerk

A 50-year-old male laborer feels a sudden sharp pain in his back, which shoots down past his right knee to his foot while lifting a heavy object. What is a common cause of this pain presentation?

An L4 to L5 disk herniation.

Lumbar Disk Herniation

- There are five lumbar nerve roots (L1 to L5) and five lumbar vertebrae
- In the lumbar region, the nerve roots exit below the pedicle of their like-numbered vertebra (unlike the cervical spine)
- Most commonly a posterolateral herniation
- Causes unilateral nerve root compression on the exiting nerve
  - For example, an L4 to L5 disk herniation causes an L5 radiculopathy
- 90% of patients improve with rest and nonsteroidal anti-inflammatory drugs alone
- Common physical examination findings
  - L2 to L3 disk (L3 nerve): Weak hip flexors
  - L3 to L4 disk (L4 nerve): Decreased knee jerk
  - L4 to L5 disk (L5 nerve): Weak dorsiflexion/foot drop, decreased sensation in first web space
  - L5 to S1 disk (S1 nerve): Weak plantar flexion, weak Achilles reflex, decreased sensation in lateral foot
- Surgery is indicated for patients with cauda equina syndrome, progressive motor deficit, and intractable pain

A L4 to L5 herniated intervertebral disk may result in foot drop.

Lumbar Disk Herniation Physical Examination Findings

	L3–L4	L4–L5	L5–S1
% of lumbar disk herniations	5–10	40–45	45–50
Compressed root	L4	L5	S1
Motor weakness	Quadriceps femoris	Tibialis anterior, extensor hallucis longus	Gastrocnemius
Decreased sensation	Medial malleolus, medial foot	Web between first and second toes, dorsum of foot	Lateral malleolus, lateral foot
Reflex diminished	Knee jerk		Achilles

A 76-year-old man with no significant past medical history develops ataxia and is found to have a ring-enhancing lesion in his right cerebellum. What is the most likely diagnosis?

Metastatic cancer is the most common brain cancer.

Brain Tumors

- Most common diagnosis of a solitary lesion in the posterior fossa of adults: Metastasis
- Most common malignancy to metastasize to the brain: Lung cancer
- Most common primary intra-axial brain tumor: Astrocytoma
    - Astrocytes have foot processes that contribute to the blood–brain barrier, and they also do potassium homeostasis
    - Treatment: Resection if possible
    - Most will degenerate to glioblastoma multiforme
- Most aggressive primary brain tumor: Glioblastoma multiforme
    - The most common primary brain tumor
    - Very poor prognosis
    - Treatment: Surgery, radiation, chemotherapy (temodar, Gliadel wafers). Steroids used to reduce swelling.
- Ependymoma
    - Tumor that involves the fourth ventricle → hydrocephalus and increased ICP
    - Treatment: Surgery, radiation
- Medulloblastoma
    - A primitive neuroectodermal tumor
    - Most commonly affects children

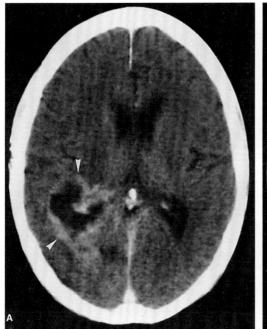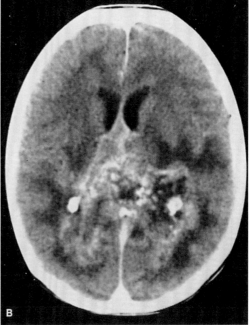

Glioblastoma multiforme. (With permission from Mulholland MW, Lillemoe KD, Doherty GM, Maier RV, Upchurch GR, eds. *Greenfield's Surgery*. 4th ed. Philadelphia, PA: Lippincott Williams & Wilkins; 2005.)

- In the fourth ventricle → hydrocephalus and increased ICP
- Symptoms: Unsteady gait (cerebellar symptoms), headaches
- Treatment: Resection if possible, radiation, chemotherapy
- Oligodendroglioma
  - Oligodendrocytes produce myelin for CNS axons
  - Slow-growing tumors that affect the cerebral hemispheres
  - Symptoms: Seizures, weakness, deficits associated with affected cerebral hemisphere
  - Treatment: Resection or radiation

A 55-year-old female presents with headaches and unilateral proptosis. An MRI demonstrates a meningioma. What is the appropriate treatment?

Resection—patients have an excellent prognosis.

Meningioma

- The most common benign intracranial tumor
- Tumor arising from the meninges
- Most common in middle-aged females
- Presents with headaches, proptosis, anosmia
- Treatment
  - Conservative monitoring for small, non-growing, asymptomatic lesions
  - Surgical resection
  - Radiotherapy

A 46-year-old woman presents with a headache and personality changes. A brain MRI demonstrates a left frontoparietal ring-enhancing lesion. What is the differential diagnosis?

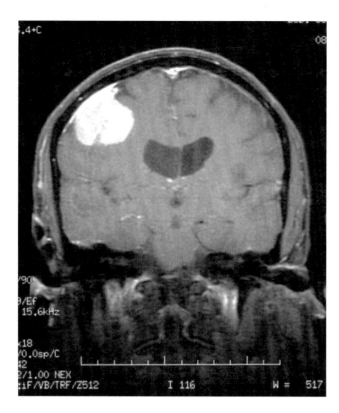

Meningioma.

Differential Diagnosis of a Ring-Enhancing Lesion in an Adult

- Metastasis
- Astrocytoma
- Abscess
- Others (lymphoma, radiation necrosis, infarction, and resolving hematoma)

Vestibular schwannoma (acoustic neuroma).

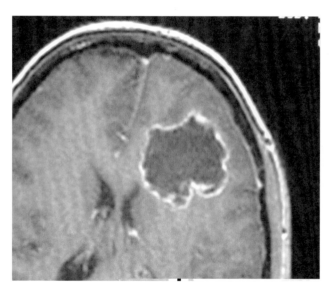

Ring-enhancing lesion.

A 45-year-old woman presents with tinnitus, disequilibrium, and left-sided hearing loss. What is the most likely diagnosis?

Vestibular Schwannoma (Acoustic Neuroma)

- Schwannoma arising from the eighth cranial nerve (vestibular division)
- Most common early symptoms: Hearing loss, tinnitus (high-pitched), disequilibrium
- Histology: Benign tumors comprised of Antoni A and B fibers
- Treatment options: Expectant, surgery, radiotherapy

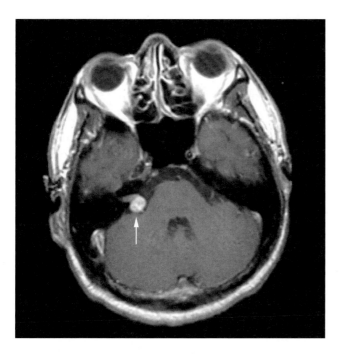

Vestibular schwannoma. (With permission from Mulholland MW, Lillemoe KD, Doherty GM, Maier RV, Upchurch GR, eds. *Greenfield's Surgery.* 4th ed. Philadelphia, PA: Lippincott Williams & Wilkins; 2005.)

A 30-year-old woman presents with a 3-week history of increasing headache and visual loss. On examination, she has a bitemporal hemianopsia. What is the most likely diagnosis?

Pituitary tumor.

Pituitary Adenoma

- Arises from the anterior pituitary
- Can be divided into functional (secreting) or non-functional (non-secreting)
  - Functional tumors usually present with symptoms caused by the physiologic effects of the excess hormones that they secrete
    - Prolactin: Amenorrhea-galactorrhea in females, impotence in males
    - Growth hormone: Acromegaly in adults, gigantism in prepubertal children
    - Adrenocorticotropic hormone: Cushing disease
  - Non-functional tumors usually do not present until they attain a sufficient size to cause neurologic deficits by mass effect (classically cause bitemporal hemianopsia)
- Treatment
  - Surgery
  - Medical options in secreting tumors (i.e., bromocriptine and cabergoline for prolactinomas; somatostatin analogues, dopamine agonists and growth hormone receptor antagonists for acromegaly
  - Radiotherapy
  - Conservative monitoring (asymptomatic lesions)

A 35-year-old AIDS patient develops a seizure and is brought to the emergency department where a head CT scan demonstrates two hypodense lesions, one in the left basal ganglia and one in the right parietal lobe. What is the most likely diagnosis?

Toxoplasmosis is a common cause of brain lesions in immunocompromised patients.

Central Nervous System Infections

- Most common brain mass lesion in AIDS patients: Toxoplasmosis
  - Differential includes lymphoma and abscess
- Most frequent CNS parasitic disease worldwide: Cysticercosis
- Most common pathogen in a brain abscess:
  - Adults: *Streptococcus*
  - Trauma patients: *Staphylococcus*
  - Infants: Gram-negative organisms
- Most frequent congenital CNS infection: Cytomegalovirus

2 | Otorhinolaryngology

Matthew L. Kashima, Bradley J. Goldstein, and Carole Fakhry

A 4-year-old child presents with intermittent drainage on his neck near the sternocleidomastoid (SCM) muscle and a history of recurrent infections. What is the most likely diagnosis?

A branchial cleft abnormality—either a cyst, sinus, or fistula.

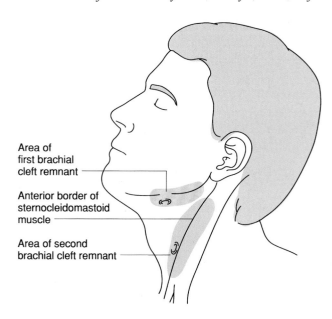

Anatomic location of branchial cleft remnants and external openings. (With permission from Mulholland MW, Lillemoe KD, Doherty GM, et al., eds. *Greenfield's Surgery.* 4th ed. Philadelphia, PA: Lippincott Williams & Wilkins; 2005.)

Area of first brachial cleft remnant

Anterior border of sternocleidomastoid muscle

Area of second brachial cleft remnant

Branchial Cleft
- A series of four arches that form in the neck early in development (4 to 6 weeks)
- Cysts are trapped remnants of clefts or pouches
- Sinuses open into the pharynx internally or the skin externally
- Fistulae have both internal and external openings
- Diagnosis: Clinical; can get CT or MRI for confirmation
- Treatment: Complete resection of the cyst and tract
- **First branchial cleft**
  - Duplication of the external auditory canal

27

- Can communicate to the oral cavity below the angle of the mandible
- Care must be taken to avoid injuring the facial nerve during resection
- **Second branchial cleft**
  - Most common (90%) of branchial cleft anomalies
  - External opening along the anterior border of SCM and internal opening at the tonsillar fossa
  - Courses between carotid vessels and over hypoglossal and glossopharyngeal nerves
- **Third branchial cleft**
  - External opening along the anterior border of SCM and internal opening at the piriform sinus
  - Courses behind carotid vessels and below the hypoglossal nerve, above the glossopharyngeal nerve

A second branchial cleft anomaly is the most common type.

An otherwise healthy child presents with a midline neck mass below the hyoid bone that is nontender. The mass moves with swallowing. What is the most likely diagnosis?

Thyroglossal duct cysts are common congenital and developmental neck masses. The differential includes thyroglossal duct cyst, dermoid cyst, teratoma, branchial cleft cyst, laryngocele, lymphangioma, and hemangioma.

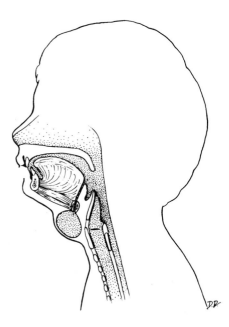

Thyroglossal duct cyst. (With permission from Fischer JE, Bland KI, Callery MP, et al., eds. *Mastery of Surgery*. 5th ed. Philadelphia, PA: Lippincott Williams & Wilkins; 2006.)

Thyroglossal Duct Cyst
- The thyroid gland is formed at the base of the tongue and migrates through the tongue to its position in the neck
- Failure of the tract to obliterate following descent leads to a thyroglossal duct cyst
- Can occur anywhere along the path of descent
- 80% are midline, and 80% are at or below the level of the hyoid bone

- A third of patients present before age 10 and about one-third of patients present after age 30
- Typically asymptomatic
- Move with swallowing and protrusion of the tongue
- Can become superinfected with upper respiratory tract infections and become tender and rapidly enlarge
- Evaluation should include imaging (CT or ultrasound) to differentiate from a thyroid mass
- An incision and drainage alone is inadequate
- Treatment is complete surgical excision of the cyst and tract to the foramen cecum at the base of the tongue and removal of the central portion of the hyoid bone (Sistrunk procedure)
- Recurrence is <10% after complete excision

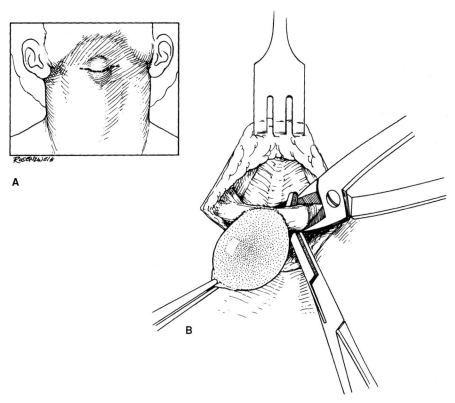

Sistrunk procedure. (With permission from Fischer JE, Bland KI, Callery MP, et al., eds. *Mastery of Surgery.* 5th ed. Philadelphia, PA: Lippincott Williams & Wilkins; 2006.)

A 1-year-old girl presents with a soft lateral neck mass that transilluminates. What is the best test to confirm the diagnosis?

History and physical examination is essential to establish the diagnosis—lymphangioma. Transillumination of the mass is characteristic.

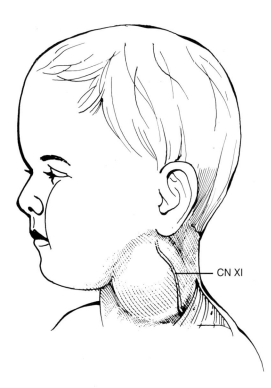

Cystic hygroma. (With permission from Fischer JE, Bland KI, Callery MP, et al., eds. *Mastery of Surgery*. 5th ed. Philadelphia, PA: Lippincott Williams & Wilkins; 2006.)

CN XI

Lymphangioma

- Developmental malformation of the lymphatics
- Divided into three categories: Simple, cavernous, and cystic hygroma
- 90% present by age 2
- Most commonly found in the neck
- Soft, painless, ill-defined mass
- If large, can cause dysphagia or respiratory symptoms
- Slowly enlarges with time
- Treatment is surgical excision
- Recurrence rate is 10%

A 1-year-old girl presents with a soft lateral neck mass that is bluish in hue. What is the best test to confirm the diagnosis?

A history and physical examination establishes the diagnosis of a hemangioma. Imaging studies will demonstrate the vascular nature (CT with contrast) and feeding vessels (MRA or angiography).

Hemangioma

- Vascular malformations can be defined as capillary, cavernous, mixed, juvenile, or proliferative
- 95% present by age 6 months
- Tend to be poorly defined, soft, compressible, cystic masses
- May have a bruit
- Initially have a period of growth followed by involution over the next 5 years
- Steroids have been shown to help arrest growth and promote resolution
- Surgical excision (possibly with embolization) is used for rare lesions that fail to resolve or for lesions that cause symptoms (CHF and Kasabach-Merritt syndrome)

One week after a total knee replacement, a 70-year-old man presents with painful, erythematous swelling over his left lower face. What is the most likely diagnosis?

Acute parotitis usually presents with fever, leukocytosis, swelling, tenderness, and foul discharge intraorally. Sialoadenitis refers to infection in one of the three, paired major salivary glands.

Sialoadenitis

- Causes of acute sialoadenitis
  - Obstruction—sialolithiasis
  - Dehydration—especially in the elderly and postoperative patients
- The most common causative organism is *Staphylococcus aureus*
- Treatment is hydration, sialogogues, antibiotics, warm compresses, and gentle massage of the affected gland
- Salivary gland stones (sialoliths) can cause obstruction leading to recurrent sialoadenitis
  - Eventually, the affected gland will burn out and scar down
  - Stones in the parotid (Stensen) or submandibular (Wharton) duct can be extracted transorally
  - Stones deeper in the gland may necessitate removal of the gland
- A parotid abscess is treated by incision and drainage—take care to incise the parotid along the course of the branches of the facial nerve

A 42-year-old woman with dental caries presents with new onset fever, neck swelling, pain, dysphagia, and a firm floor of the mouth. What is the most likely diagnosis?

Ludwig angina is a severe infection of the floor of the mouth in the submandibular and submental spaces. Spread of infection occurs along fascial planes.

Ludwig Angina

- Infection typically of dental origin
- Spreads around the mylohyoid muscle into the submandibular space
- Infection past the mylohyoid progresses rapidly
- Presents with swelling and displacement of the tongue superiorly and posteriorly, trismus, odynophagia, woody induration of the neck, as well as induration of the floor of the mouth
- Usually not a discrete abscess (absence of frank pus)
- Treatment is with IV antibiotics, tracheostomy (occasionally), and wide drainage
- Complications include loss of airway, septic emboli, septic shock, and aspiration
- The "danger space" is located between the prevertebral and alar divisions of the cervical fascia because of the easy spread of infection from this location to the mediastinum

A 22-year-old man arrives to the emergency department with a Glasgow coma scale (GCS) of 15, pulse of 110, blood pressure of 120/60, and a stab wound to the lateral neck above the level of the mandible. What is the next step in management?

Angiography should be performed for a Zone 3 injury that lacks indications for immediate neck exploration.

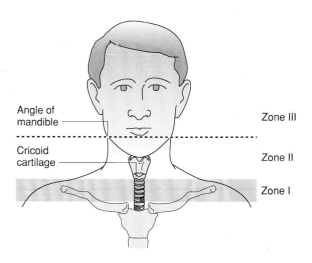

Zones of the neck. (With permission from Mulholland MW, Lillemoe KD, Doherty GM, et al., eds. *Greenfield's Surgery*. 4th ed. Philadelphia, PA: Lippincott Williams & Wilkins; 2005.)

Neck Zones

- Zone 1: Manubrium to cricoid cartilage
  - Most lethal when carotid is injured
  - Esophageal injuries can lead to mediastinitis
- Zone 2: Cricoid cartilage to angle of mandible
  - Most frequently injured
- Zone 3: Angle of mandible to skull base
  - Least frequently injured
- Carotid artery is injured in 6% of cases
- Indications for a neck exploration in trauma patients
  - Severe, active bleeding
  - Expanding hematoma
  - Progressing neurologic deficit
  - Loss of pulse
  - Hemoptysis/hematemesis
  - Subcutaneous emphysema, dyspnea, or stridor

There is some controversy about how to best manage penetrating neck trauma. Zone 1 and Zone 3 injuries are usually evaluated with arteriography to assess for occult vascular injury. Stable Zone 2 injuries are the easiest to follow with clinical examinations. Examination should include fiberoptic laryngoscopy.

A 23-year-old presents with epistaxis after being inadvertently elbowed during a basketball game. What is the appropriate treatment?

First, stop the bleeding by holding pressure over the nasal alae for 15 minutes without letting go. The patient should be seated with his head forward and allowed to spit any blood that accumulates in his mouth or throat. This position helps prevent aspiration and swallowing of blood, which can cause coughing and emesis.

Epistaxis

- 90% lifetime prevalence rate
- 90% are anterior

- Risk factors: Dryness, rhinosinusitis, digital trauma, nasal fracture, anticoagulation, thrombocytopenia, hypertension, nasal mass
- Most common site: Little's area (Kiesselbach plexus) in the anterior septum

Treatment

- Position patient as above and hold pressure for 15 minutes
- If still bleeding, blow nose to remove any clots, apply topical decongestant (e.g., oxymetazoline 0.05%), and reapply pressure
- If still bleeding, pack nose anteriorly using surgicel, gelfoam, or vaseline-impregnated gauze
- If still bleeding, consult otolaryngology for visualization
- Consider packing the other side of the nose and/or placing posterior packing (e.g., Foley catheter and Epistat)
- If still bleeding, the patient may need cauterization, operative intervention (ligation of the internal maxillary artery or external carotid), or embolization

Nasal Fracture

- Presents with pain, crepitance over the dorsum of the nose, epistaxis, and nasal deformity
- Workup includes history and physical examination, including examination of the nasal septum to rule out the presence of a septal hematoma
- Obtain CT scan of nose and face to exclude other injuries to the facial skeleton
- Treatment
  - Closed reduction
    - Can manipulate fracture and realign nose without using open incisions
    - Immediate reduction (less than 3 hours from time of injury) allows for fracture repair before swelling can obscure the contours of the face
    - Delayed reduction (5 to 14 days after injury) allows for fracture repair after swelling has resolved, but before the bones have healed
  - Open septorhinoplasty
    - For fractures that fail a closed reduction procedure or that present more than 2 weeks after the onset of injury
    - Open approach allows for nasal recontouring as well as the option of refracturing the nasal bone to produce an optimal outcome
- Complications
  - Cosmetic deformity
  - Cerebrospinal fluid (CSF) leak
  - Nasal airway obstruction
  - Chronic rhinosinusitis
  - Septal hematoma
    - Can lead to a septal abscess with resorption of septal cartilage, resulting in a saddle nose deformity or septal perforation

---

A 50-year-old man presents with a painless mass near the angle of his mandible. What is the most likely diagnosis? What is the appropriate treatment?

This is most likely a mass in the tail of the parotid gland. The most common parotid mass is a pleomorphic adenoma (benign mixed tumor). These tumors are treated with superficial parotidectomy, sparing the facial nerve.

Workup of Parotid Mass

- Tumors usually present as painless masses, but can present with facial paralysis if the facial nerve is involved
- Use CT scan or MRI to determine the location in either the superficial or deep parotid lobe
  - The parotid gland is divided into superficial and deep lobes by the facial nerve
- Begin with a fine needle aspiration (FNA)
  - Open biopsy should be avoided to prevent implantation of tumor into the wound
- Treatment is removal of the parotid tissue surrounding the lesion
  - Superficial parotidectomy if the mass is superficial to the facial nerve
  - Total parotidectomy if the lesion is deep to the facial nerve
- The facial nerve should be spared unless the nerve is invaded by tumor
- Document nerve function preoperatively to ensure facial nerve function is preserved postoperatively

Parotid Tumors

- The majority (80%) of salivary gland tumors originate in the parotid gland
  - Tumors in smaller glands are more likely to be malignant
  - Risk factors for malignancy include tobacco use and radiation exposure
- Most parotid lesions are benign (80%)
  - Pleomorphic adenoma is the most common benign mass (65%)
  - The second most common benign parotid mass is a Warthin tumor
    - Up to 10% of patients will have bilateral lesions
    - Associated with a history of smoking
  - A monomorphic adenoma is the least common
- The most common malignant parotid lesion is mucoepidermoid carcinoma, followed by adenoid cystic carcinoma
- The treatment for malignant parotid lesions includes removal of the lesion with sparing of the facial nerve (if it is not involved) and neck dissection for large tumors or tumors with aggressive histology
- The great auricular nerve is the most commonly injured nerve in parotid surgery, which leads to decreased sensation of the auricle

---

Following a parotidectomy, a patient complains of gustatory sweating. What is the next step in management?

Gustatory sweating (Frey syndrome) is a common complication of parotid surgery. Treatment includes reassurance, topical antiperspirants, topical anticholinergics, and botulinum toxin injection.

Complications of Parotidectomy

- Frey syndrome
  - Occurs in 30% to 60% of patients but is only symptomatic in 10%
  - Due to aberrant regeneration of the secretomotor parasympathetic fibers of the auriculotemporal nerve into the severed sympathetic fibers that supply the sweat glands of the overlying skin
  - Treatment is with topical anticholinergics or botulinum toxin injection

- Sialocele
  - Usually self-limited but may require serial aspiration or a pressure dressing
- Facial weakness/paralysis
  - Temporary facial weakness occurs in 10% to 30% of patients following parotidectomy
  - Permanent facial paralysis occurs in less than 3%
  - Upper division weakness resulting in incomplete eye closure must be addressed with ocular protection (e.g., moisture chamber, drops, and ointment) to prevent corneal ulcers
  - A gold weight for the upper lid may be necessary for passive eye closure if the weakness is permanent
  - Other procedures for facial reanimation include static facial slings, cranial nerve VII to XII transposition, and cranial nerve VII to VII cross facial innervation using a nerve graft

---

A 68-year-old man is diagnosed with a tumor of the minor salivary gland. What is the likelihood that it is malignant?

The smaller the salivary gland, the more likely the neoplasm is malignant: 20% of parotid gland tumors, 50% of submandibular gland tumors, and at least 60% of minor salivary gland tumors are malignant.

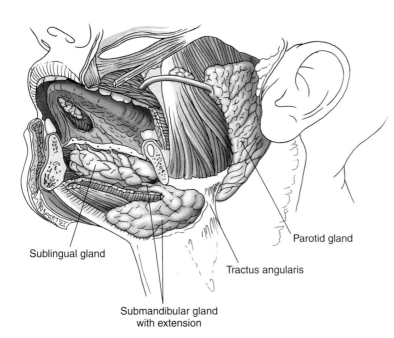

Sublingual gland

Tractus angularis

Submandibular gland with extension

Parotid gland

Parotid and salivary gland anatomy. (With permission from Fischer JE, Bland KI, Callery MP, et al., eds. *Mastery of Surgery.* 5th ed. Philadelphia, PA: Lippincott Williams & Wilkins; 2006.)

Salivary Gland Malignancies
- Comprise 3% of head and neck malignancies
- Sometimes related to history of radiation exposure

Mucoepidermoid Carcinoma
- Most common malignant salivary tumor
- 10% of all parotid tumors
- Prevalence highest in the fifth decade of life
- Women more commonly affected than men
- Classified as low-, intermediate-, or high-grade lesions
- Five-year survival is 70% for low-grade lesions and 50% for high-grade lesions

Adenoid Cystic Carcinoma

- Comprise 10% of all salivary neoplasms
- 3% of parotid tumors, 15% of submandibular tumors, and 30% of minor salivary gland tumors are adenoid cystic carcinomas
- Two-thirds are found in the minor salivary glands
- Is the most common malignancy of the submandibular, sublingual, and minor salivary glands
- Perineural invasion is common and can occur early—requires surgery and postoperative radiation
- Adenoid cystic carcinoma of the minor salivary glands of the palate may require maxillectomy for excision

Acinic Cell Carcinoma

- Peak incidence in the fifth decade of life
- Women slightly more commonly affected than men
- The majority are found in the parotid gland with most of the remaining tumors in the submandibular gland
- Comprise 15% of malignant parotid tumors
- Five-year survival is 80%

Malignant Mixed Tumors

- Develop from pleomorphic adenomas, a phenomenon known as carcinoma ex-pleomorphic adenoma
- 75% occur in the parotid gland
- Local invasion as well as locoregional and distant metastases are common
- Five-year survival is less than 10%

Nerves at risk for injury during a submandibular gland excision include the hypoglossal nerve, the lingual nerve, and the marginal mandibular branch of the facial nerve.

A 52-year-old woman presents with a new lateral neck mass. What is the next step in management?

An FNA biopsy is an excellent initial test following complete history and physical examination. A neck mass in an adult is cancer until proven otherwise.

Evaluation of a Non-thyroid Neck Mass

- FNA and CT scan with IV contrast are good first steps
- Avoid open biopsy, since this may spill tumor cells and disrupt surgical planes
- Avoid FNA if mass is pulsatile or if imaging is consistent with carotid body tumor

Differential Diagnosis of a Non-thyroid Neck Mass

- Metastatic squamous cell carcinoma from a primary site in the upper aerodigestive tract (i.e., tonsils, tongue base, nasopharynx, hypopharynx, larynx, scalp, unknown head and neck primary)
- Other metastases (thyroid carcinoma, melanoma, and lung)
- Lymphoma, carotid body tumor, vagal schwannoma, branchial cleft cyst, thyroglossal duct cyst, and infection

> A 61-year-old man presents with a new lateral neck mass. An FNA reveals squamous cell carcinoma. His physical examination is otherwise normal. CT and MRI are normal and a panendoscopy is unremarkable. What is the next step in management?

A neck dissection or radiation therapy may be required for a squamous cell carcinoma in the neck with an unknown primary site.

Squamous Cell Carcinoma in a Neck Mass with an Unknown Primary Site

- Begin with a thorough head and neck examination
- Perform an FNA biopsy of the mass
- Use CT scan or MRI (and occasionally PET scan) to look for evidence of primary site (e.g., tonsil or tongue base asymmetry)
- Perform panendoscopy in the operating room, which includes palpation, laryngoscopy, esophagoscopy, and bronchoscopy, with directed biopsies of the nasopharynx, tongue base, epiglottis, true and false vocal folds, piriform sinuses, post-cricoid region, and tonsils. If biopsies are negative, tonsillectomies are recommended
- Spiral chest CT may replace bronchoscopy
- Do not accept a negative FNA if suspicion for malignancy is high—repeat FNA due to possible sampling error
- An open biopsy can be performed at the time of panendoscopy
- Be prepared to perform a neck dissection if cancer is found on frozen section
- Human papilloma virus (HPV) and Epstein Barr virus detection from primary or nodal tissue are recommended

If no primary malignancy is found, the neck is treated with surgery or radiation, and the most likely primary sites are treated with radiation therapy to Waldeyer ring (the lymphoid tissues that form a ring around the opening of the throat: Tonsils laterally, adenoids superiorly, and lingual tonsil at the base).

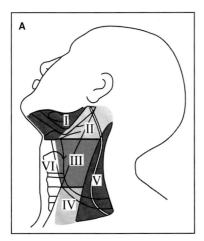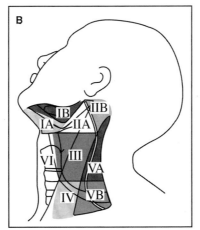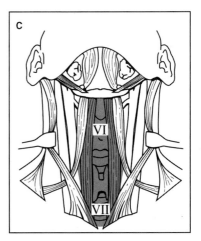

Cervical lymph node levels. (With permission from Fischer JE, Bland KI, Callery MP, et al., eds. *Mastery of Surgery.* 5th ed. Philadelphia, PA: Lippincott Williams & Wilkins; 2006.)

Neck Dissection

- Anterior cervical triangle: Anterior border of SCM inferiorly, inferior border of the mandible superiorly, and midline of the neck medially
- Posterior cervical triangle: Posterior border of SCM anteriorly, trapezius muscle posteriorly, and clavicle inferiorly

- Levels of neck dissection
    - Contents of submental and submandibular triangles
    - Anterior cervical triangle from skull base to carotid bifurcation
    - Anterior cervical triangle from carotid bifurcation to omohyoid muscle
    - Anterior cervical triangle from omohyoid muscle to clavicle
    - Posterior cervical triangle
    - Paratracheal and pretracheal nodes
- Radical neck dissection is removal of lymph node levels I to V, SCM, spinal accessory nerve (CN XI), omohyoid, ipsilateral thyroid, cervical branch of the facial nerve, and internal jugular vein
    - The majority of the morbidity from radical neck dissection is from CN XI resection
- Modified radical neck dissections spare the SCM, IJ, and CN XI
- Selective neck dissections involve removal of one or more levels and are generally performed to address primary draining nodes in N0 disease
- CN XI can be identified at the skull base exiting the jugular foramen and crossing lateral to the transverse process of C2
- Care must be taken to preserve the phrenic and vagus nerves

Risk Factors for Squamous Cell Carcinoma

- Tobacco and alcohol use can work synergistically to increase cancer risk
- HPV infection appears to be a common finding in pharynx cancers in non-smokers, especially base of tongue and tonsil cancer
- Leukoplakia of the pharynx or oral cavity often contains only dysplasia but may harbor carcinoma or carcinoma in situ and should be biopsied
- Erythroplakia carries a higher risk of malignancy
- Plummer-Vinson syndrome increases the risk of tongue and hypopharynx cancer
- Epstein-Barr virus increases the risk of nasopharyngeal cancer
- The majority (~90%) of oral cavity tumors are squamous cell cancers

---

A 75-year-old man with a 100 pack-year smoking history presents with hoarseness. What diagnostic test will reveal his lesion?

Indirect or fiberoptic laryngoscopy will demonstrate the site and extent of a glottic lesion, as well as the degree of cord mobility.

Laryngeal Cancer

- 4:1 male to female ratio
- Incidence highest in the sixth and seventh decades of life
- Principal risk factor is cigarette smoking
- 90% are squamous cell carcinoma
- Additional risk factors include chronic laryngotracheal reflux, inhalant exposure, and previous neck irradiation
- Presents as persistent hoarseness (glottic tumors), dysphagia, odynophagia, referred otalgia, hemoptysis, weight loss, or airway obstruction/stridor
- Can be supraglottic (40%), glottic (59%), or subglottic (1%)
- The *supraglottic* and *subglottic areas* have rich bilateral lymphatic drainage and high rates of regional lymph node metastases. Tumors in these areas are treated with surgery and radiation

- The *glottic area* is devoid of lymphatics; therefore, tumors confined to the glottis are associated with a low incidence of metastasis to locoregional lymph nodes
- Panendoscopy with biopsy is important in evaluation
- CT scan, MRI, and chest X-ray are routine
- PET-CT is becoming more common in evaluating lesions
- Surgery, radiation, chemoradiation, and combined modalities are used for treatment
- Early-stage tumors can be treated with radiation and salvage surgery
- "Organ preservation" surgery (supraglottic/supracricoid/partial laryngectomy) is useful for certain tumors
- Advanced-stage tumors require laryngectomy, a modified neck dissection, and adjuvant chemoradiation
- It is important to address the patient's nutritional status and the need for a feeding tube prior to treatment

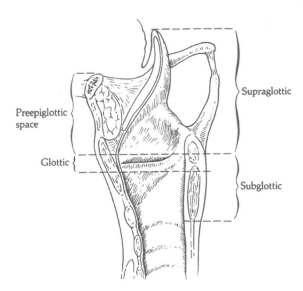

Major subdivisions of the larynx. (With permission from Fischer JE, Bland KI, Callery MP, et al., eds. *Mastery of Surgery*. 5th ed. Philadelphia, PA: Lippincott Williams & Wilkins; 2006.)

A 55-year-old man presents with an ulcerative lesion on the lower lip. What is the most likely histopathology of this lesion?

Greater than 95% of lip lesions are squamous cell carcinoma.

Lip Cancer
- The lower lip is frequently involved (probably due to sun exposure)
- Lower lip lesions are usually squamous cell carcinoma
- Upper lip lesions are usually basal cell carcinoma
- Most lip cancers are treated with surgical excision
- Defects of up to one-third may be closed primarily
- Local flaps are used for larger defects
- Free tissue transfer is used occasionally

Oral Cavity

- 90% are squamous cell carcinoma
- Other cancers include minor salivary gland malignancies, lymphomas, sarcomas, and melanomas
- Risk factors are tobacco (chewed and smoked), alcohol, poor oral hygiene, and chewing betel nuts (common in Southeast Asian communities)
- Workup includes a thorough head and neck examination, panendoscopy, biopsy, and CT/MRI
- Surgery followed by radiation is used to treat bulky tumors or tumors of significant depth
- Reconstructive options include primary closure, healing secondarily, skin graft, microvascular free flap, and a regional flap (pectoralis and latissimus)

For oral cavity cancers in general, neck dissection is performed for palpable metastases, or when the risk of occult metastases is greater than 20%. A neck dissection is often performed in conjunction with excision of primary tumors.

A 40-year-old man with HIV presents with a new cervical neck mass. What is the most likely diagnosis?

Cervical adenopathy in HIV-infected patients is common. Idiopathic follicular hyperplasia is the most common lymph node finding. An FNA biopsy is necessary to rule out malignancy, of which lymphoma is the most common type.

Cervical Adenopathy in the Human Immunodeficiency Virus Patient

- Differential diagnosis
  - Infection (atypical mycobacterium, PCP, lymphoma, tuberculosis, toxoplasmosis, and cat scratch disease)
  - Benign neoplasm (salivary gland disease, benign cervical adenopathy, and lymphoepithelial cysts)
  - Malignant neoplasm (Kaposi sarcoma, lymphoma, squamous cell carcinoma, and metastatic disease)
- Evaluate adenopathy with an FNA
- Perform an open biopsy only if the FNA is non-diagnostic and the patient has constitutional symptoms, localized adenopathy and/or a dominant nodule, or cytopenia
- Kaposi sarcoma may involve skin, oral mucosa, or lymph nodes
  - Treatment is local excision and radiotherapy
- Lymphoepithelial cysts are benign, multiloculated cysts that occur in the tail of the parotid
  - The cysts are frequently bilateral
  - Treatment is observation
  - Cysts will recur after aspiration and surgical excision

A 13-year-old boy presents with acute onset dysphagia and voice change ("hot potato voice"). On examination, he is found to have uvular deviation to the right side and bulging of the left anterior tonsillar pillar.

Peritonsillar abscess is most commonly caused by local spread from acute tonsillitis.

Peritonsillar Abscess

- Symptoms include fever, dysphagia, and voice change ("hot potato voice")
- A polymicrobial infection
- A needle aspiration of the abscess can be done and a specimen for culture obtained. If this fails, do tonsillar incision and drainage. Treat with antibiotics, hydration and analgesics

3 Cardiac Surgery

George Berberian

> Which conduit has the best long-term patency following coronary artery bypass surgery?

The internal mammary artery has the best long-term patency. The internal mammary artery is the first branch of the subclavian artery.

Vascular Anatomy

- The right coronary artery supplies
  - The right atrium
  - The right ventricle
  - The anterolateral left ventricle
  - The interventricular septum (posterior descending artery)
  - The sinoatrial (SA) and atrioventricular (AV) nodes
- The left coronary artery
  - Left anterior descending branch supplies
    - Interventricular septum
    - Anterolateral left ventricle
  - Circumflex branch supplies
    - Posterolateral left ventricle
- Dominance
  - Determined by the coronary artery from which the posterior descending artery originates
  - 90% of patients are right dominant
- The 10-year patency of an internal mammary graft is excellent (85%)

Coronary Artery Disease

- The most common cause of death in the United States
- Medical optimization: β-blocker, angiotensin-converting enzyme inhibitor
- Coronary artery bypass grafting is indicated for
  - ST elevation myocardial infarction (MI) with failed percutaneous intervention, hemodynamic instability, cardiogenic shock, or other MI complication
  - Low ejection fraction (EF) secondary to ischemia

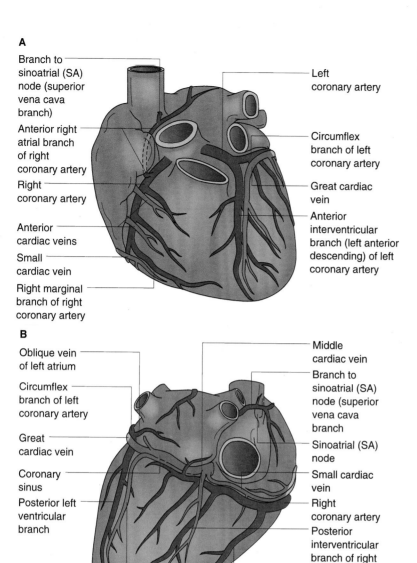

A

Branch to sinoatrial (SA) node (superior vena cava branch)

Anterior right atrial branch of right coronary artery

Right coronary artery

Anterior cardiac veins

Small cardiac vein

Right marginal branch of right coronary artery

Left coronary artery

Circumflex branch of left coronary artery

Great cardiac vein

Anterior interventricular branch (left anterior descending) of left coronary artery

B

Oblique vein of left atrium

Circumflex branch of left coronary artery

Great cardiac vein

Coronary sinus

Posterior left ventricular branch

Posterior vein of left ventricle

Middle cardiac vein

Branch to sinoatrial (SA) node (superior vena cava branch

Sinoatrial (SA) node

Small cardiac vein

Right coronary artery

Posterior interventricular branch of right coronary artery (posterior descending artery)

Right marginal artery

Coronary artery anatomy. (A) Anterior view. (B) Posterior view. (With permission from Mulholland MW, Lillemoe KD, Doherty GM, et al., eds. *Greenfield's Surgery*. 4th ed. Philadelphia, PA: Lippincott Williams & Wilkins; 2005.)

- Left main coronary artery disease
- Three-vessel disease
- Two-vessel disease with proximal left anterior descending artery disease and EF <50%

A 22-year-old man presents to the emergency department (ED) with a stab wound to the chest. He is hypotensive. A focused assessment with sonography for trauma (FAST) ultrasound examination of the heart demonstrates collapse of the right atrium. What is the differential diagnosis?

The finding of right atrial collapse suggests a tension pneumothorax or cardiac tamponade. Both conditions may also present with jugular venous distention. The absence of breath sounds over one lung mandates the emergent placement of a large-bore needle (or a chest tube, if available) to decompress the tension pneumothorax. The diagnosis of cardiac tamponade can be confirmed with the sonographic finding of pericardial blood.

Cardiovascular Trauma

- The right ventricle is the most commonly injured chamber in both blunt and penetrating cardiac trauma
- The right atrium is a low-pressure chamber and collapses with tension pneumothorax or cardiac tamponade
- A tension pneumothorax decreases venous return by compressing the superior and inferior vena cava
  - A chest X-ray (CXR) should *not* be performed because it wastes time
  - Emergent chest decompression is indicated
- Penetrating cardiac injury
  - Often presents with tamponade
  - Emergent pericardiocentesis is needed for cardiac tamponade unless an ED thoracotomy is indicated
  - ED thoracotomy
    - Blunt trauma—use only if pulse lost in the emergency room (ER)
    - Penetrating trauma—use only if pulse lost en route to ER or in ER
    - Left anterolateral thoracotomy at fourth interspace
    - Open pericardium anterior to phrenic nerve to relieve tamponade
    - Start cardiac massage and attempt to control bleeding from injury
- Blunt cardiac injury
  - If there is a new murmur, ectopy, or increased cardiac enzymes → emergent echo
  - Otherwise, admit for serial enzymes and cardiac monitoring
- Aortic injury
  - 15% of deaths from motor vehicle accidents
  - Due to rapid deceleration → disruption at points of aortic fixation, such as the ligamentum arteriosum
  - Diagnosis
    - Unequal radial pulses if subclavian takeoff is involved
    - CXR: Widened mediastinum, loss of aortic knob
  - Treat with antihypertensives until definitive surgical repair

---

Following a lower extremity vascular bypass procedure, a patient is noted to be slightly hypothermic. A pulmonary artery catheter reveals a pulmonary capillary wedge pressure of 20, a cardiac index of 1.2, and a systemic vascular resistance of 1,400. What treatment is indicated?

These findings are most consistent with postoperative heart failure or a postoperative MI. Dobutamine is the treatment of choice for postoperative heart failure presenting with low cardiac output.

Cardiogenic Shock/Heart Failure

- Postoperative cardiac failure is suggested by:
  - Increased central venous pressure
  - Increased pulmonary artery wedge pressure
  - Decreased cardiac output (which may manifest as decreased urine output)
- A dobutamine or dopamine infusion is indicated to treat cardiogenic shock

Vasoactive Agents

- Receptors
  - α_1—vascular smooth muscle constriction; gluconeogenesis, glycolysis
  - β_1—myocardial contraction and SA rate
  - β_2—relaxes vascular and bronchial smooth muscle; $\uparrow$ insulin, glucagon, and renin
  - Dopamine—relaxes renal and splanchnic smooth muscle
- Inotropes

Drug	Mechanism of action	Heart Rate (HR)	Pulmonary Capillary Pressure (PCP)	Cardiac Index (CI)	Systemic Vascular Resistance (SVR)	Mean Arterial Pressure (MAP)	Dose (μg/kg/min)
Dobutamine	β_1, β_2	$\uparrow$	$\downarrow$	$\uparrow$	$\downarrow$	$--$	3–15
Milrinone	Phosphodiesterase $\rightarrow$ NO release and $\rightarrow$ $\uparrow$ cAMP $\rightarrow$ $\uparrow$ Ca flux and $\uparrow$ myocardial activity	$\uparrow$	$\downarrow$	$\uparrow$	$\downarrow$	$\downarrow$	0.1–0.75

- Mixed inotropes/vasoconstrictors

Drug	Mechanism of action	HR	PCP	CI	SVR	MAP	Dose (μg/kg/min)
Norepinephrine (Levophed)	β_1, β_2, α_1 – Low dose $\rightarrow$ β_1 $\rightarrow$ $\uparrow$contractility –High dose $\rightarrow$ α_1 $\rightarrow$ potent vasoconstrictor of splanchnics	$\uparrow$	$\uparrow$	$\uparrow$	$\uparrow$	$\uparrow$	0.02–0.25
Epinephrine	β_1, β_2, α_1 – Low dose $\rightarrow$ β_1, β_2 $\rightarrow$ $\uparrow$ contractility and vasodilation – High dose $\rightarrow$ α_1 $\rightarrow$ vasoconstriction	$\uparrow$	$--$	$\uparrow$	$\uparrow$	$\uparrow$	0.02–0.25
Dopamine	Dopamine, β_1, β_2, α_1	$\uparrow$	$--$	$\uparrow$	$--$	$--$	3–15

- Vasoconstrictors

Drug	Mechanism of action	HR	PCP	CI	SVR	MAP	Dose
Phenylephrine (Neo-Synephrine)	α_1	$--$	$\uparrow$	$--$	$\uparrow$	$\uparrow$	0–9 μg/kg/min
Vasopressin	Arginine vasopressin (AVP)	$--$	$--$	$--$	$\uparrow$	$\uparrow$	0.01–0.1 U/min

- Vasodilators
  - Nitroprusside can $\rightarrow$ cyanide toxicity

Drug	Mechanism of action	HR	PCP	CI	SVR	MAP	Dose (μg/kg/min)
Nitroglycerin	NO → smooth muscle relaxation *Primarily venous dilation*	−−	↑	−−	↓	↓	0–3
Nitroprusside	Arginine vasopressin (AVP)	−−	−−	−−	↓	↓	0–9

What is the mechanism of an intra-aortic balloon pump?

A balloon pump augments diastolic blood flow and reduces afterload.

Intra-aortic Balloon Pump

- Can be placed at the bedside
  - The tip of the catheter should be just distal to the left subclavian 1 to 2 cm below the top of the arch
- Reduces afterload by inflating during diastole (40 milliseconds before the T-wave) and deflating during the P-wave (systole) → increased perfusion to the coronary arteries
- The indications for an intra-aortic balloon pump include
  - Acute MI with shock
  - Acute mitral insufficiency

A 56-year-old man is found to have a new holosystolic murmur 5 days after an acute MI. What is the next step in management?

A transesophageal echocardiogram should be performed for any suspicious findings following an acute MI. Given a new systolic murmur, it is important to rule out mitral regurgitation (MR) and a ventricular septal defect (VSD).

Acute Myocardial Infarction

- Complications after an acute MI usually present 3 to 7 days later and include
  - MR from a ruptured papillary muscle
  - VSD
  - Ventricular free wall rupture
- Can present as a new holosystolic murmur

What is the greatest risk factor in a patient's history for estimating preoperative cardiac risk?

An MI within 6 months prior.

- All elective surgeries should be postponed until 6 months post-MI
- β-Blockers (such as propranolol) are associated with improved cardiac outcomes:

- They should always be started postoperatively in people who have been on β-blockers preoperatively
- They should *not* be started postoperatively on people not on β-blockers preoperatively due to increased risk of stroke

---

A 41-year-old woman develops new-onset atrial fibrillation following a pulmonary lobectomy. Her vital signs are normal. What is the next step in management?

Treatment should center on heart rate control and evaluation for an underlying cause. Postoperative atrial fibrillation in a stable patient is usually transient and self-limited.

Atrial Fibrillation

- Treatment depends on the patient's blood pressure
    - If hemodynamically stable:
        - Calcium-channel blockers (verapamil)
        - β-Blockers (metoprolol or esmolol)
        - Antiarrhythmics (amiodarone)
    - If hemodynamically unstable, treat with emergent defibrillation
- Correct any electrolyte abnormalities
- Look for underlying causes such as MI, pneumothorax, pulmonary embolus, sepsis, volume overload, and shock

---

A 79-year-old woman has persistent chest pain, hypertension, a systolic ejection murmur that is decreased with standing, and episodes of syncope. What is the most likely diagnosis?

Aortic stenosis.

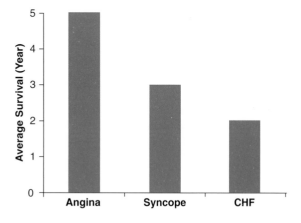

Survival by aortic stenosis symptom.

Aortic Stenosis

- Symptoms
    - Angina (most common presenting symptom)
    - Syncope
    - Congestive heart failure (portends the worst prognosis)

- Signs
    - Mid-systolic ejection murmur that radiates to the neck
    - Murmur decreased with standing or straining
- Most common acquired valve disease
- Due to calcification of the aortic valve
    - Bicuspid aortic valve
    - Rheumatic fever
- Associated with decreased left ventricle compliance
- Indications for valve replacement (any of the following)
    - Any of the above symptoms
    - Aortic valve area <0.75 cm^2
        - Usually have a pressure gradient >50 mmHg
    - Perform coronary catheterization if age >40 or angina

Aortic Regurgitation
- Symptoms: Congestive heart failure (CHF)
- Signs: Diastolic decrescendo murmur
- Can be caused by endocarditis, aortic dissection, or bicuspid aortic valve
- Indications for repair (either of the following)
    - Class II heart failure (shortness of breath on exertion)
    - Decreased ventricular function

Mitral Stenosis
- Symptoms
    - Pulmonary congestion
    - Atrial fibrillation
    - Atrial thrombus
- Signs: Mid-diastolic murmur
- Most commonly secondary to rheumatic fever
- Indications for valvuloplasty or replacement
    - Symptoms or mitral valve area <1 cm^2

Mitral Regurgitation
- Symptoms: CHF
- Signs: Pansystolic murmur
- Can be caused by endocarditis, recent MI with chorda rupture, myxomatous valve
- Indications for repair (either of the following)
    - Class II heart failure (shortness of breath on exertion)
    - Decreased ventricular function

Bioprosthetic Valves
- No need for anticoagulation
- Have a shorter life span
- Indications
    - Patients who desire pregnancy

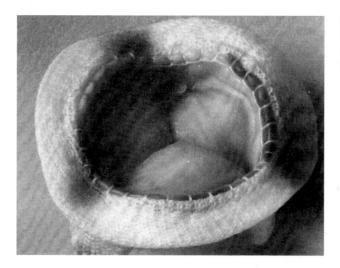

Bioprosthetic valve. (With permission from Mulholland MW, Lillemoe KD, Doherty GM, et al., eds. *Greenfield's Surgery*. 4th ed. Philadelphia, PA: Lippincott Williams & Wilkins; 2005.)

- Patients with contraindication to anticoagulation
- Older patients who are unlikely to require another valve in their lifetime and have frequent falls
- Contraindications
  - In children due to rapid calcification
  - Chronic renal dialysis

A 45-year-old female presents with myalgias, weight loss, anorexia, and fever. She has a history of rheumatic heart disease and recently underwent a tooth extraction for a dental abscess. On exam, she has splinter hemorrhages and indurated palmar nodules. What is her most likely diagnosis?

The most likely diagnosis is endocarditis.

Endocarditis

- Risk factors: Native valve disease (including mitral valve prolapse with regurgitation), prosthetic valves, rheumatic heart disease, congenital cardiac malformations, IV drug use
  - First-generation cephalosporins are indicated in these patients for pre-procedural endocarditis prophylaxis
  - Aortic valve is the most common site of prosthetic valve infections
  - Mitral valve is the most common site of native valve infections
- Pathogens
  - Native valve
    - *Streptococcus viridans*—most common
    - *Staphylococcus aureus*
    - *Enterococcus*
  - Prosthetic valve
    - *Staph. epidermidis*
    - *Strep. viridans*
- Pathophysiology
  - Initial endocardial injury → platelet aggregation and non-bacterial valvular vegetations
  - Transient bacteremia of any source seeds the vegetation
  - Bacterial overgrowth then ensues

- Signs
  - Petechiae
  - Splinter hemorrhages
  - Roth spots: Vasculitis of retinal arteries
  - Osler nodes: Indurated palmar nodules
  - Janeway lesions: Red macules on distal extremities
  - Distal septic emboli
- Indications for valve replacement
  - CHF
  - Embolic disease
  - Persistent sepsis despite antibiotics
  - Abscess

What is the most common congenital heart defect?

A ventricular septal defect is the most common congenital heart defect; approximately 50% close spontaneously.

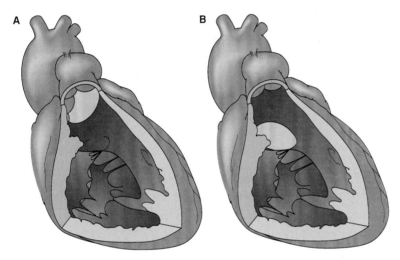
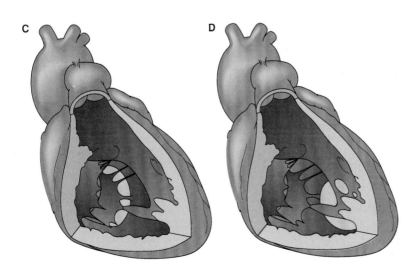

Ventricular septal defects.
(A) Subpulmonary VSD.
(B) Membranous VSD.
(C) Atrioventricular (AV) canal type VSD. (D) Muscular VSD. (With permission from Mulholland MW, Lillemoe KD, Doherty GM, et al., eds. *Greenfield's Surgery.* 4th ed. Philadelphia, PA: Lippincott Williams & Wilkins; 2005.)

Ventricular Septal Defect

- A left-to-right shunt
- An operation is indicated for severe symptoms or a failure to thrive
- The operation is usually deferred until age 1 to 2 years unless the defect is significant and the condition worsens

Reversal of any left-to-right shunt because of chronic pulmonary hypertension results in an Eisenmenger syndrome, an irreversible and lethal condition that manifests as cyanosis.

What type of atrial septal defect is the most common?

Ostium secundum.

Atrial Septal Defect

- A left-to-right shunt
- The incidence of an atrial septal defect is increased in patients with Down syndrome
- Ostium secundum is the most common type
- Elective repair is indicated at age 3 to 4 years

A 23-year-old man presents with symptoms of congestive heart failure and a CXR demonstrating rib notching. What is the likely diagnosis?

Coarctation of the aorta can present in early adulthood as congestive heart failure or hypertension (with frequent headaches).

Coarctation of the Aorta

- An affected infant with coarctation of the aorta may appear normal at birth
- Rib notching may be seen on CXR from bony erosion due to dilated intercostal collaterals
- The most common site of coarctation is near the ligamentum arteriosum
- A pulse discrepancy (decreased lower extremity pulses) may be found

---

A 3-month-old girl is frequently noted to be in the squatting position. Her mother notes that the baby has also had intermittent "blue spells." What is the most likely diagnosis?

Tetralogy of Fallot often presents as cyanosis in the first 6 months of life.

Tetralogy of Fallot

- The most common cyanotic congenital heart lesion
- Is comprised of four defects
  - Right ventricular outflow obstruction
  - Right ventricular hypertrophy
  - Ventricular septal defect (right-to-left shunt)
  - Overriding aorta

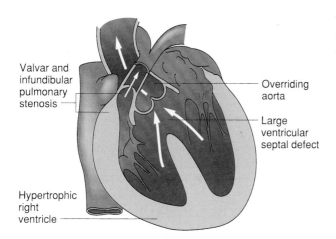

Tetralogy of Fallot. (With permission from Mulholland MW, Lillemoe KD, Doherty GM, et al., eds. *Greenfield's Surgery.* 4th ed. Philadelphia, PA: Lippincott Williams & Wilkins; 2005.)

Valvar and infundibular pulmonary stenosis

Overriding aorta

Large ventricular septal defect

Hypertrophic right ventricle

- Pulmonary blood flow is dependent on a patent ductus arteriosus
- Squatting may relieve dyspnea by increasing SVR, which decreases the right-to-left shunt

---

A newborn baby boy is noted to be cyanotic at birth. In the immediate neonatal period, he has persistent poor oxygen saturation. Physical examination demonstrates a systolic murmur and a loud single heart sound. What treatment is required?

Transposition of the great arteries requires surgical intervention in the newborn period.

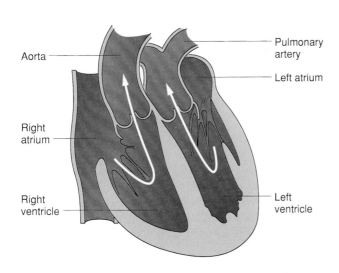

Aorta

Right atrium

Right ventricle

Pulmonary artery

Left atrium

Left ventricle

Transposition of the great arteries. (With permission from Mulholland MW, Lillemoe KD, Doherty GM, et al., eds. *Greenfield's Surgery.* 4th ed. Philadelphia, PA: Lippincott Williams & Wilkins; 2005.)

Transposition of the Great Arteries

- A right-to-left shunt
- The aorta usually arises anteriorly from the right ventricle
- The neonate relies on oxygenated and deoxygenated blood mixing via an atrial septal defect and/or a ventricular septal defect
- Give prostaglandin E_2 to keep the ductus arteriosus open (indomethacin is used to close the ductus arteriosus)
- Definitive treatment is the arterial switch operation with reimplantation of the coronary arteries

A newborn presents with significant congestive heart failure and a massively enlarged heart. What is the most likely diagnosis?

Truncus arteriosus.

Truncus Arteriosus

- A right-to-left shunt
- Characterized by the presence of a single arterial trunk arising from both ventricles
- Surgical repair is performed when the patient is stable

4 | Thoracic Surgery

Sunil Singhal

A 56-year-old man presents to the emergency room, coughing up several cups of thick bloody sputum. What is the most appropriate first step in managing massive hemoptysis?

Intubate the patient and perform a rigid bronchoscopy.

Massive Hemoptysis

- Greater than 600 mL of blood loss in 24 hours
- Causes
  - Necrotizing pneumonia
  - Tuberculosis
  - Cystic fibrosis
  - Neoplastic lesions
  - Wegener granulomatosis
  - Inflammatory lesions
- Management should always begin with securing the airway
- Use rigid bronchoscopy to localize the site of bleeding
- Control the source of bleeding

Rigid bronchoscopy is preferred over flexible bronchoscopy because it permits selective intubation of the non-bleeding side, suctioning of blood, and the best visual field. The patient should be positioned in a decubitus position with the healthy, non-bleeding side in the superior position to avoid aspiration.

A 58-year-old female is found to have a 1-cm peripheral lung nodule during a preoperative chest X-ray (CXR) for an elective umbilical hernia repair. What is the next step in management?

Review an old CXR for comparison. A chest CT is required to evaluate any new mass or a change in size.

Solitary Pulmonary Nodule

- Defined as a lesion <3 cm in size
- 5% are malignant (in people over 60 years of age, approximately half are malignant)

- Once discovered, the first step is to review old chest radiographs to determine the age of the nodule
  - Lesions unchanged for more than 2 years should be followed with yearly chest radiographs
- A CXR should be reviewed for evidence of calcification, which suggests benign disease and may be observed with a repeat CXR 3 months later
- If there is no evidence of calcification or the mass is changing in size, a chest CT should be obtained
  - If a CT scan reveals any suspicious morphology or mediastinal lymph node enlargement, a tissue diagnosis should be made
    - CT findings suggestive of malignancy include corona radiate (spiculations), lobulations, irregularity of the mass
  - Tissue diagnosis can be made with diagnostic bronchoscopy, mediastinoscopy, percutaneous biopsy, or thoracoscopic biopsy
  - A nodule that is not suspicious for malignancy or is under 0.5 cm in size can be followed with a repeat CT scan in 6 months

Most calcified solitary pulmonary nodules (SPNs) are benign, representing granulomas.

A 39-year-old asthmatic but otherwise healthy farmer from Ohio is noted to have an episode of hemoptysis. CXR reveals a hilar mass. What fungal infection is most likely?

Histoplasmosis.

Fungal Infections

- Histoplasmosis
  - The most common fungal infection in the United States
  - Is particularly endemic to the Mississippi river basin
  - Fusion of the mediastinal lymph nodes can result in a single large mass that becomes encapsulated (mediastinal granuloma)
  - Most infections are self-limited and do not require treatment
  - Advanced disease (fibrosing mediastinitis) is due to a high degree of exposure and has a poor outcome
- Aspergillosis
  - Tends to colonize in pre-existing pulmonary cavities and develop a "fungus ball" (aspergilloma)
  - Surgery is the treatment of choice in immunocompetent individuals
- Blastomycosis
  - Unique in that patients develop simultaneous pulmonary and cutaneous manifestations
- Actinomycosis
  - Patients develop an abscess with yellow-brown particles resembling sulfur granules
  - Classically presents in patients with poor oral hygiene who experience an indolent, but progressive course of fever, night sweats, weight loss, and blood-streaked sputum

---

A 46-year-old driver in a motor vehicle crash is noted to have an opacification over a broken anterior right sixth rib. He is otherwise hemodynamically stable, without hemoptysis or a pleural effusion. What is the most likely diagnosis?

Pulmonary contusion.

Pulmonary Contusion

- Self-limited bruise of the lung parenchyma
- Rule out any active bleeding
- Treat with supplemental oxygen, close monitoring for respiratory failure, vigorous chest physiotherapy, and pain control
- Consider an thoracic epidural for anesthesia

A 26-year-old male develops streptococcal pneumonia. Despite intravenous antibiotics, he continues to spike temperatures and has a leukocytosis. A CT scan of the chest reveals a loculated pleural fluid collection. What is the next appropriate step?

A chest tube thoracostomy is indicated for the treatment of an empyema.

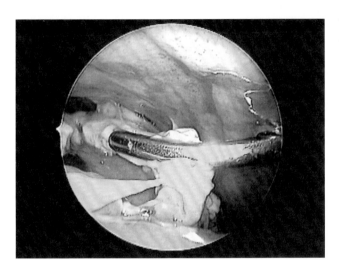

Video-assisted thoracoscopic surgery treatment of an empyema. (With permission from Mulholland MW, Lillemoe KD, Doherty GM, et al., eds. *Greenfield's Surgery*. 4th ed. Philadelphia, PA: Lippincott Williams & Wilkins; 2005.)

Empyema

- Pus in the pleural space
- Characteristics of pleural fluid with empyema: pH < 7.0, glucose < 40 mg/dL, protein > 3 g/dL, LDH > 1,000 IU/L
- The most common etiology is pneumonia (called a parapneumonic effusion)
- Exudative phase (<24 hours): Treat with intravenous antibiotics and thoracentesis
- Fibropurulent phase (24 to 72 hours): Treat with intravenous antibiotics, chest tube thoracostomy, and consider intrapleural fibrinolytic agents (i.e., streptokinase)
- Organized phase (>72 hours): Treat with intravenous antibiotics, consider chest tube thoracostomy, and intrapleural fibrinolytic agents
  - More likely to require video-assisted thoracoscopic surgery (VATS) or limited thoracotomy with rib resection
  - Complicated cases will require decortication (i.e., removal of constricting peel over the lung) and a muscle transposition flap

Staphylococcus and *Streptococcus* are the most common organisms cultured from an empyema.

Evaluation of Pleural Fluid

Test	Transudate	Exudate	Empyema
WBC	<1,000	>1,000	>1,000
pH	7.45–7.55	≤7.45	<7.30
Pleural fluid protein to serum ratio	<0.5	>0.5	>0.5
Pleural fluid LDH to serum ratio	<0.6	>0.6	>0.6

An 8-year-old student in primary school develops progressive wheezing unresponsive to inhaled nebulizers. Bronchopulmonary evaluation demonstrates a tracheal lesion. What is the most likely diagnosis?

Benign tracheal papilloma.

Benign Tracheal Papilloma

- Most common in children
- Usually multifocal
- Associated with human papilloma virus 6 and 11
- Treat with endoscopic laser ablation
- High tendency for recurrence

A 17-year-old man develops sudden shortness of breath while watching TV. He has no medical history of lung disease or recent trauma. A CXR demonstrates a large right pneumothorax. What is the most likely etiology?

A ruptured apical bleb is the most common etiology of a non-traumatic, non-iatrogenic pneumothorax.

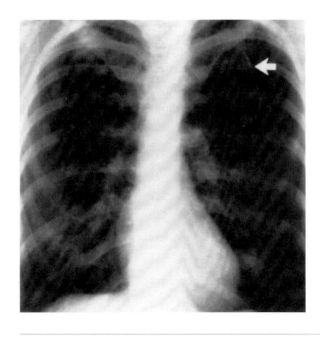

Pneumothorax. (With permission from Mulholland MW, Lillemoe KD, Doherty GM, et al., eds. *Greenfield's Surgery*. 4th ed. Philadelphia, PA: Lippincott Williams & Wilkins; 2005.)

Primary Spontaneous Pneumothorax

- Occurs due to the rupture of small apical blebs (a bleb is <2 cm whereas a bulla is >2 cm in size).
- Typically occurs in tall, thin men between the ages of 20 to 35 years
- A physical exam should be directed to rule out Marfan disease
- Typically presents with chest pain and dyspnea
- Obtain a CT scan to establish the size of the pneumothorax and delineate associated parenchymal disease
- Indications for surgery
  - Recurrence after first episode (most common indication)
  - First episode, complicated by persistent air leak or hemothorax
  - Failure of the lung to re-expand
  - Tension pneumothorax on the first episode
  - Bilateral pneumothorax on the first episode
  - Absence of medical facilities in isolated regions
  - Occupational hazard (i.e., pilot, deep sea diver, etc.)

A 39-year-old is in a motor vehicle accident. CXR reveals an incidental 2-cm pulmonary mass with popcorn calcifications. What is the most likely diagnosis?

Pulmonary hamartoma.

Pulmonary Hamartoma

- Round lesions located in the periphery of the lung
- Typically slow growing
- Represent 10% of all pulmonary nodules
- The majority are discovered incidentally, but they can also present with pneumonia, atelectasis, or hemoptysis
- Diagnosed by CXR ("popcorn" calcification), spiral CT, bronchoscopy, and FNA (fine needle aspiration)
- Treated with enucleation or wedge resection

A 64-year-old smoker is found to have a mass obstructing the left mainstem bronchus on radiographic studies. During bronchoscopic examination under general anesthesia, a biopsy specimen is taken. The patient immediately develops hemorrhage from this site. What is the next step in management?

Management of a Hemorrhagic Bronchial Biopsy Site

- Advance the bronchoscope to the mainstem bronchus proximal to the site of hemorrhage
- Advance the endotracheal tube over the bronchoscope to diminish spillage to the contralateral lung
- Working through the bronchoscope lumen, apply topical epinephrine (0.2 mg of epinephrine in 500 cc of lactated ringers)
- Consider cauterization, tamponade with epinephrine soaked gauze, or selective balloon tamponade

You have been carefully following a patient with an SPN in your thoracic surgery clinic. What is the most likely pathology of a lung nodule based on doubling time?

Doubling Time of Nodule Size

- <20 days, most likely infectious in nature
- 20 to 400 days, most likely a pulmonary malignancy
- >400 days, likely a benign lung mass

Six weeks after extubation following a prolonged ICU course, a 28-year-old man reports shortness of breath on exertion. A CXR is normal. What is the most likely diagnosis?

Post-intubation stenosis.

Post-intubation Stenosis

- Presents as dyspnea on exertion 1 to 6 weeks after extubation
- Symptomatic with luminal narrowing of >50%
- Diagnosed by bronchoscopy and CT scan
- Treatments include dilation using rigid bronchoscopy, laser resection, internal stents, tracheal reconstruction, segmental resection and primary anastomosis, and permanent tracheostomy

What is the lifetime risk of developing lung cancer in smokers?

10%.

Tobacco Use

- 25% of all Americans smoke
- The relative risk of smokers to non-smokers in developing lung cancer is 13
- 90% of lung cancer is attributable to tobacco use
- The overall 5-year survival for lung cancer is 10%
- After lung cancer, the other most common cancer in smokers is head and neck cancer

A 72-year-old patient undergoes a tracheostomy and gastrostomy tube after a cerebrovascular accident. Three weeks later, while awaiting rehabilitation placement, he becomes acutely hypotensive and develops profuse bleeding from his tracheostomy site. What is the next step in management?

Place a finger in through the tracheostomy site and put pressure over the artery to control the bleeding. Then, as soon as possible, perform emergent intubation and proceed to the operating room for evaluation of a possible tracheoinnominate artery fistula.

Tracheoinnominate Artery Fistula

- Management centers on control of the airway, control of bleeding, and resuscitation of the patient
- Hyperinflate the tracheostomy balloon

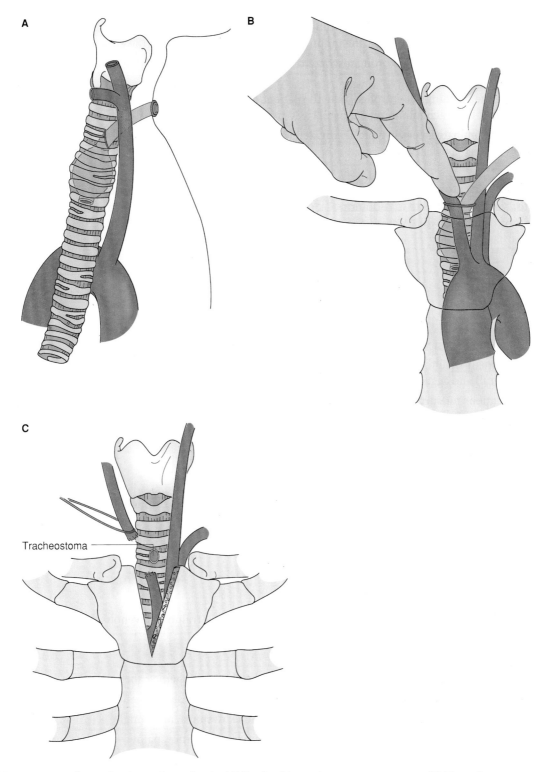

Tracheostoma

Management of a tracheoinnominate fistula. (A) Tracheal innominate artery anatomy. (B) Manually compress the innominate artery. (C) The innominate artery is typically divided with no reconstruction. (With permission from Mulholland MW, Lillemoe KD, Doherty GM, et al., eds. *Greenfield's Surgery*. 4th ed. Philadelphia, PA: Lippincott Williams & Wilkins; 2005.)

- Place an endotracheal tube above the tracheostomy
- If hyperinflating the tracheostomy tube fails to control the bleeding, remove the tracheostomy tube, and manually compress the innominate artery while advancing the endotracheal tube
- Alternatively, use a rigid bronchoscope to compress the tracheostomy balloon against the innominate artery
- Once the bleeding is controlled, take the patient emergently to the operating suite for surgical repair of the tracheoinnominate fistula
- The innominate artery is typically divided with no reconstruction

---

An 18-year-old intoxicated college student presents to the emergency department after a motor vehicle crash. He is requiring 4 L of oxygen via nasal cannula and has paradoxical motion of his chest wall. What is the most likely diagnosis?

Flail chest.

Flail Chest

- Fracture of at least three ribs, each in a separate location resulting in paradoxical motion of a segment of chest wall
- Treatment should focus on pain control with a patient-controlled analgesia (intravenous or epidural) and aggressive pulmonary toilet
- Indications for surgery include failure to wean from mechanical ventilation and severe cosmetic deformity
- Surgically managed by internal fixation (wire sutures, intramedullary wires, Judet staples) or external fixation (metal plate)

A 58-year-old retired carpenter presents with facial flushing, right upper arm edema, dyspnea, and a cough. What is the most likely diagnosis?

Superior vena cava (SVC) syndrome.

Superior Vena Cava Syndrome

- Partial or complete obstruction of the SVC with possible intraluminal venous thrombosis
- More common in men between the ages of 50 and 70 years
- 95% are due to malignancy
    - Most common associated malignancy is small cell bronchogenic cancer
    - Also associated with infectious, catheter-related, or other rare causes
- May present with facial fullness or flushing, headache, dyspnea, and cough
- Less common complaints include edema of the upper extremities, pain, dysphagia, and syncope
- Physical findings include prominent distended and tortuous venous systems in the face, neck, and upper trunk; facial cyanosis; and pleural effusion
- Once diagnosed by CT scan, a tissue diagnosis can be made by bronchoscopy, FNA biopsy, or mediastinotomy
- Surgical intervention is NOT recommended except in select individuals with a benign etiology
- Steroids can be temporizing
- Chemotherapy, radiation therapy, or both can effectively relieve the signs and symptoms arising from malignant disease

A 35-year-old female nurse's aide presents to her primary care doctor with neck and shoulder pain with intermittent paresthesias in the medial aspects of her arm and her fourth and fifth fingers. Physical exam findings reveal that her symptoms can be reproduced by lifting her arms over her head. Chest radiograph and shoulder X-rays reveal a cervical rib. What is the next step in management?

Surgery is not the first step in the management of thoracic outlet syndrome. The patient should be placed on a physical therapy regimen prior to consideration for surgery.

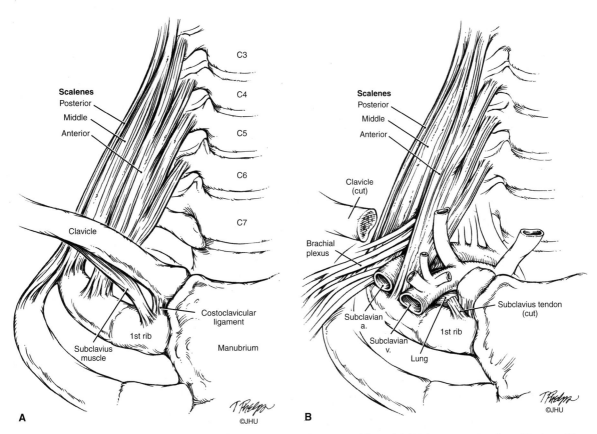

Anatomy of scalenes, brachial plexus, subclavian artery and vein, and first rib. (With permission from Fischer JE, Bland KI, Callery MP, et al., eds. *Mastery of Surgery*. 5th ed. Philadelphia, PA: Lippincott Williams & Wilkins; 2006.)

Thoracic Outlet Syndrome

- Compression of the brachial plexus (90%), subclavian artery, or subclavian vein against the cervical rib, the anterior scalene, and/or the middle scalene muscle
- Cervical and chest radiographs can be diagnostic
- For concerns of arterial compression or venous compromise, vascular studies are indicated
- Medical management is typically 85% successful (exercise to improve posture and weight reduction to relieve pressure)
- Surgery typically entails rib resection and release of the scalene muscles
- Indications for surgery include
  - Failure of conservative treatment
  - Arterial complications (occlusion, aneurysm, or distal emboli)
  - Venous thrombosis

Thoracic outlet syndrome is most commonly neurogenic (not vascular) and can often be treated medically.

A 51-year-old female develops progressive right-sided pleuritic chest pain. CXR and CT scan are suspicious for the presence of a pleural-based tumor. What is the most likely diagnosis?

Metastatic tumors (lung and breast) are the most common pleural tumors (90%). Mesothelioma is the most common primary malignant pleural tumor.

Malignant Mesothelioma

- Neoplastic mesothelial cells expand in the pleural space and encase the lung
- Most often caused by the combination of asbestos (85%) exposure and tobacco abuse
- Presents as dyspnea and chest pain (90% of patients)
- Diagnosis is made with a CT scan and open/thoracoscopic biopsy (FNA and pleural fluid analysis are typically non-diagnostic)
- Early stage disease is treated with an extrapleural pneumonectomy
- Advanced disease is treated with palliation (pleurectomy and/or chemoradiation)
- Median survival is <1 year

A 58-year-old female admits to several months of worsening cough, shortness of breath, and now, blood-tinged sputum. She undergoes bronchoscopy and is discovered to have a mass in the left upper lobe. A biopsy of this mass reveals features consistent with a neuroendocrine tumor. What is the most likely diagnosis?

Pulmonary neuroendocrine tumors include typical carcinoid tumors (most common and least aggressive), atypical carcinoid (intermediately aggressive), and small cell lung cancer (aggressive).

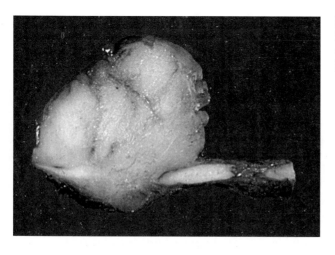

Lung carcinoid. (With permission from Mulholland MW, Lillemoe KD, Doherty GM, et al., eds. *Greenfield's Surgery*. 4th ed. Philadelphia, PA: Lippincott Williams & Wilkins; 2005.)

Typical Carcinoid Tumor

- 5% of all lung tumors
- Neuroendocrine tumor
- Well-differentiated and slow-growing
- Metastases are rare

- The majority are biologically inactive, although they are capable of producing peptides and hormones—serum chromogranin A levels can be measured
- Usually symptomatic due to endobronchial obstruction can present with recurrent pneumonia, wheezing, chest pain, or hemoptysis
- 75% are visible on bronchoscopy
- Treatment is surgical resection

Four days after a transhiatal esophagectomy for curative resection of an esophageal adenocarcinoma, the patient develops pleuritic chest pain. CXR reveals a left pleural effusion. Thoracentesis reveals several hundred milliliters of a milky white fluid. What is the next step in management?

The patient most likely sustained an iatrogenic injury to the thoracic duct. A chylothorax can sometimes be managed with chest drainage and total parental nutrition (TPN). A persistent thoracic duct leak may require surgical oversewing.

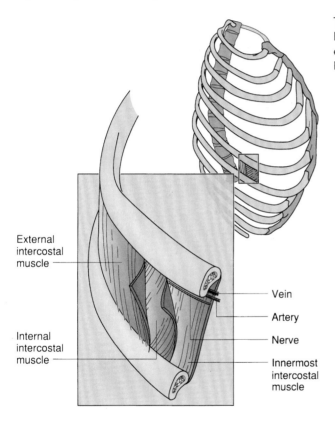

Thoracic duct anatomy. (With permission from Mulholland MW, Lillemoe KD, Doherty GM, et al., eds. *Greenfield's Surgery.* 4th ed. Philadelphia, PA: Lippincott Williams & Wilkins; 2005.)

External intercostal muscle

Internal intercostal muscle

Vein

Artery

Nerve

Innermost intercostal muscle

Chylothorax

- Commonly results from injury to the thoracic duct during thoracic surgery
  - Injury above T6 → left-sided chylothorax
  - Injury below T6 → right-sided chylothorax
- Treatment
  - Conservative treatment
    - Chest tube placement
    - NPO/TPN or low fat diet for 3 to 4 weeks
  - MRI ductogram and interventional radiology for coiling of cisterna chyla

- Surgical therapy—indicated if conservative therapy fails
  - Ligation of thoracic duct on the right side low in mediastinum—if not malignant
  - For malignant causes, perform mechanical or talc pleurodesis

If conservative measures fail after 3 to 4 weeks, the patient will require surgery to ligate the thoracic duct.

A 42-year-old female presents to her primary care doctor with diplopia and difficulty in chewing as the day progresses. Chest radiograph reveals an anterior mediastinal mass. What is the most likely diagnosis?

Thymoma.

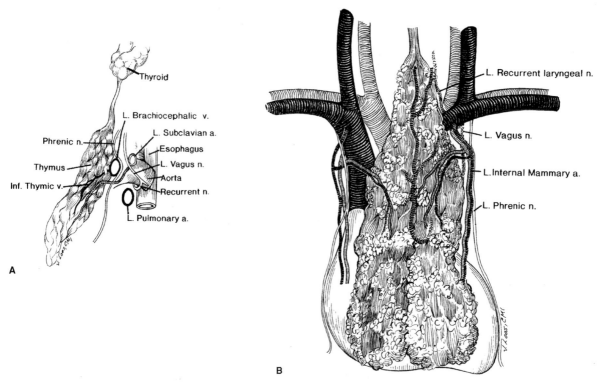

Normal anatomy of thymus. (With permission from Fischer JE, Bland KI, Callery MP, et al., eds. *Mastery of Surgery.* 5th ed. Philadelphia, PA: Lippincott Williams & Wilkins; 2006.)

Thymoma

- Myasthenia gravis is an autoimmune disorder characterized by progressive loss of skeletal muscle strength with sustained activity/repetitive stimulation
- In 80% of cases, the disease is mediated by antibodies against the nicotinic receptor of acetylcholine at the neuromuscular junction
- Myasthenic crisis is a rapid deterioration in neuromuscular function with respiratory compromise due to ventilatory muscle insufficiency or weakness of the upper airway musculature
- 10% of all patients with myasthenia gravis have a thymoma
- 50% of all patients with a thymoma have myasthenia gravis
- Thymomas are typically well-differentiated and encapsulated

- If pathology reveals that the thymoma invades through the capsule, it is considered malignant
- Treatment is total thymectomy, either by a transcervical approach or median sternotomy
- Malignancy is diagnosed clinically by invasion of the surrounding structures (35%)
- Excise en bloc with the tumor if possible
- Thymomas in myasthenia gravis patients need special perioperative preparation: Plasmapheresis to decrease acetylcholine receptors, steroids, and perioperative tensilon
- Malignant thymomas require postoperative radiation
- After thymectomy, complete response (no symptoms without medication) is seen in about 45% of patients
- More than 80% of patients experience at least some improvement in disease symptoms after thymectomy
- Symptoms can improve 3 months to decades after treatment

> What is the most common cause of acute mediastinitis?

Median sternotomy following cardiac surgery.

Acute Mediastinitis

- Causes
  - Sternotomy
  - Esophageal disruption
  - Spread of infection from the oropharynx, neck, lung, pleura, ribs, or subphrenic region
  - Blunt/penetrating trauma
- Principles of management
  - Intravenous antibiotics
  - Search for a causative organism
  - Pain control
- Surgical intervention (wide debridement and drainage tube placement) may be required for severe infections secondary to esophageal disruption and postoperative cardiac surgery

> An 18-year-old college student develops chest pain. A chest radiograph reveals an anterior mediastinal mass. What is the next step in management?

A hematological workup and CT scan. The most likely differential diagnosis is a lymphoma versus a germ cell tumor.

Evaluation of a Mediastinal Mass

- Complete blood count with differential
- Tumor markers: α-fetoprotein and β-human chorionic gonadotropin
- CT scan (preferred over MRI)
- FNA
- If FNA non-diagnostic, will require mediastinoscopy or VATS

Mediastinal Tumors by Compartment

- Anterior (thymus)—most common site for a mediastinal tumor (the "5 Ts")
  - Thymoma (#1)

- Thyroid cancer and goiters
- T-cell lymphoma
- Teratoma (and other germ cell tumors)
- Parathyroid adenomas
- Middle (heart, trachea, ascending aorta)
  - Bronchogenic cysts
    - Are posterior to carina
    - Arise from abnormal foregut or tracheobronchial tree buds
    - Resect if symptomatic in an adult or asymptomatic in children
  - Pericardial cysts
  - Lymphoma
- Posterior (esophagus, descending aorta)
  - Enteric cysts
  - Neurogenic tumors
  - Lymphoma

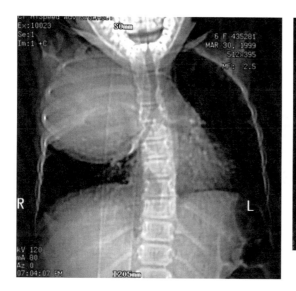 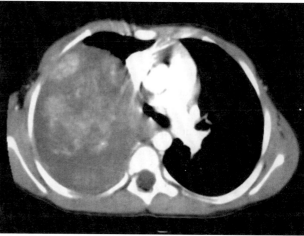

Large neurogenic tumor (paraganglioma). (With permission from Mulholland MW, Lillemoe KD, Doherty GM, et al., eds. *Greenfield's Surgery.* 4th ed. Philadelphia, PA: Lippincott Williams & Wilkins; 2005.)

A 40-year-old man presents with bruises of his chest wall from playing rugby. He continues to have tenderness over the site for a week. His primary care doctor performs a CXR, which reveals a radiopaque mass in his fifth rib with "popcorn" calcifications. What is his most likely diagnosis?

Chondrosarcoma.

Chondrosarcoma

- Most common malignant neoplasm of the chest wall (>50%)
- The most common locations are the ribs (80%) and the sternum (20%)
- Typically diagnosed by excisional biopsy
- Starts in the medulla of the bone and eventually erodes through the cortex

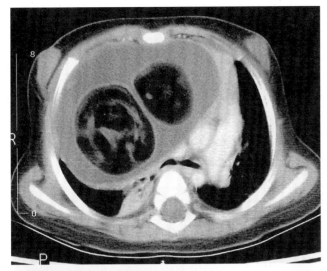

Mediastinal teratoma. (With permission from Mulholland MW, Lillemoe KD, Doherty GM, et al., eds. *Greenfield's Surgery.* 4th ed. Philadelphia, PA: Lippincott Williams & Wilkins; 2005.)

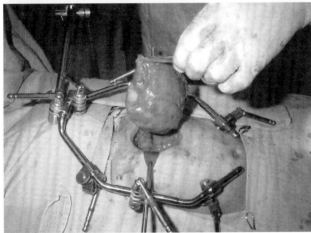

- Treat with wide local excision and 4 cm margins and typically requires chest wall reconstruction
- Prognosis depends on tumor grade, size, and location

Osteochondroma
- Most common benign tumor of the chest wall
- Excise with 2 cm margins

A 58-year-old man with a history of heavy tobacco use presents with hiccups and dyspnea on exertion. Chest radiograph reveals elevation of the right hemidiaphragm. What is the most likely diagnosis?

Phrenic nerve invasion by a primary lung tumor.

Phrenic Nerve Invasion
- Tumors on the medial side of the lung can invade mediastinal structures and the phrenic nerve
- Phrenic nerve involvement may also cause referred shoulder pain due to its common origin from the C3 to C5 nerve roots

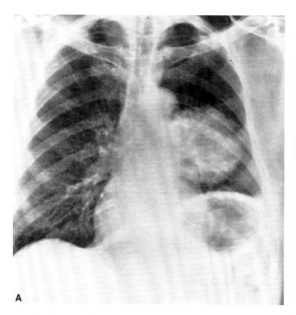
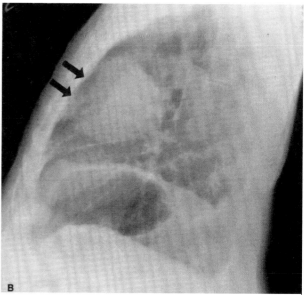
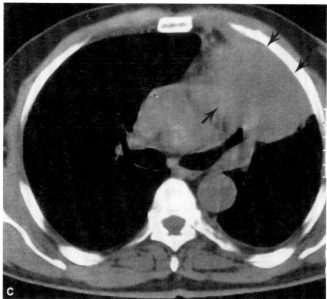

Large lung mass with phrenic nerve invasion. (With permission from Mulholland MW, Lillemoe KD, Doherty GM, et al., eds. *Greenfield's Surgery.* 4th ed. Philadelphia, PA: Lippincott Williams & Wilkins; 2005.)

What is the most common symptom at the time of presentation in a patient with lung cancer?

95% of patients with lung cancer are symptomatic at the time of presentation. Symptoms are caused by local tumor growth, chest wall invasion, mediastinal invasion, metastatic disease, or tumor-related paraneoplastic syndrome. Dry cough is the most common presenting symptom.

Presentation of Lung Cancer

- Those arising in large airways or centrally located can produce local symptoms including cough, localized wheezing, hemoptysis, focal atelectasis, dyspnea, and post-obstructive pneumonitis
- A cavitating tumor or post-obstructive pneumonitis can produce symptoms of fevers, chills, and productive cough
- Tumors arising in small airways or the periphery are usually asymptomatic

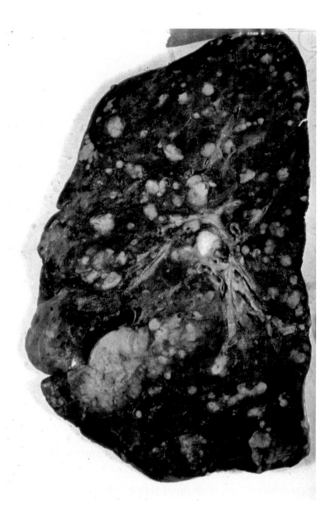

Metastatic carcinoma of the lung. (With permission from Mulholland MW, Lillemoe KD, Doherty GM, et al., eds. *Greenfield's Surgery.* 4th ed. Philadelphia, PA: Lippincott Williams & Wilkins; 2005.)

- Systemic symptoms include fatigue, weight loss, anorexia, cachexia, and fever
- Mediastinal invasion can cause recurrent laryngeal nerve injury on the left (voice cord paralysis) or phrenic nerve injury on the right (diaphragmatic paralysis)

Metastatic Tumors to the Lung

- Most common metastatic tumors in the lung: Colon, breast, renal
- Criteria for pulmonary resection
  - Metastatic disease is limited to the lung (single or multiple lesions)
  - Primary carcinoma is controlled
  - Metastases can be resected with adequate pulmonary reserve postoperatively
- Most important prognostic indicator is the interval from the primary tumor to the discovery of the metastases

A 48-year-old woman presents with a 2-cm peripheral lung nodule. A biopsy demonstrates lung adenocarcinoma. There is evidence of tumor invasion into the visceral pleura, but there are no signs of nodal metastasis. What is the appropriate management?

The tumor stage is T2 N0 M0 (Stage IB). Pulmonary resection is indicated for non-small cell lung cancer stages I–IIIA.

TNM Staging for Non-small Cell Lung Cancer

- Useful for evaluating candidacy for surgical resection
- Tumor staging (T)
  - Tis: Carcinoma in situ
  - T1: No larger than 3 cm
  - T2: The cancer has one or more of the following features:
    - Larger than 3 cm
    - Involves a main bronchus
    - Extends into the visceral pleura
  - T3: The cancer has one or more of the following features:
    - Spread to chest wall, diaphragm, mediastinal pleura, or parietal pericardium
    - Invades a main bronchus and is closer than 2 cm to the carina
    - Airway obstruction with pneumonia or total lung atelectasis
  - T4: The cancer has one or more of the following features:
    - Spread to mediastinum, heart, trachea, esophagus, vertebral body, or carina
    - Two or more separate tumor nodules in the same lobe
    - Malignant pleural effusion
- Nodal staging (N)
  - N0: No spread to lymph nodes
  - N1: Nodes within the lung and/or ipsilateral hilar lymph nodes
  - N2: Spread to subcarinal lymph nodes, pulmonary ligament, para-esophageal lymph nodes, para-aortic lymph nodes, aortic and aortic window lymph nodes, pretracheal and retrotracheal lymph nodes, upper paratracheal and lower paratracheal lymph nodes
  - N3: Contralateral mediastinal or hilar lymph nodes or any scalene or supraclavicular lymph nodes
- Metastasis staging (M)
  - M0: No spread to distant organs or areas
  - M1: Distant spread
  - Approximately 5% to 10% of all patients with lung cancer will have metastasis to the liver or adrenal glands at presentation

Stage Grouping for Non-small Cell Lung Cancer

Stage	T	N	M
Stage 0	Tis (in situ)	N0	M0
Stage IA	T1	N0	M0
Stage IB	T2	N0	M0
Stage IIA	T1	N1	M0
Stage IIB	T2	N1	M0
	T3	N0	M0
Stage IIIA	T1-2	N2	M0
	T3	N1-2	M0
Stage IIIB	Any T	N3	M0
	T4	Any N	M0
Stage IV	Any T	Any N	M1

A 72-year-old long-standing smoker presents with right-sided shoulder pain and unilateral ptosis. What is the most likely diagnosis?

A superior sulcus tumor ("Pancoast tumor").

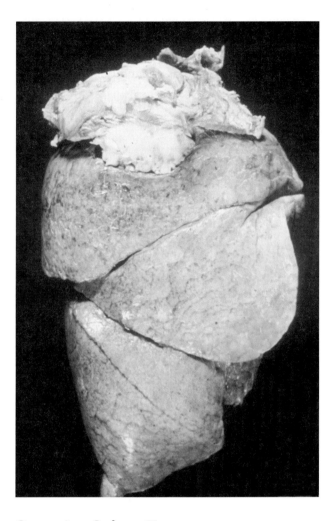

Pancoast tumor. (With permission from Mulholland MW, Lillemoe KD, Doherty GM, et al., eds. *Greenfield's Surgery.* 4th ed. Philadelphia, PA: Lippincott Williams & Wilkins; 2005.)

Superior Sulcus Tumor

- A clinical syndrome due to tumor growth in the superior sulcus at the lung apex, resulting in invasion of local neural structures
- Signs and symptoms
  - Pain in the shoulder or medial portion of the scapula is the most common symptom (>90%)
  - Horner syndrome: Ptosis, miosis, hemianhydrosis, enophthalmos
  - Radicular pain with or without muscle wasting in the distribution of:
    - The ulnar nerve to the elbow (T1 distribution) and/or
    - The medial forearm and hand (C8 distribution)
- The pathology includes squamous cell carcinoma (50%), adenocarcinoma (25%), and large cell carcinoma (25%)
- CT and MRI define the extent of involvement and invasion of adjacent structures
- Treatment is radiation therapy first, followed by tumor and chest wall resection

A 52-year-old with an 80 pack-year smoking history has a centrally located lung mass. He is scheduled to undergo transbronchial biopsy. What will the histopathology most likely reveal?

Centrally located tumors tend to be squamous cell carcinoma or small cell lung cancer (squamous cell tumors are more common). Peripherally located tumors tend to be adenocarcinoma or large cell carcinoma.

A 52-year-old man undergoes a CT-guided FNA of a 3-cm malignant appearing pulmonary mass. What is the most likely histopathology?

Non-small cell lung cancer.

Non-small Cell Lung Cancer

- Most common type of lung cancer (75%)
- Non-small cell lung cancer can be subdivided into adenocarcinoma, squamous cell carcinoma, and large cell carcinoma
- Adenocarcinoma
    - The most common type—25% to 35% of lung cancers
    - From mucous glands
    - Peripheral location
    - Greater chance of distant metastases
- Squamous cell carcinoma
    - 25% to 30% of lung cancers
    - From bronchial epithelium
    - Central location
    - Distant metastases are less common than with other types
- Large cell carcinoma
    - 10% of lung cancers
    - Central or peripheral location

A 55-year-old female with a 6-cm hilar mass is diagnosed with small cell lung cancer. What is the most common therapy for small cell lung cancer?

Chemotherapy.

Small Cell Lung Cancer

- Small cell lung cancer is staged as either limited disease or extensive disease
- Limited disease is based on a locally contained tumor that can be radiated in a single portal
- Extensive disease refers to disseminated tumor
- Chemotherapy is the first-line treatment for both limited and extensive diseases
- Radiotherapy is used as an adjuvant in limited disease
- Surgery has a very limited role in the management of small cell lung cancer

> A patient is discovered to have a newly diagnosed lung cancer. What is the likelihood this patient has distant metastases?

40%.

> A 72-year-old woman with localized lung cancer undergoes preoperative pulmonary function testing. Her FEV_1 is predicted to be 0.6. Her PaO_2 is 47 and her $PaCO_2$ is 59. What should be the recommendation for surgery?

A predicted FEV1 less than 0.8 and significantly abnormal blood gas values contraindicate a pulmonary resection.

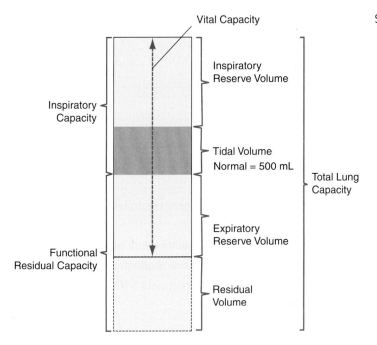

Spirometric parameters.

Spirometric Parameters

- Total lung capacity = volume in the lungs after a maximal inspiration
- Vital capacity = maximum volume that can be expired after a maximal inspiration
- Tidal volume = volume of gas inspired or expired during a normal or unforced breath
- Functional residual capacity = volume remaining in the lungs after a normal expiration
- Residual volume = volume remaining in the lungs after a maximal expiration (cannot be measured directly with a spirometer)

Other Spirometric Parameters

- Expiratory reserve volume = the maximal volume of gas that can be expired after a normal expiration
- Inspiratory reserve volume = the maximal volume of gas that can be inspired after a normal inspiration
- Inspiratory capacity = the maximal volume of air that can be inspired from the end expiratory level
- Minute ventilation (L/minute) = respiratory rate multiplied by tidal volume

Contraindications to Pulmonary Resection

- Distant or regional metastases
- FEV_1 predicted to be less than 0.8 L
- Split lung function tests can predict if the diseased lung can be removed without significant reduction in the remaining pulmonary function
- Gas exchange: Carbon monoxide diffusion capacity (DLCO) < 40% predicted (11 to 12 mL/minute/mmHg CO), PaO_2 < 50 mmHg (room air), and $PaCO_2$ > 45 mmHg (room air) are predictors of mortality following pulmonary resection

Chronic smoking leads to a decreased FEV_1, FEV_1/FVC, and total lung capacity. Residual lung volume may be increased.

A 52-year-old female smoker presents to the emergency department with seizures. Laboratory data reveal a plasma sodium of 117 mEq/L. Chest radiograph demonstrates a left hilar mass. What is the most likely diagnosis?

This patient has syndrome of inappropriate antidiuretic hormone (SIADH) secondary to small cell lung cancer.

Syndrome of Inappropriate Antidiuretic Hormone

- Diagnosis is based on:
  - Hyponatremia
  - Low serum osmolality (<275 mOsm/kg)
  - High urine sodium excretion (>25 mEq/L)
  - An inappropriately high urine osmolality (urine osmolality > serum osmolality)
- Occurs in 10% of all patients with small cell lung cancer
- Treatment involves correction of plasma sodium with hypertonic saline combined with diuretics
- Once in a less severe range (Na^+ > 125 mEq/L), fluid restriction alone is adequate
- Patients with relapsed tumors and recurrent SIADH may require treatment with demeclocycline

---

A 67-year-old female with no significant past medical history presents to the emergency department with hemoptysis and on further workup is found to have a peripheral lung mass. While in the hospital for workup, she develops flank pain and is found to have a kidney stone. She is also complaining of vague abdominal pain and cramping. What further workup should be done?

The patient has symptoms of hypercalcemia, which can be seen in squamous cell cancer secondary to release of parathyroid hormone related protein (PTHrP).

Paraneoplastic Syndromes Associated with Lung Cancer

- Hypercalcemia
  - In squamous cell cancer
  - Due to secretion of PTHrP
- SIADH
  - In small cell lung cancer
  - Due to inappropriate secretion of ADH

- Cushing syndrome
  - In small cell lung cancer
  - Due to adrenocorticotropic hormone (ACTH) analog production → patient will fail dexamethasone suppression test
- Eaton-Lambert syndrome
  - In small cell lung cancer
  - Caused by antibodies against calcium channels
  - Causes weakness that improves with effort

Despite increasing the degree of inspiratory oxygen in a postoperative gastric bypass patient, he continues to have episodes of oxygen desaturation. Positive end-expiratory pressure (PEEP) is instituted with improved arterial oxygen saturation. What is the primary mechanism by which PEEP improves oxygenation?

Alveolar recruitment.

Indications for Positive End-Expiratory Pressure
- To recruit alveoli by increasing the functional residual capacity
- To protect against lung injury due to closing of atelectatic units
- To improve cardiac performance during heart failure by increasing mean intrathoracic pressure

Complications of Positive End-Expiratory Pressure
- Decreased cardiac output when there are concurrent high airway pressures
- Barotrauma and a resultant pneumothorax
- Fluid retention
- Intracranial hypertension

A 43-year-old alcoholic undergoes an endoscopic retrograde cholangiopancreatography for chronic pancreatitis. Within 8 hours of the procedure he develops left-sided pleuritic chest pain. CXR reveals pneumomediastinum and a left-sided pleural effusion. What is the most appropriate next diagnostic study?

A gastrograffin swallow study should be performed to rule out an esophageal perforation.

Esophageal Rupture
- A known complication of upper endoscopy
- In a patient with a normal esophagus that has ruptured into the pleural space, immediate surgical repair is mandatory
- Open thoracotomy through the right chest is typically performed; however, for lower esophageal tears, the left chest approach can provide adequate exposure
- Depending on the size of the rupture, extent of spillage, and the patient's comorbidities, the esophagus can be repaired primarily versus diversion through a "spit fistula"
- The contaminated region must be adequately drained with chest tubes

5 | Orthopedic Surgery

Caroline Chebli

A 14-year-old boy sustains a supracondylar humerus fracture. He has diminished pulses distal to the fracture. Which artery is most likely injured?

Brachial artery injury is classically associated with supracondylar humerus fractures.

Common Neurovascular Injuries Associated with Orthopedic Injuries

- Anterior shoulder dislocation: Axillary nerve injury
  - Weakness of deltoid—weak arm abduction
  - Decreased sensation to lateral upper arm
- Supracondylar fracture of the humerus: Median nerve and brachial artery
  - Anterior Interosseous nerve branch injury most common
  - Weakness of thenar muscles—cannot do "thumbs up"
  - Weakness of wrist flexion, pronation
  - Decreased sensation of radial aspect of palm and radial 3½ fingers
- Midshaft fracture of the humerus: Radial nerve injury
  - 18% of humerus fractures are associated with radial nerve injury
  - The nerve can be lacerated, trapped in the fracture site, or most commonly, contused
  - In closed fractures, 75% to 90% of radial nerve injuries will recover within 3 to 4 months—if there is no return of nerve function at this time, surgical exploration is recommended
  - With open fractures, radial nerve exploration should be done primarily
  - If the fracture is reduced and radial nerve function disappears, immediate exploration and release of the nerve is recommended
- Posterior dislocation of the knee: Popliteal artery
  - 50% of knee dislocations are reduced prior to presentation in the emergency room
  - In the absence of an obvious vascular injury (decreased or absent distal pulses, an expanding pulsatile hematoma, a palpable thrill), which requires immediate vascular surgical treatment, the next step is measurement of an ABI
  - An ankle-brachial index (ABI) > 0.9 is highly sensitive and specific for ruling out vascular injury
- Distal radius fracture: Median nerve injury
- Fibular neck injury: Common peroneal nerve
  - Foot drop

> Following a crush injury to the right lower extremity, a patient is noted to have weak pulses, a swollen lower extremity with tense skin, and severe pain on passive motion. What is the next step in management?

An emergent fasciotomy should be performed for extremity compartment syndrome.

Extremity Compartment Syndrome

- Most common in the anterior compartment of the lower extremity and manifests as a foot drop
- Use a Stryker monitor to measure compartment pressures
    - Compartment syndrome present if:
        - Absolute pressure is >30 mmHg
        - Diastolic blood pressure minus measured compartment pressure is <30 mmHg
- "5 P's"
    - Pain out of proportion to physical exam (pain on passive movement)
    - Pallor
    - Pulselessness
    - Paralysis
    - Paresthesia

Pain out of proportion to physical exam is the hallmark of extremity compartment syndrome.

> A 19-year-old male motocross racer is in the final stretch of the race when his forearms go numb and he feels his hands loosen on the grips. The intensity of the pain makes it impossible for him to pull the brake lever to stop. He crashes his bike and does not finish the race. What is the most likely diagnosis?

Chronic exertional compartment syndrome (CECS).

Chronic Exertional Compartment Syndrome

- During strenuous exercise, such as motocross racing, the muscle volume increases due to increased blood flow to the area
- The increase in muscle volume occurs within a non-expanding compartment
- The increase in pressure causes a decrease in arteriole blood flow while reducing venous return
- The muscle does not receive enough oxygen to supply its demand and becomes ischemic causing pain
- The history is very consistent: the pain starts as a dull ache, which progresses until the activity is stopped. The pain is predictable and reproducible.
- Diagnosis of CECS is with resting and post exercise compartment P at 1 and 5 minutes post exercise
    - Resting P ≥15 mmHg
    - 1 minute post exercise P ≥30 mmHg
    - 5 minutes post exercise P ≥20 mmHg
- For lower extremity CECS, compartment releases are a successful cure. For forearm CECS, little is known regarding surgical compartment releases

- The forearm consists of three compartments
  - Volar
    - Muscles: The wrist and finger flexors including the flexor digitorum superficialis (FDS), flexor carpi radialis, flexor pollicis longus, flexor digitorum profundus (FDP), and flexor carpi ulnaris
    - Nerves: Ulnar nerve, median nerve, superficial branch of the radial nerve, anterior interosseous nerve
    - Arteries: Ulnar artery, median artery, anterior interosseous artery
  - Dorsal
    - Muscles: Finger and thumb extensors and long thumb abductor
    - Nerves: Posterior interosseous nerve
    - Arteries: Posterior interosseous artery
  - Lateral compartment
    - Muscles: Extensor carpi radialis brevis, extensor carpi radialis, and brachioradialis

---

A 32-year-old man is involved in a motorcycle collision and sustains an open tibia fracture. What is the appropriate treatment for this type of fracture?

All open fractures should be treated with emergent operative debridement and stabilization.

Treatment of Open Fractures
- Irrigation and debridement
- Culture all wounds, then begin IV antibiotics
- Tetanus prophylaxis
- Stabilization of fracture

The greatest risk factor for developing nonunion is smoking.

A 40-year-old male is removing rust from his metal shed using a solution containing hydrofluoric acid. He inadvertently spills some on his hand. He copiously irrigates the area with water and subsequently presents to the emergency room an hour later due to increasing pain. What is the correct immediate management?

Immediate irrigation with water for 20 minutes then apply topical calcium gluconate gel to affected area for 30 minutes. If pain persists after 1 to 2 hours, proceed to local infiltration of calcium gluconate. If this is unsuccessful, arterial infusion of calcium gluconate is indicated.

Hydrofluoric Acid Burn
- Upon contact with the skin, the acid causes immediate pain with blistering and edema within 1 to 2 hours
- Patients have pain out of proportion to appearance of burn
- Hydrofluoric acid penetrates tissue causing local and systemic damage
- The fluoride anion dissociates and causes necrosis of soft tissue, bony erosion, and electrolyte abnormalities by binding Ca and Mg
- With application of calcium gluconate gel, Ca binds F and it precipitates out as salt
- In extreme cases where systemic toxicity is present, severe metabolic abnormalities are possible—hypocalcemia is the most common

A father picks up his 2-year-old daughter by her hands and swings her around. Afterward, she refuses to use her right arm and is holding her arm slightly flexed, pronated, and close to her body. What is the most likely diagnosis?

This is a classic history for nursemaid's elbow, a common pediatric orthopedic injury.

Nursemaid's Elbow

- The radial head can be reduced by flexing the arm to 90 degrees, supinating the arm, applying a posteriorly directed force on the radial head, and extending the elbow
- Sometimes an audible clunk can be heard
- No immobilization is necessary for the first dislocation

A 6-year-old girl falls onto her outstretched hand and complains of pain in her wrist. What are two types of fractures commonly seen in children?

A "greenstick fracture" is an incomplete fracture where the cortex is disrupted on one side only. A "torus fracture" is a buckle of cortex on one side of the metaphysis of long bones. Both types of fractures are found almost exclusively in children.

A 5-year-old boy presents with a humerus fracture of the right arm. An X-ray demonstrates a spiral fracture. What is the most likely diagnosis?

Child abuse is common and must be seriously considered in any spiral fractures of long bones in children (humerus, tibia, femur).

What are the three types of peripheral nerve injury?

Neuropraxia, axonotmesis, and neurotmesis.

Peripheral Nerve Injuries

- Neuropraxia
  - Physiologic interruption of nerve conduction
  - Stretch injury
  - Good prognosis—recovery usually in 6 to 8 weeks
- Axonotmesis
  - Axonal and myelin loss with intact Schwann cell sheath
  - Axon undergoes Wallerian degeneration
  - Sensory loss with axonal regeneration proximal to distal at 1 mm/day
  - Fair prognosis
- Neurotmesis
  - Complete division of nerve
  - Spontaneous recovery is impossible

- If untreated, scar tissue blocks the nerve from regenerating and may result in a painful neuroma due to formation of a mass of misdirected axons
- Repaired by a precise apposition of nerve ends

Regenerating axons grow at a rate of approximately 1 mm per day.

A 50-year-old male is involved in a motor vehicle crash and is brought to the emergency department complaining of pain in his cervical spine. On physical exam, he is noted to have 4/5 strength in his biceps muscles bilaterally. What is the next course of action in the treatment of this patient?

Do a CT of the cervical spine to ensure that there are no indications for emergent spine decompression (fracture or dislocation, soft tissue or bony compression of the cord). If there are none, begin IV steroids per protocol.

Spinal Cord Trauma

- The IV steroid protocol is only indicated for blunt spinal cord injury per the NACIS (National Acute Spinal Cord Injury Studies) II and III trials
- For acute non-penetrating SCI <3 hours after injury, give a 24-hour regimen of high-dose methylprednisolone with a 30 mg/kg bolus followed by a 5.4 mg/kg infusion for 23 hours
- For acute non-penetrating SCI between 3 to 8 hours after injury, give a 48-hour steroid regimen with a 30 mg/kg bolus followed by a 5.4 mg/kg infusion for 23 hours
- For acute non-penetrating SCI >8 hours after injury, methylprednisolone should not be used
- For acute penetrating SCI, methylprednisolone is not recommended

A progressive neurologic deficit is an indication for surgery.

A 25-year-old female driver who was involved in a motor vehicle collision is brought to the emergency department. On physical exam, she is found to have pain in her upper lumbar spine. What is the most common injury associated with this mechanism?

Chance fractures are frequently found in patients complaining of back pain following motor vehicle accidents.

Chance Fracture

- Pure bony injury extending from posterior to anterior through the spinous process, pedicles, and vertebral body, respectively
- Associated with seatbelt injury
- Caused by flexion–distraction forces
- Given the mechanism involved, it is imperative to rule out an abdominal injury

What is the radiographic presentation of a spondylolisthesis?

Spondylolisthesis is a structural defect of the pars interarticularis causing an anterior subluxation (or slippage) of the superior vertebral body on the inferior one.

A 21-year-old male was snowboarding near Camp Muir at Mount Rainier (altitude of 10,000 feet) when he became lost in a white out snowstorm. After several hours, he was rescued and evaluated. He was found to have frostbite in both feet. What is the correct initial management of his problem?

Rapid rewarming by submersion in warm water 104 to 107.6 degrees for 15 to 30 minutes.

Frostbite

- A thermal injury to tissue that is classified by the depth of damage to the skin
  - First degree: Central whitish area surrounded by erythema
  - Second degree: Present with blisters within 24 hours
  - Third degree: Blisters that progress to eschars
  - Fourth degree: Tissue necrosis
  - All frostbite presents the same initially and the extent of damage cannot be known until thawing has occurred
- Treatment
  - Once in an environment where there is no risk of refreezing, rewarming is safe to initiate
  - Once rewarming has been accomplished, pad and splint the injured extremity
  - At this point, administer tetanus prophylaxis and analgesia
  - Monitor the limb closely for signs of compartment syndrome
  - IV or intra-arterial administration of tPA within 24 hours of injury can reduce the need for amputation
  - Demarcation occurs at 1 to 3 months from injury and debridements are performed during this period

When surgically acquiring a posterior iliac crest bone graft, which vessel must be coagulated?

The superior gluteal artery.

A 35-year-old woman with a medical history significant for diabetes has a sudden onset of pain in her right knee. There is no history of trauma. She is mildly febrile and is unable to bear weight on her right lower extremity due to pain. What is the next most important step in her management?

A knee joint aspiration should be performed in any patient with signs and symptoms of infection.

Organisms in Septic Arthritis

- *Staphylococcus aureus* (most common)
- Hemolytic streptococci

Gonococcal Arthritis

- More common in females
- Migrating polyarthralgia
- Commonly involves the knee, elbow, or wrist
- Treatment consists of 2 weeks of penicillin and joint immobilization

Septic arthritis is diagnosed on gram stain and culture of the aspirated joint fluid.

What is the most common site of skeletal tuberculosis?

The spine (i.e., Pott disease) is the most common site of skeletal tuberculosis and usually involves the thoracic anterior vertebral body.

Spinal Tuberculosis

- Presents as worsening pain at night with an insidious onset
- The thoracic spine is the most common location
- Treatment is antibiotics, rest, and bracing
- Surgical indications include a neurologic deficit, spinal instability, or progressive kyphosis

A 60-year-old man has just finished a meal consisting of wine, cheese, and steak. The next morning he is awakened by an intense, burning pain in his great toe. What is the most likely diagnosis?

Gout commonly presents at the first metatarsal phalangeal (MTP) joint.

Gout

- Negative birefringence of rod-shaped urate crystals under polarized light is diagnostic
- An acute attack usually presents in the first MTP joint
- Treat acute flare up with rest and nonsteroidal anti-inflammatory drugs (NSAIDs)
- Colchicine and allopurinol take time to work and are used as maintenance therapy

Congenital Pyrophosphate Disorder

- Disorder of pyrophosphate metabolism in older patients
- Aspirated joint fluid reveals short, blunt, rhomboid-shaped crystals with weakly positive birefringence
- The knee is the most common location for acute attacks

A 40-year-old woman has had some aching in both hands for some years. Recently, she has noted her fingers drifting ulnarly. What is the most likely diagnosis?

Rheumatoid arthritis is a common cause of ulnar deviation of the fingers.

Rheumatoid Arthritis

- Peak incidence in fourth and fifth decades
- More common in females
- Rheumatoid factor is positive in 90% of patients
- Treat with steroids or immune modulators

Osteoarthritis

- The primary symptom is joint pain
- Osteoarthritis (OA) results in decreased joint mobility due to articular cartilage destruction, loss of joint space, capsular contracture, and osteophytes

- Bouchard nodes = OA of the proximal interphalangeal (PIP) joint
- Heberden nodes = OA of the distal interphalangeal (DIP) joint
- Treat conservatively with rest and immobilization of joint and NSAIDs

An obese 13-year-old boy is playing football when he is suddenly unable to bear weight on his left lower extremity. On physical exam, you note his foot is externally rotated and any attempt to internally rotate his hip causes pain. What is the most likely diagnosis?

A slipped capital femoral epiphysis (SCFE) is common in adolescent males (11 to 15 years of age).

Slipped Capital Femoral Epiphysis
- A separation of the capital femoral epiphysis through the growth plate
- There is a zone of provisional calcification present
- There may be medial and posterior displacement of the capital epiphysis
- SCFE presents as hip pain with motion
    - The pain is often referred to the knee
    - The patient may be unable to rotate the hip internally
- X-ray looks like a ice cream cone with the scoop falling off of the cone
- 25% are bilateral
- There is an increased risk of developing avascular necrosis (AVN) of the femoral head
- Treatment is in situ pinning

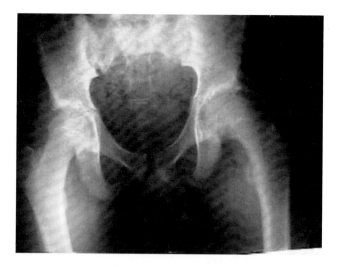

Slipped capital femoral epiphysis.

A mother notices her 6-year-old son ambulating with a limp. He occasionally complains of hip pain and will rest to relieve the pain. Radiographs show flattening of the femoral head. What is the most likely diagnosis?

Leg-Calve-Perthes disease commonly occurs in boys 4 to 8 years of age.

Leg-Calve-Perthes Disease
- Avascular necrosis of the proximal femoral epiphysis
- Acute onset of hip pain with a limp and loss of hip motion

- X-ray shows flattening of the femoral head
- Easily confused with septic arthritis
- Treatment is maintenance of range of motion with limited exercise
- Femoral head will remodel without sequelae most of the time

> A 14-year-old male soccer player presents with anterior knee pain. On physical exam, he is tender over his tibial tuberosity. What is the most likely diagnosis?

Osgood-Schlatter disease is one of the most common causes of knee pain in the adolescent and is caused by traction apophysitis of the tibial tuberosity.

Osgood-Schlatter Disease
- Tibial tubercle apophysitis caused by traction injury from patellar tendon
- Symptoms: Pain in front of knee
- Diagnosis: X-ray with irregular shape or fragmenting of the tibial tubercle
- Treatment
  - Mild symptoms: Activity limitation
  - Severe symptoms: Cast for 6 weeks followed by activity limitation

> A 49-year-old man with poorly controlled diabetes presents with painful flatfoot in his right lower extremity. X-rays demonstrate the classic "bag of bones" appearance indicating multiple unhealed fractures. What is the most likely diagnosis?

A Charcot foot is a common problem among diabetics and is caused by the associated neuropathy.

Charcot Joint
- Joint destruction caused by an inability to sense the required distribution of weight at the affected joint
- Associated with underlying neurologic disorders
- Diabetes is the most common cause of neuropathy

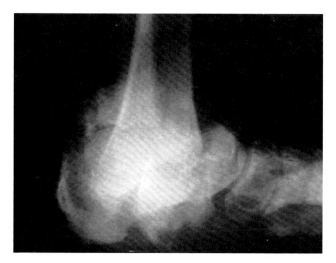

Charcot ankle.

An 89-year-old female trips and falls over her bed at home. She presents to the emergency room with a laceration on her eye, questionable loss of consciousness, and a flexed and externally rotated right leg. Further workup reveals a negative head CT scan and a right femoral neck fracture. What is the appropriate thromboprophylaxis for this patient?

Low molecular weight heparin or low-dose unfractionated heparin.

Deep Vein Thrombosis
- 50% of deep vein thrombosis have been prevented by the effective use of thromboprophylaxis
- If surgery is to be delayed, preoperative anticoagulation is recommended
  - Either low-dose molecular weight heparin (LMWH) or unfractionated heparin can be used
- Postoperative prophylaxis should be initiated with fondaparinux, LMWH, warfarin, or low-dose unfractionated heparin for 10 to 35 days after surgery
- Aspirin alone is not considered effective prophylaxis

What muscles make up the rotator cuff?

The acronym SITS describes the muscles.

Rotator Cuff Muscles
- S: Supraspinatus
- I: Infraspinatus
- T: Teres minor
- S: Subscapularis

A 31-year-old mother of two children notices her right hand falls asleep whenever she is performing any overhead activities. EMG/NCV studies are normal. What are two tests to diagnose thoracic outlet syndrome (TOS)?

An Adson maneuver or a Wright test may reproduce symptoms of thoracic outlet syndrome.

Tests for Thoracic Outlet Syndrome
- Adson maneuver
  - Elevation of first rib by placing shoulder in slight abduction and extension
  - Contraction of the scalene muscles and rotation of the head to the affected side to stretch/extend the neck
  - When the patient inhales while in this position, diminished pulse or reproduction of symptoms indicates presence of TOS
- Wright test
  - External rotation, abduction, and extension of arm with the neck rotated away causes a diminished pulse and reproduction of symptoms

What ligaments are disrupted in an acromioclavicular separation?

The coracoclavicular and acromioclavicular ligaments.

Clavicle Fractures

- The most common site is the middle third of the clavicle
- Treatment is a sling and gentle range of motion (as pain allows)
- Main risk with this fracture is vascular impingement
- 97% heal without any other intervention
- If <2 cm of shortening or compromise of overlying skin, recommend surgical treatment

Proximal Humerus Fractures

- Most commonly located at the surgical neck
- Treatment is closed reduction and immobilization
- An anatomic neck fracture (above the tuberosities) is associated with avascular necrosis

What tendon is involved in "tennis elbow" (lateral epicondylitis)?

The extensor carpi radialis brevis.

A 32-year-old man develops wrist pain after falling on his outstretched hand. He has tenderness over the anatomic snuffbox. What is the most likely diagnosis?

A scaphoid fracture is classically associated with pain in the anatomic snuff box of the wrist.

Scaphoid Fracture

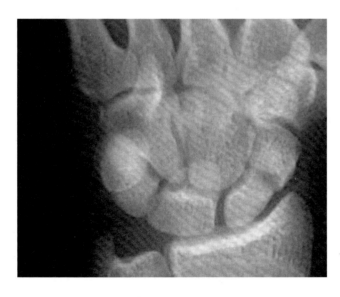

Scaphoid fracture.

- May not be detected on initial X-rays
- A bone scan or MRI may be necessary for diagnosis
- Treatment is with a long arm thumb "spica" cast
- Repeat an X-ray in 3 weeks

Colle Fracture

- Fracture of the distal radius
- Usually happens after a fall on an outstretched hand
- Treatment: Closed reduction

Scaphoid fractures are associated with a high incidence of avascular necrosis because the blood supply enters the scaphoid distally.

A 12-year-old girl falls off a swing set onto her right arm. X-rays show a fracture of her proximal ulna. What should also be noted on the X-ray?

A dislocated radial head is associated with a proximal ulnar fracture.

Monteggia Fracture

- A well-described fracture of the proximal ulna with radial head dislocation
- Caused by a fall on an outstretched hand
- Treatment: Open reduction internal fixation

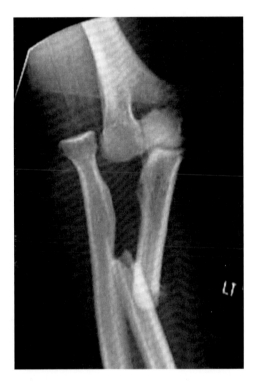

Monteggia fracture.

What is the most common cause of failure of a carpal tunnel release?

An incomplete release.

Carpal Tunnel Syndrome

- Entrapment of the median nerve at the wrist (carpal canal)
- Usually idiopathic but can be caused by a distal radius fracture

- Thenar atrophy
- Positive Tinel sign and positive Phalen maneuver
- Initial treatment with splinting, NSAIDs, and possible carpal tunnel injection

Median Nerve Innervation
- First and second lumbricals
- Thenar muscles except ulnar head of the flexor digitorum brevis (FDB)
- Skin of palmar 3½ fingers

Ulnar Nerve Innervation
- Hypothenar muscles
- All interossei muscles
- Third and fourth lumbricals and ulnar FDB
- Sensory to all of fifth finger, ½ of fourth finger, and dorsal hand

Radial Nerve Innervation
- Wrist extension, finger extension, thumb extension, triceps (no hand muscles)
- Sensory to first 3½ fingers on dorsal side
- Saturday night palsy
  - Wrist drop, decreased sensation of dorsum of hand, and posterolateral forearm
  - Due to laying with arm over a chair for an extended period

---

A 35-year-old laborer notes that upon waking from sleep his ring finger is locked in flexion. He also notes a tender nodule at the base of his ring finger. What is the most likely diagnosis?

He has a trigger finger.

Stenosing Tenosynovitis ("Trigger finger")
- Caused by the passage of a swollen flexor tendon sheath beneath the A1 pulley
- Finger can lock in either flexion or extension
- Conservative treatment is with NSAIDs and injection
- If conservative treatment fails, then release the A1 pulley

---

A 50-year-old secretary is having difficulty in opening jars due to wrist pain. She has tenderness over her radial wrist. What test is used to diagnose de Quervain's disease?

A Finkelstein test is performed by placing the thumb in a fist and deviating the wrist to the ulnar side. This test exacerbates the tenosynovitis of the first dorsal compartment of the hand (abductor pollicis longus and extensor pollicis brevis).

What is the most common site of a ganglion cyst?

Ganglion cysts often occur at the scapholunate joint on the dorsum of the wrist.

Giant Cell Tumor of the Tendon Sheath

- Benign
- Arises from the short vinculum near the interphalangeal joint (IPJ)
- Both FDP and FDS are involved

Inclusion Cyst

- Implantation of epithelium into subcutaneous tissue
- Treatment: Cyst excision

A 20-year-old woman is skiing and falls. Her thumb was caught and is forced into abduction by her ski pole. What injury is caused by this mechanism of injury?

A gamekeeper thumb.

Gamekeeper Thumb

- Disruption of the ulnar collateral ligament of the metacarpophalangeal (MCP) joint of the thumb by an abduction force
- Results in valgus instability of the MCP joint
- Treatment requires open repair of the ligament because the adductor aponeurosis becomes interposed
- Common in skiers

A man is cutting vegetables when the knife slips and he cuts his finger over his middle phalanx. He is unable to extend his PIP joint. Without treatment, what will be the sequela of this injury?

A permanent deformity.

Boutonniere Deformity

- Caused by disruption of the central extensor tendon near its insertion into the base of the middle phalanx
- The lateral bands displace toward the palm and become PIP joint flexors
- As a result, the PIP joint flexes with DIP joint extension
- Treatment: Immobilization of the PIP joint in extension for 6 weeks with the DIP joint free to flex

---

A 20-year-old basketball player jams his long finger. He is unable to extend the distal phalanx of his long finger. What is his injury?

A mallet deformity.

Mallet Deformity

- Injury to the extensor tendon insertion into the dorsum of the distal phalanx
- Treat with dorsal splinting of the DIP joint in extension for 6 to 8 weeks

---

What is the most common organism found in hand infections?

Staph. aureus (80%).

A teenager is involved in a fist fight and is brought to the emergency department complaining of pain over his fifth metacarpal head. You notice an area of skin that is open. What is the most common organism found in human bite wounds?

Eikenella corrodens is the most common organism in human bite wounds. The wound must be treated with irrigation, debridement, and antibiotics.

Boxer Fracture

- Fracture of the distal metacarpal of the fifth finger
- Caused by hitting an object with a clenched fist
- Presents with pain, swelling, and loss of knuckle prominence
- Often associated with a human bite
- Treatment is closed reduction and splinting of finger with MCP joint at 90 degrees to keep the collateral ligaments on stretch and prevent extension contracture

A 28-year-old man with a history of IV drug use presents to the emergency department with a painful index finger. He is unable to extend his finger due to pain and swelling. What is the next step in management?

Emergent incision and drainage. Flexor tenosynovitis is a surgical emergency.

Flexor Tenosynovitis

- An infection of the fingertip pulp
- Presents with fusiform swelling, flexed position of the finger, and tenderness over flexor tendon sheath
- Flexion or extension causes pain
- Treatment is emergent incision and drainage

Paronychia

- Infection of the nail plate/terminal joint space of finger
- Usually caused by *Staph. aureus*
- Treat with incision over medial or lateral border for drainage

High-Pressure Solvent Injection Injury of a Hand

- A high-pressure solvent injection should be treated with urgent wide surgical opening of the digit to prevent rapid progression of the inflammatory response, compartment syndrome, and loss of the finger

Phenol Burn Injury

- Should be treated with topical propylethylene glycol

How should an amputated limb be treated in the acute trauma setting?

Wrap the amputated part in sterile gauze, place in a plastic bag, and submerge the bag in ice water. If properly cooled after injury, the digit may be viable for up to 24 hours.

Following surgery for a radius and ulnar bone fracture, a patient has been complaining of increasing pain in her forearm and has required an increasing amount of pain medication. What is the next step in management?

Reassess for a compartment syndrome by examining the patient for pain with passive finger extension. Compartment syndrome may also present with paresthesias in the median and ulnar nerve distributions.

What is the sequela of an undiagnosed forearm compartment syndrome?

A Volkmann contracture.

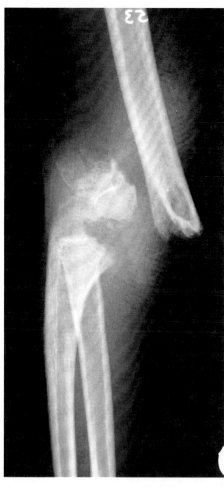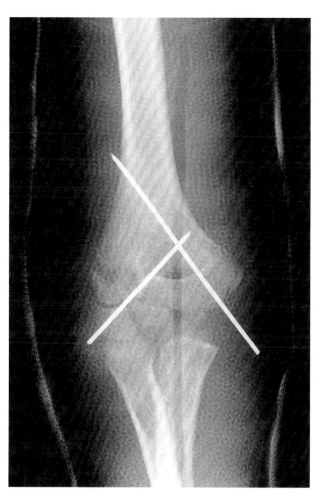

Supracondylar fracture of the humerus that can result in a Volkmann contracture if not fixed appropriately. (With permission from Mulholland MW, Lillemoe KD, Doherty GM, et al., eds. *Greenfield's Surgery.* 4th ed. Philadelphia, PA: Lippincott Williams & Wilkins; 2005.)

Volkmann Ischemic Contracture

- Results from an untreated forearm compartment syndrome
- Secondary to compromise of the anterior interosseous artery
- The degeneration of the FDP and flexor pollicis longus (deep flexor compartment) causes a fixed flexion contracture of the wrist and fingers and neuropathy of the median and ulnar nerves

A 50-year-old man notices over a period of years that he has a thick band of tissue over the palm of his fifth metacarpal. Slowly, his finger is beginning to flex, and it is interfering with his ability to grasp objects. What is the most likely diagnosis?

A Dupuytren contracture can present with a nodule in the palmer fascia of the fourth or fifth digits.

Dupuytren Contracture
- Proliferation of myofibroblasts
- More common in men of northern European origin
- Autosomal dominant inheritance but exogenous factors also contribute
- Begins with nodule formation in the palmer fascia in line with the pretendinous bands
- Treat with open fasciotomy and excision of the palmer fascia

Dupuytren's Contracture

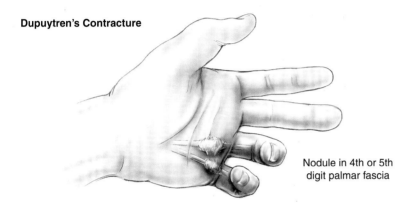

Nodule in 4th or 5th digit palmar fascia

What type of collagen comprises articular cartilage?

Type II collagen.

What is the most common type of collagen in bone?

Type I collagen.

Six months following a closed reduction and pinning for a femoral neck fracture, a 40-year-old man experiences worsening groin pain. What is a complication of femoral neck fractures?

Avascular necrosis; this complication can be treated with anatomic reduction and internal fixation or hemiarthroplasty.

A college football player experiences a blow to the outside of his right leg as it is firmly planted in the ground. He feels a pop and his knee buckles. He has a positive anterior drawer and Lachman test. Which ligament is most likely injured?

Anterior cruciate ligament (ACL).

Knee Injuries

- Medial collateral ligament (MCL) tear: Valgus force to knee
- Anterior cruciate ligament (ACL) tear: Hyperextension injury of knee or forced internal rotation of tibia
  - Perform a Lachman test to diagnose an ACL tear
- Posterior cruciate ligament (PCL) tear: Direct blow to anterior tibia with knee flexed
  - Perform a posterior drawer test to diagnose a PCL tear
- Meniscus tears: Medial meniscus injury is more common

A 30-year-old male is playing basketball when he feels a pop in his left heel. What is the test to diagnose an Achilles tendon rupture?

Place the patient prone with knee flexed, squeezing the calf. If there is plantar flexion of the foot, the Achilles tendon is intact. This is called the Thompson test.

A 1-month-old infant is noted to have a hip click on physical exam. She has unequal thigh skin folds and unequal leg lengths when her hips and knees are flexed. What is the most likely diagnosis?

Hip dysplasia.

Developmental Dysplasia of the Hip

- Risk factors include being first-born, a breech presentation at birth, and female gender
- 10% are bilateral
- Diagnose with physical exam (rotating hip) and ultrasound
- Treatment: Pavlik harness, which keeps the legs abducted and the femoral head in the acetabulum

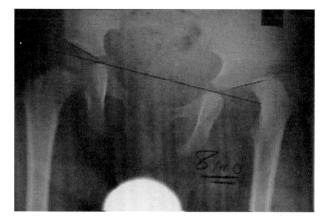

Developmental dysplasia of the hip.

A 2-month-old infant presents to the office with talipes equinovarus (congenital clubfoot). What is the initial step in management?

Manipulation with serial casting is the initial step in management. If unsuccessful or recurrent, then a soft tissue release should be performed.

What is the etiology of torticollis?

An ischemic event within the midportion of the sternocleidomastoid muscle, usually traumatic and seen within the first 2 weeks of life.

Pediatric Congenital Hand Disorders

- Congenital radioulnar synostosis
  - Fusion of the proximal radius and ulna
  - Unable to pronate or supinate forearm
- Madelung deformity
  - Subluxation of the wrist due to defective growth of ulnar and distal third of radius
  - Treat with an osteotomy
- Syndactyly
  - Most common congenital hand anomaly
  - Simple: Absence of a bony connection
  - Complex: Presence of a bony connection
  - Complete: Joined to tip of finger
  - Incomplete: Joined short of tip of finger

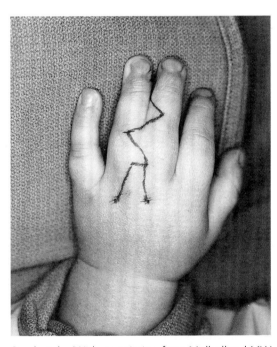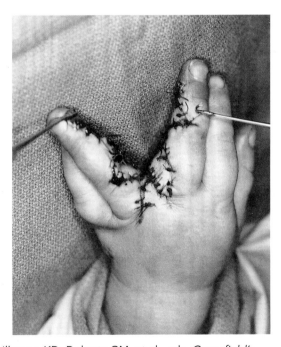

Syndactyly. (With permission from Mulholland MW, Lillemoe KD, Doherty GM, et al., eds. *Greenfield's Surgery.* 4th ed. Philadelphia, PA: Lippincott Williams & Wilkins; 2005.)

Cleidocranial Dysostosis

- Autosomal dominant inheritance
- Aplasia of the clavicle
- Increased transverse cranial diameter
- Delayed closure of the fontanelles
- Child can approximate the tips of the shoulders in front of the chin

A 14-year-old girl is referred by her school nurse for a slight curvature of the spine. What is the diagnosis?

Scoliosis is commonly found in prepubertal females.

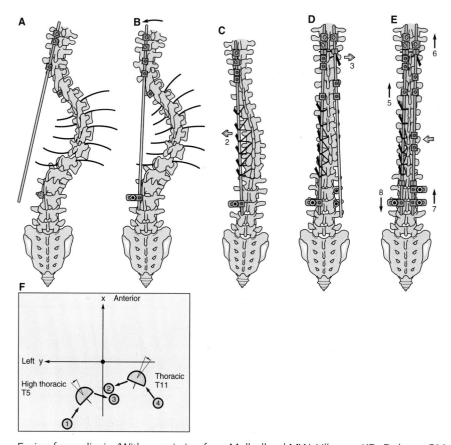

Fusion for scoliosis. (With permission from Mulholland MW, Lillemoe KD, Doherty GM, et al., eds. *Greenfield's Surgery.* 4th ed. Philadelphia, PA: Lippincott Williams & Wilkins; 2005.)

Scoliosis

- Seen in prepubertal females
- Usually idiopathic
- Right thoracic curve most common
- Curves 20 to 40 degrees: Use brace to slow progression until skeletal maturity
- Curves >40 degrees: Consider spinal fusion

What is the best study to evaluate soft tissue tumors?

MRI.

What is the most common primary bone tumor?

Multiple myeloma (bone scan is negative so it is important to do skeletal survey).

A 12-year-old boy has been experiencing pain in the middle of his back for the last few weeks that awakens him from sleep. His mother notes that Motrin relieves the pain for a while but he is requiring increasing amounts. An X-ray reveals a 1-cm lytic area with a central radiodense nidus. What is the most likely diagnosis?

Osteoid osteomas most commonly present in teenagers as night "bone" pain that is relieved by salicylates.

Osteoid Osteoma

- Most common in second decade
- Presents as night pain relieved by salicylates
- Commonly occurs in the posterior elements of the spine and may present as scoliosis

A 23-year-old man presents with a hard and firm lower thigh mass. An X-ray demonstrates a sunburst appearance at the distal femur. What is the most likely diagnosis and the treatment required?

The most likely diagnosis is an osteosarcoma, which will require neoadjuvant therapy followed by an en bloc resection if there are no signs of distant metastases.

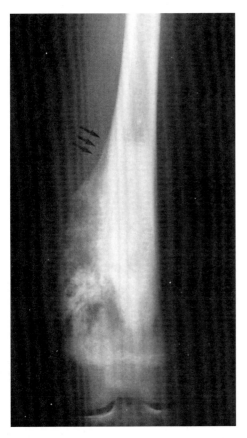

Osteosarcoma with Codman triangle. (With permission from Mulholland MW, Lillemoe KD, Doherty GM, et al., eds. *Greenfield's Surgery.* 4th ed. Philadelphia, PA: Lippincott Williams & Wilkins; 2005.)

Osteosarcoma

- Most commonly seen in the second decade of life
- X-ray shows a destructive lesion of the metaphysis with matrix ossification
- X-ray may demonstrate a "Codman triangle" with cortical destruction (sunburst appearance)
- The distal femur is the most common site (followed by the proximal tibia)
- Spreads hematogenously (metastasis to lungs is most common)
- Treat with neoadjuvant chemotherapy then reevaluate for limb salvage
- Must do en bloc surgical resection and reconstruction vs. amputation
- Can arise from Paget bone disease in older patients

A 15-year-old man is kicked in the distal femur while playing soccer. X-rays do not reveal a fracture; however, there is a lesion with a stippled calcification noted. The patient has been asymptomatic until his above noted injury. What is the most likely diagnosis?

An enchondroma.

Enchondroma

- Benign neoplasm arising from cartilaginous elements in the bone that undergo calcification
- Multiple enchondromas are possible (Ollier disease)
- Multiple enchondromas can occur with soft tissue hemangiomas (Maffucci syndrome)
- Malignant degeneration is associated with multiple enchondromas

Chondroblastoma

- Most commonly seen in the first and second decades before closure of the epiphyses
- X-ray findings of an osteolytic epiphyseal lesion with calcium deposits
- Treat with curettage and bone grafting

Chondrosarcoma

- Malignant bone lesion that occurs in adults
- Most commonly affects the shoulder, pelvic girdles, knee, and spine
- Pain or a mass is usually present
- Treatment is with wide resection only

Giant Cell Tumor

- X-ray demonstrates an eccentric lytic lesion in the epiphysis and metaphysic
- Knee and distal radius are most commonly affected
- Treat with curettage and chemical cauterization (phenol)
- Can recur and metastasize to the lungs

A 14-year-old little league pitcher experiences a sudden onset of pain in his right shoulder while pitching in a game. X-rays reveal a lesion in the proximal humerus with a central lytic area, thinned cortices, and expansion of the bone. What is the most likely diagnosis?

The proximal humerus is the most common site for a unicameral bone cyst.

Unicameral Bone Cyst

- Also commonly seen in the proximal femur and distal tibia
- Occurs during active bone growth
- Treat with methyl prednisolone acetate injection
- Recalcitrant lesions should be treated with curettage and bone grafting

---

An 18-year-old woman notices pain and swelling in her proximal tibia for the last few months. She has no significant history of injury to this area. X-rays show an eccentric, lytic, expansile lesion in the metaphysis of her tibia. What is the most likely diagnosis?

An aneurysmal bone cyst.

Aneurysmal Bone Cyst

- Osteolytic lesion found in the metaphysis of long bones
- Histologically, there are characteristic blood-filled cavernous spaces within fibrous tissue and no endothelial lining
- Treat with curettage and bone grafting

A 10-year-old child is experiencing pain around her knee as well as fevers. Laboratory studies show an elevated sedimentation rate, white blood cell count, leukocytosis, and anemia. X-rays show a large destructive lesion involving the metaphysis and diaphysis of her tibia with an onion skin appearance to the cortex. What is the most likely diagnosis?

An Ewing tumor.

Ewing Tumor

- Arises from the diaphyseal marrow of long bones
- Patients are usually under 20 years old
- Onion skinning parallel to the shaft of the bone visible on X-ray
- Lymphatic and hematogenous spread
- Metastasize to the lung

A 60-year-old woman with a long-standing history of lower back pain begins having obstipation. On rectal exam, she is noted to have loss of rectal tone and a palpable mass. X-rays show a destructive lesion in her sacrum and a CT scan shows midline destruction of her sacrum as well as a soft tissue mass. What is the most likely diagnosis?

A chordoma.

Chordoma

- A malignant neoplasm
- Found at the ends of the vertebral column (spheno-occipital region and sacrum)
- Arises from embryonic remnants of the notochord
- Treatment is complete surgical excision

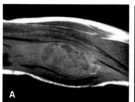 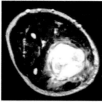 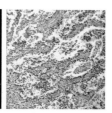

Resection of a rhabdomyosarcoma. (With permission from Fischer JE, Bland KI, Callery MP, et al., eds. *Mastery of Surgery.* 5th ed. Philadelphia, PA: Lippincott Williams & Wilkins; 2006.)

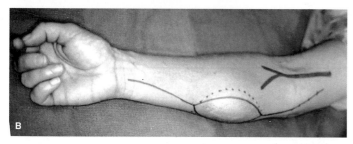

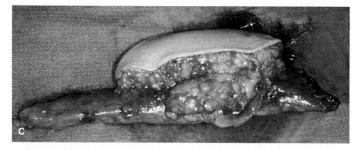

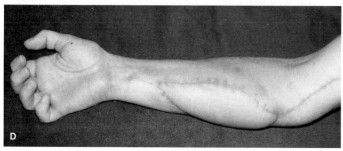

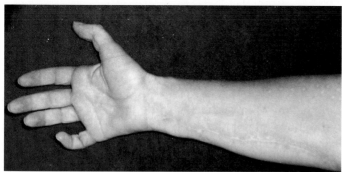

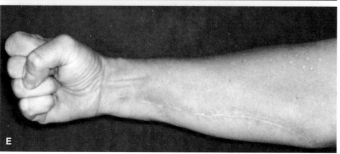

Rhabdomyosarcoma

- Patients <20 years of age
- Arises from striated muscle cells
- Hematogenous spread
- Treatment is chemotherapy and wide local excision

A 65-year-old man with a 20 pack-year history of tobacco abuse presents to your office with a complaint of right groin pain. An X-ray shows mild arthritis and a lytic lesion in his right hip. What is the most likely diagnosis?

Metastatic disease.

Most Common Cancers That Metastasize to Bone

1. Breast
2. Prostate
3. Thyroid
4. Lung
5. Kidney

A bone scan is the most sensitive test for metastatic disease in bone.

6 | Vascular Surgery

Peter R. Nelson

A 72-year-old man presents 2 weeks after a stroke resulting in right arm and leg weakness and expressive aphasia. He is found by duplex ultrasound to have 80% to 99% left carotid stenosis and a <50% right carotid stenosis. What is the next step in management?

Confirm that the patient is on antiplatelet therapy with ASA/dipyridamole or clopidogrel, initiate statin therapy, and plan for a left carotid endarterectomy (CEA) as soon as stroke symptoms have stabilized or resolved.

Carotid Endartectomy

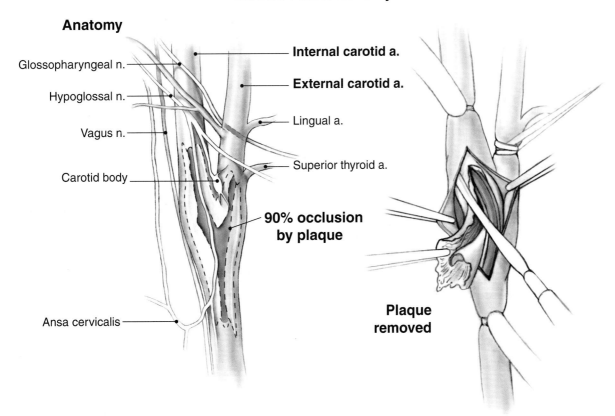

Anatomy

Glossopharyngeal n.

Hypoglossal n.

Vagus n.

Carotid body

Ansa cervicalis

Internal carotid a.

External carotid a.

Lingual a.

Superior thyroid a.

90% occlusion by plaque

Plaque removed

Indications for CEA

- Symptomatic patients with >70% stenosis
- Symptomatic patients with 50% to 69% stenosis, with ulceration or when all other sources (i.e., cardiac embolus) have been ruled out
- Asymptomatic good medical risk patients with >80% stenosis

Carotid Disease

- Can present as a transient ischemic attack (TIA)
  - A neurologic event that resolves completely within 24 hours
  - Symptoms that last >24 hours constitute a stroke, which requires further brain imaging
- Timing of CEA
  - Proceed when residual symptoms stabilize or resolve completely
  - An immediate CEA is indicated for a "crescendo" or evolving TIA/cerebrovascular accident (CVA) (frequent, worsening, or fluctuating neurological findings)
  - The traditional 6-week delay may only be necessary in patients with a large, disabling CVA
- An endarterectomy with patch angioplasty (autogenous vein or prosthetic patch) leads to better outcomes than primary arterial closure
- An eversion endarterectomy may have similar outcomes

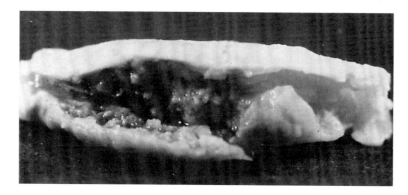

Carotid artery plaque. (With permission from Mulholland MW, Lillemoe KD, Doherty GM, Maier RV, Upchurch GR, eds. *Greenfield's Surgery.* 4th ed. Philadelphia, PA: Lippincott Williams & Wilkins; 2005.)

Complications of Carotid Endarterectomy

- Airway compression from an expanding hematoma
- Vagus nerve (laryngeal branch) injury causes *vocal cord paralysis* and *hoarseness*
- Hypoglossal nerve injury causes *tongue deviation* toward the side of surgery
- Any postoperative dyspnea or change in neurologic exam warrants emergent re-operation

Amaurosis fugax (transient monocular blindness) results from an embolus to the ophthalmic artery, a branch of the internal carotid artery, and is an indication for CEA.

A 76-year-old man with a significant cardiac history presents with a left hemispheric TIA. He has had a previous left CEA in the remote past and a carotid duplex now shows a critical (80% to 99%) recurrent stenosis. How should this be managed?

Consider a left carotid angioplasty with stenting using an embolic protection device.

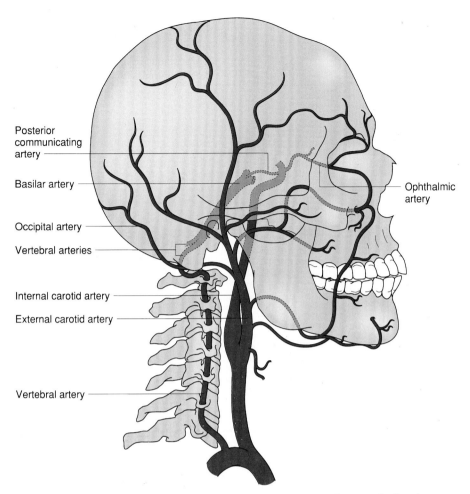

Posterior communicating artery

Basilar artery

Occipital artery

Vertebral arteries

Internal carotid artery

External carotid artery

Vertebral artery

Ophthalmic artery

Normal carotid and vertebral artery anatomy. (With permission from Mulholland MW, Lillemoe KD, Doherty GM, Maier RV, Upchurch GR, eds. *Greenfield's Surgery*. 4th ed. Philadelphia, PA: Lippincott Williams & Wilkins; 2005.)

Carotid Angioplasty and Stenting

- Carotid angioplasty and stenting (CAS) is restricted to:
  - High-risk symptomatic patients <80 years of age with ≥70% stenosis
  - High-risk symptomatic patients <80 years of age with 50% to 70% stenosis
  - High-risk asymptomatic patients <80 years of age with >80% lesions
- High anatomic/surgical risk factors
  - Redo carotid intervention
  - Radiation-induced stenosis
  - Prior radical neck dissection
  - A surgically inaccessible lesion (above C2)
  - Common carotid lesion below clavicle
  - Contralateral vocal cord palsy
  - Contralateral internal carotid occlusion
  - Tracheostomy
- Embolic protection with either a balloon, filter, or reversal of flow device is needed
- CT angiography with 3D reconstruction is useful to delineate the aortic arch and carotid anatomy for procedural planning

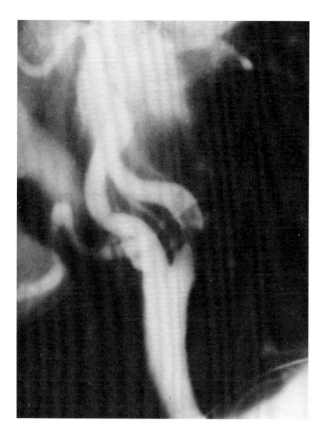

Angiogram demonstrating an isolated atherosclerotic lesion. (With permission from Mulholland MW, Lillemoe KD, Doherty GM, Maier RV, Upchurch GR, eds. *Greenfield's Surgery.* 4th ed. Philadelphia, PA: Lippincott Williams & Wilkins; 2005.)

- Pre-procedure loading with clopidogrel for 7 to 10 days and continued therapy for at least 30 days post-intervention is recommended
- Anatomic challenges to performing a CAS include difficult arch anatomy (i.e., elongated, tortuous, and/or diseased arch; bovine arch), significant common carotid disease, heavily calcified lesions, and a tortuous internal carotid artery
- A redo CEA is considered in these situations but often requires interposition grafting and has a higher risk of cranial nerve injury

Carotid stenting should be considered in symptomatic patients (>50% stenosis) or asymptomatic patients (>80% stenosis) if they have medical problems or anatomic abnormalities that make them high risk for CEA.

A 35-year-old man with a past medical history of Ehlers-Danlos syndrome presents with new-onset headache, neck pain, Horner's syndrome, and amaurosis fugax of the left eye. What is the diagnosis and best initial management?

The patient had a spontaneous carotid dissection. Anticoagulation is the first-line treatment for most extracranial carotid artery dissections. He should then be followed with serial duplex ultrasound exams.

Carotid Artery Dissection

- Presents with ipsilateral neck pain and embolic symptoms in patients with collagen vascular disorders
- May be spontaneous (60% to 70%) or traumatic (30% to 40%)
- Duplex ultrasound may be a reasonable first diagnostic test and can often identify a flap or thrombus just distal to the carotid bulb with highly resistive waveforms
- The diagnostic gold standard is arteriography; however, noninvasive imaging with MR or CT angiography is often adequate to make the diagnosis while also providing axial imaging to rule out hemorrhage

- The classic radiographic finding is a tapered stenosis or occlusion of the internal carotid artery associated with an aneurysm at the base of the skull
- The treatment for a patient with spontaneous dissection with minimal or no neurological deficits is anticoagulation (acutely with unfractionated heparin; long term with warfarin) and antiplatelet therapy (ASA)
- Surgery or percutaneous intervention
  - Considered in patients with active ongoing symptoms or with a contraindication to anticoagulation
  - Depends on the location and extent of the dissection
  - Can perform interposition grafting, ICA ligation, or EC-IC bypass
  - Often challenging and fraught with complications in patients with collagen vascular disorders

Most carotid dissections recanalize and heal completely within a few months of initiating anticoagulation therapy and do not require surgical intervention.

A 43-year-old Caucasian female undergoes evaluation following two episodes of TIA. Cerebral angiography reveals a "string of beads" appearance of the internal carotid arteries bilaterally. What is the most likely diagnosis?

A "string of beads" appearance on the arteriogram of a young or middle-aged woman is characteristic of fibromuscular dysplasia (FMD).

Fibromuscular Dysplasia

- Typically affects Caucasian women (~90%) in the 4th or 5th decade of life
- Bilateral in 65% of cases
- Associated with intracranial aneurysms in 10% to 50% of cases
- Pathology shows medial fibroplasia in 80% to 95% of cases
- Approximately 10% of cases are symptomatic and present with TIA, stroke, or amaurosis fugax
- Diagnosis can be suggested by duplex ultrasound, CT, or MR angiography, but is confirmed by arteriography, particularly if intervention is warranted
- Asymptomatic patients are treated with antiplatelet therapy, monitoring for hypertension, and evaluation for the presence of an intracranial aneurysm
- Surgical options in symptomatic patients include open graduated internal dilatation and open balloon angioplasty
- Renal FMD
  - Occurs in 8% to 40% of patients with carotid FMD
  - Overall more common and typically presents with hypertension
  - May require initial or simultaneous treatment with percutaneous angioplasty alone (without stenting) to prevent complications of hypertension

FMD can involve the renal, carotid, external iliac, splenic, hepatic, vertebral, or axillary arteries.

A 69-year-old man with an incidental finding of a 4.3-cm abdominal aortic aneurysm (AAA) presents to the office. He has no complaints and a normal physical exam. What is the next step in his management?

Repeat the CT scan in 1 year or repeat an ultrasound in 6 months to assess the growth of the aneurysm. In the meantime, provide counseling regarding the typical symptoms related to an AAA.

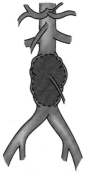
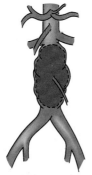
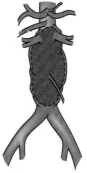

Infrarenal   Juxtarenal   Suprarenal

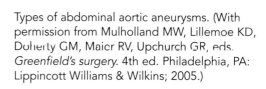

Types of abdominal aortic aneurysms. (With permission from Mulholland MW, Lillemoe KD, Doherty GM, Maier RV, Upchurch GR, eds. *Greenfield's surgery.* 4th ed. Philadelphia, PA: Lippincott Williams & Wilkins; 2005.)

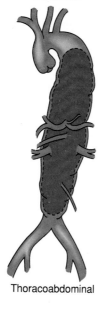

Thoracoabdominal

Abdominal Aortic Aneurysm

- Most commonly found in the infrarenal aorta
- Results from degeneration of the wall with loss of elastin and weakening of collagen
- Most commonly secondary to atherosclerosis
- Average growth rate of approximately 10% per year
- Most are asymptomatic and found incidentally on abdominal imaging
  - May also present as back/abdominal pain or an abdominal mass on examination
- Risk of rupture (per year)
  - <5 cm: 1% to 4%
  - 5 to 6 cm: 5% to 8%
  - 6 to 7 cm: 8% to 15%
  - 7 to 8 cm: 15% to 30%
  - >8 cm: 30% to 50%
- Indications for elective repair (either endovascular or open) are diameter >5.5 cm, presence of symptoms, or growth >1.0 cm/year or 0.5 cm in 6 months
- Open repair can be accomplished through either an anterior or retroperitoneal approach and involves either a tube graft or bifurcated aortobiiliac repair (generally if iliac arteries are >2.5 cm)
  - Impotence is a common complication of an open repair (>30%)

- Endovascular repair ideally requires
  - Neck diameter ≤32 mm
  - Neck length >10 mm
  - Neck angulation ≤60 degrees
  - Common iliac diameters ≤20 mm
  - External iliac diameters ≥7 mm
- Endovascular repair has a lower short-term morbidity and mortality compared to open repair, but mortality is equal at 2 years
- As with most vascular procedures, cardiac complications are the most common cause of perioperative morbidity and mortality
- Cardiac and renal complications are the most common cause of death beyond 30 days postoperatively

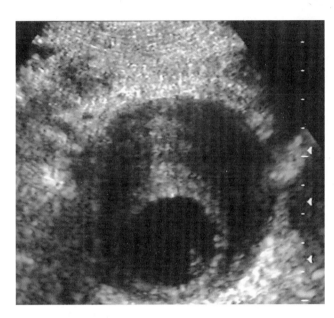

Ultrasound of an AAA. (With permission from Mulholland MW, Lillemoe KD, Doherty GM, Maier RV, Upchurch GR, eds. *Greenfield's Surgery*. 4th ed. Philadelphia, PA: Lippincott Williams & Wilkins; 2005.)

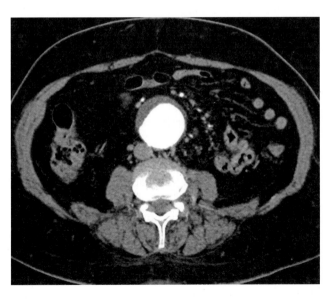

Large abdominal aortic aneurysm. (With permission from Mulholland MW, Lillemoe KD, Doherty GM, Maier RV, Upchurch GR, eds. *Greenfield's Surgery*. 4th ed. Philadelphia, PA: Lippincott Williams & Wilkins; 2005.)

Screening is now approved for AAA in populations at risk (i.e., males >55 years old who have ever smoked, and men or women >55 years old with a family history of aneurysms).

A 75-year-old man with a history of hypertension presents to the emergency department with acute-onset severe abdominal and lower back pain. His physical exam reveals a markedly distended and diffusely tender abdomen. His vital signs on presentation include a blood pressure of 70/40 mmHg and a heart rate of 130 bpm. Two large-bore IVs are in place. What should be the next step in management?

A high suspicion for a ruptured AAA necessitates an emergent exploration. As with any unstable patient with a surgical abdomen, a CT scan should not delay operative exploration.

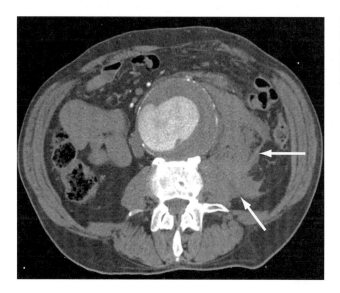

Ruptured AAA. (With permission from Mulholland MW, Lillemoe KD, Doherty GM, Maier RV, Upchurch GR, eds. *Greenfield's Surgery*. 4th ed. Philadelphia, PA: Lippincott Williams & Wilkins; 2005.)

Ruptured Abdominal Aortic Aneurysm

- The classic triad of signs/symptoms include severe acute abdominal and/or back pain, hypotension, and a pulsatile abdominal mass
  - 95% of cases will demonstrate at least one of these three findings
  - <50% will have all three findings
- Operative mortality is approximately 50%, while overall mortality from a ruptured AAA is historically approximately 80%
- Proximal control can be achieved by incising the diaphragmatic crus to expose and clamp the supraceliac aorta
  - A nasogastric tube is essential to help distinguish the aorta from the esophagus at this level
- The most common location for rupture is the left retroperitoneum below the renal vessels
- Most emergent cases can be managed with a tube graft repair
- If the patient is stable enough on presentation to permit a CT scan, the anatomy can be evaluated for endovascular repair
- Endovascular repair, when appropriate, is feasible and may reduce operative mortality rates to 20% to 30%
- Postoperative management should focus on resuscitation, monitoring for postoperative hemorrhage, and aggressive management to prevent renal failure

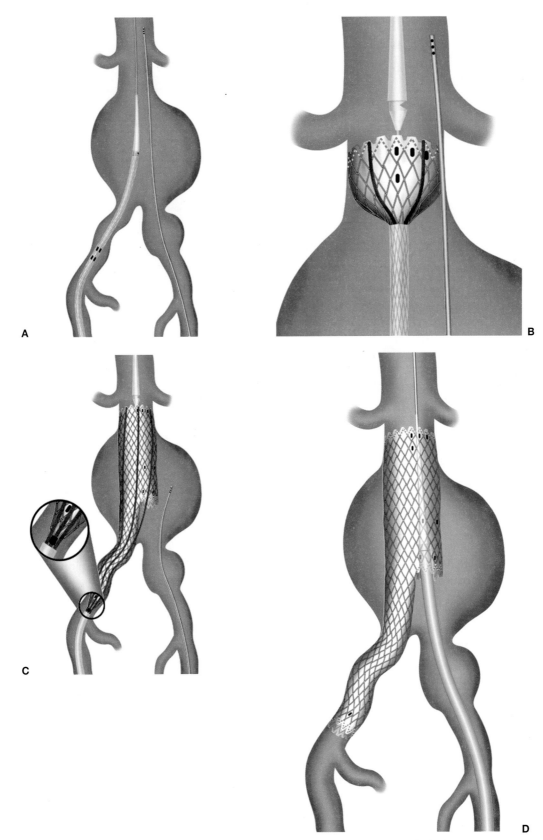

Endovascular repair of an AAA. (A) insertion of aortic endograft. (B) initial graft deployment at levels of renal arteries. (C) completion of main body device with ipsilateral limb. (D) insertion of contralateral limb component. (E) placing contralateral limb. (F) completed deployment. (With permission from Mulholland MW, Lillemoe KD, Doherty GM, Maier RV, Upchurch GR, eds. *Greenfield's Surgery.* 4th ed. Philadelphia, PA: Lippincott Williams & Wilkins; 2005.)

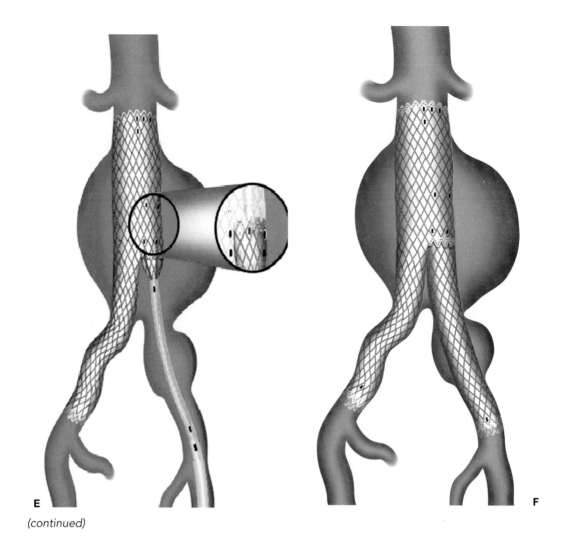

E   F

(continued)

A retroaortic left renal vein is an anatomic variation that is susceptible to injury during aortic exposure and cross-clamping during an open AAA repair.

A 77-year-old male presents with a pulsatile abdominal mass, weight loss, and generalized malaise. A physical exam reveals a widened abdominal aorta, measuring approximately 6 cm in size. Laboratory data are all normal except an elevated erythrocyte sedimentation rate. What is the diagnosis and how should you proceed from here?

An inflammatory AAA should be evaluated with a CT scan, followed by surgical repair.

Inflammatory Abdominal Aortic Aneurysm

- Characteristic enhancing rim around the aortic wall (signet ring appearance) on CT scan
- Not caused by an infectious organism
- Most common in males in the 7th decade of life
- Presents with abdominal pain, weight loss, myalgias, and an elevated erythrocyte sedimentation rate
- The inflammatory reaction often involves adjacent structures (duodenum (>90%), ureters, vena cava, and left renal vein), complicating dissection, and open repair

- Repair is typically via an open retroperitoneal approach; however, growing experience with endovascular repair shows promise for technical feasibility with prompt resolution of inflammation and associated symptoms
- The inflammatory process resolves after graft placement

A retroperitoneal approach is advantageous for repair of inflammatory aneurysms to avoid injury to the duodenum and other adjacent structures.

On postoperative day one following an aortic aneurysm repair, a 63-year-old female is noted to have melena. What is the next step in management?

In the early postoperative period following an aortic aneurysm repair, any patient with bloody or melanotic stool, or severe diarrhea requires an immediate rigid or flexible sigmoidoscopy. Broad-spectrum IV antibiotics and fluid resuscitation should also be started for presumed ischemic colitis.

Ischemic Colitis Following Aortic Aneurysm Repair
- Complicates 1% to 6% of AAA repair cases
- Presents with abdominal pain, distension, diarrhea, lower GI bleeding, or melanotic stool
- Laboratory values may reveal acidosis, leukocytosis, and thrombocytopenia
- A high index of suspicion is essential to making the diagnosis
- Risk factors
  - Known mesenteric vascular occlusive disease
  - Intraoperative ligation of the inferior mesenteric artery (IMA)
  - Advanced age
  - Prior colectomy with interruption of the mesenteric circulation
  - Pelvic irradiation
  - Internal iliac artery occlusion or exclusion
  - Perioperative hypotension
- A sigmoidoscopy can diagnose mucosal ischemia
- The treatment depends on the degree of colon ischemia
  - Mild ischemic colitis (mucosal) can be managed with bowel rest, broad-spectrum antibiotics, fluid resuscitation, consideration for parenteral nutrition, and serial endoscopy (if warranted)
  - Full thickness bowel necrosis, peritonitis, or sepsis requires colectomy with a proximal diverting colostomy or ileostomy; a primary colonic anastomosis is not recommended
  - The rectum is generally spared in this setting because of its blood supply from the internal iliac artery
  - Long-term surveillance of colonic function is prudent due to the increased incidence of colonic stricture at areas of partial thickness ischemia

During an AAA repair, the inferior mesenteric artery is identified and either ligated (if chronically occluded or if pulsatile back-bleeding is present) or re-implanted (if patent but with minimal back-bleeding suggesting poor collaterals).

A 58-year-old male presents to the emergency department with hematemesis. His past surgical history is significant for an aortic aneurysm repair 5 years ago. What is the next diagnostic step?

Any upper or lower GI bleeding in a patient with a remote history of prior aortic reconstruction should be investigated with an upper endoscopy for an aortoenteric fistula.

Aortoenteric Fistula

- An aortoenteric fistula complicates 0.4% to 2.4% of aortic reconstructions
- A herald bleed followed by a variable period of stability is a common presentation
- An EGD to visualize the 3rd and 4th portions of the duodenum is the primary diagnostic study, often requiring a long pediatric colonoscope to get the distance needed for visualization
- A normal EGD exam does not rule out the presence of an aortic graft infection
- A CT scan may support the diagnosis by demonstrating perigraft fluid or gas, an anastomotic pseudoaneurysm, focal bowel wall thickening, or extravasation of oral contrast
- Any infected prosthetic (gram stain infected material) requires removal
- Treatment options
  - A two-stage extra-anatomic axillobifemoral bypass through non-infected tissue planes with subsequent aortic graft excision, bowel repair, and aortic stump closure
  - Direct inline aortic replacement with autogenous femoral vein graft repair (neo-aortoiliac system)
  - Alternative in situ repairs including antibiotic (i.e., rifampin) soaked prosthetic grafts or cadaveric homografts

Despite management of the aortic stump by oversewing healthy aortic tissue and providing coverage with an omental flap, muscle flap, or serosal patches, stump blowout still occurs in up to one-third of cases.

A 65-year-old male is 10 years post-endovascular repair for an AAA. On a screening CT to evaluate for endoleak, he is found to have a large blush of contrast outside of the lumen of the graft at its distal attachment. What is the next step in management?

The patient has a type I endoleak and will require immediate operative repair.

Endoleak

- Patients should be screened annually with CT scans after endovascular repair to assess for endoleak
- Type I: Have a leak at the proximal (IA) or distal (IB) attachment of the graft
  - Requires immediate repair
- Type II: Have persistent flow in the aneurysm through low pressure collaterals including the lumbar or inferior mesenteric arteries
  - Does not require repair unless the aneurysm is enlarging
- Type III: Have a leak between modular components of a graft
  - Requires immediate repair
- Type IV: Fabric porosity

Endoleak management should take into account the status of the aneurysm sac remodeling.

A 76-year-old female is referred to a vascular surgeon after her primary care physician identifies a thoracic aortic aneurysm that measures 7 cm. What is the best management for her and what is her risk of rupture?

The natural history of thoracic aneurysms is not as well delineated as for abdominal aneurysms. Most surgeons will offer repair to medically fit patients once the aneurysm has reached 6 cm in maximal diameter.

Thoracoabdominal Aortic Aneurysm

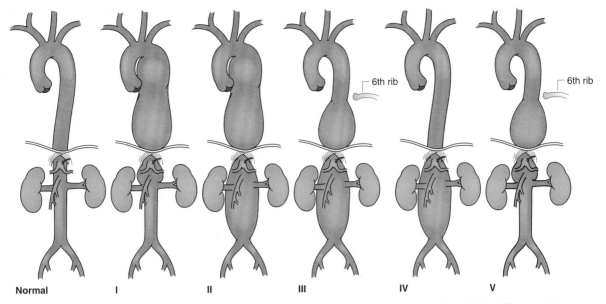

Types of thoracoabdominal aortic aneurysms (TAAAs). (With permission from Mulholland MW, Lillemoe KD, Doherty GM, Maier RV, Upchurch GR, eds. *Greenfield's Surgery.* 4th ed. Philadelphia, PA: Lippincott Williams & Wilkins; 2005.)

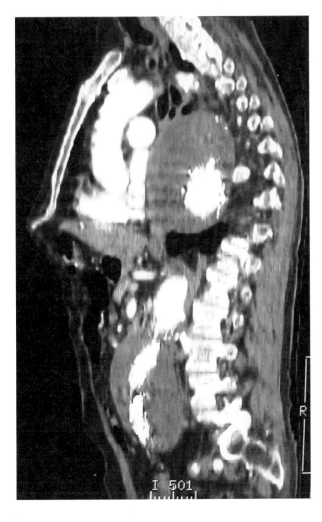

CT of a type II TAAA. (With permission from Mulholland MW, Lillemoe KD, Doherty GM, Maier RV, Upchurch GR, eds. *Greenfield's Surgery.* 4th ed. Philadelphia, PA: Lippincott Williams & Wilkins; 2005.)

- Crawford classification:
  - Type I: Extends from distal to the left subclavian artery to the renal arteries
  - Type II: Extends from distal to the left subclavian artery to the aortic bifurcation
  - Type III: Involves the distal half of the descending thoracic aorta with variable involvement of the abdominal aorta
  - Type IV (total abdominal aneurysm): Involves the infradiaphragmatic aorta to the aortic bifurcation
  - Type V: Involves the distal descending thoracic aorta to the renal arteries
- Open TAAA repair involves thoracoabdominal exposure and replacement of the involved thoracic and abdominal aorta with a polyester synthetic graft, along with reimplantation of the T9-L2 intercostal and visceral branches, adjunctive hypothermic distal perfusion, and spinal drainage
- Elective TAAA repair is associated with significant mortality (4% to 21%) and morbidity, including paralysis attributed to spinal ischemia (5% to 10%); rates are even higher for urgent/emergent repair
- Experience is evolving with hybrid open visceral revascularization (debranching) followed by thoracoabdominal aortic stent grafting and fenestrated/branched endografts

If there is no abdominal component (isolated thoracic aneurysm), thoracic endovascular aortic repair (TEVAR) is a viable option.

A 56-year-old man presents through the emergency department with back pain that he describes as "tearing." A CT scan obtained shows a thoracic aortic dissection that begins distal to the left subclavian artery. What is the management of this patient and when should surgical therapy be employed?

Confirm perfusion of the aortic branches (iliac arteries, renal arteries, and mesenteric arteries). Admit the patient to the ICU for monitoring and aggressive blood pressure control (SBP < 120 mmHg).

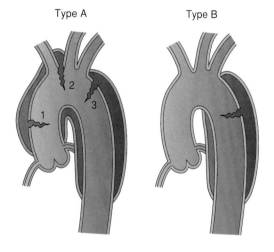

Type A   Type B

Stanford classification of aortic dissections. (With permission from Mulholland MW, Lillemoe KD, Doherty GM, Maier RV, Upchurch GR, eds. *Greenfield's Surgery*. 4th ed. Philadelphia, PA: Lippincott Williams & Wilkins; 2005.)

Thoracic Aortic Dissection

- Stanford classification
  - Type A involves the ascending aorta and is a cardiac surgical emergency to prevent retrograde dissection causing hemopericardium and pericardial tamponade or acute malperfusion of the coronary arteries
  - Type B does not involve ascending aorta and is usually initially managed with aggressive blood pressure control

- Indications for operative intervention with Type B aneurysms
  - Malperfusion of a branch vessel
  - Rupture of the descending aorta
  - Persistent pain due to the dissection or its extension
  - Inability to medically control blood pressure
  - Aneurysmal degeneration (>6 cm) of the dissected aorta
- Open repair for Type B dissection involves thoracoabdominal exposure and replacement of the descending thoracic aorta with a polyester synthetic graft, along with adjunctive hypothermic distal/visceral perfusion, reimplantation of the T9-L2 intercostal arteries, and spinal drainage
- An operative mortality of 10% to 20% and paraplegia rates of 20% to 30% have been reported for open repair

Thoracic aortic endografting (TEVAR) is evolving in the management of throacic dissection especially with signs of malperfusion.

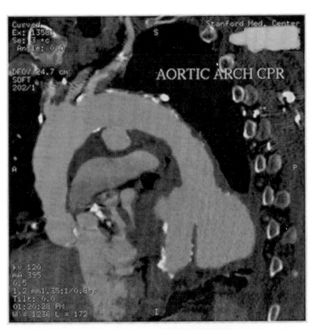

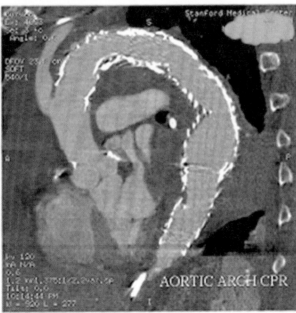

Angiogram of a TAA (A) pre-aneurysm repair and (B) post-stent graft repair. (With permission from Mulholland MW, Lillemoe KD, Doherty GM, Maier RV, Upchurch GR, eds. *Greenfield's Surgery*. 4th ed. Philadelphia, PA: Lippincott Williams & Wilkins; 2005.)

One-third of patients with descending thoracic aortic dissections will ultimately need operative intervention.

A 62-year-old man with a history of an AAA repair 4 years ago presents with a pulsatile mass in the right popliteal fossa. A duplex ultrasound confirms a popliteal artery aneurysm. What is the likelihood of discovering a popliteal artery aneurysm on the other leg?

Popliteal artery aneurysms are bilateral in approximately two-thirds of cases.

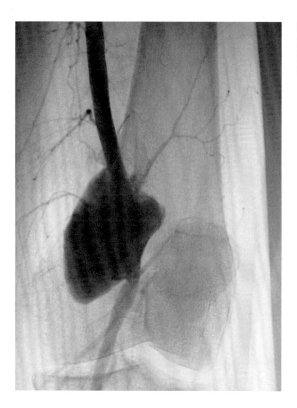

Popliteal artery aneurysm. (With permission from Mulholland MW, Lillemoe KD, Doherty GM, Maier RV, Upchurch GR, eds. *Greenfield's Surgery.* 4th ed. Philadelphia, PA: Lippincott Williams & Wilkins; 2005.)

Popliteal Artery Aneurysm

- Most common peripheral aneurysm
- Occurs predominantly in men
- 80% will have an additional extrapopliteal aneurysm, and there is a 30% to 60% incidence of having an associated AAA
- Can easily be detected on physical examination as a prominent popliteal pulse
- The diagnosis is confirmed by duplex ultrasound, which is the initial diagnostic test of choice
- Without intervention, 40% to 60% will eventually develop symptoms
- Typically presents with an acute thrombosis or distal embolization
  - Generally does NOT present with rupture
- A lower extremity angiogram is important before any surgical intervention to define the anatomy, particularly the status of perfusion/patency of distal vessels (distal runoff)
- Surgery is indicated for the presence of symptoms, size >2 cm, or any evidence of mural thrombus within the aneurysm on duplex scan

- Surgical options include ligation/exclusion of the aneurysm with:
  - Surgical bypass using an autogenous vein from a medial approach for extensive aneurysms not limited to the popliteal fossa
  - Surgical bypass using an autogenous vein from a posterior approach for aneurysms limited to the popliteal fossa with significant mass effect
  - Endovascular repair using covered stent grafts
- Delayed mass effect requiring a subsequent staged aneurysm decompression is uncommon (approximately 4% of cases)
- For patients with an acute thrombosis, thrombolysis followed by repair improves limb salvage rates through the identification of distal bypass targets
- Amputation rates for acute popliteal artery aneurysm thrombosis are as high as 80%

Surgery is indicated for asymptomatic aneurysms >2 cm and all symptomatic aneurysms.

A 78-year-old woman is found to have calcifications in the left upper quadrant on an abdominal X-ray. A CT scan confirms the presence of a 4-cm splenic artery aneurysm. What is the next step in management?

In women beyond child-bearing age, no further therapy is needed unless the patient is symptomatic.

Splenic Artery Aneurysm

- The most common visceral artery aneurysm
- Commonly associated with multiple pregnancies, portal hypertension, and pancreatitis
- Can be first detected on a plain X-ray demonstrating a signet ring appearance of associated calcification
- Presents clinically with left upper quadrant (LUQ) or epigastric pain or bleeding following rupture
- A "double rupture" refers to an initial bleed into the lesser sac, followed by free rupture into the peritoneum
- Indications for resection include size >2 cm in a woman of childbearing age or in patients with any associated symptoms
- Rupture during pregnancy usually occurs in the 3rd trimester and is associated with a high mortality
- Treatment options include an open or laparoscopic repair, aneurysm resection, splenectomy, or endovascular embolization (in patients with high operative risk)

Splenic artery aneurysms should be repaired in young women of child-bearing age because of the risk of rupture during pregnancy and its high associated mortality.

An 80-year-old woman presents complaining of abdominal pain 15 minutes following every meal, which has lead to food avoidance and weight loss of 30 pounds. What is the next step in management?

A duplex ultrasound of her mesenteric vessels followed by consideration for diagnostic arteriography.

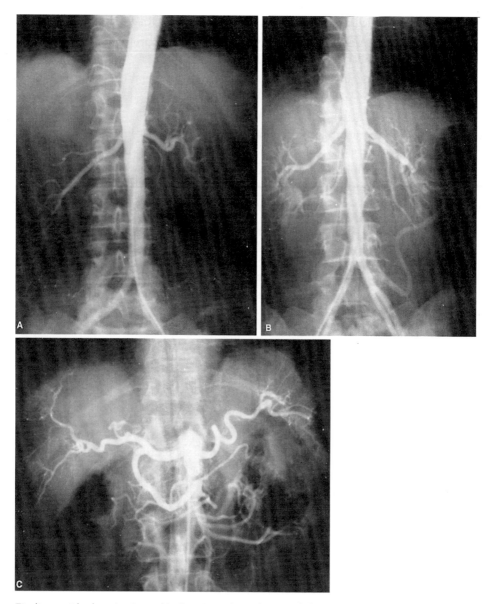

Findings with chronic visceral ischemia with occlusion of the SMA and IMA with collateral flow through the celiac. (With permission from Mulholland MW, Lillemoe KD, Doherty GM, Maier RV, Upchurch GR, eds. *Greenfield's Surgery*. 4th ed. Philadelphia, PA: Lippincott Williams & Wilkins; 2005.)

Chronic Mesenteric Ischemia

- Predominantly found in women
- Bimodal age distribution
  - 5th to 6th decades in heavy smokers
  - 7th to 8th decades in typical vasculopathies
- The prevalence of >50% mesenteric arterial stenosis is 6% to 10% on autopsy studies with the majority being asymptomatic
- Cardinal signs of chronic mesenteric ischemia include postprandial abdominal pain, significant (10 to 15 kg or more) weight loss, and sitophobia ("fear of food")
- Duplex ultrasonography is the initial non-invasive diagnostic study of choice with sensitivity and specificity reported in the 90% to 96% range

- Advances in MR and CT angiography make them reasonable alternatives, with additional information provided by axial imaging
- Digital subtraction angiography remains the standard for definitive imaging in patients with convincing symptoms and suggestive non-invasive imaging
- Preoperative hyperalimentation is controversial in these malnourished patients with no reported benefit and the added risk of a line-related infection
- Open mesenteric bypass
  - Antegrade aortomesenteric bypass to both the celiac artery and SMA for "complete" revascularization
  - Retrograde iliac-SMA "C-loop" bypass for single vessel revascularization
  - Early patency rates are comparable: 93% and 95%, respectively
  - Synthetic and autogenous conduits offer similar patency rates: 89% and 95%, respectively
    - Only vein grafts should be used in cases where any bowel resection may be required
  - Overall symptom-free survival: 70% to 86%
  - Perioperative mortality: <10%
- Percutaneous revascularization with angioplasty and stenting:
  - Reported technical success: 80% to 96%
  - Initial clinical response: 70% to 100%
  - Primary patency rates: 60% to 70%
  - Primary-assisted patency: 70% to 88%
  - May have higher symptomatic recurrence rate than open bypass but generally amenable to repeat percutaneous intervention

A high index of suspicion for chronic mesenteric ischemia is critical to making a prompt diagnosis and expediting intervention.

An 85-year-old male with a history of atrial fibrillation who has not been anticoagulated due to his significant fall risk presents complaining of severe abdominal pain. On exam, his abdomen is distended, but his exam does not correlate with his symptoms. He is hemodynamically unstable and has a leukocytosis of 20. What is the next step in management?

Aggressive resuscitation and exploratory laparotomy to evaluate for mesenteric ischemia.

Acute Mesenteric Ischemia
- Classically presents with pain out of proportion to exam
- Arterial
  - Embolic
    - Most common type
    - Mostly emboli from the left atrium or ventricle
    - Most commonly, emboli lodge in the SMA distal to the middle colic artery
    - The proximal jejunum and transverse colon are spared
  - Thrombotic
    - Most commonly occludes at the origin of the SMA
    - The entire small bowel, ascending and transverse colon are at risk
  - Non-occlusive
    - In critically ill patients on pressors
    - Can affect any region of the bowel

- Venous
  - Seen with hypercoagulable states, vasculitis, and portal hypertension
  - Most commonly involves the SMV
- Management
  - Embolic/thrombotic: Embolectomy or bypass with resection of infarcted bowel
  - Non-occlusive: Intra-arterial papaverine, glucagon, and nitrates; cessation of pressors
  - Venous: Anticoagulation with heparin and Coumadin

Prompt diagnosis and emergent intervention for acute mesenteric ischemia is warranted.

A 59-year-old male letter carrier presents with complaints of bilateral calf heaviness and weakness after walking 200 yards, requiring him to stop and rest. What is the best initial management for this patient?

The treatment of intermittent claudication (as defined below) is non-surgical: conservative therapy with smoking cessation, structured exercise, attention to hypertension, diabetes, and hypercholesterolemia (statins), and antiplatelet therapy. Surgery is occasionally indicated for rare cases of significant life-debilitating claudication, but with mixed results.

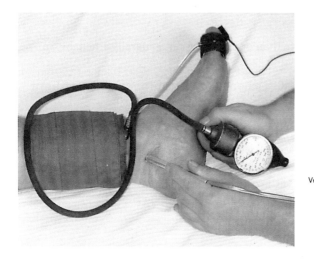

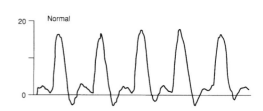

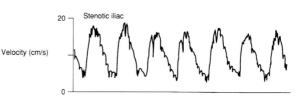

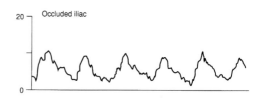

Screening for peripheral arterial disease. (With permission from Mulholland MW, Lillemoe KD, Doherty GM, Maier RV, Upchurch GR, eds. *Greenfield's Surgery.* 4th ed. Philadelphia, PA: Lippincott Williams & Wilkins; 2005.)

Intermittent Claudication

- Reproducible exercise-induced muscle aching, weakness, or pain in the same muscle group that is relieved by rest
- Claudication means "to limp"
- Symptoms occur at the same predictable distance each time

- Symptoms need to be distinguished from those caused by other conditions such as diabetic neuropathy, neurogenic radiculopathy from lumbar disc or degenerative disease, arthritic conditions, or generalized muscle fatigue from deconditioning
- In unusual cases of young otherwise healthy individuals without significant cardiovascular risk factors, rare diagnoses such as popliteal entrapment syndrome, cystic adventitial disease, a persistent sciatic artery or vasculitis should be entertained
- Vasculogenic claudication should be confirmed through history, physical exam, and non-invasive testing including stress ankle-brachial indices (ABIs)
- With strict attention to smoking cessation, exercise, and risk-factor modification, symptoms will improve in 80% of claudicants
- Structured exercise should consist of a minimum of 30 minutes of walking daily, or at least 3 days a week, to achieve significant benefit
    - Exercise bicycles, swimming, or other forms of exercise may also provide benefit through general cardiovascular improvements
- Adjunctive pharmacologic therapy with cilostazol, a type-III phosphodiesterase inhibitor, provides symptomatic relief in approximately 50% of patients
- Based on a chronic stable natural history, <20% of claudicants will require surgical intervention, and <10% will ever require a major amputation
- Claudication is a marker for generalized cardiovascular disease with mortality rates in this population of 30% to 50% at 5 years due to cardiovascular causes
- Intervention options for claudicants who clearly fail conservative therapy and have significant life-debilitating disease
    - Percutaneous intervention (i.e., angioplasty/stenting) in the iliac, superficial femoral, or rarely tibial locations
    - A femoropopliteal bypass with an autogenous vein graft
- It is rare for a patient to meet the indications for surgery

Intermittent claudication is essentially a non-surgical condition for which smoking cessation, exercise, and risk-factor modification is the best treatment.

A 73-year-old diabetic male presents with complaints of left foot pain at night that wakes him and forces him to hang his foot over the side of the bed for relief. What is the best initial management for this patient?

Following a thorough history and physical examination, proceed to arteriography to delineate his arterial anatomy in preparation for a potential revascularization procedure.

Critical Limb Ischemia
- Critical limb ischemia is defined as arterial insufficiency leading to rest pain or tissue loss (non-healing ulceration) with a significant risk of limb loss if untreated (25% for rest pain, 75% for tissue loss at 1 year)
- Attention should be paid to cardiovascular risk factors and smoking cessation, followed by expeditious determination regarding revascularization
- Digital-subtraction arteriography remains the standard for arterial imaging; however, advances in CT angiography, MR angiography, and duplex arterial mapping make them non-invasive alternatives in centers with appropriate expertise
- A primary amputation should be considered in patients who are non-ambulatory, who have a non-salvageable foot, or who have no revascularization options

- Revascularization requires an adequate inflow source, an adequate outflow target with continuity to the foot, and an appropriate conduit
  - The optimal conduit for infrainguinal revascularization is an autogenous greater saphenous vein, if available
  - Less durable alternatives include a composite arm vein, a prosthetic graft with distal vein cuff, or a cryopreserved vascular graft
  - Meticulous technique when handling the arteries and conduit along with a command of distal arterial anatomy are critical keys to success
- Bypass patency rates of 60% at 5 years are generally reported for vein bypass procedures
  - Postoperative surveillance using duplex ultrasonography is critical to maintaining acceptable long-term primary-assisted patency rates
- Surgical site infection rates as high as 40% have been reported for lower extremity revascularization procedures, which warrants compulsive attention to antibiotic prophylaxis and wound and tissue handling

An aggressive revascularization program with appropriate patient selection, meticulous technique, and compulsive postoperative surveillance can lead to long-term functional limb-salvage rates in excess of 80%.

A 24-year-old female is seen in the emergency room after a motocross accident caused a posterior knee dislocation. After manual reduction of the knee by the orthopedic surgeons, she has a diminished pulse in the ipsilateral foot, but no motor-sensory deficits. Does this person need vascular imaging?

Any hard sign of vascular injury mandates definitive vascular imaging.

Peripheral Vascular Trauma
- Several orthopedic injuries are classically associated with vascular injury
  - Posterior knee dislocations are associated with a 40% incidence of popliteal artery injury
- Any diminished or absent distal extremity pulse or an ABI <0.90 should warrant arterial imaging
- Signs of acute extremity ischemia include pain, pulselessness, pallor, poikilothermia, paresthesia, and paralysis
- Although angiography is still the gold-standard, CT angiography or duplex arterial imaging may be a reliable substitute in centers with appropriate capabilities
- The popliteal vein is often injured with the popliteal artery; if the repair is simple (end-to-end anastomosis), it should also be repaired
- Repair options for a radiographically proven arterial injury:
  - Femoral popliteal artery bypass through a medial approach using an autogenous vein from the contralateral (uninjured) leg
  - Interposition bypass graft through a posterior approach using an autogenous vein from the contralateral (uninjured) leg
  - A percutaneous endovascular repair with a self-expanding stent or stent graft may be considered in select cases
  - A temporary shunt can be considered if the degree of soft tissue or bony injury warrants reconstruction prior to revascularization
- The pulse should be checked before and after any orthopedic manipulation, and the dressings or casts applied should be fashioned to facilitate distal perfusion monitoring
- Antiplatelet therapy should be initiated as soon as it is safe from a bleeding risk standpoint

Hard signs of vascular injury include active hemorrhage, an expanding hematoma, loss of a pulse, or other signs of decreased distal perfusion.

A 68-year-old female complains of right groin swelling 1 day after a cardiac catheterization via a right common femoral artery cannulation. What is the best imaging technique for this patient?

Local access complications are the most common source of morbidity from arterial cardiovascular interventions. Duplex ultrasonography is a sensitive, noninvasive tool to make the diagnosis.

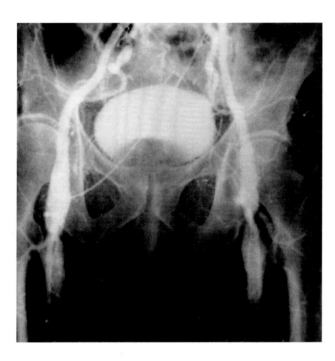

Bilateral femoral artery aneurysms. (With permission from Mulholland MW, Lillemoe KD, Doherty GM, Maier RV, Upchurch GR, eds. *Greenfield's Surgery.* 4th ed. Philadelphia, PA: Lippincott Williams & Wilkins; 2005.)

Femoral Artery Pseudoaneurysm

- A pseudoaneurysm is a "hole" in an arterial wall with the extravasating blood being contained by the surrounding tissue
- The vast majority are small and will thrombose spontaneously
  - Systemic anticoagulation and antiplatelet therapy will prolong the time to closure
- Color duplex imaging should be used to determine the size of the pseudoaneurysm, the width of the communication to the artery, the length of the tract feeding the aneurysm, and the flow within the femoral artery and vein
- An arteriovenous fistula may also result from iatrogenic access trauma and is less likely to heal spontaneously and therefore may require operative or endovascular repair if symptomatic
- Pseudoaneurysms needing intervention may be repaired with any of several methods
  - Operative closure of the arteriotomy with direct suture or patch angioplasty
  - Ultrasound-guided compression under conscious sedation
  - Ultrasound-guided thrombin injection under local anesthetic
- A thrombin injection requires clear ultrasound visualization, a punctate connection to the artery, and a long narrow neck to ensure success and minimize the risk of native artery thrombosis and distal ischemia

- Maintain an awareness of the use of arterial closure devices and their possible complications, including infection

Indications for operative intervention for pseudoaneurysms include hemodynamic instability, physical expansion or rupture, decreased distal perfusion or embolization, femoral nerve palsy, overlying skin compromise, or failure of alternative methods.

Three days following a left femoral to popliteal artery bypass, a 53-year-old man develops a pulmonary embolism and is treated with systemic anticoagulation. On postoperative day seven, his hands are noted to be discolored and his urine output diminishes. What is the next step in management?

Discontinuation of heparin administration is the initial management of presumed heparin-induced thrombocytopenia (HIT).

Heparin-Induced Thrombocytopenia

- Occurs with low molecular weight heparin (LMWH) and subcutaneous or intravenous heparin therapy, including heparin flushes for intravenous catheters
- Type I HIT, a nonimmune transient mild thrombocytopenia, occurs in up to 10% of patients after 3 to 5 days of heparin therapy and resolves spontaneously following its discontinuation
- Type II, immune HIT, causes platelet aggregation with severe, acute thrombocytopenia 5 to 8 days after first exposure (or immediately upon re-exposure) leading to end-organ thrombosis and rarely bleeding
- Due to antiplatelet IgG to a heparin-platelet protein (usually platelet factor IV)
- Forms a white clot (platelet aggregation)
- Suspect HIT when there is an absolute platelet count <100,000/mm^3, a 30% decrease in platelet count from baseline, or a falling platelet count
- A heparin-associated antibody test can confirm the diagnosis
- Treatment includes cessation of heparin therapy and anticoagulation with alternative anticoagulants (hirudin or argatroban) followed by warfarin therapy.
- Morbidity and mortality rates with HIT (as high as 61% and 23%, respectively) can be reduced to 7% and 1%, respectively, with prompt recognition and treatment

The treatment of HIT is immediate discontinuation of heparin, before any other intervention.

A pregnant 19-year-old woman has acute shortness of breath and is evaluated with a V-Q scan which shows a high-probability for a pulmonary embolus. Interestingly, she has been on LMWH for several weeks for a known deep venous thrombosis (DVT). What is the next step in her management?

Placement of an inferior vena cava (IVC) filter is indicated given that she likely had a thromboembolic event while on anticoagulation therapy. An IVC filter is placed at the level of L2 to L3.

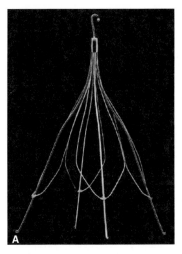
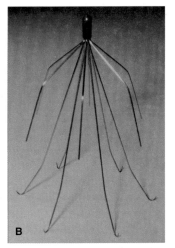
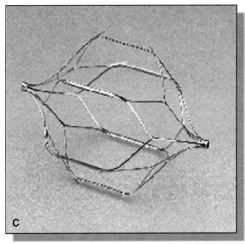

Retrievable IVC filters. (With permission from Fischer JE, Bland KI, Callery MP, et al., eds. *Mastery of Surgery.* 5th ed. Philadelphia, PA: Lippincott Williams & Wilkins; 2006.)

Inferior Vena Cava Filter Placement

- Indications
    - Bleeding complications from anticoagulation therapy for DVT
    - Presence of DVT with a contraindication to anticoagulation (i.e., gastrointestinal bleeding, recent neurosurgery, head trauma)
    - A thromboembolic event despite adequate anticoagulation
    - Recurrent pulmonary embolus with marginal pulmonary reserve
    - The presence of multiple risk factors for thrombosis (e.g., morbid obesity, paralysis, multiple trauma, hypercoagulable state)
- IVC filters are normally placed in the infrarenal IVC at the L2 to L3 vertebral level
    - In pregnancy, imaging should be performed to delineate compression of the IVC by the gravid uterus, which sometimes requires placement in a suprarenal location.
- Complete venography at the time of IVC filter placement will identify venous anomalies in approximately 10% of cases
- Bedside IVC filter placement has been described using either transabdominal duplex ultrasound or intravascular ultrasound
- Optional IVC filters are now available for use in situations where only temporary filtration is required (i.e., perioperatively, recovery from trauma) and can be removed when safe resumption of anticoagulation is possible
- IVC thrombosis/occlusion is a rare complication of IVC filters and may not require treatment, but consideration for catheter-directed thrombolysis may be prudent in symptomatic patients

IVC filter placement does not replace anticoagulation for the treatment of thrombophlebitis. The transition from heparin to warfarin should be initiated as soon as it can be safely administered.

7 | Transplantation

Talia B. Baker and David Axelrod

> During a routine kidney transplant, the organ turns blue and swells up immediately after re-perfusion. Why?

Hyperacute rejection of the organ due to preformed antibodies, which can be prevented by pre-transplant cross match.

Types of Rejection

Hyperacute Rejection (Minutes to Hours)

- Mediated by preformed antibodies to donor antigens
- Antibodies bind to the organ, activate complement and cytotoxic T cells (CD8), and induce vascular thrombosis
- Occurs within minutes to hours after re-perfusion of the organ
- Requires removal of the graft
- Usually prevented by cross matching to detect donor-specific antibodies in the recipient (see below)

Accelerated Rejection (<1 Week)

- Caused by sensitized T cells to donor antigens
- Produces a secondary immune response
- Treatment: Increased immunosuppression, pulse steroids, and possibly antibody therapy (i.e., OKT3)

Acute Rejection (1 Week to 1 Month)

- Mediated by recipient T cells
- Cytotoxic and helper T cells recognize donor-derived proteins expressed on MHC II proteins on antigen-presenting cells (macrophages, B cells)
- T cells bind using an antigen-specific T-cell receptor and once activated secrete IL-2 promoting T-cell proliferation (CD4 and CD8) and endothelial cell destruction
- Reversible with increased immunosuppression, pulse steroids, or anti-lymphocyte therapy

Chronic Rejection (Months to Years)

- Long-term changes in the graft leading to graft fibrosis, vascular damage, and organ dysfunction
- Exact mechanism varies by organ, but likely involves alloantigen-dependant and alloantigen-independent mechanisms

- Partially a type IV hypersensitivity reaction (sensitized T cells)
- Antibody formation, monocytes, and cytotoxic T cells also have a role
- Not reversible with immune suppression, although chronic rejection is more common in patients who experience multiple episodes of acute rejection

> What is the major cause of graft loss in heart and kidney allografts?

Chronic rejection.

Chronic Rejection

Despite vast improvements in immunosuppression, chronic rejection is still the major cause of graft loss in hearts and kidneys (but not livers)

- Lesions resemble changes seen in patients with atherosclerosis with cellular proliferation and deposition of collagen, ground substance, and lipid
- Characteristic lesions of chronic rejection result from repetitive endothelial injury by host antibody or antibody–antigen complexes and complement with proliferation of the intima

> A kidney becomes available for transplantation. However, it is a poor human leukocyte antigens (HLA) tissue typing match, there are positive T cells on the cross match test, and there it has a cold ischemic time of 38 hours. Are any of these factors absolute contraindications to using this organ for transplantation?

While these factors are not favorable for a successful transplantation of the organ, they are not absolute contraindications.

ABO Incompatibility
ABO Blood Group Determination

- ABO blood group antigens are carbohydrate moieties
- They are expressed on endothelial cells that are potential targets of recipient preformed cytotoxic anti-ABO antibodies
- Transplantation across incompatible blood groups may result in humoral (antibody)-mediated hyperacute rejection (except livers where blood group incompatible transplants are possible)
- ABO incompatible transplant can be performed *only* in properly pre-conditioned patients who have undergone plasmapheresis

MHC Antigens: (Encoded by Genes on Chromosome 6 and Designated Human Leukocyte Antigens)

MHC Class I (A, B, and C)	MHC Class II (DR, DP, DQ)
• CD8 T-cell activation	• CD4 T-cell activation
• Present on all nucleated cells	• On antigen-presenting cells—B cells, monocytes, dendritic cells
• Single chain with five domains	• Two chains with four domains each
• Target for cytotoxic T cells	• Activator for helper T cells

Panel Reactive Antibody

- Serum screening for preformed antibodies using a panel of typing cells
- Techniques identical to cross match
- Expressed as a percentage of cells with which the patient's serum reacts (0% to 100%)
- Sensitization (or increased panel reactive antibody) occurs as a consequence of prior pregnancy, blood transfusion, or transplant

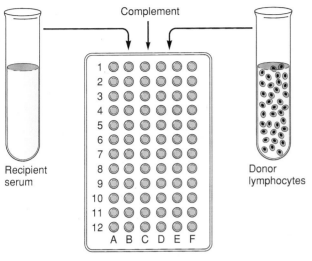

Lymphocytotoxicity cross match. (With permission from Mulholland MW, Lillemoe KD, Doherty GM, et al., eds. *Greenfield's Surgery.* 4th ed. Philadelphia, PA: Lippincott Williams & Wilkins; 2005.)

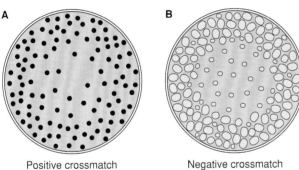

Cross Match

- Refers to any test for the detection of recipient sensitization against donor HLA
- Presensitization to HLA antibodies occurs only with previous exposure to foreign HLA from blood transfusions, pregnancy, or prior transplantation
- Cross matching to exclude the presence of antibodies to donor leukocytes must be carried out immediately prior to transplantation
- Hyperacute or accelerated rejection frequently occurs if transplantation is performed with a strongly positive cross match (e.g., a positive HLA I IgG cross match)

Methods

1. *Complement-dependent lymphocytotoxicity cross match*—Utilizes recipient serum, donor cells (T cells, B cells, or monocytes), and complement. If specific donor antibodies are present, antibody binding leads to fixation of complement and lysis of donor lymphocytes. Most commonly used cross match tests utilize mixed lymphocyte populations (most being T cells), therefore a strong cross match indicates antibodies to HLA I.
2. *Flow cytometry (FC)*—much more specific and sensitive

> Is successful kidney/pancreas transplant associated with stabilization of proliferative retinopathy?

Yes—stabilization or even improvement.

Simultaneous Kidney/Pancreas Transplant

- Successful pancreas transplant approximates euglycemia with normalization of glycosylated hemoglobin
- Stabilizes or improves diabetic retinopathy
- Improves both autonomic and peripheral diabetic neuropathy, but requires months to years to be demonstrable
- Prevents recurrence of diabetic nephropathy in transplanted kidneys
- Decreases orthostatic hypotension
- Not associated with reversal of peripheral vascular disease or coronary artery disease
- Overall graft survival rates are up to 90%

Technique of Pancreas Transplant

- Pancreas is anastomosed to the common iliac artery and vein
- Duodenal drainage is most commonly enteric; however, can be into bladder to monitor urinary amylase
- Bladder drainage is associated with hematuria, renal stones, and bicarbonate loss

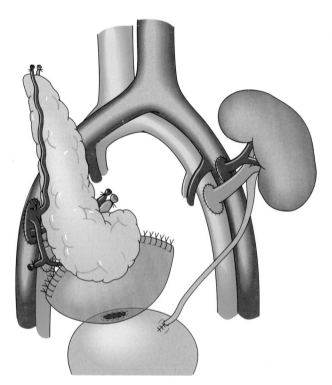

Simultaneous kidney–pancreas transplant with urinary anastomosis. (With permission from Mulholland MW, Lillemoe KD, Doherty GM, et al., eds. *Greenfield's Surgery.* 4th ed. Philadelphia, PA: Lippincott Williams & Wilkins; 2005.)

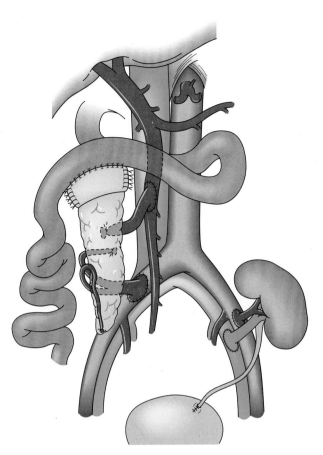

Simultaneous kidney–pancreas transplant with enteric drainage. (With permission from Mulholland MW, Lillemoe KD, Doherty GM, et al., eds. *Greenfield's Surgery*. 4th ed. Philadelphia, PA: Lippincott Williams & Wilkins; 2005.)

The acceptable maximal cold ischemia time is shortest in which organ/s?

Heart and lungs.

Preservation of Donor Organs

- Hypothermia (4°C to 7°C) to decrease metabolism
- Preservation solutions designed to improve cell wall stability—University of Wisconsin solution (high K and hyperosmolar)
- Cold ischemia time
    - Heart/Lung: 0 to 4 hours (ASAP)
    - Pancreas: 0 to 12 hours (up to 24)
    - Liver: 0 to 12 hours (up to 24)
    - Kidney: 0 to 48 hours (72 with perfusion)

What are the criteria to establish brain death?

No pupillary response to light
No corneal reflex
No eye movement with doll's eyes or caloric testing
No motor response to supraorbital pain
No cough reflex
Apnea

- Each year, there are 11,000 to 14,000 cadaveric organ donors
- Most donors are victims of trauma, cerebrovascular accidents, cerebral anoxia, or non-metastasizing brain tumors
- In 2% of cases, patients are declared dead after cardiovascular death in cases in which brain death criteria have not been met

Prerequisites for Diagnosis of Brain Death

- All appropriate diagnostic and therapeutic procedures have been performed and the patient's condition is irreversible
- With hypothermia, the patient must be rewarmed to normothermia
- In cases of alcohol ingestion, at least 8 hours must elapse

Clinical Exam for Brain Death

- Apnea test documenting no respiratory drive despite a $PaCO_2 > 50$
- Absence of cephalic reflexes (pupillary, corneal, oculo-auditory, oculovestibular, oculocephalic, cough, pharyngeal, and swallowing)

Confirmatory Test (May Be Required in Some States)

- No blood flow to brain on a nuclear medicine perfusion scan
- Lack of brain activity on an electroencephalography (EEG)

Donor Exclusion Criteria

- HIV infection
- Malignancy (except some isolated CNS malignancy)
- Bacterial sepsis
- Hepatitis B surface antigen positive

Relative Contraindications for Organ Donation

- Advanced age
- IV drug use/abuse
- Extensive trauma

What is the mechanism of action of the commonly used immunosuppressive medications?

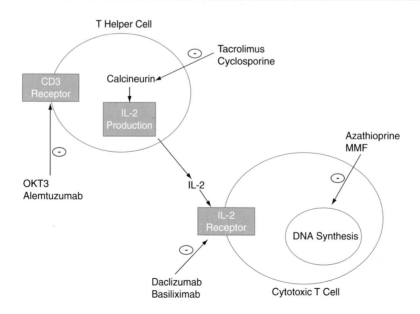

Class	Example	Mechanism of action	Toxicity
Calcineurin inhibitors	Tacrolimus (Prograf) Cyclosporine (Neoral, Gengraf)	Inhibits IL-2 production by activated T cells, reducing cellular proliferation	Nephrotoxic, neurotoxic, hair loss (tacro), hair gain (cyclo), diabetes (tacro)
Anti-metabolites	Azathioprine (Imuran) Mycophenolate mofetil (CellCept)	Inhibits DNA synthesis by blocking nucleotide synthesis	Leukopenia, anemia, diarrhea
Steroids	Prednisone	Block cytokine production, inhibit dendritic cell function	Hypertension, weight gain, osteonecrosis, impaired wound healing, etc.
IL-2 receptor inhibitors	Daclizumab (Zenapax) Basiliximab (Simulect)	Humanized antibodies the bind to IL-2 receptor and block T-cell proliferation. Used for induction therapy	Requires intravenous infusions, but no toxicity
Regulatory kinase inhibitor	Sirolimus (Rapamune)	Inhibits the TOR protein leading to cellular arrest at the G_1 stage	Hypercholesterolemia, hypertriglyceridemia, impaired wound healing
Anti-lymphocyte antibodies (monoclonal)	Muromobab-CD3 (OKT3) Alemtuzumab (Campath)	Bind to lymphocyte receptors (OKT3:CD3) (Campath: CD-52) leading primarily to T-cell lysis	Rash, increased risk of malignancy, viral infections (CMV)
Polyclonal antibodies	Anti-thymocyte globulin (ATGAM, Thymoglobulin)	Non-specific lysis and clearance of coated B and T cells	Serum sickness, increase risk of viral infections, increased risk of malignancy
Graft radiation	External beam radiotherapy	DNA strand breakage leading to impaired proliferation	Rarely used, skin damage, impaired wound healing

Use of Immunosuppression

Induction
Given at the time of transplant to reduce the risk of acute cellular rejection
- Monoclonal and polyclonal antibody preparations
- IL-2 receptor inhibitors

Maintenance
Provided to decrease incidence of acute rejection over the life of the graft
- Steroids
- Calcineurin inhibitors
- Anti-metabolites
- Sirolimus

Treatment of Rejection

- Steroids
- Monoclonal and polyclonal antibody therapy
- Graft irradiation

Complications of Long-term Immunosuppression

- Nephrotoxicity in patients treated with cyclosporine or tacrolimus contribute to late renal allograft loss and native renal failure in patients receiving extra-renal organs (heart, liver, lung)
- Post-transplant lymphoproliferative disorder: B-cell proliferation with spectrum from benign proliferation that responds to lowering of immunosuppression to malignant B-cell lymphoma requiring chemotherapy. Associated with Epstein Barr virus (EBV).
- Cardiovascular disease: Particularly common in renal transplant patients and patients taking rapamycin

---

A 24-year-old woman presents 3 weeks after kidney transplant with fever of 102 degree. What is the most likely cause?

Bacterial infection.

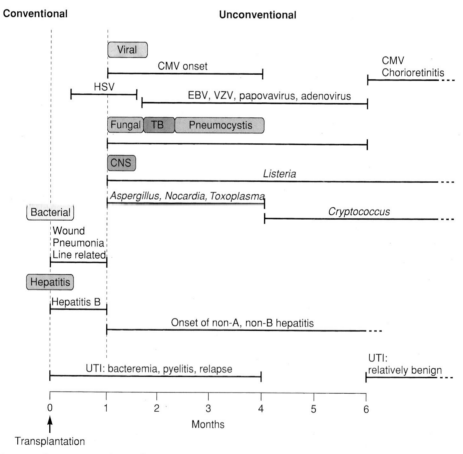

Timing of post-transplant infections. (With permission from Mulholland MW, Lillemoe KD, Doherty GM, et al., eds. *Greenfield's Surgery.* 4th ed. Philadelphia, PA: Lippincott Williams & Wilkins; 2005.)

Fever in Transplant Recipient

Management of Immunosuppressed Patient with Fever

- History and physical exam with a focus on wound infection, graft tenderness, dysuria, cough, rash, and diarrhea
- Labs/Tests: Urinalysis, chest X-ray, CBC, chemistry, blood cultures
- Empiric antibiotics until culture results return
  - *Up to 1 month post-transplant:* Most commonly caused by bacterial infection in wound, lung, urinary tract, central line associated bacteremia, *Clostridium difficile* colitis
  - *Two to 6 months post-transplant:* Highest risk of opportunistic infections including cytomegalovirus (CMV), *Pneumocystis carinii pneumonitis* (PCP), invasive aspergillosis, disseminated toxoplasmosis, disseminated varicella zoster. Also, patients are at risk of re-activated tuberculosis
  - *Greater than 6 months:* Bacterial infections, cryptococcosis, norcardiosis, herpes zoster
  - *During antibody therapy for rejection:* Opportunistic and viral infections more likely

---

A 33-year-old man is 6 weeks status post-cadaveric renal transplantation. Immunosuppression was induced with Simulect, tacrolimus, Cellcept, and steroids. The transplanted kidney functioned immediately and the patient was discharged with a creatinine of 0.9 mg/dL. The patient returns to clinic with a temperature of 40°C and shortness of breath. His WBC is 1.8. His creatinine is elevated to 1.4, and his bilirubin and transaminases are slightly elevated. His tacrolimus blood level is 8.2 ng/mL. What diagnosis most compatible with the above findings?

Cytomegalovirus infection—the most common infection in transplant recipients after the first month. The highest risk in transplants is for CMV donor +/recipient −.

Clinical Presentation of Cytomegalovirus

- Ranges from asymptomatic viremia to lethal disseminated disease
- Mild to moderate disease: Fever, malaise, headache, arthralgia, and myalgias
- Labs: Leukopenia and thrombocytopenia
- End-organ involvement correlates with type of transplant
  - Liver txp: Hepatitis (elevated transaminases, gamma-glutamyl transpeptidase (GGT), alkaline phosphatase, and minimal increase in bilirubin)
  - Kidney txp: Glomerulopathy
  - Pancreas txp: Pancreatitis
  - Lung/heart txp: Pneumonitis (bilateral interstitial, unilobar, and nodular infiltrates)

Other organs affected: Eyes (retinitis), gut (colitis, gastritis, esophagitis), CNS (encephalitis, polyradiculopathy)

Diagnosis: CMV blood antigenemia vs. quantitative CMV PCR assay

Treatment: Ganciclovir (IV)/Valganciclovir (PO)

Prevention: Prophylaxis for 3 months post-transplant is usual standard of care

---

Transplantation and the use of immunosuppressive medications increase the risk of what types of malignancy?

Skin cancer, Kaposi sarcoma, lymphoma.

Malignancies Whose Risks Are Increased in Post-transplant Patients

- Skin cancer: >20 times increased risk
  - Squamous cell and melanoma (basal cell CA is more frequent in general population)
- Kaposi's sarcoma: May respond to decreased immunosuppression
- Lymphoma: B-cell lymphoma non-Hodgkin type
- Post-transplant lymphoproliferative disease (PTLD)
  - Highest incidence in children
  - 95% associated with EBV
  - Highest risk in EBV +/donor to EBV—recipient
  - Usually extranodal presentation
  - Responds to decrease or cessation of immunosuppression/chemotherapy or XRT are often necessary

Malignancies That Have Little or No Increased Incidence in Post-transplant Patients

- Colon
- Breast
- Prostate
- Lung

What diseases recur in allografts after renal transplantation and can lead to graft loss?

Focal segmental glomerulosclerosis (FSGS), membranous proliferative glomerulonephritis (MPGN), systemic lupus erythematosus (SLE), hemolytic uremic syndrome. Recurrent disease in kidney transplant accounts for <2% of all graft loss.

Diseases That May Recur and Cause Graft Loss (% = Likelihood of Graft Loss)

- FSGS: 40%
- MPGN: 30%
- SLE: 5% to 30%—*transplantation should be delayed until disease is no longer active*
- Hemolytic uremic syndrome: 50%

Diseases That May Recur but Rarely Cause Graft Loss

- Anti-GBM disease: <2%—*delay transplant until anti-GBM antibodies have disappeared*
- Alport syndrome: Rare
- Diabetic nephropathy: ~100% will recur, but rarely causes graft loss (<2%)
- IgA nephropathy: <10%

Seven days after cadaveric renal transplant, a patient develops a fever to 101°F, pain and tenderness over the incision and oliguria. Serum Cr has risen from 1.5 to 1.9 mg/dL. What is the first non invasive test that should be done to evaluate this patient?

Ultrasound or nuclear medicine renal scan. If these are normal, obtain allograft biopsy to exclude acute rejection.

Technique of Kidney Transplant

- Kidney implanted in iliac fossa
- Anastomosed to external iliac vessels usually via a retroperitoneal approach

---

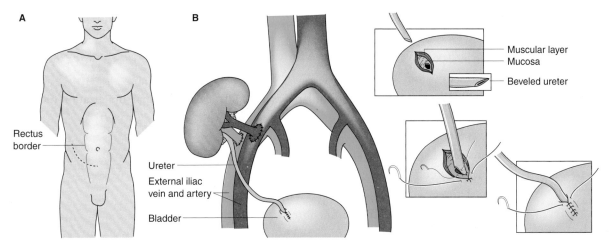

Kidney transplant technique. (With permission from Mulholland MW, Lillemoe KD, Doherty GM, et al., eds. *Greenfield's Surgery*. 4th ed. Philadelphia, PA: Lippincott Williams & Wilkins; 2005.)

Complications of Kidney Transplant

- Early
    - Bleeding: Rarely requires a blood transfusion, but may compress renal vessels
    - Venous thrombosis: Often leads to graft loss
    - Wound infection: Bacterial and treated with antibiotics
    - Urine leak: Treated with drainage and stenting with possible re-operation

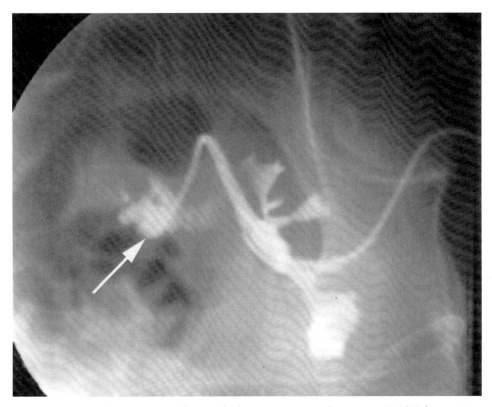

Percutaneous nephrostogram with urine leak at ureterovesical anastomosis. (With permission from Mulholland MW, Lillemoe KD, Doherty GM, et al., eds. *Greenfield's Surgery*. 4th ed. Philadelphia, PA: Lippincott Williams & Wilkins; 2005.)

- Late
  - Lymphocele
    - Incidence: 0.06% to 18%
    - Most present within 3 months
    - Treat with percutaneous drainage or laparoscopic intraperitoneal marsupialization (90% successful)
  - Renal artery stenosis
    - Presents with hypertension and increase in Cr
    - Treat with percutaneous stent placement
  - Ureteral stricture
    - Presents with increased Cr, hydronephrosis
    - Treat with percutaneous stenting with possible re-implantation

---

An 18-year-old male with a history of depression presents with lethargy, confusion, and new onset jaundice. What is the most likely cause?

Tylenol overdose.

Causes of Acute Liver Failure in US

- Acetaminophen toxicity (20%)
- Cryptogenic (15%)
- Drug induced failure (12%)
- Acute hepatitis B (10%)
- Hepatitis A (7%)
- Others: Wilson disease, fatty liver of pregnancy, Budd-Chiari syndrome, mushroom intoxication, ischemic injury, autoimmune hepatitis, herpes virus, adenovirus

Initial Evaluation

- Mental status exam to assess degree of encephalopathy
- Physical exam
- Labs: CBC, LFTs, PT/PTT, factor V level, hepatitis serologies
- RUQ ultrasound to rule out vascular thrombosis

Management of Patient with Acute Liver Failure

- Transfer to transplant center for evaluation
- ICU admission with intubation for Stage 3 encephalopathy (confusion, reactive only to verbal stimuli)
- Lactulose administration to produce 3 to 4 bowel movements per day
- Broad spectrum antibiotics as prophylaxis
- GI ulcer prophylaxis with H_2 blockers
- Central venous monitoring if renal function deteriorates or hemodynamic instability
- Intracranial pressure monitor (ICP) monitoring once patient is intubated with Stage 4 encephalopathy (deep coma)—use mannitol to decrease ICP as needed until serum osmolality >320
- May need recombinant factor VII to correct coagulopathy
- In case of acetaminophen toxicity, begin IV acetylcysteine (Mucomyst) as soon as possible

Criteria for Listing Patient for Transplant in Acute Liver Failure
Kings College Criteria

Acetaminophen toxicity	Non-acetaminophen toxicity
pH <7.30 after resuscitation	INR >6.5
Or	*Or 3 of the 5 criteria below*
INR >6.5	Age <10 or >40
Cr >3mg/dl	Etiology: Cryptogenic, drugs
Encephalopathy III-IV	Duration of jaundice before encephalopathy >7 days
	INR >3.5
	Serum bilirubin >17.5 mg%

A 48-year-old male with a history of IV drug use and alcohol abuse presents with 2 months of ascites, jaundice, and confusion. What are some of the etiologies that can result in decompensation in this patient?

GI bleed from varices, spontaneous bacterial peritonitis (SBP), malignancy.

Cirrhotic liver disease produces four major complications: Portal hypertension, ascites, encephalopathy, and malignancy. In patients with cirrhotic liver disease, multiple etiologies can result in decompensation including a GI bleed from varices, the development of SBP, or the development of malignancy.

Etiology of Chronic End-stage Liver Failure in Adults

- Hepatocellular diseases: Viral hepatitis (B and C), autoimmune, alcohol, obesity (non-alcoholic steatohepatitis NASH), chronic Budd-Chiari (hepatic vein thrombosis)
- Cholestatic liver disease: Primary biliary cirrhosis, primary sclerosing cholangitis, secondary biliary cirrhosis
- Congenital/metabolic diseases: Wilson disease, alpha-1 antitrypsin deficiency, glycogen storage disease type I, familial amyloidotic polyneuropathy, polycystic liver disease

Management of Portal Hypertension/Esophageal Varices

- Esophagogastroduodenoscopy with banding to control varices
- β-blocker therapy to reduce risk of bleeding
- Surgical shunt (distal splenorenal) for patients with Child A cirrhosis and minimal ascites
- Transjugular intrahepatic portocaval shunt (TIPS) for patients with advanced cirrhosis who are potential transplant candidates
- In non-transplant candidates who are not candidates for shunt, perform esophageal devascularization procedure (Suguira)
- For acute, life-threatening bleeds: ICU admission, large bore IVs, immediate endoscopy with banding if possible, Sengtaken-Blakemore tube for tamponade if necessary, octreotide infusion, urgent TIPS. Emergent surgical shunt associated with very high mortality.
- Surgical shunts can worsen encephalopathy

Management of Hepatic Encephalopathy

- Correct underlying etiology (GI bleeding, infection, electrolyte abnormalities)
- Lactulose: Works by decreasing GI bacterial load and nitrogen absorption—mostly works in the colon
- Zinc sulfate 300 mg PO BID to increase urea synthesis in liver

Management of Ascites

- Fluid (<1 L/day) and sodium (2 to 4 g/day) restriction
- Diuretic therapy with spironolactone (100 to 400 mg/day) and lasix (20 to 160 mg/day)
- Large volume paracentesis with albumin infusion if >6 L removed
- TIPS for refractory ascites in transplant candidates
- SBP: Diagnosed on tap with >250 WBC/mL. Prophylaxis indicated in patients with prior episode of SBP or ascites with low albumin (<1 gm/dL) using fluoroquinolones.

Management of Malignancy

- Patients with cirrhosis should have regular screening with ultrasound, triphasic CT, or MRI to assess for the development of tumor
- Serum AFP measurements every 3 to 6 months (> 200 ng/mL), although this test has a low sensitivity
- See section below on treatment of malignancy

What are the indications/contraindications for adult liver transplant?

Patients Should Be Considered for Liver Transplant When They Have Any of the Following

- Decompensated cirrhosis with a model for end-stage liver disease (MELD) score >7
- The presence of unresectable, locally advanced hepatocellular carcinoma (HCC)
- Quality of life-limiting complications of end stage liver disease including severe pruritus, encephalopathy, or recurrent variceal bleeding

Absolute Contraindications for Liver Transplant

- Extra-hepatic malignancy
- Uncontrolled extra-hepatic infection
- Significantly elevated pulmonary artery pressures (mean >50 mmHg)
- Irreversible brain damage

Relative Contraindications to Liver Transplant

- Advanced age
- Large intrahepatic hepatocellular carcinoma >5 cm or >3 lesions
- HIV unless very well controlled on therapy and as part of a clinical trial
- Active alcohol use within 6 months
- Lack of adequate social/financial support

What is the outcome of liver transplant for acute and chronic liver disease?

Overall patient survival following liver transplant is 86% at 1 year 72% at 5 years.
Overall graft survival is 81% at 1 year and 64% at 5 years.

Patient Survival by Etiology

Etiology of liver disease	5-Year survival (%)
Acute hepatic failure	69
Cholestatic liver disease (PSC or PBC)	81
Non-cholestatic liver disease (hepatitis B and C)	70
Malignancy	59
Biliary atresia	80

What treatment options are available for a patient with localized HCC?

- Primary therapy for HCC is resection in patients without significant cirrhosis in whom >20% hepatic mass can be preserved
- In cirrhosis patients, resection may result in hepatic decompensation; therefore, local therapy or transplantation is indicated

Local Therapy Options

- Alcohol ablation
- Cryotherapy
- Radiofrequency ablation
- Intra-arterial chemoembolization

In patients with HCC meeting the following criteria, transplantation is indicated and a MELD bonus is award to increase the likelihood of transplantation. The 5-year patient survival in these patients is 85%.

- One lesion <5 cm or three lesions all <3 cm
- Absence of metastatic disease
- Absence of major vascular invasion

What is the management of a 6-week-old infant with persistent jaundice?

Kasai portoenterostomy.

Most frequent cause of end stage liver disease in children is extra-hepatic biliary atresia. Diagnosed in 1 in 15,000 newborns, 10% of whom have associated abnormalities (e.g., polysplenia, malrotation). Initial treatment is a Kasai portoenterostomy; however, most patients will eventually need a transplant.

Indications for Pediatric Liver Transplantation

- Failed Kasai procedure with cholestasis
- Recurrent cholangitis
- Cirrhosis resulting in growth failure, ascites, variceal bleeding, hypersplenism resulting in thrombocytopenia
- Fulminant hepatic failure
- Neonatal liver failure

- Inborn errors of metabolism (tyrosinemia, glycogen storage disease, Crigler-Najjar syndrome, etc.)
- Unresectable intrahepatic tumors (hepatoblastoma)

> True/false: A "fixed" elevated pulmonary vascular resistance (PVR) is a contraindication for heart transplant.

True.

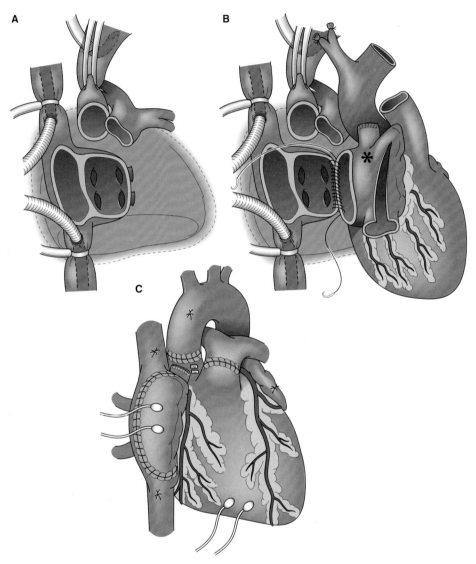

Traditional method of anastomosis for cardiac transplant. (With permission from Mulholland MW, Lillemoe KD, Doherty GM, et al., eds. *Greenfield's Surgery.* 4th ed. Philadelphia, PA: Lippincott Williams & Wilkins; 2005.)

Longstanding left ventricular failure may produce pulmonary vascular remodeling and "fixed" elevations in PVR (>6 woods units). Heart transplantation into a recipient with increased PVR *unresponsive to vasodilator therapy* predictably leads to right ventricular failure of the transplanted heart and death. However, these patients CAN be considered for combined heart–lung transplant.

Indications for Heart Transplantation

1. End-stage heart failure refractory to maximal medical management
2. A estimated survival without transplant of <6 to 12 months
3. Not amenable to other conventional therapy

Medical Management for Patients with End-stage Cardiac Failure

Stage 1

- Exercise
- Fluid (2 L/day) and Na (2 g/day) restriction
- Digoxin, loop diuretics, ACE inhibitors

Stage 2

- Hemodynamic monitoring
- IV nitroprusside/diuretics
- Anticoagulation
- Ultrafiltration

Stage 3

- IV inotropic support with dobutamine or milrinone

Stage 4

Mechanical support (indications: Cardiac index < 2.0, MAP < 60 mmHg, worsening hepatic and renal function)

- Intra-aortic balloon pump
- Ventricular assist device
- Total artificial heart

8 Pediatric Surgery

Richard J. Hendrickson and Denis D. Bensard

A 5-year-old boy has severe inspiratory stridor. What is the next step in management?

Inspiratory stridor is an airway emergency in children. Immediate intubation in an operating room is the treatment of choice.

Epiglottitis

- *Haemophilus influenzae* is the most common organism
- A lateral X-ray may show edema of the epiglottis (bird's beak)
- Orotracheal intubation should be performed in the OR
- If unable to intubate due to swelling, perform an open tracheostomy

Never nasotracheally intubate a child because the angle between the superior and inferior glottis is too large.

A newborn infant has excessive salivation, choking, and regurgitation with feeding. What is the most likely diagnosis?

This can be a classic presentation of a tracheoesophageal fistula (TEF).

Tracheoesophageal Fistula

- Results from the abnormal ingrowth of ectodermal ridges during the 4th week of gestation
- Approximately 25% to 40% of neonates with TEF are premature or low-birth weight
- A maternal history of polyhydramnios is common
- Approximately 50% of neonates with TEF have an associated anomaly
  - Cardiovascular (most common)
  - GI malformations
  - GU anomalies
  - Skeletal
  - CNS
- Associated with VACTERL (vertebral, anorectal, cardiac, tracheoesophageal, renal, limb) abnormalities

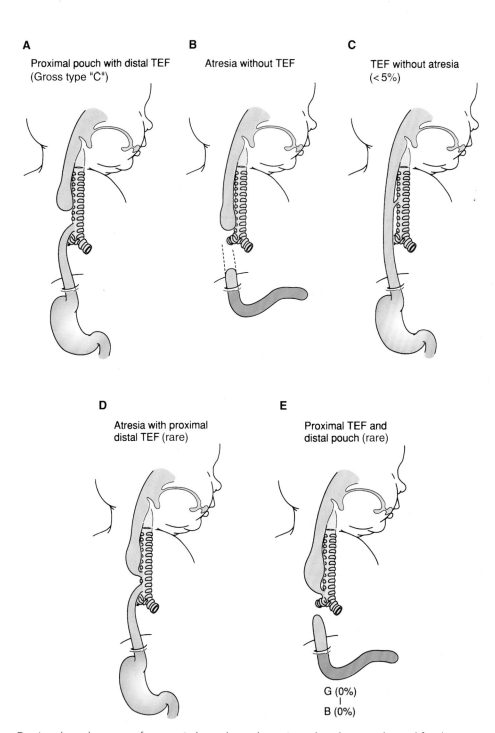

A Proximal pouch with distal TEF (Gross type "C")

B Atresia without TEF

C TEF without atresia (< 5%)

D Atresia with proximal distal TEF (rare)

E Proximal TEF and distal pouch (rare)

G (0%)
|
B (0%)

Depicted are the types of congenital esophageal atresia and tracheoesophageal fistula. (A) Proximal esophageal atresia with distal tracheoesophageal fistula (Gross Type C). (B) Isolated esophageal atresia without tracheoesophageal fistula. (C) Tracheoesophageal fistula without esophageal atresia. (D) Esophageal atresia with proximal and distal tracheoesophageal fistula (rare). (E) Proximal tracheoesophageal fistula with distal esophageal atresia (rare). (With permission from Mulholland MW, Lillemoe KD, Doherty GM, et al., eds. *Greenfield's Surgery.* 4th ed. Philadelphia, PA: Lippincott Williams & Wilkins; 2005.)

- There are five types of TEF:
  - Proximal esophageal atresia with distal TEF (85%)
  - Isolated esophageal atresia
  - H-type TEF without esophageal atresia

- Proximal TEF with distal esophageal atresia
- Proximal and distal TEF

Most Common Type of Tracheoesophageal Fistula

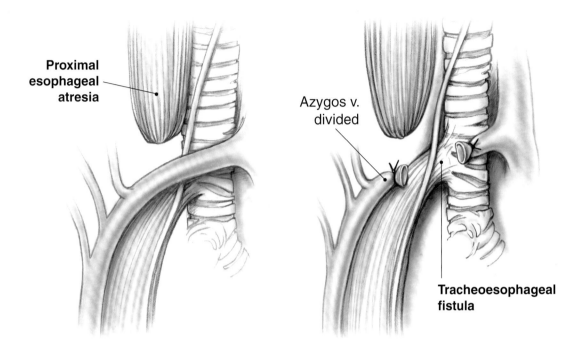

- Diagnosis
  - Inability to pass a nasogastric tube is suspicious for TEF
  - Chest X-ray can help determine the length of the esophageal gap
  - Abdominal X-ray with air in the stomach excludes an isolated esophageal atresia
- Treatment
  - Right extra-pleural thoracotomy through the fourth intercostal space or thoracoscopic trans-pleural repair
  - The proximal esophagus is richly supplied by vessels from the thyrocervical trunk
  - The distal esophagus has a more tenuous segmental supply from the intercostal arteries
  - The operation includes TEF ligation and transection, and restoration of esophageal continuity via an end-to-end anastomosis
  - On postoperative day 5 to 7, an esophagram is obtained and if no leak is identified, then oral feeds are started and the chest drain is removed
- Early complications (5% to 15%)
  - Anastomotic disruption (secondary to poor blood supply and tension)
  - Recurrent TEF
  - Tracheomalacia
- Late complications
  - Anastomotic stricture (25%)
  - Gastroesophageal reflux (50%)
  - Esophageal dysmotility (100%)

Proximal esophageal atresia with distal TEF is the most common type of TEF.

> Which immunoglobulin is secreted in breast milk?

IgA is the most common antibody in breast milk, the gut, saliva, and most bodily secretions.

> Which immunoglobulin does not cross the blood-placenta barrier?

IgM is large and does not cross the placenta (remember M for Magnum).

> An 8-year-old boy presents following a bicycle crash with a ruptured spleen. What is the best indicator of early shock?

Tachycardia in childhood is defined as a heart rate >150 for a neonate, >120 in the first year, and >100 after 1 year. It is the best indicator of shock.

Fluid Resuscitation in Children
- 20 cc/kg of crystalloid bolus for trauma
- If shock persists after a second bolus, then administer blood (10 cc/kg)
- An acceptable urine output is 2 to 4 cc/kg/hr in children
- Children have a lower glomerular filtration rate compared to adults

> A healthy infant presents with bilious emesis, abdominal distention, and shock. What is the most likely diagnosis?

The presentation with shock suggests malrotation with midgut volvulus—a surgical emergency. In fact, bilious emesis in a newborn is malrotation until proven otherwise.

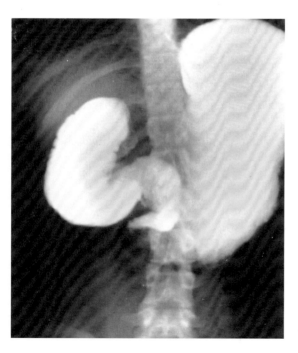

Malrotation. An upper gastrointestinal imaging study is shown that demonstrates contrast in the stomach and proximal duodenum. The distal duodenum does not cross midline and there is an abrupt cut-off consistent with the diagnosis of malrotation with midgut volvulus. (With permission from Mulholland MW, Lillemoe KD, Doherty GM, et al., eds. *Greenfield's Surgery.* 4th ed. Philadelphia, PA: Lippincott Williams & Wilkins; 2005.)

Malrotation

- During the 6 to 12th week of gestation, the intestine undergoes evisceration, elongation, and eventual return to the peritoneum in a 270 degree counterclockwise rotation with fixation
- Malrotation is associated with abnormal rotation and fixation
- Ladds bands extend from the colon to the duodenum, causing duodenal obstruction and biliary emesis
- Midgut volvulus refers to the narrow-based mesentery twisting around the superior mesenteric artery (usually clockwise)
- This results in intestinal obstruction and vascular occlusion
- Most develop symptoms in the first month of life
- If the patient is stable and the diagnosis is in question, then perform an UGI (gold standard test), which will demonstrate:
  - Bird's beak appearance of third part of duodenum
  - Ligament of Treitz is to the right of midline
- Midgut volvulus is a surgical emergency
  - Volume resuscitation is essential
  - If the patient is in shock, no diagnostic studies are warranted
  - Immediate surgical exploration is required to avoid loss of small intestine and possible death
  - Surgical treatment is the Ladd's procedure
    - Division of abnormal peritoneal bands
    - Correction of malrotation
    - Restoration of a broad-based mesentery
    - Appendectomy (because cecum is in the left upper quadrant)

An upper GI contrast series should only be performed if malrotation is suspected in the absence of midgut volvulus or shock—conditions which mandate emergent surgical exploration because of possible vascular compromise.

A full-term neonate with Down syndrome has bilious emesis during the first day of life. The newborn's abdominal exam is normal. What is the most likely diagnosis?

Duodenal atresia is most likely in this patient.

Duodenal Atresia

- Failure of recanalization during the 8th to 10th week of gestation
- Characterized by bilious emesis
- No abdominal distention
- Usually presents within the first 24 hours of life
- Trisomy 21 is present in approximately 25% of infants with duodenal atresia
- 85% of atresias are distal to the ampulla of Vater
- Rule out an anorectal malformation and check for patent anus
- "Double bubble" sign on abdominal X-ray
  - Air within the stomach and first and second portions of duodenum
  - If there is no distal air, the diagnosis is secure and no further studies are indicated
  - If there is distal air, an urgent UGI should be performed to rule out midgut volvulus

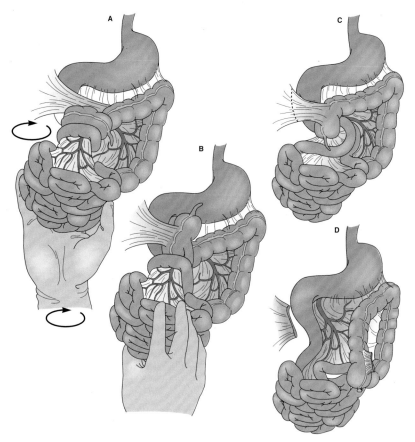

Ladd procedure. (A and B) Detorsion of midgut. (C and D) Division of Ladd's bands (peritoneal attachments) of cecum to abdominal cavity. (With permission from Mulholland MW, Lillemoe KD, Doherty GM, et al., eds. *Greenfield's Surgery*. 4th ed. Philadelphia, PA: Lippincott Williams & Wilkins; 2005.)

- Surgical treatment is a duodenoduodenostomy. The repair may be performed by upper transverse laparotomy incision or laparoscopic technique.

Duodenal atresia often presents in the first 24 hours of life as bilious emesis without abdominal distention.

A 3-day-old full-term infant has bilious emesis and abdominal distention. What is the differential diagnosis?

The differential diagnosis includes intestinal atresia, malrotation, meconium ileus, Hirschsprung disease, and imperforate anus.

Jejunoileal Atresia
- Caused by an in utero mesenteric vascular accident
- Usually presents with bilious emesis within the first 2 to 3 days of life
- Associated with cystic fibrosis in 10% of cases
- Abdominal distention is usually present with a distal atresia
  - Abdominal X-ray demonstrates multiple distended loops of bowel with air–fluid levels
  - Contrast enema demonstrates a microcolon and no reflux into dilated intestines
  - Contrast enema can also show multiple areas of involvement (10% of cases)

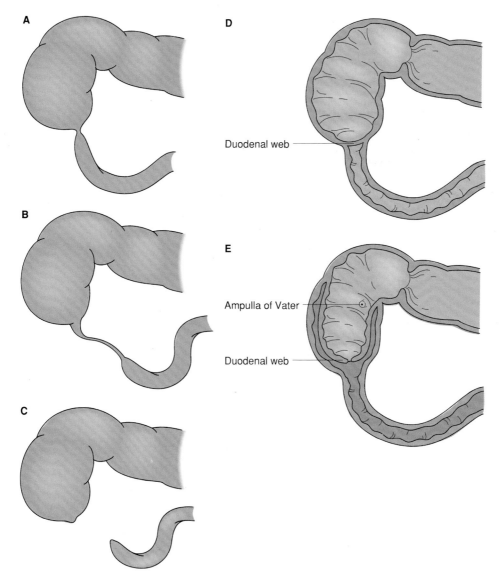

Anatomic forms of duodenal atresia. (A) Short segment atresia with patent lumen. (B) Long segment atresia with patent lumen. (C) Complete atresia with discontinuity. (D) Distal duodenal web. (E) Proximal duodenal web. (With permission from Mulholland MW, Lillemoe KD, Doherty GM, Maier RV, Upchurch GR, eds. *Greenfield's Surgery*. 4th ed. Philadelphia, PA: Lippincott Williams & Wilkins; 2005.)

- Surgical correction involves an end-to-end anastomosis
  - A tapering enteroplasty can be used for a bowel size discrepancy
  - Resection of the bulbous proximal end may be necessary
  - Preserve length to avoid short gut syndrome

Colonic Atresia

- Caused by an in utero mesenteric vascular accident
- Similar in presentation to jejunoileal atresia
- Abdominal distention is present
- X-ray shows multiple dilated loops of intestine with air–fluid levels
- It can be difficult to distinguish between small and large intestine

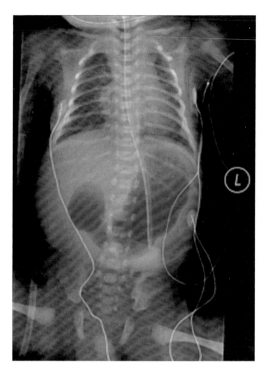

Plain abdominal radiograph of an infant with duodenal atresia. Air is seen in a dilated stomach and proximal duodenum. This finding is commonly referred to as a "double bubble sign". It is important to note that air is not seen in the distal gastrointestinal tract. If air is seen in the distal gastrointestinal tract then duodenal stenosis or malrotation with midgut volvulus should be considered and a contrast imaging study may be indicated.

- Contrast enema demonstrates microcolon with a cutoff usually in the proximal colon
- Surgical correction involves an end-to-end anastomosis as above

Intestinal atresia can be associated with gastroschisis.

A newborn with cystic fibrosis presents with mild abdominal distention. An X-ray demonstrates a "ground glass" appearing mass on the right side of the abdomen. What is the next step in management?

A gastrografin enema is usually successful in treating simple meconium ileus (MI). Complicated cases may require surgery.

Meconium Ileus

- Obstruction of the terminal ileum by a highly viscid and tenacious meconium
- Approximately 15% of neonates with meconium ileus have cystic fibrosis
- A chloride sweat test should be performed to rule out cystic fibrosis
- Simple meconium ileus can usually be treated with:
    - Gastrografin enemas
    - *N*-Acetylcysteine enemas
    - Rectal irrigation
- Complex meconium ileus (with atresia, perforation, or volvulus) or patients refractory to conservative therapy require surgical treatment
    - Enterotomy or limited intestinal resection with evacuation of meconium
    - An enterostomy may also be necessary

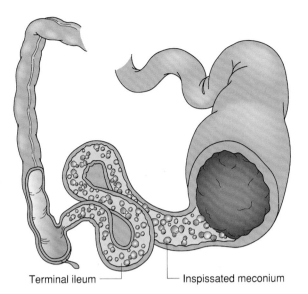

Uncomplicated meconium ileus. The proximal intestinal lumen is obstructed with the abnormal inspissated meconium which obstructs the distal ileum. The colon is small due to the in-utero proximal obstruction. (With permission from Mulholland MW, Lillemoe KD, Doherty GM, Maier RV, Upchurch GR, eds. *Greenfield's Surgery.* 4th ed. Philadelphia, PA: Lippincott Williams & Wilkins; 2005.)

Terminal ileum ———| |——— Inspissated meconium

N-Acetylcysteine enemas can be used for meconium ileus.

A full-term neonate has bilious emesis during the first and second days of life. The newborn's abdominal exam reveals marked distention. An abdominal X-ray is significant for dilated loops of small bowel. A contrast enema reveals a narrow rectum, compared to the sigmoid. The baby failed to evacuate the contrast the following day. What is the next step in management?

A bedside suction rectal biopsy at least 2 cm above the dentate line is the gold standard test for infants suspected to have Hirschsprung disease.

Hirschsprung Disease

- Failure of the normal migration of neural crest cells
- Absent ganglia in the myenteric and submucosal plexus
- The absence of ganglia always begins in the distal rectum and extends proximally
- 80% to 85% of cases are limited to the rectosigmoid
- Presents as bilious emesis, feeding intolerance, and abdominal distention
- Associated with failure to pass meconium within the first 48 hours of life
- A contrast enema demonstrates a contracted rectum with proximally dilated large bowel
- Failure to evacuate rectal contrast at 24 hours can be diagnostic
- Suction rectal biopsy is required to confirm absence of ganglion cells and nerve hypertrophy
- Surgical treatment
  - Soave endorectal pull through with removal of the diseased aganglionic distal bowel and a coloanal anastomosis
  - Children who present acutely ill may need a staged procedure with a diverting colostomy
  - Remember to do frozen intraoperative biopsies to help determine the anatomic location of the transition zone
  - Even though the diseased bowel has been removed, enterocolitis may still occur, requiring rectal irrigations and broad spectrum antibiotics

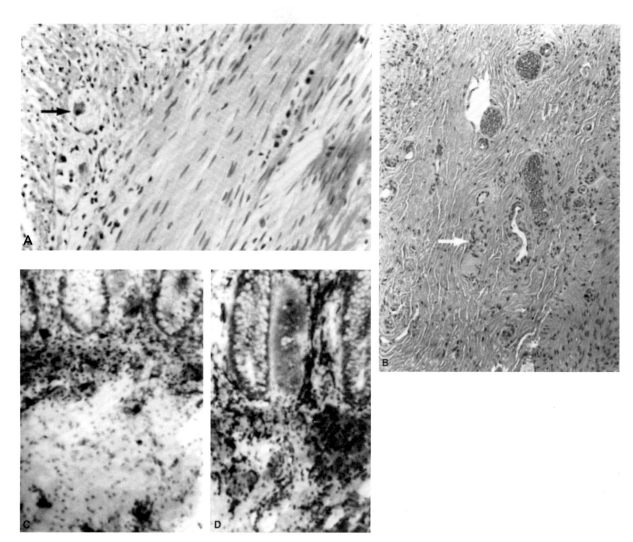

Rectal biopsy in patient with Hirschsprung disease. (A) Normal rectal biopsy with ganglion cells indicated by arrow (hematoxylin-eosin). (B) Rectal biopsy specimen with aganglionosis (hematoxylin-eosin). Note the characteristic thickened nerve fiber (*arrow*). (C) Normal rectal biopsy using acetylcholinesterase histochemical staining. (D) Similarly stained specimen from a patient with Hirschsprung disease. Many thickened submucosal nerve fibers stain densely black. (With permission from Mulholland MW, Lillemoe KD, Doherty GM, Maier RV, Upchurch GR, eds. *Greenfield's Surgery.* 4th ed. Philadelphia, PA: Lippincott Williams & Wilkins; 2005.)

Hirschsprung disease often presents in the first 24 hours of life as bilious emesis with abdominal distention.

Imperforate Anus

- Congenital defect with the anus absent or misplaced
- Usually forms an anterior fistulous tract
- May be associated with a cloacal deformity
- Divided into "high" and "low" malformations (relative to levator muscle)
- High/cloacal anomalies (fistula to bladder, vagina, or prostatic urethra) are initially treated with an end sigmoid colostomy, followed by a posterior sagittal anorectoplasty (PSARP) and genitourinary reconstruction if a cloacal anomaly is present
- Low anomalies are treated with a PSARP
- Preoperative anal dilatation may be required to avoid stricture

A colostomy is not generally needed to treat a low (below levator muscle) imperforate anus.

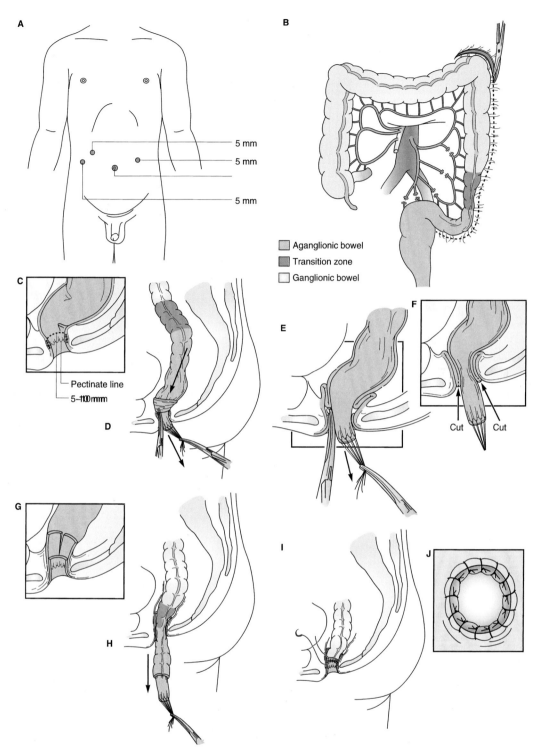

Laparoscopic-assisted pull-through for Hirschsprung disease. (A) Sites for operative trocar placement. (B) Division of colon and rectal mesentery with mobilization of proximal colon. (C) Circumferential incision in rectal mucosa 5 to 10 mm cephalad to the pectinate line. (D) Mucosal traction sutures to facilitate further dissection from rectal muscular cuff. (E) Transanal submucosal dissection is continued cephalad to meet the caudal extent of the transperitoneal rectal dissection. (F) Circumferential incision of rectal muscular cuff. (G) Rectal muscular cuff is split posteriorly to accommodate the pull-through segment (the pull-through segment is not shown here to clarify this maneuver). (H) Rectum and sigmoid colon are pulled through the rectal muscular cuff to the anastomotic site. (I) Colon is transected at appropriate site with confirmation of ganglion cells by frozen section. (J) Transanal, end-to-end single layer colorectal anastomosis. (With permission from Mulholland MW, Lillemoe KD, Doherty GM, Maier RV, Upchurch GR, eds. *Greenfield's Surgery.* 4th ed. Philadelphia, PA: Lippincott Williams & Wilkins; 2005.)

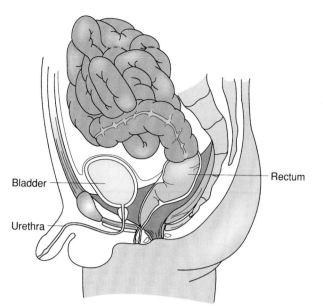

Bladder

Urethra

Rectum

Male infant with low imperforate anus and perineal fistula. Note that the fistula is anterior to the striated muscle complex. (With permission from Mulholland MW, Lillemoe KD, Doherty GM, Maier RV, Upchurch GR, eds. *Greenfield's Surgery.* 4th ed. Philadelphia, PA: Lippincott Williams & Wilkins; 2005.)

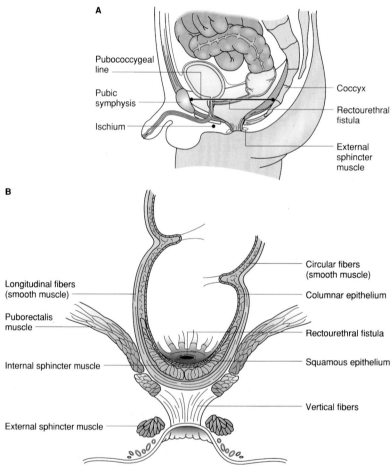

A

Pubococcygeal line

Pubic symphysis

Ischium

Coccyx

Rectourethral fistula

External sphincter muscle

B

Longitudinal fibers (smooth muscle)

Puborectalis muscle

Internal sphincter muscle

External sphincter muscle

Circular fibers (smooth muscle)

Columnar epithelium

Rectourethral fistula

Squamous epithelium

Vertical fibers

High imperforate anus and rectourethral fistula. (A) Male infant with high imperforate anus, showing the pubococcygeal line, ischium, and striated muscle complex. The rectal pouch ends cephalad to the pubococcygeal line. This location of the rectourethral fistula is typical. (B) Coronal view showing incomplete development of the rectal pouch within the striated muscle complex. The rectourethral fistula is shown. (With permission from Mulholland MW, Lillemoe KD, Doherty GM, Maier RV, Upchurch GR, eds. *Greenfield's Surgery.* 4th ed. Philadelphia, PA: Lippincott Williams & Wilkins; 2005.)

A 7-day-old premature neonate has emesis, abdominal distention, and bloody stools. What is the differential diagnosis?

Necrotizing enterocolitis (NEC) and malrotation.

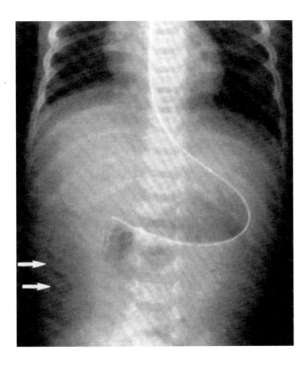

An abdominal radiograph of an infant with necrotizing enterocolitis. The *arrows* demonstrate air within the intestinal wall or pneumatosis intestinalis. (With permission from Mulholland MW, Lillemoe KD, Doherty GM, Maier RV, Upchurch GR, eds. *Greenfield's Surgery.* 4th ed. Philadelphia, PA: Lippincott Williams & Wilkins; 2005.)

Necrotizing Enterocolitis

- More common in premature infants after initiation of feeding
- Abdominal X-rays often demonstrate pneumatosis intestinalis or portal vein gas
- Treatment is conservative: NPO, gastric decompression, antibiotics, serial X-rays
- Medical management is successful in about 50% of cases
- Indications for surgery
  - Free air
  - Abdominal wall erythema/cellulitis (this indication often appears on exams)
  - Worsening acidosis
  - Hyperkalemia
  - Palpable mass
  - Worsening abdominal distention
  - Overall deterioration
- Surgery often involves resection of the affected intestine and creation of an end ileostomy and mucous fistula
- If the neonate survives, then a bowel reanastomosis is performed around 4 to 6 weeks postoperatively, after a contrast study is done to rule out strictures
- NEC is the most common cause of short gut syndrome in childhood

Erythema over the infant's abdomen is an ominous sign and is an indication for surgery in patients with NEC.

A 4-week-old infant presents with non-bilious projectile vomiting. What is the most likely electrolyte disturbance?

Hypertrophic pyloric stenosis (HPS) presents with non-bilious vomiting and a resultant hypokalemic, hypochloremic, metabolic alkalosis (a metabolic disturbance typical of vomiting patients). Once the serum potassium gets to a critical low value, the kidneys compensate by releasing hydrogen ions instead of potassium with exchange of sodium. This will lead to a "paradoxical aciduria" (i.e., eliminating hydrogen ions instead of potassium within the renal sodium/potassium channel).

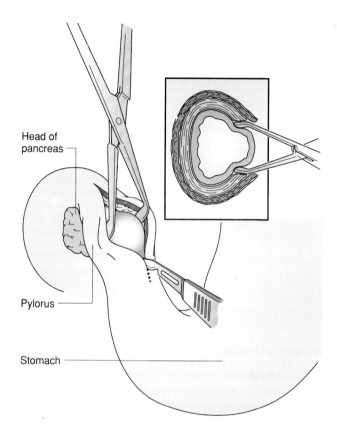

Head of pancreas

Pylorus

Stomach

Pyloromyotomy for hypertrophic pyloric stenosis. The serosa of the thickened pylorus is incised sharply. The hypertrophied muscle fibers are fractured using a pyloric spreader taking care to not injure the underlying mucosa. (With permission from Mulholland MW, Lillemoe KD, Doherty GM, Maier RV, Upchurch GR, eds. *Greenfield's Surgery.* 4th ed. Philadelphia, PA: Lippincott Williams & Wilkins; 2005.)

Hypertrophic Pyloric Stenosis

- Idiopathic thickening and elongation of the pylorus that causes gastric outlet obstruction
- Typical age of presentation is 3 to 6 weeks old
- Typical presentation is a healthy infant who initially fed normally, then develops non-bilious "projectile" emesis after feeding
- Is four times more common in males
- An "olive" is palpable in about 50% of infants
- Mild jaundice occurs in 5% of cases due to reduced glucuronyl transferase activity
- Diagnosis is confirmed by ultrasound
- Criteria are pyloric diameter >1.4 cm, pyloric wall >0.4 cm, pyloric channel (length of pylorus) >1.6 cm
- Emesis (not just in kids) causes a hypokalemic, hypochloremic metabolic alkalosis
- Fredet-Ramstedt pyloromyotomy is the treatment of choice (open or laparoscopic)
- Surgery is not an emergency, and should be performed only after fluid and electrolyte abnormalities are corrected

A healthy 11-month-old boy presents 1 week after having a cold with sudden emesis, severe crampy abdominal pain, and bloody stools. What is the next diagnostic step?

Intussusception is the most common cause of intestinal obstruction in early childhood and classically presents between ages 3 months and 3 years. An air contrast enema is both diagnostic and therapeutic.

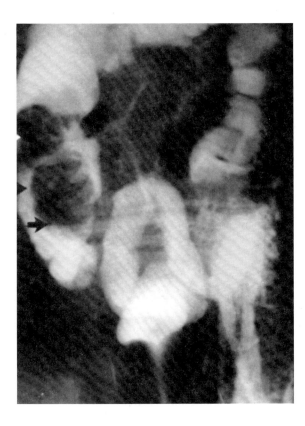

Contrast enema demonstrating ileocolic intussusception. While air enema is now routinely used for reduction of idiopathic ileo-colonic intussusception the contrast in this picture demonstrates the filling defects in the colon produced by the inspissated ileum. (With permission from Mulholland MW, Lillemoe KD, Doherty GM, Maier RV, Upchurch GR, eds. *Greenfield's Surgery.* 4th ed. Philadelphia, PA: Lippincott Williams & Wilkins; 2005.)

Intussusception

- Most cases occur before the age of 3 years
- Etiology is thought to be due to lymphoid hyperplasia in the terminal ileum after a viral illness
  - Can also be seen with Meckel diverticulum, polyps, or masses, which act as a lead point
  - Intussusception in adults commonly has a malignancy as the lead point
- Most commonly occurs at the ileocecal junction
- The proximal bowel (intussusceptum) invaginates into the distal bowel (intussuscipien) causing swelling, obstruction, and possible vascular compromise
- Controlled hydrostatic air contrast enema is successful in treating about 90% of cases with no subsequent surgery needed
- Indications for surgery
  - Unsuccessful hydrostatic reduction
  - Third episode
  - Peritonitis
  - Duration >12 hours

- Surgery involves reduction, appendectomy, and bowel resection for pathology
- Recurrence after radiographic or surgical treatment is about 5%

Intussusception is classically associated with "currant jelly" stool in a child between 3 months and 3 years old.

> A healthy 2-year-old boy presents with painless bloody stools. What is the most likely diagnosis?

Meckel diverticulum can cause symptoms similar to diverticulosis, diverticulitis, or obstruction.

Meckel Diverticulum
- The most common cause of GI bleed in children (50% of all painless lower GI bleeds in children <2)
- Due to patent vitelline (omphalomesenteric) duct remnant
- True diverticula
- Commonly have ectopic gastric (60% to 80%) or pancreatic mucosa (5% to 10%)
- Located on anti-mesenteric border
- A technetium-99 pertechnetate "Meckel" scan can assist with diagnosis and localization
    - Pre-test administration of glucagons and pentagastrin can further improve sensitivity
- Segmental resection is indicated for symptoms
- Rule of 2's
    - 2% of the population
    - 2% are symptomatic
    - 2 times more common in boys
    - 2 feet proximal to ileocecal valve
    - 2 years of age or less at presentation
    - 2 presentations (bleeding or obstruction)
    - 2 tissue types—pancreatic (most common) or gastric (ulcerates and bleeds)

Meckel diverticulum is the most common cause of lower GI bleeding in children.

> A 1-month-old infant has acholic stools and persistent jaundice. What is the most likely diagnosis?

Biliary atresia is the most common cause of neonatal jaundice requiring surgery.

Biliary Atresia
- Jaundice in the newborn that persists >2 weeks is no longer considered physiologic.
    - Unconjugated hyperbilirubinemia
        - Most commonly secondary to low glucuronyltransferase activity in the newborn, which is benign
        - Also consider Crigler-Najjar and Gilbert syndromes

- Conjugated hyperbilirubinemia
  - Signify disease of the liver or biliary tract
  - Common causes in infants include biliary atresia, choledochal cysts, and cholestasis
- Early diagnosis (before age 2 months) is critical to early intervention (before age 3 months) and improved outcome
- Hallmark findings
  - Bile duct proliferation
  - Cholestasis with plugging
  - Inflammatory cell infiltrate
  - Progression to cirrhosis
  - Must rule out hepatocellular dysfunction due to infectious, hematologic, metabolic, or genetic disorders
- Ultrasound helps to determine bile duct size, whether a gallbladder is present, and fluid collections from perforation of biliary tree
  - Bile ducts are not enlarged in biliary atresia
- If biliary atresia is suspected, then a limited right upper quadrant incision is used for local exploration and liver biopsy
- The initial goal of surgery is to establish a diagnosis
  - If a gallbladder is identified, then perform a cholangiogram
  - If cholangiography demonstrates a patent but hypoplastic biliary system, the incision is closed
    - Consider the differential diagnosis for hepatocellular jaundice (neonatal hepatitis, Alagille syndrome, cystic fibrosis, alpha 1-anti-trypsin deficiency)
  - If a patent gallbladder or extrahepatic biliary tree cannot be identified, the incision is elongated and a Kasai (portoenterostomy) operation should be performed
    - The fibrotic gallbladder and extrahepatic biliary tree is dissected up to the porta hepatis and resected
    - A Roux-en-Y is created and the roux jejunal limb is sutured to the transected porta hepatis to help reestablish bile flow from the minute bile ducts
  - If the cholangiogram demonstrates a choledochal cyst, then the cyst is excised as discussed previously
  - Liver transplantation is reserved for:
    - Progression to decompensated liver disease
    - Failed Kasai operation (no bile drainage)
    - Cases where the disease is diagnosed late

Diagnosis and intervention for biliary atresia before 2 to 3 months of age is important in preventing progressive liver injury. Upon exploration, the initial goal of surgery is to obtain or confirm the diagnosis.

A neonate is born with an abdominal wall defect to the right of the umbilicus. The eviscerated intestines appear thickened and do not have a peritoneal covering. What is the diagnosis?

This description is consistent with gastroschisis.

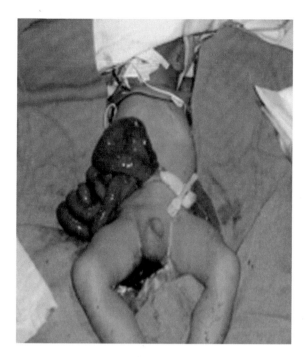

Gastroschisis. Note the eviscerated bowel to the right of the umbiliculus and the absence of a peritoneal covering.

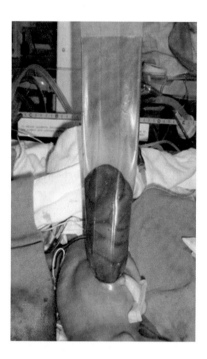

Silo for the initial treatment of gastroschisis. In the same infant the eviscerated bowel has been placed into a silicone bag (silo) with a flexible ring. After the intestine has been placed into the silo the flexible ring is deployed into the abdomen. The silo is suspended over the infant and the bowel is reduced over the ensuing 3–7 days. Once the bowel has been fully reduced the silo is removed and the defect closed operatively.

Gastroschisis

- Intrauterine rupture of the umbilical vein (there is 1 vein and 2 arteries)
- Eviscerated intestines have no peritoneal covering
- Abdominal wall defect to the right of the umbilicus (usually 2 to 5 cm in size)
- Intestines are usually thickened, edematous, and foreshortened
- Associated anomalies are not common (except intestinal atresia in 10% to 15%)
- Preoperative management includes volume resuscitation, gastric decompression, confirmation of bowel viability, and protective dressings

- Treatment
    - Attempt primary reduction; if unsuccessful then use a Silastic "silo"
    - A "silo" allows for a bedside staged closure to be followed by a primary closure
    - During surgical exploration, confirm the presence or absence of intestinal atresia
    - Post-op ileus is common and TPN can be life-saving

Gastroschisis, in contrast to omphalocele, is rarely associated with other congenital anomalies, with the exception of intestinal atresia, which is present in 10% to 15% of cases.

A baby is born with an abdominal wall defect. The exposed intestine and liver have an intact peritoneal covering and appear normal. What is the diagnosis?

An omphalocele has an intact peritoneal covering.

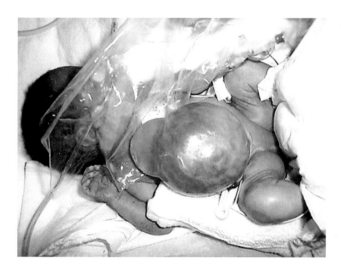

An infant with omphalocele is shown. In this case there is a large abdominal defect with an intact peritoneal covering.

What is the likelihood of an associated anomaly with an omphalocele?

Omphalocele is associated with a 40% to 80% incidence of another congenital anomaly.

Omphalocele
- Defect through the umbilicus (usually 4 to 10 cm in size)
- Peritoneal covering over intestines (and occasionally organs—usually liver)
- The intestines appear normal
- Associated anomalies are common: Cardiac (most common), pericardial, sternal, diaphragmatic, musculoskeletal, GI, and GU
- Associated with Beckwith-Wiedemann syndrome (omphalocele, hyperinsulinemia, and macroglossia)
- Pentalogy of Cantrell: Omphalocele, cardiac defects, pericardium defects, sternal defects, diaphragmatic septum transversum
- Preoperative management includes volume resuscitation, gastric decompression, and identification of associated anomalies

- Primary reduction is optimal, but if the defect is too large then a staged closure is indicated
- The outcome of these patients is related more to the associated anomalies than the omphalocele defect itself

Cardiac defects are the most commonly associated anomaly with omphalocele.

A few hours after birth, a newborn develops dyspnea, retractions, and cyanosis. What is the most likely diagnosis?

The most frequent presentation of congenital diaphragmatic hernia (CDH) is respiratory distress secondary to hypoxemia. Following delivery, a honeymoon period of a few hours to a day may precede symptoms.

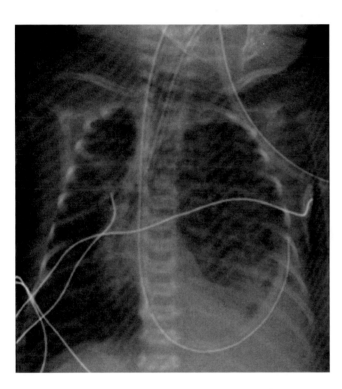

A radiograph of an infant with congenital diaphragmatic hernia. Note the nasogastric tube within the herniated stomach in the left chest. There is also mediastinal shift to the right from the herniated abdominal viscera.

Congenital Diaphragmatic Hernia

- There are two types:
    - Bochdalek (posterolateral) is the most common (80% are on the left)
    - Morgagni (anteromedial)
- Chest radiograph demonstrates loops of intestine or a gastric bubble in the thorax
- A nasogastric tube will help confirm the diagnosis, with the tip of the NG tube in the stomach located in the ipsilateral thorax
- Resuscitation and stabilization are essential prior to surgical repair
- Those infants not responding to medical therapy (inhalation nitric oxide, oscillator, etc.) may require extracorporeal membrane oxygenation (ECMO)
- Beware of a contralateral pneumothorax during aggressive ventilation
- Open surgical repair is via a laparotomy using a subcostal incision, with reduction of the eviscerated intestine and organs (spleen on the left) and closure of the defect. In some centers

- the preferred approach is now thoracoscopic with comparable results to the traditional open approach
  - Primary repair of the diaphragm is optimal, but a patch may be necessary to avoid excessive tension on the repair

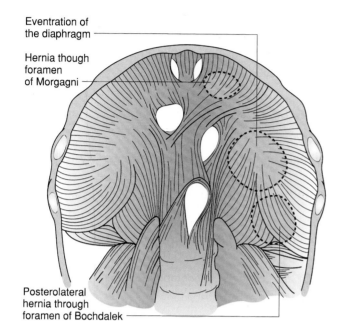

Eventration of the diaphragm

Hernia though foramen of Morgagni

Posterolateral hernia through foramen of Bochdalek

Positions of congenital diaphragmatic hernias. Several congenital anomalies of the diaphragm may occur during development. The most common is the posterior lateral defect through the foramen of Bochdalek. Less common is an anteromedial defect through the foramen of Morgagni. Eventration of the diaphragm is not a true hernia but rather weakening of the central tendon of the diaphragm. (With permission from Mulholland MW, Lillemoe KD, Doherty GM, Maier RV, Upchurch GR, eds. *Greenfield's Surgery.* 4th ed. Philadelphia, PA: Lippincott Williams & Wilkins; 2005.)

A congenital diaphragmatic hernia is not a surgical emergency—resuscitation and stabilization are essential prior to surgery.

A 2-year-old boy complains of belly pain and lack of appetite. Physical examination is significant for a large abdominal mass as well as opsoclonus and myoclonus. What is the most likely diagnosis?

Neuroblastoma is the most common malignant solid abdominal tumor in children. It presents with a large abdominal mass and opsoclonus/myoclonus ("dancing eyes/dancing feet").

Neuroblastoma

- Derived from neural crest tissue
  - May arise anywhere along the sympathetic ganglia
  - Most common location is adrenal medulla (50%)
- Average age at presentation is 1 to 2 years
- Commonly extends across the midline
- Ocular involvement may present as "raccoon eyes"
- Calcifications are visible on X-ray
- Most cases have elevated catecholamines, vanillylmandelic acid, and metanephrines
- Due to the production of hormones, children may present with flushing, hypertension, watery diarrhea, periorbital ecchymosis, and abnormal ocular movements
- Age at presentation is the major prognostic factor
  - Patients <1 year old have an overall survival >70%
  - Patients >1 year old have an overall survival <35%

- Good prognostic features
    - Tumors with <10 copies of N-myc gene
    - Aneuploid tumors
    - Low mitosis-karyorrhexis index
    - Normal lactate dehydrogenase and catecholamine levels
- Rarely metastasizes
- Primary surgical excision is the treatment of choice if technically feasible; otherwise, biopsy and do chemotherapy
- Can re-attempt resection post-chemotherapy

The N-myc gene is associated with neuroblastoma.

A 4-year-old girl is noted to have an abdominal mass by her mother while bathing. Physical examination confirms a mass as well as hypertension. Further history taking identifies a recent history of hematuria. What is the most likely diagnosis?

Wilms' tumor is the second most common malignant solid abdominal tumor in children.

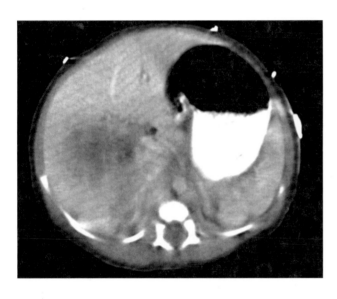

A computed tomography scan of a child with a large Wilms' tumor of the left kidney.

Wilms' Tumor (Nephroblastoma)
- Derived from the kidney
- Most common malignant renal tumor of childhood
- 3 to 4 years old at presentation
- 10% are bilateral
- Associated with various syndromes
    - WAGR—Wilms' tumor, aniridia, genitourinary malformations, mental retardation
    - Beckwith-Wiedemann syndrome
    - Denys-Drash syndrome—Wilms' tumor, intersex disorders
- X-ray calcifications are not present
- Prognosis is based on tumor grade

- Treatment
  - Nephrectomy if unilateral
  - Partial nephrectomy and chemotherapy if bilateral

> A premature newborn is noted to have only one palpable testicle. What is the next step in management?

Cryptorchidism
- An undescended testicle
- Is seen most commonly in premature and low birth weight infants
- Diagnosis: Absence of palpable testicles
- Treatment
  - Reassess in 6 months as many testes will later spontaneously descend
  - If testes do not descend, need to retrieve them and fix them in the scrotal sac or remove them
  - These patients require yearly testicular exams as they have much higher rates of testicular germ cell cancer

Hydrocele
- A fluid collection in the patent processus vaginalis
- Communicating hydroceles
  - Processus vaginalis is patent into the peritoneal cavity
  - Can develop an incarcerated inguinal hernia
  - Should be excised
- Non-communicating hydroceles
  - There is no communication between the fluid collection and the peritoneal cavity
  - Most will resolve spontaneously

> A 2-year-old boy with a history of Beckwith-Wiedemann syndrome is noted to have increasing abdominal girth. On exam, he has hepatomegaly. What is his diagnosis?

Hepatoblastoma is an embryonal tumor that is associated with Beckwith-Wiedemann syndrome and is most commonly found in children <3 years of age.

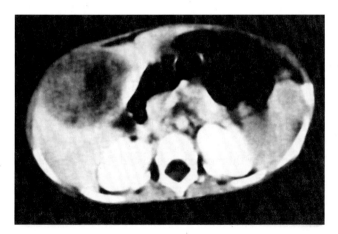

A computed tomography scan of the abdomen demonstrating an infant with hepatoblastoma of the right hepatic lobe. (With permission from Mulholland MW, Lillemoe KD, Doherty GM, Maier RV, Upchurch GR, eds. *Greenfield's Surgery*. 4th ed. Philadelphia, PA: Lippincott Williams & Wilkins; 2005.)

Hepatoblastoma

- Embryonal tumor
- Associated with Beckwith-Wiedemann syndrome and Familial adenomatous polyposis
- Symptoms: Increased abdominal girth, precocious puberty (secondary to hCG production)
- Diagnosis: Elevated α-fetoprotein, MRI, and biopsy
- Treatment: Resection and chemotherapy

A 12-year-old boy presents for evaluation of his indented sternum. What is the next step in management?

Pectus excavatum is best repaired surgically after the age of 5 years.

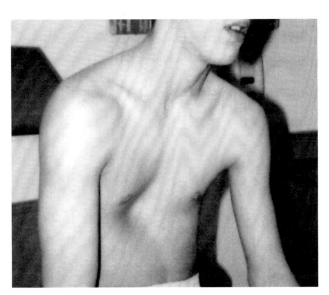 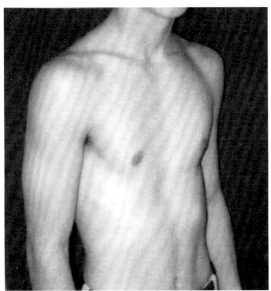

Pectus excavatum pre- and post-op. Note pre-operatively that the sternum is depressed and the costal margins flared. The defect results from abnormal cartilage development. Correction with placement of a substernal bar results in correction of the sternal depression with remodeling of the abnormal cartilage. (With permission from Mulholland MW, Lillemoe KD, Doherty GM, Maier RV, Upchurch GR, eds. *Greenfield's Surgery*. 4th ed. Philadelphia, PA: Lippincott Williams & Wilkins; 2005.)

Pectus Excavatum

- Often presents within the first year of life
- More common in boys
- Due to posterior angulation of the sternum below the second costal cartilage and posterior angulation of the costal cartilages to meet the sternum
- May be associated with scoliosis, Marfan's, and mitral valve prolapse
- Is associated with decreased exercise tolerance secondary to decreased lung volumes
- Obtain pulmonary function tests and an echocardiogram
- Surgical repair includes the open "Ravitch" procedure or thoracoscopic-assisted "Nuss" procedure
    - Ravitch procedure—sternal osteotomy with cartilage resection
    - Nuss procedure—insertion of a sternal bar
    - Surgery is most often performed for cosmesis

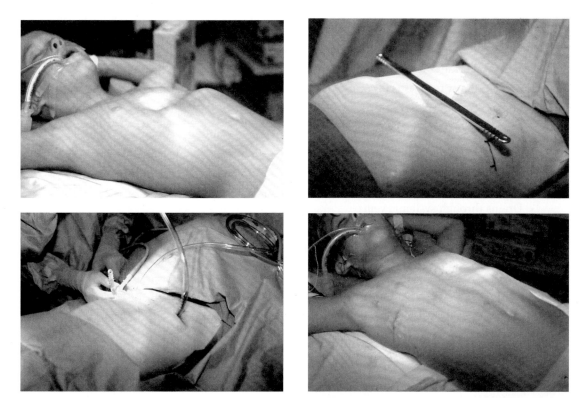

Thoracoscopically assisted Lorenz Bar insertion (Nuss procedure). (A) The patient is positioned with the arms upward to allow access to the chest bilaterally. (B) A Lorenz bar of appropriate length is selected. (C) Bilateral incisions are made. A thoracosope is introduced into the right hemithorax. The Lorenz bar is bent into a curved shaped to correct the defect. The modified Lorenz bar is tunneled subcutaneously and then inserted into the left hemithorax just lateral to the sternum. The bar is carefully passed anterior to the mediastinal contents and below the sternum with thoracoscopic guidance. Once across the mediastinum the bar is brought through the left hemithorax and subcutaneous tunnel on the left. Once completed the bar is rotated 180 degrees correcting the deformity. (D) Immediate postoperative appearance. (With permission from Mulholland MW, Lillemoe KD, Doherty GM, Maier RV, Upchurch GR, eds. *Greenfield's Surgery*. 4th ed. Philadelphia, PA: Lippincott Williams & Wilkins; 2005.)

Surgical repair of pectus excavatum should not be performed before age 5.

A child is diagnosed with pulmonary sequestration following an episode of pneumonia. What is the next step in management?

Intralobar pulmonary sequestration should be treated with a segmentectomy or lobectomy. The extralobar type generally does not require surgery.

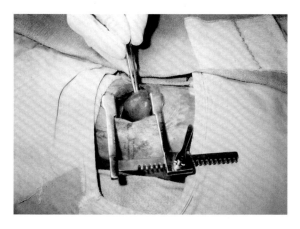

Excision of pulmonary sequestration. A muscle sparing thoracotomy has been performed. The abnormal lung sequestration is mobilized through the incision and resected. (With permission from Mulholland MW, Lillemoe KD, Doherty GM, Maier RV, Upchurch GR, eds. *Greenfield's Surgery*. 4th ed. Philadelphia, PA: Lippincott Williams & Wilkins; 2005.)

Pulmonary Sequestration

- Does not communicate with the tracheobronchial tree
- Most have aberrant blood supply from the aorta
- More common at the posterior or medial aspects of left lower lobe (LLL)
- Intralobar sequestration
    - Drain through the pulmonary veins
    - Not associated with other anomalies
    - Resect for infectious and bleeding risks
- Extralobar sequestration
    - Drains through systemic veins
    - Associated with other anomalies
    - Observe (usually asymptomatic) and delayed resection at 6 to 9 months of age

---

On a routine chest X-ray, an area of hyperlucency is identified at the left upper lobe of the lung. What is the next best step in management?

Asymptomatic congenital lobar overinflation should be managed conservatively with observation.

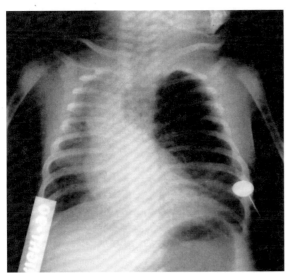

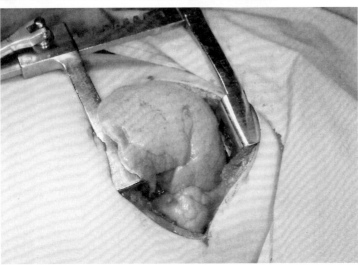

Congenital lobar overinflation. A plain chest radiograph demonstrates a hyperinflated left upper lobe of the lung with mediastinal shift to the right. The lower photograph demonstrates the hyperinflated lobe herniating through the chest incision. (With permission from Mulholland MW, Lillemoe KD, Doherty GM, Maier RV, Upchurch GR, eds. *Greenfield's Surgery.* 4th ed. Philadelphia, PA: Lippincott Williams & Wilkins; 2005.)

Congenital Lobar Overinflation

- Localized area of air trapping within the parenchyma ("emphysema")
  - Due to cartilage malformation
  - Leads to hyper-expansion of the involved portion
- Hyperlucency on chest X-ray
- The left upper lobe (LUL) is the most common location
- Most are found incidentally in asymptomatic patients
- Occasionally symptoms may mimic signs of a tension pneumothorax with mediastinal shift on chest X-ray

Placing a chest tube into an area of congenital lobar emphysema can be lethal and should be avoided despite the clinical similarities to a tension pneumothorax.

A newborn presents with a multicystic lung mass and respiratory distress. What is the next best step in management?

A symptomatic congenital cystic adenomatoid malformation (CCAM) requires pulmonary resection.

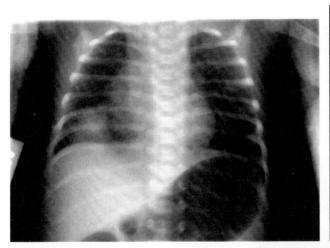
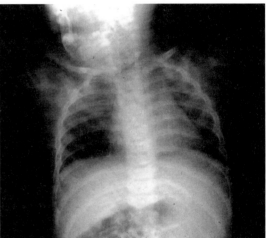
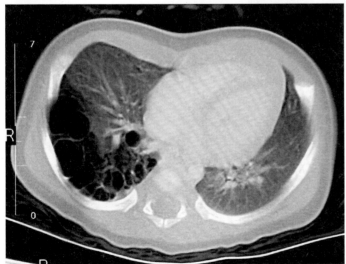

Congenital cystic adenomatoid malformation (CCAM). (A) Newborn chest radiograph of CCAM. Note that immediately after birth, the mass is fluid-filled and appears as a density in the right hemithorax. (B) Chest radiograph of the same child at 5 months of age prior to surgical excision. Now the lesion appears cystic due to air entrapment within the CCAM. (C) The computed tomography of the lesion demonstrates the abnormal area of the lung characterized by large air filled cysts. (With permission from Mulholland MW, Lillemoe KD, Doherty GM, Maier RV, Upchurch GR, eds. *Greenfield's Surgery*. 4th ed. Philadelphia, PA: Lippincott Williams & Wilkins; 2005.)

Congenital Cystic Pulmonary Adenomatoid Malformation

- Multicystic hamartoma of lung, formerly referred to as CCAM
- Bronchial (airway) communication is present
- The presence of symptoms is an indication for pulmonary resection in the newborn period
- In asymptomatic infants, surgery is delayed until 6 to 9 months of age
- Lobectomy rather than segmentectomy remains the recommended procedure

---

A 7-year-old girl presents with dysphagia. A CT scan demonstrates a mediastinal mass. What is the most likely diagnosis?

T-cell lymphoma.

Mediastinal Masses in Children

- T-cell lymphoma (most common)
- Teratoma
- Tumor (neuroblastoma, neurofibroma, ganglioneuroma, germ cell tumors)
- Thymic mass
- Bronchogenic cyst

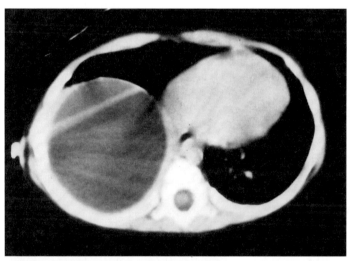

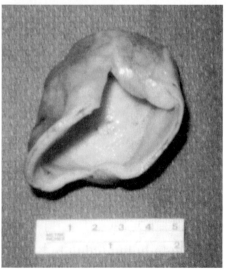

Enterogenous cyst. This represents another abnormality in the spectrum of bronchopulmonary foregut malformations. (A) Computerized tomography demonstrating a large mass occupying the right hemithorax. (B) Surgical specimen. (With permission from Mulholland MW, Lillemoe KD, Doherty GM, Maier RV, Upchurch GR, eds. *Greenfield's Surgery.* 4th ed. Philadelphia, PA: Lippincott Williams & Wilkins; 2005.)

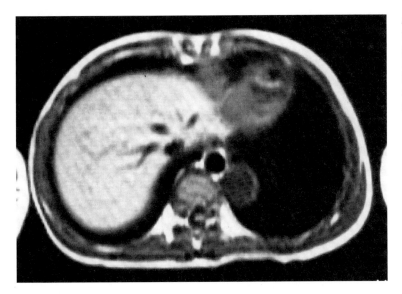

A computed tomography of a child with a bronchogenic cyst. (With permission from Mulholland MW, Lillemoe KD, Doherty GM, Maier RV, Upchurch GR, eds. *Greenfield's Surgery.* 4th ed. Philadelphia, PA: Lippincott Williams & Wilkins; 2005.)

What is the most common malignancy in children?

The most common childhood malignancy is leukemia (ALL), and the prognosis with appropriate therapy is good.

9 | Urologic Surgery

Karen E. Boyle

A 68-year-old male presents with the sensation of incomplete emptying and a decreased urinary stream. On examination he has a suprapubic mass and on digital rectal examination (DRE) his prostate is 70 cc in volume. A post-void residual is 500 cc. What is the most likely treatment required?

An α-1 antagonist or 5-α reductase inhibitor is indicated to treat benign prostatic hyperplasia (BPH) and outlet obstruction.

Benign Prostatic Hyperplasia

- BPH is the most common nonmalignant neoplastic process afflicting men
- BPH causes irritative symptoms (nocturia, urgency, and frequency) and obstructive symptoms (decreased urinary stream and hesitancy)
- BPH develops in the transition zone of the prostate, causing bladder outlet obstruction
- Clinical assessment tools include flow rate, post void residual, serum creatinine, and renal ultrasound findings

Treatment of Benign Prostatic Hyperplasia

- Tamsulosin (Flomax), rapaflo, uroxatral are the primary medical therapy for BPH
  - Selective oral α-1 antagonist
  - Does not affect prostate volume
  - Clinical improvement in 2 to 4 weeks
- Finasteride (Proscar) or Avodart are 5-α reductase inhibitors
  - Work by decreasing intraprostatic dihydrotestosterone
  - Can reduce total gland volume by 20% to 25%
  - Finasteride works well for patients with large glands and hematuria secondary to BPH
  - Clinical improvement in 2 to 6 months
- Minimally invasive procedures
  - PVP Greenlight laser transurethral resection of the prostate (TURP)
  - Transurethral microwave thermotherapy
  - Transurethral needle ablation

- Surgeries
  - TURP
  - Simple open prostatectomy—used only for *very* large glands
- Indications for surgery
  - Recurrent episodes of urinary retention
  - Recurrent urinary tract infections
  - Renal insufficiency
  - Bladder calculi
  - A large median prostate lobe
  - Severe debilitating symptoms
  - Failure of more conservative/minimally invasive measures

A 56-year-old male presents with a prostate-specific antigen (PSA) of 4.0. He has no urinary complaints and is feeling well. His past medical history is negative. His father has a history of prostate cancer. On DRE his prostate is 20 cc in volume and smooth with no nodules palpable. What is the next step in management?

Discuss the risks and benefits of prostate cancer screening and detection tests. The next step is to perform a transrectal ultrasound (TRUS)-guided 12-core needle biopsy of the prostate.

Prostate Cancer

- Most common cancer in men
- Adenocarcinoma is the most common type (>90%)
- Primarily develops in the peripheral portion of prostate gland, which makes it appreciable on DRE
- Risk factors
  - Age is the most significant risk factor
  - A family history of prostate cancer is important (a first-degree relative with the disease implies a two fold increased risk)
  - African American race
- PSA is used in conjunction with DRE to help provide early detection of disease
  - The use of routine PSA to screen for prostate cancer has now fallen out of favor
  - PSA is used to detect biochemical disease recurrence following treatment
  - Patients with an elevated PSA and/or abnormal DRE are recommended to undergo TRUS-guided prostate biopsy
- A metastatic workup should be performed in select patients based upon the clinical picture
  - Workup is usually comprised of a bone scan and CT or MRI
  - Prostate bone metastases are osteoblastic and will be hyperdense on X-ray or CT

Treatment of Prostate Cancer

- Patients with suspected localized prostate cancer and a greater than 10-year expected survival should undergo definitive therapy
  - Definitive therapy consists of brachytherapy, external beam radiation therapy, or radical retropubic prostatectomy (performed open, laparoscopic, or robotic-assisted laparoscopic)
  - At the time of prostatectomy, depending upon Gleason grade/score a pelvic lymphadenectomy may be performed first
  - Complications: Incontinence, impotence

- Post-prostatectomy, PSA should drop to 0 after 3 weeks—if it does not, have a high index of suspicion for metastases
- In patients with significant comorbidities and/or more extensive disease, consider watchful waiting or systemic therapy (e.g., androgen deprivation therapy and "hormonal therapy")

Bone is the most common location for metastases in prostate cancer and can manifest as back pain or an increased serum alkaline phosphatase level.

A 32-year-old female presents to the emergency room with left-sided flank pain. She has had decreased oral intake for 2 days and recently began to have worsening nausea and emesis. Her past medical history is negative. On examination she is febrile to 38.7, tachycardic, and appears uncomfortable. Her WBC is 10, creatinine is 1.2, and BUN is 45. You suspect an obstructive ureteral calculus. Which diagnostic test should be performed next?

The patient should have a pregnancy test as well as a non-contrast spiral CT of the abdomen and pelvis using a stone protocol.

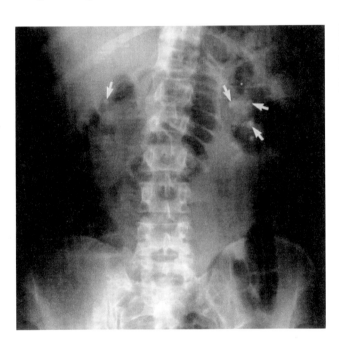

Renal calculi. (With permission from Mulholland MW, Lillemoe KD, Doherty GM, Maier RV, Upchurch GR, eds. *Greenfield's Surgery.* 4th ed. Philadelphia, PA: Lippincott Williams & Wilkins; 2005.)

Urinary Calculi

- Calcium stones (calcium oxalate + calcium phosphate) are the most common type (70%)
  - Associated with hyperparathyroidism, hyperoxaluria
  - Treat with hydration or management as below for larger stones
- Staghorn calculi are large, infected renal calculi
  - Composed of Mg–ammonium phosphate (struvite) and Ca phosphate
  - Due to infection with urease-producing bacteria (Proteus mirabilis)
  - Forming the renal calyx and pelvis as a branched staghorn
  - Treatment: Antibiotics and hydration
- Cystine stones
  - Caused by defect in transport of cysteine
  - Treatment: Hydration, urine alkalinization

- Uric acid stones
  - Associated with gout, Lesch-Nyhan (high purine turnover), myeloproliferative disorders
  - Treatment: Hydration, urine alkalinization
- 90% of stones are radiopaque and seen on KUB X-ray
- Uric acid stones are radiolucent
- Manifestations of stones
  - Asymptomatic (non-obstructive renal stones)
  - Flank pain: Colicky flank pain that radiates to the lateral abdomen (proximal ureteral stones) or pain that radiates into the groin and genitals (distal ureteral stones)
  - Microscopic or gross hematuria

Obstructive pyelonephritis/sepsis

Normal Ureter and Vascular Anatomy

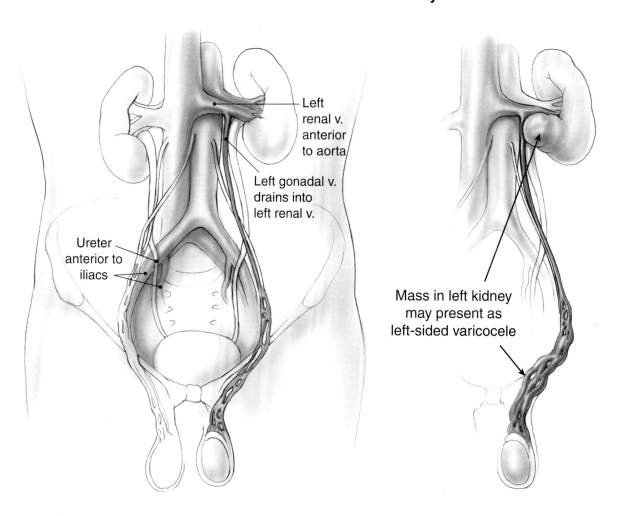

Left renal v. anterior to aorta

Left gonadal v. drains into left renal v.

Ureter anterior to iliacs

Mass in left kidney may present as left-sided varicocele

Treatment of Urinary Calculi

- Ureteral stones at three distinct points:
  - The ureteropelvic junction (UPJ)
  - The pelvic brim where the ureter crosses the iliac vessels
  - The ureterovesical junction

- Most stones (90%) are less than 4 mm in diameter and pass spontaneously
  - Stones less than 4 to 5 mm can be observed to see if they will pass spontaneously
  - Hydration, analgesia, and urine straining constitute expectant management
- Larger stones are less likely to pass (>7 mm stones have about 20% to 30% chance of passing)
- Non-obstructive renal stones less than 2.5 cm can be managed by extracorporeal shock-wave lithotripsy
- Larger renal stones require percutaneous nephrolithotomy (PCNL)
- Staghorn calculi require percutaneous removal
- Surgery is indicated in patients for:
  - Severe pain not controlled with oral analgesia
  - Complete obstruction of a solitary kidney
  - Large stones with obstruction, infection, and hydronephrosis
- Surgical options include: Cystoscopy with stent placement, ureteroscopy with laser lithotripsy, and PCNL

White blood cell casts are a marker of pyelonephritis or glomerulonephritis

A 58-year-old male presents to clinic with new-onset painless, gross hematuria. He does not have symptoms of dysuria, urgency or frequency. His past medical history is significant for tobacco use for 30 years and hypertension. He takes metoprolol and has no drug allergies. His physical examination is notable for a 20 cc prostate that is benign to palpation. His last PSA was 0.3. What is the next step in management?

A CT scan with IV contrast, cystoscopy, and urine cytology should be performed to evaluate the patient for bladder cancer.

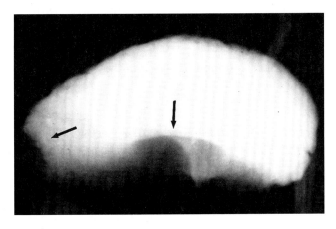

IVP demonstrating bladder filling defect in a patient with bladder cancer. (With permission from Mulholland MW, Lillemoe KD, Doherty GM, Maier RV, Upchurch GR, eds. *Greenfield's Surgery.* 4th ed. Philadelphia, PA: Lippincott Williams & Wilkins; 2005.)

Bladder Cancer
- Painless gross hematuria is the most common presentation
- Other presentations include microscopic hematuria and irritative voiding symptoms
- Risk factors include cigarette smoking, age, and exposure to aniline dyes, cyclophosphamide, and phenacetin
- Cigarette smoking is strongly associated with bladder cancer

- Bladder cancer pathology
  - Transitional cell carcinoma (>90%)
  - Squamous cell carcinoma (5% to 7%, associated with Schistosomiasis and chronic infections)
  - Adenocarcinoma/urachal carcinoma (1% to 2%)
- Multifocal disease can affect the entire urothelium (renal pelvis, ureter, bladder, and urethra)
- Disease does not usually progress in a step-wise pattern from papillary to muscle invasive
- Obtain urine cytology, cystoscopy, and an upper tract evaluation with a CT scan or IVP
- Perform a transurethral resection of bladder tumor (TURBT) for tissue diagnosis

Treatment of Bladder Cancer

- Superficial bladder cancer and carcinoma in situ (CIS) can be treated with:
  - Intravesical chemotherapy with Mitomycin C
  - Intravesical immunotherapy with Bacillus Calmette-Guerin (BCG), a live attenuated strain of mycobacterium
- Perform a radical cystectomy with urinary diversion for:
  - BCG failure in CIS
  - Muscle-invasive disease
- Urinary diversion commonly utilizes the ileum for creation of a neobladder (attached to the native urethra) or an ileal conduit with a urinary stoma
- Neoadjuvant chemotherapy can be attempted to downstage tumors from unresectable to resectable
- Chemotherapy is used for advanced disease
- 50% of patients with muscle-invasive bladder cancer will progress to metastatic disease even after curative local therapy

For bladder cancer that has not invaded the muscle, TURBT and BCG is the initial therapy. Cystectomy, chemotherapy, and radiation therapy are reserved for cases with muscular invasion.

Six hours following a TURP procedure for bladder cancer, a patient is found in the recovery room to be having seizures. What is the most likely etiology?

Hyponatremia secondary to copious bladder irrigation (post-TURP syndrome). Airway protection should be the first priority in any seizure patient. Management should then focus on correcting the hyponatremia.

Post-transurethral Resection of the Prostate Syndrome

- Hyponatremia following any procedure with bladder irrigation
- Can manifest as seizures/cerebral edema
- Treated by correcting hyponatremia (but not too rapidly to avoid central pontine myelinolysis)

A 45-year-old female presents with an incidentally discovered 6 cm renal mass on a CT scan. The mass enhances with IV contrast. What is the most likely diagnosis?

Renal cell carcinoma (RCC).

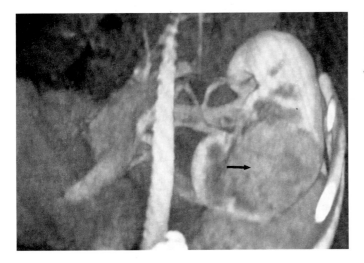

Renal cell carcinoma. (With permission from Mulholland MW, Lillemoe KD, Doherty GM, Maier RV, Upchurch GR, eds. *Greenfield's Surgery*. 4th ed. Philadelphia, PA: Lippincott Williams & Wilkins; 2005.)

Renal Masses

- A solid renal mass with negative Hounsfield units usually represents fat/angiomyolipoma
- A solid renal mass with positive Hounsfield units (enhancing post contrast) is most commonly RCC
- A simple cyst is benign, round, smooth, and thin walled
  - Simple cysts typically are low density (−20 Hounsfield units) and have no contrast enhancement on CT
  - No treatment is required
- A complex renal cyst should be considered suspicious for malignancy
  - Suspicious features include internal septations, calcium deposits, an irregular wall, and areas of contrast enhancement
- Non-renal cancers can metastasize to the kidney (breast is most common)

All complex cysts with any suspicious features should be removed.

Renal Cell Carcinoma

- Occurs in "younger" adults (40 to 60 years of age)
- Greater than 50% of RCCs are detected incidentally
- The classic presentation triad is pain, hematuria, and flank mass
- Other presenting signs and symptoms include pain, weight loss, fever, erythrocytosis (secondary to increased erythropoietin levels), left-sided varicocele, and hypertension
- Paraneoplastic syndromes are present in 20% of patients with RCC
  - Hypercalcemia
  - Hypertension
  - Polycythemia
  - Stauffer syndrome
    - Nonmetastatic hepatic dysfunction
    - Seen in up to 20% of cases
    - Lab tests reveal elevated alkaline phosphatase, prothrombin time, bilirubin, and transaminases
    - Need to rule out liver metastases
    - Hepatic function normalizes after nephrectomy in 60% to 70%

- Treatment is radical nephrectomy including removal of Gerota's fascia and regional lymph nodes
- RCC can directly extend into the renal vein, up the IVC, and into the atrium—cancers going up into the IVC can still be resected
- An isolated lung or liver metastasis should be resected
- Partial nephrectomy (renal sparing surgery) can be used for small peripheral lesions or in patients with solitary kidneys or bilateral tumors
- Surgery can be performed open, laparoscopic, or robotic

A left-sided varicocele can be a presentation of a left renal cell cancer since the left gonadal vein drains directly into the left renal vein.

A 20-year-old man presents to the emergency department following a motor vehicle crash. He is oriented but hypotensive, complaining of mild abdominal discomfort. After two large-bore IVs are secured, an exploratory laparotomy is performed. The right kidney is noted to have significant bleeding with multiple lacerations involving the hilum. During the exploration the patient continues to be unstable. What is the next step in management?

A nephrectomy should be performed because of the life-threatening nature of the hemorrhage. Inspection of the contralateral kidney is advised before closing.

Renal Trauma

- >99% have hematuria
- 60% to 90% of all renal injuries result from blunt trauma
- All blunt trauma patients with gross hematuria, microscopic hematuria and shock, rapid deceleration injury/clinical indicators should undergo a CT scan with IV contrast
- All penetrating trauma with hematuria requires an imaging study
- The degree of hematuria may not correlate to the severity of injury
- A CT scan can document vessel injury and extravasation
- Unless there is hilar injury with vessel damage or collecting duct disruption, most injuries will resolve with non-operative management
- A nephrectomy should be performed for life-threatening bleeding (i.e., hemodynamic instability)
- Renal vein trauma can be treated with simple ligation of the renal vein if the patient is unstable
  - Venous outflow through the lumbar and adrenal branches will often suffice
- Use absorbable sutures in the renal or ureteral system to minimize the risk of kidney stone formation

---

A young male patient presents to the emergency department following a high-velocity motor vehicle crash. He is hemodynamically stable and is assessed and imaged in the trauma bay accordingly. Pertinent findings on examination include a mildly tender abdomen, an abrasion to his left flank, and gross hematuria. A CT scan is obtained that demonstrates a hematoma around the left kidney and an apparent kidney laceration, described as Grade II renal injury. His hematocrit is 40. Other lab values are within normal limits. He continues to have a stable heart rate and blood pressure. What is the next step in management?

Observation and supportive treatment.

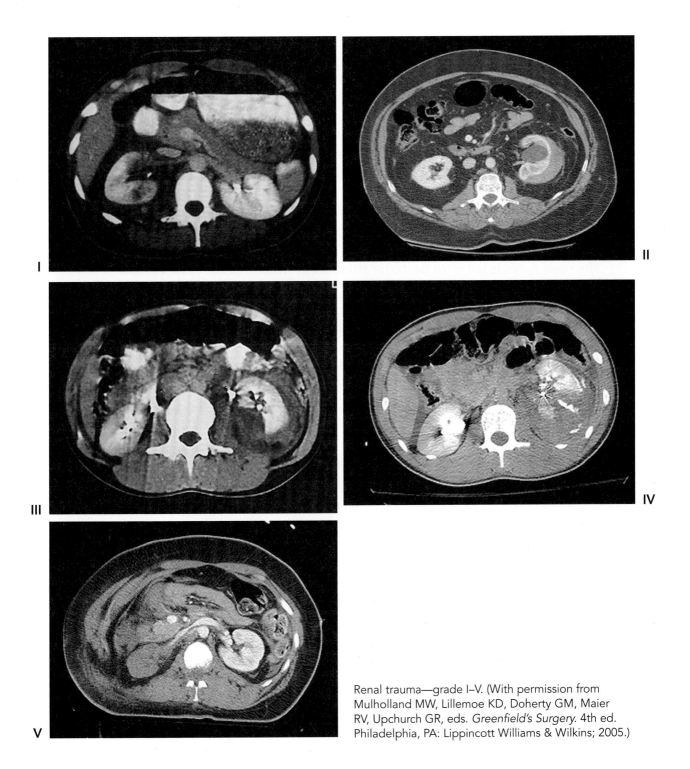

I, II, III, IV, V

Renal trauma—grade I–V. (With permission from Mulholland MW, Lillemoe KD, Doherty GM, Maier RV, Upchurch GR, eds. *Greenfield's Surgery*. 4th ed. Philadelphia, PA: Lippincott Williams & Wilkins; 2005.)

Management of Renal Trauma

- American Association for the Surgery of Trauma Organ Injury Scale for the Kidney
    - Grade I: Subcapsular, nonexpanding hematoma; no parenchymal laceration
    - Grade II: Nonexpanding perirenal hematoma confined to the renal retroperitoneum, laceration of renal cortex <1 cm parenchymal depth, no urinary extravasation
    - Grade III: Laceration of renal cortex >1 cm parenchymal depth with collecting system rupture or urinary extravasation

- Grade IV: Parenchymal laceration extending through the renal cortex, medulla, collecting system, main renal artery, or vein injury with contained hemorrhage
- Grade V: Completely shattered kidney, avulsion of renal hilum, devascularized kidney
- Grade I–III renal trauma should be managed conservatively with bed rest, antibiotics, serial hematocrits, and a repeat CT at 48–72 hours
  - Urinary extravasation requires ureteral stent placement
- Grade IV or V renal trauma usually requires surgical exploration
- Upon inspection during a laparotomy for penetrating trauma, Gerota's fascia should NOT be opened unless there is an expanding hematoma or major kidney injury
- Before performing a nephrectomy for trauma, a single shot IVP by giving an IV contrast bolus can confirm a functioning contralateral kidney

Remember that the right renal artery lies behind the vena cava and the right renal vein. The renal pelvis is the most posterior structure in relation to the renal vessels.

A 22-year-old intoxicated man presents to the emergency department following a motor vehicle crash. He is intubated and has two large-bore IVs. Overall, he is in stable condition with normal vital signs. He has no obvious injuries. Following placement of a foley catheter, blood is noted in the collection bag. What is the next step in management?

A cystogram should be performed to rule out a bladder injury. It is important to include a post-void film to rule out extravasation.

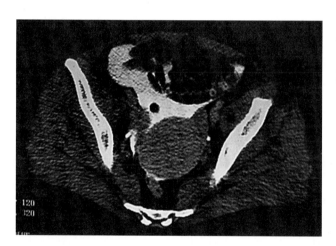

Intraperitoneal bladder injury. (With permission from Mulholland MW, Lillemoe KD, Doherty GM, Maier RV, Upchurch GR, eds. *Greenfield's Surgery.* 4th ed. Philadelphia, PA: Lippincott Williams & Wilkins; 2005.)

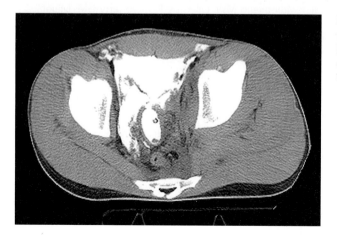

Extraperitoneal bladder injury. (With permission from Mulholland MW, Lillemoe KD, Doherty GM, Maier RV, Upchurch GR, eds. *Greenfield's Surgery.* 4th ed. Philadelphia, PA: Lippincott Williams & Wilkins; 2005.)

Bladder Trauma

- Commonly associated with major abdominal injuries (35%)
- Blunt trauma is most commonly extraperitoneal (80%); intraperitoneal trauma is less common (20%)
- Extraperitoneal ruptures can be managed with an indwelling foley catheter unless associated injury exists
- Intraperitoneal ruptures require exploration and repair
- Obtain a cystogram using an 18F foley filled under gravity with at least 300 cc of 30% contrast. Clamp the foley and obtain AP and oblique films. Always obtain a post-drainage film.
- CT cystography (fill bladder retrograde as in plain film cystography) is a good test when available (can replace plain film cystogram)
- Keep the patient maximally drained (using a foley, suprapubic tube, or pelvic drain) following repair

A young female presents to the emergency department having sustained multiple gunshot wounds to her abdomen and pelvis. She is taken for an emergent exploration. When the foley is placed, her urine is noted to be blood-tinged. What is the next step in management?

Proceed with exploration and, when appropriate, inspect the kidneys, ureters, and bladder for injury.

Ureteral Trauma

- Penetrating trauma causes ureteral injury more commonly than blunt trauma
- Usually associated with other injuries
- Hematuria is often absent
- No single test is reliable
- If available, a pre-op CT scan with IV contrast and delayed images can suggest injury
- In the OR, an IV methylene blue bolus with lasix can be given

Management of Ureteral Injuries

- Blood supply is segmental: Originates medially for the upper 2/3 and laterally for the lower 1/3
- Techniques for an abdominal ureteral injury
  - Spatulate
  - Stent
  - Tension free ureteroureterostomy
- Techniques for a pelvic ureteral repair
  - Psoas hitch
  - Downward nephropexy
  - Reimplantation into the bladder
- Use an absorbable interrupted suture over a stent
- Management of a ureteral contusion
  - Stent (the bladder can be opened to place a stent under direct vision)
- Other (less commonly used) maneuvers include a Boari flap, transureteroureterostomy, renal autotransplant, and an ileal ureter
- Delayed diagnosis
  - <5 days: Consider repair
  - >5 days: Control urinary extravasation with a ureteral stent, urinary diversion, and drainage of any urinoma; definitive repair in 6 weeks

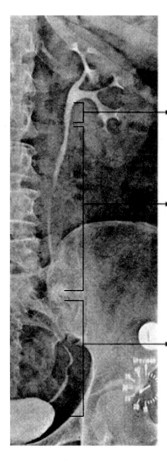

Ureteral reconstruction. (With permission from Mulholland MW, Lillemoe KD, Doherty GM, Maier RV, Upchurch GR, eds. *Greenfield's Surgery.* 4th ed. Philadelphia, PA: Lippincott Williams & Wilkins; 2005.)

Ureteropelvic Junction
Reanastomosis

Proximal and Mid Ureter
Short defects: End-to-end anastomosis
Long defects: Vesicopsoas hitch, Boari flap, or transureteroureterostomy

Distal Ureter
Short defects: Reimplantation
Long defects: Vesicopsoas hitch or Boari flap reimplantation

A 42-year-old male presents to the emergency department following a straddle injury. He has blood at his meatus and is unable to urinate. He has a palpable suprapubic mass. On examination he has a hematoma of his penis, scrotum, and perineum. What is the next step in management?

A retrograde urethrogram is indicated before placement of a foley catheter when a urethral injury is suspected.

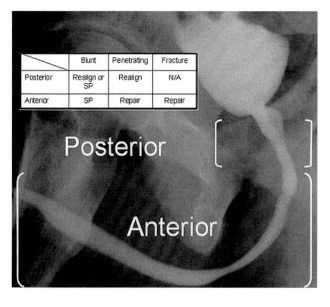

	Blunt	Penetrating	Fracture
Posterior	Realign or SP	Realign	N/A
Anterior	SP	Repair	Repair

Posterior

Anterior

Retrograde urethrogram. (With permission from Mulholland MW, Lillemoe KD, Doherty GM, Maier RV, Upchurch GR, eds. *Greenfield's Surgery.* 4th ed. Philadelphia, PA: Lippincott Williams & Wilkins; 2005.)

Urethral Trauma

- Usually involves the posterior urethra (90%)
- Occurs in 4% to 14% of pelvic fractures (most commonly associated with bilateral pubic rami fractures)
- Indications for a retrograde urethrogram
  - Blood at the meatus
  - High-riding (freely mobile) prostate on DRE
  - Inability to urinate (palpable full bladder)
  - Perineal hematoma
- Retrograde urethrogram: 14F foley placed 1 to 2 cm into the urethra, inflate balloon 1 to 2 cc to secure, 30% hypaque injected. Obtain lateral decubitus films.

Treatment of Urethral Trauma

- Posterior urethral injuries are treated with primary endoscopic realignment using cystoscopy and wire vs. suprapubic tube
  - Primary open realignment should NOT be performed for posterior injuries (it is associated with an increased rate of impotence, incontinence, stricture)
- Anterior urethral injury requires an open anastomotic repair

---

A 20-year-old male presents with a mass in his testicle found on a school sports physical. He is otherwise healthy and takes no medications. On examination his right testicle is normal and his left testicle has a firm mass in the inferior pole that does not transilluminate. What is the next step in management?

Transscrotal ultrasound of the testicles and laboratory tests for tumor markers.

Testicular Cancer

- A solid, firm intratesticular mass is testicular cancer until proven otherwise
- Cryptorchidism, or an undescended testicle, is a risk factor
  - The risk is also increased in the contralateral (normally descended) testicle
- Affects young men 20 to 40 years of age (testicular lymphoma is seen men over 50 years)
- 95% are germ cell tumors, either seminoma or non-seminoma (yolk sac, embryonal, choriocarcinoma, teratoma)
- Obtain tumor markers: α-fetoprotein (AFP), β-hCG, and LDH (correlates with tumor bulk).
  - 10% of seminomas and 90% of non-seminomatous cancer have elevated tumor markers
- Treatment is radical orchiectomy via an *inguinal* approach
  - Leave a long tie on the spermatic cord for identification during a possible retroperitoneal lymph node dissection (RPLND)
  - Do NOT biopsy these masses as it can cause seeing of a tumor
- Obtain a CT scan of abdomen and pelvis and a CXR to rule out metastatic disease
- Once a pathologic diagnosis from an orchiectomy is obtained, treatment depends on tumor type
  - Seminoma
    - Does not produce AFP
      - If pathology confirms a seminoma and the AFP is elevated, it is a mixed germ cell tumor and is treated as a non-seminomatous cancer
    - Spreads to the retroperitoneal and periaortic lymph nodes
    - Seminomas are uniquely radiosensitive (even with metastatic disease)
    - Seminomas are treated with orchiectomy and radiation therapy to the retroperitoneum

- Chemotherapy is reserved for patients with regional or distant metastases (cisplastin is commonly used)
  - Non-seminomatous germ cell tumor
    - Radioresistant
    - Spreads to the lungs
    - Treat with orchiectomy and an RPLND
    - Chemotherapy (cisplastin) is used for advanced disease

Never biopsy a testicular mass: Perform an orchiectomy via an inguinal incision so as not to alter lymphatic drainage.

A 35-year-old male was kicked in the scrotum during a soccer game. He has exquisite tenderness of his right testicle and it is swollen with significant ecchymosis. What is the next step in management?

A testicular rupture should be suspected based on the mechanism and presentation. An emergent scrotal exploration for an acute scrotum is indicated.

Testicular Trauma

- Blunt trauma results in testicular rupture in approximately 50% of cases
- Presents as scrotal pain, ecchymosis, and hematocele
- For an unimpressive clinical picture and normal ultrasound, manage conservatively with analgesics and scrotal elevation
- For an acutely tender scrotum and/or a suspicion of testicular rupture, explore!
- A normal scrotal ultrasound should not dictate the decision to explore; the decision should be based on the physical examination
- Nonoperative management of significant testicular injuries results in a higher rate of subsequent orchiectomy

A 16-year-old male presents with left scrotal pain that began 4 hours ago. He denies trauma to his genitalia, and the pain has been progressively worsening over time. He also is complaining of nausea. On examination his left testicle is acutely tender, displaced, and swollen. What is the next step in management?

A testicular torsion should be suspected and an emergent scrotal exploration for an acute scrotum is indicated.

Testicular Torsion

- Torsion of the testicle is the most common cause of acute scrotal pain in boys
- Suspect torsion in any patient with acute scrotal pain, swelling, or a high transverse-lying testis
- A scrotal ultrasound with color Doppler can confirm the diagnosis if the clinical diagnosis is unclear; however, do not wait for an ultrasound if testicular torsion is suspected—take the patient immediately to surgery
- Testicles should be explored within 6 hours to increase the salvage rate
- If the testicle is viable after torsion is reduced, orchiopexy should be performed
- If the testis is infarcted, an orchiectomy should be performed
- Orchiopexy of the contralateral testis is debated

An orchiopexy should always be performed following de-torsion of a testis.

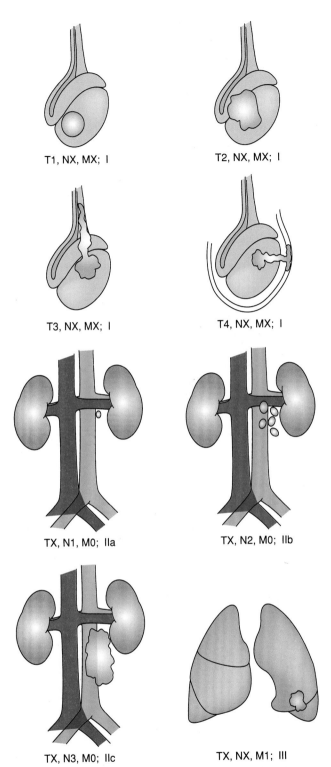

Staging of testicular cancer. (With permission from Mulholland MW, Lillemoe KD, Doherty GM, Maier RV, Upchurch GR, eds. *Greenfield's Surgery*. 4th ed. Philadelphia, PA: Lippincott Williams & Wilkins; 2005.)

T1, NX, MX; I

T2, NX, MX; I

T3, NX, MX; I

T4, NX, MX; I

TX, N1, M0; IIa

TX, N2, M0; IIb

TX, N3, M0; IIc

TX, NX, M1; III

Several months following a complicated abdominal perineal resection, a patient continues to have urinary retention. What is the most likely etiology?

Following radical pelvic surgery, voiding dysfunction can result from pelvic plexus injury.

Voiding Dysfunction from Radical Pelvic Surgery

- Patients can present with urinary incontinence or varying degrees of urinary retention
- Caused by injury to the pelvic plexus
- Requires clean intermittent catheterization
- Most dysfunctions are transient, but it can take 6 to 12 months for bladder function to improve
- Obtain a urodynamic study to assess bladder function

A 49-year-old female with a recently diagnosed history of multiple sclerosis presents with incontinence. She is able to void, but feels that she never fully empties her bladder. What tests should be performed for further examination?

Urodynamic studies.

Urinary Incontinence

- Stress incontinence
  - Occurs when the intra-abdominal pressure exceeds that of the urethral sphincter
  - Patients will often complain of incontinence after coughing
  - Treatment
    - Conservative: Kegel exercises
    - Surgical: Suburethral sling, retropubic urethropexy
- Urge incontinence
  - Due to detrusor muscle hyperactivity
  - Treatment
    - Conservative: Kegel exercises, decrease caffeine intake
    - Medication: Oxybutynin (anticholinergic)
    - Surgery: Augmentation cystoplasty (a segment of the bowel is used to augment the size of the bladder)
- Overflow incontinence
  - Inability to fully empty bladder
  - Risk factures: BPH, diseases of the spinal cord
  - Treatment
    - Medications to treat BPH
    - TURP
    - Intermittent catheterization

A 30-year-old female received an abdominal CT scan to evaluate her complaints of vague gastrointestinal discomfort. On the CT scan, large bilateral renal cysts are present which distort the normal renal contour. What the diagnosis is?

Autosomal dominant polycystic kidney disease (ADPKD).

Renal Cystic Disease

- Polycystic kidney disease
  - ADPKD is usually diagnosed in adults
  - It is generally progressive and is a common cause of end-stage renal disease

- On gross examination there are multiple, irregular, bilateral cysts
- Pancreatic and hepatic cysts can also occur
- ADPKD is associated with cerebral berry aneurysms
- 50% of infants who present with ADPKD will expire due to respiratory failure or sepsis
- Autosomal recessive polycystic kidney disease (ARPKD)
  - Presents in infancy/childhood
  - No gross cysts, only dilated collecting ducts and periportal fibrosis
  - Most often fatal due to pulmonary hypoplasia
- Multicystic dysplastic kidney
  - Common cause of an abdominal mass in a newborn
  - Can be seen on prenatal ultrasound
  - Distinguished from UPJ obstruction using ultrasound
  - The cysts of the multicystic kidney do not communicate
  - The contralateral kidney can have vesicoureteral reflux (30%)

A newborn male infant has a palpable left-sided abdominal mass. An ultrasound demonstrates UPJ obstruction. What is the next step in management?

Pyeloplasty is the treatment of choice for UPJ obstruction.

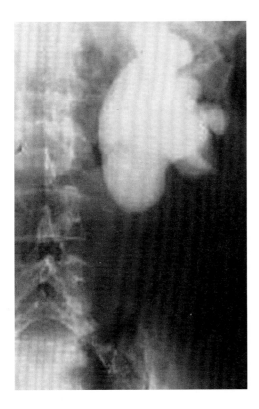

IVP showing hydronephrosis secondary to UPJ obstruction. (With permission from Mulholland MW, Lillemoe KD, Doherty GM, Maier RV, Upchurch GR, eds. *Greenfield's Surgery.* 4th ed. Philadelphia, PA: Lippincott Williams & Wilkins; 2005.)

Ureteropelvic Junction Obstruction

- Blockage of the ureter where it meets the renal pelvis; usually congenital from either an abnormality of the muscle itself or a crossing vessel
- Presents as an abdominal mass in a newborn

- Can be seen on prenatal ultrasound
- Can present later in life with flank pain or infection
- The diagnosis is made using ultrasound and a diuretic renal scan
- The treatment is pyeloplasty (surgical repair of the obstructed renal pelvis)

A 4-year-old female presents with a fever and left-sided pyelonephritis. Which imaging study is best to evaluate for vesicoureteral reflux?

A voiding cystourethrogram (VCUG).

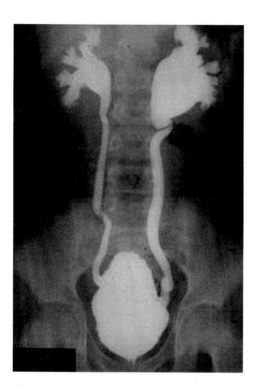

Voiding cystourethrogram showing bilateral VUR. (With permission from Mulholland MW, Lillemoe KD, Doherty GM, Maier RV, Upchurch GR, eds. *Greenfield's Surgery.* 4th ed. Philadelphia, PA: Lippincott Williams & Wilkins; 2005.)

Vesicoureteral Reflux

- Congenital condition caused by the ureteral bud coming off too close to the urogenital sinus on the mesonephric duct
  - The ureter has a short intravesical (intramural) length
  - The ureteral orifice is usually cephalad and lateral to its normal position at the trigone
- Urine travels retrograde from the bladder into the ureter and often into the kidney
- Evaluate for vesicoureteral reflux using ultrasound and VCUG in:
  - Any child with a febrile urinary infection
  - Any boy with a urinary infection
  - Any girl with recurrent urinary infections
- Hereditary, so be suspicious in siblings and screen with imaging studies
- Low grade reflux can be conservatively treated with observation and antibiotic prophylaxis with close follow-up; treat any voiding dysfunction

High-grade vesicoureteral reflux requires surgical intervention with ureteral re-implantation.

10 | Obstetrics and Gynecology

Ruchi Garg

> A 21-year-old gravida 1, para 0 female with a 15-week twin gestation presents with persistent nausea, vomiting, and intense right-sided abdominal pain accompanied by fevers and chills for 2 days. What is the most likely diagnosis?

Acute appendicitis is the most common surgical complication during pregnancy.

Surgical Issues in Pregnancy

- **Acute appendicitis**
  - Associated with obstetrical complications of preterm labor, spontaneous abortion and/or maternal mortality
  - Most classic signs of appendicitis (i.e., RLQ pain, rebound tenderness, obturator, psoas and/or Rovsing signs) are absent in pregnancy
  - Ultrasonography is a useful diagnostic tool
  - Laparoscopy may be used if the diagnosis is uncertain
- **Acute cholecystitis**
  - Second most common surgical complication of pregnancy
  - Pregnancy predisposes to cholelithiasis due to increased gallbladder volume, decreased intestinal motility, and delayed gallbladder emptying
  - Presentation is similar to non-pregnant patients
- **Adnexal/ovarian torsion or ruptured corpus luteum**
  - Rule out ectopic pregnancy
  - Treatment is surgical detorsion
  - An adnexectomy should be performed if necrosis is evident
- **Trauma in pregnancy**
  - The mother should be stabilized first!
  - Perform a CT scan if the patient is stable (ultrasonography is less useful in assessing injuries)
  - Laboratory tests should include an Rh status
  - A postmortem cesarean section may be performed if the fetus is viable

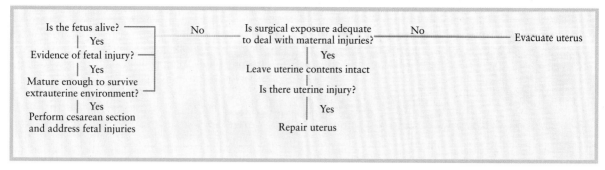

Algorithm for addressing maternal injuries with a gravid uterus. (With permission from Mulholland MW, Lillemoe KD, Doherty GM, Maier RV, Upchurch GR, eds. *Greenfield's Surgery*. 4th ed. Philadelphia, PA: Lippincott Williams & Wilkins; 2005.)

A 35-year-old gravida 5, para 4004 at 34 weeks of gestation presents with a complaint of bleeding (similar to menstrual bleeding) noted on her bed when she awoke in the morning. What is the next step in management?

Obtain a detailed history especially with regards to hypertension, drug abuse, and trauma, and perform a transabdominal pelvic ultrasound to determine the location of the placenta (transvaginal ultrasound is contraindicated).

Third Trimester Bleeding

- Affects 2% to 6% of all pregnancies
- Vaginal spotting may be secondary to massive hemorrhage
- Differential diagnosis: Vasa previa, placenta previa, abruptio placenta (placental abruption)

Vasa Previa

- Umbilical vein insertion into placental membranes instead of the central region of the placenta
- Bleeding occurs when one of these vessels ruptures near the internal os
- Associated with fetal hemorrhage leading to emergent delivery via cesarean section

Placenta Previa

- Implantation of the placenta partially or completely over the cervical os
- Presents as painless bright red vaginal bleeding
- Do NOT perform a vaginal exam! (speculum exam is ok)
- Achieve maternal and fetal hemodynamic stability followed by delivery (vaginal or cesarean)

A 28-year-old woman at 20 weeks of gestation presents to the emergency department following a motor vehicle crash. She is now having abdominal pain, severe lower abdominal tenderness, and contractions. Her physical examination is significant for blood in the vagina, uterine contractions, and a fetal heart rate of 75 bpm. What diagnostic step can confirm a placental abruption?

A Kleihauer-Betke test can confirm placental abruption. It detects fetal blood in the maternal circulation.

Placental Abruption

- Deceleration injury where the placenta separates from the uterus
- Can present as vaginal bleeding, abdominal tenderness, contractions, or fetal distress
- Non-trauma-related causes/risk factors include advanced maternal age, smoking, cocaine use, maternal hypertension, multiparity, and chorioamnionitis
- High fetal mortality
- Can test for the presence of fetal blood in the maternal circulation (Kleihauer-Betke test) to confirm the diagnosis
- Achieve maternal and fetal hemodynamic stability followed by delivery as indicated (vaginal or cesarean)

A 31-year-old pregnant woman presents to the emergency department following a motor vehicle crash. She is Rh-positive. She has multiple injuries but none involving the abdomen or pelvis. On ultrasound, the uterus is intact. What is the recommended management of her Rh-positive status?

Rh immunoglobulin therapy is only indicated in the pregnant, Rh-negative trauma patient.

Trauma in Pregnancy

- Blood loss can be significant without signs of shock due to increased blood volume in pregnancy
- Emergent C-section can be performed for worsening maternal condition
- All pregnant Rh-negative trauma patients should be considered for Rh immunoglobulin therapy unless the injury is remote from the uterus

Uterine Rupture

- The most common location is the posterior fundus
- Delivery of the baby may be indicated based on viability
- Aggressive resuscitation often required until uterus clamps down after delivery

An 18-year-old female presents with a history of foul-smelling discharge for 2 days with a sudden onset of lower abdominal pain for 1 day along with some nausea and vomiting. Her past medical history is remarkable for a sexual history of five partners and multiple sexually transmitted diseases. She has not had an appendectomy. What are the possible surgical emergencies that should be ruled out prior to making the above diagnosis?

While pelvic inflammatory disease (PID) is the most likely etiology of her illness, acute appendicitis and ectopic pregnancy must be immediately ruled out.

Pelvic Inflammatory Disease

- Most commonly multibacterial (e.g., *Neisseria gonorrhoeae*, *Chlamydia trachomatis*, bacterial vaginosis, *Escherichia coli*, *Actinomyces israelii*, *Mycoplasma hominis*)
- Absolute diagnostic criteria include bilateral adnexal pain and cervical motion tenderness
- Relative criteria include elevated WBC, erythrocyte sedimentation rate, vaginal discharge, and fevers
- Pelvic ultrasound is useful to look for hydrosalpinx, pyosalpinx, or a tubo-ovarian abscess

- Differential diagnosis: Ovarian torsion, appendicitis, ectopic pregnancy, diverticulitis, Crohn's disease, urinary tract infection, pyelonephritis, and nephrolithiasis in the differential diagnosis
- Outpatient treatment typically cefoxitin plus probenecid/doxycycline
- Inpatient treatment reserved for patients unable to tolerate oral intake or with complications
- Sequelae
  - Infertility due to tubal damage or adhesions
  - Tubo-ovarian abscess
    - Diagnosed by ultrasound
    - Treated with antibiotics
    - If does not resolve, proceed to surgical resection or radiological drain placement in premenopausal women
    - In postmenopausal women, perform a TAH-BSO because of the high incidence of cancer

---

A 22-year-old female was seen and diagnosed with a left ectopic pregnancy with some complex fluid in the cul-de-sac, but left against medical advice 4 hours ago with a hematocrit of 26. She has now returned with worsening pain and a hematocrit of 22. What is the next step in management?

Emergent operative salpingectomy or salpingostomy. An ectopic pregnancy is a true surgical emergency.

Ectopic Pregnancy

- A pregnancy implanted anywhere but the uterus (most commonly in the fallopian tubes)
- Risk factors include PID, previous ectopic pregnancy, presence of an intrauterine device (IUD), and diethylstilbestrol (DES) exposure
- Presents with a positive β-hCG and abdominal pain
- Ruptured ectopic pregnancies may present with shoulder pain, abdominal distention, and shock
- A physical exam may reveal a palpable adnexal mass (sometimes visible as an early fetus on ultrasound)
- Criteria for methotrexate treatment
  - Hemodynamically stable (no evidence of rupture)
  - Quantitative β-hCG <15,000
  - No evidence of liver or renal disease
  - Size <3.5 cm
  - Patient can be relied upon to take the medication
  - Pregnancy is not an intra-uterine
- If criteria for methotrexate treatment are not met, a surgical resection (salpingostomy or salpingectomy) is indicated
- Remember to look at the other fallopian tube at the time of surgery

---

A 26-year-old woman with regular menses is noted to have a firm mass in the cul-de-sac on a rectovaginal exam. The mass is slightly tender to palpation. Transvaginal ultrasonography reveals a 3 × 3 cm complex mass. What is the most appropriate next step in evaluation?

Follow up transvaginal ultrasonography in 3 months. CA-125 has a low sensitivity in premenopausal woman and should be ordered sparingly. OVA-1 test can be ordered in premenopausal women to triage and appropriately refer this patient.

Benign Ovarian Mass

- Ovarian masses less than 5 cm are generally benign
- Other signs of benign masses include simple cysts and unilateral cysts
- Common among premenopausal ovulating women
- Freely mobile

If discovered incidentally during a non-gynecological operation, do NOT perform a hysterectomy, bilateral salpingo-oophorectomy, or biopsy of the mass. If consent is already available and the mass has been discussed with the patient preoperatively, then a unilateral salpingo-oophorectomy may be appropriate.

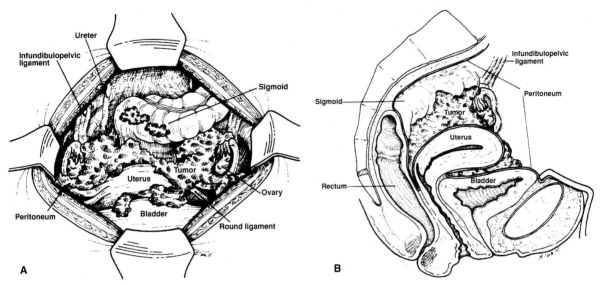

Anatomy of an ovarian tumor. (With permission from Fischer JE, Bland KI, Callery MP, et al., eds. *Mastery of Surgery.* 5th ed. Philadelphia, PA: Lippincott Williams & Wilkins; 2006.)

Ovarian Tumors

- A corpus luteum cyst (follicular cyst) spontaneously resolves within 3 months
- Granulosa theca cell tumor
  - 25% malignant
  - Produces sex hormones (excess estrogen) that may result in precocious puberty
  - 50% associated with endometrial hyperplasia and 5% to 15% associated with endometrial cancer
    - Patient may present with abnormal vaginal bleeding
  - Inhibin levels may be elevated
- Mucinous cystadenoma
  - 30% malignant
  - Notorious for their capacity to grow to a very large size
- Serous cystadenoma
  - 10% malignant (serous cystadenocarcinoma)
  - Most common benign neoplasm of the ovary
- Sertoli-Leydig tumor
  - Secretes testosterone

- Symptoms: Virilization → hirsutism, temporal balding, hypertrophy of the clitoris, hoarseness, and breast atrophy
  - Benign cystic teratomas (a.k.a., mature teratoma or dermoid)
    - Most common between 10 and 20 years
    - Most common ovarian tumor in pregnancy
    - 15% bilateral
    - Can reach 20 cm in size
      - Rarely malignant (5%)
  - The most common malignant form is dysgerminoma with a 5-year survival rate of 70%
    - Symptoms
      - Precocious pseudo-puberty
    - Diagnosis
      - May secrete hCG or α-fetoprotein (AFP)
      - Positive pregnancy test in the absence of pregnancy
    - Treat with surgical resection in premenopausal women (if histology shows malignancy, operative staging is required)
    - Treat with an oophorectomy in postmenopausal women
    - Remember to examine the contralateral ovary
  - Choriocarcinoma
    - Malignant trophoblastic proliferation
    - Follows a hydatidiform molar pregnancy
    - Secretes hCG
    - Treatment: Chemotherapy; total hysterectomy if necessary
  - Dysgerminoma (germ cell tumor)
    - Comprise less than 5% of all ovarian cancers; however, in children and adolescents, more than 60% of ovarian neoplasms are germ cell tumors and 1/3 are malignant
    - Lymphatic spread
    - Seminomas are the most radiosensitive

An ovarian vein thrombosis diagnosed by CT scan should be treated with anticoagulation therapy.

A 50-year-old woman presents with a complaint of sudden-onset excruciating left lower quadrant pain that is intermittent and worse with movement. She does not report any other complaints. She does report having been told that she has ovarian cysts and diverticulosis. The workup was only significant for a 7-cm complex cyst on the left ovary with good blood flow seen on pelvic ultrasound. What is the next step in management?

Surgical resection of the cyst. The consent for the procedure should include consent for staging for an ovarian malignancy, if discovered.

Ovarian Cancer

- Staging of ovarian cancer
  - I: Growth limited to ovaries
  - II: Growth involving one or both ovaries with pelvic extension

- III: Cancer with peritoneal implants outside the pelvis; positive retroperitoneal or inguinal nodes; superficial liver metastases; or tumor limited to the true pelvis but with histologically proven extension to the small bowel or omentum
  - IV: Distant metastases, parenchymal liver extension, or positive pleural effusion cytology
- Epidemiology
  - 75% 5-year survival with stage I disease
  - 10% to 25% 5-year survival with stage III disease
- Surgical staging includes
  - Peritoneal washings
  - Total hysterectomy with removal of both tubes and ovaries
  - Omentectomy
  - Diaphragmatic and peritoneal biopsies
  - Lymph node dissection
  - ± Appendectomy
- Debulking surgery may yield an improved survival benefit when used in conjunction with chemotherapy
- Meigs syndrome
  - Hydrothorax, ascites, ovarian cancer
  - Patients present with shortness of breath and abdominal distention
  - Treatment: Pleural catheter
- Pseudomyxoma peritonei
  - Spread of mucinous tumors to peritoneal surfaces
  - Results in the abdomen being filled with mucin
  - Patients are at high risk for small bowel obstruction

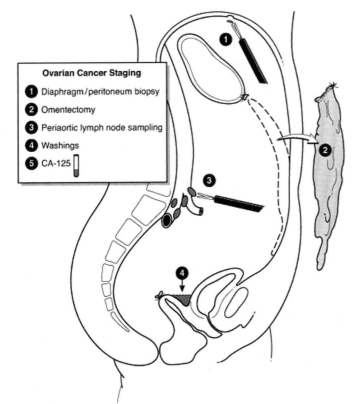

Maneuvers in ovarian cancer staging.

Ovarian Cancer Staging
1. Diaphragm/peritoneum biopsy
2. Omentectomy
3. Periaortic lymph node sampling
4. Washings
5. CA-125

> A 30-year-old female has a history of chronic pelvic pain and is now having difficulty with infertility. She has no history of sexually transmitted diseases or PID and has only had one sexual partner. She has normal periods. What is the next step in diagnosis?

Her symptoms are consistent with endometriosis, which can lead to chronic pelvic pain and infertility. Initial diagnosis can be made with ultrasound or MRI. If these are not conclusive, an exploratory laparoscopy can be performed.

Endometrioma/Endometriosis

- Symptoms include cyclical or constant pain due to adhesions and infertility
- Diagnosis is made by surgical biopsy
  - Grossly, lesions resemble "chocolate cysts"
  - Pathology must show two out of three criteria: Endometrial glands, endometrial stroma, or hemosiderin-laden macrophages
- Treatment includes nonsteroidal anti-inflammatory drugs, oral contraceptives, lupron (GnRH agonist) for 3 to 6 months, laser ablation, lysis of adhesions (for infertility), or hysterectomy

> A 23-year-old woman is diagnosed with invasive cervical cancer. What virus types are highly associated with cervical cancer?

HPV is associated with 99.6% of cervical cancers. Human papillomavirus (HPV) types 16 and 18 are associated with 70% of cervical cancers. Vaginal and vulvar cancers are also associated with these strains.

Cervical Cancer

- Second most common cancer of the female reproductive system
- A Pap smear is only about 50% sensitive (and there is a 15% to 20% false negative rate)
- Mean age for women with invasive cervical cancer is 45 to 55 years
- Most common presenting symptom is postcoital, painless vaginal bleeding
- Staging based on physical exam, cystoscopy, proctoscopy, CXR, and IVP
  - I: Limited to the cervix
  - II: Spread to the vagina but does not involve the lower 1/3
    - IIa: Spread to upper 2/3 of the vagina
    - IIb: Involves the parametria
  - III: Spread to the lower 1/3 of the vagina
    - IIIa: Spread to lower 1/3 of the vagina
    - IIIb: Extends to pelvic sidewall and/or hydronephrosis
  - IV: Distant spread
    - IVa: Spread to bladder or rectum
    - IVb: Distant metastasis
- The obturator lymph nodes are often the first nodes involved
- The pretreatment evaluation for stage IIB or higher includes CXR, IVP or cystoscopy, sigmoidoscopy, CT or PET scan
- Treatment
  - Surgical

- Simple hysterectomy or radical hysterectomy for stage I
- Oophorectomy only if patient >50 years of age or has ovarian pathology
- Consider a pelvic exenteration for recurrent central disease
- Chemoradiation or radiation alone
  - Used for patients who are not good surgical candidates and who have advanced disease (stages II–IV)
  - Radiation alone can be used in post-hysterectomy patients with high-risk features for recurrence
  - The most commonly used chemotherapy agent is cisplatin
  - Whole pelvic radiation with additional brachytherapy is commonly used

Vaginal Cancer

- Fewer than 2% of gynecologic malignancies
- Usually in the upper half of the vagina
- Clear cell vaginal adenocarcinoma is associated with DES exposure in utero
- Diagnosis usually made by an abnormal Pap smear and colposcopic evaluation
- The treatment is a partial vaginectomy or total vaginectomy and/or radiation
- 5-year survival is 40% to 55%

Vulvar Cancer

- Predominantly in older women
- Criteria for local excision
  - <2 cm in diameter
  - <1 mm deep
  - Negative nodes (biopsy all palpable lymph nodes >1 cm)
- If criteria for local excision not met, perform radical vulvectomy with unilateral or bilateral inguinal or femoral lymph node dissection
- Complications of surgery include lymphedema, urinary or stress incontinence, cystocele, and rectocele
- The 5-year survival for patients with stage I and II disease treated by surgery is 90%

During an exploration for a colon cancer in a 55-year-old female, a large, firm mass is found in the left ovary. What is the next step in management?

If appropriate consents are available then perform a unilateral salpingo-oophorectomy and send the ovaries to pathology to rule out a Krukenberg tumor versus primary ovarian malignancy.

Krukenberg Tumor

- A malignancy metastatic to the ovary from the GI tract, breast, or uterus
- Usually bilateral and freely mobile
- Retains the shape of the ovaries and can be very large
- Histology shows mucin-secreting signet ring cells
- 5% of what preoperatively appears to be ovarian malignancies are actually metastases from other tumors

All patients with a suspected ovarian malignancy and GI symptoms should undergo an upper GI series, barium enema, or endoscopy prior to laparotomy.

A 17-year-old nulligravid adolescent girl is operated on for presumed appendicitis. Intraoperatively she is found to have a twisted right ovarian solid mass about 6 × 6 cm in size. A salpingo-oophorectomy is performed and a frozen section analysis reveals a malignant ovarian germ cell tumor. There is no other gross evidence of disease. What is the next step in operative management?

Surgical staging with preservation of the uterus and the contralateral tube and ovary should be performed.

Germ Cell Tumors

- Mean age at diagnosis is 21
- Types
  - Pure dysgerminoma (most common)
  - Immature teratoma
  - Endodermal sinus tumor
  - Mixed type
- 60% stage I at diagnosis and 30% stage III/IV at diagnosis
- Spreads to peritoneum and lymph nodes
- Types of germ cell tumors
  - Immature teratoma
    - ±AFP/LDH
    - 95% with abdominal pain
  - Dysgerminoma
    - 90% cure rate
    - ↑LDH
    - ±hCG
    - Multinucleated syncytiotrophoblastic giant cells, lymphocytes
  - Gonadoblastoma
    - Check chromosomes—46XX
    - Streak ovaries—BSO
  - Endodermal sinus tumors (yolk sac tumor)
    - AFP, ±LDH, hCG
  - Embryonal and polyembryonal
    - hCG, AFP
  - Monodermal teratomas
    - Thyroid, carcinoid, and neuroectodermal
  - Treat all with adjuvant therapy except for stage I dysgerminoma and stage I grade I immature teratoma
  - Chemotherapy regimens
    - VAC—vincristine, actinomycin-D, cyclophosphamide
    - PVB—Cisplatin, vinblastin, bleomycin
    - BEP—Cisplatin, etoposide, bleomycin—equal efficacy as PVB with less toxicity
  - 80% to 90% resume normal menses after treatment
  - 95% cure with stage I and 75% cure in advanced stage
  - Most recurrences within 24 months

> A 54-year-old postmenopausal woman who has not used hormonal therapy has had persistent spotting for the past 8 months. What is the most appropriate next step in management?

An endometrial biopsy to rule out malignancy should be performed. Endometrial cancer is the most common gynecologic malignancy.

Endometrial Cancer

- 80% of women diagnosed are postmenopausal (5% are under age 40)
- Most women diagnosed have stage I disease with a 5-year survival rate of at least 75%
- Risk factors
  - Late menopause
  - Nulliparity
  - Unopposed estrogen
  - Obesity
  - Hypertension
  - Diabetes
- Hallmark symptom: Abnormal vaginal bleeding (i.e., postmenopausal bleeding, intermenstrual bleeding, or heavy menses)
- An office endometrial biopsy with a pipelle or an intraoperative fractional dilation and curettage can be diagnostic
- Pelvic ultrasound is useful to evaluate the endometrium
- The recommended therapy is total hysterectomy with removal of both tubes and ovaries, peritoneal washings, and lymph node dissection
- Adjuvant chemotherapy and tumor-directed radiation is given to patients with metastases to pelvic lymph nodes, poorly differentiated tumors, invasion deep into the myometrium, or occult cervical involvement

> A 64-year-old postmenopausal woman presents with excruciating pain and an inability to void. This occurred after she felt some pressure and noted a prolapsing necrotic mass from her vagina. What is the most likely diagnosis?

A prolapsing necrotic mass in a postmenopausal woman suggests uterine sarcoma.

Uterine Sarcoma

- Poor prognosis
- Presenting symptom is vaginal bleeding
- Tissue may protrude/prolapse through the cervical os
- Recommended therapy is total hysterectomy with removal of both tubes and ovaries, peritoneal washings, and lymph node dissection
- Postoperative radiation and/or chemotherapy as indicated
- 5-year survival is approximately 30%

Gestational Trophoblastic Disease

- Spectrum of tumors including complete hydatidiform mole, partial hydatidiform mole, placental site trophoblastic tumor, and choriocarcinoma
- Complete mole

- Lacks fetal tissue
- 46XX
- All chromosomes are of paternal origin
- Partial mole
  - Identifiable fetal parts
  - Triploid karyotype due to an extra set of chromosomes of paternal origin
- Usually presents with abnormal vaginal bleeding
- "Snowstorm" pattern on ultrasound
- The treatment is uterine evacuation with suction curettage
  - Need to be prepared with type and cross
  - Check Rh status
  - Administer pitocin as the evacuation is begun
- Follow β-hCG levels until zero
- May need chemotherapy
  - Actinomycin-D
  - Methotrexate
  - EMACO (for advanced or resistant disease)—etoposide, methotrexate, actinomycin-D, cyclophosphamide, Oncovin

11 Thyroid and Parathyroid

Rebecca S. Sippel and Herbert Chen

A 45-year-old woman presents with a palpable thyroid nodule. What is the next step in management?

A fine needle aspiration (FNA) is an excellent initial test to evaluate a thyroid nodule.

Fine Needle Aspiration (FNA) of Neck Mass

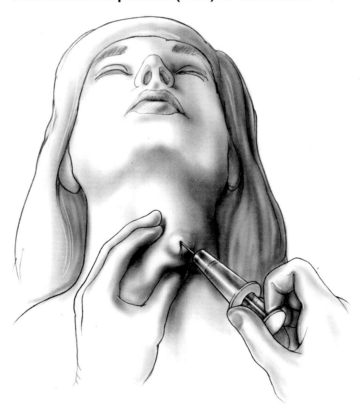

FNA of a thyroid nodule is performed with a fine gauge needle. This can be performed by palpation, but is best done under ultrasound guidance.

Thyroid Nodule Evaluation

- History
  - Family history (goiter, MEN, thyroid cancer)
  - History of radiation
  - Symptoms: Hyper/hypothyroid, compressive symptoms
- Physical exam
  - Characteristics of the nodule and the gland
  - Voice changes
  - Lymph node status
- Diagnostic tests
  - Ultrasound to document size and to look for additional nodules
  - FNA, ideally under ultrasound guidance
  - Thyroid scintigraphy if there is a concern of hyperthyroidism (suppressed TSH)
  - Blood tests depending on history (T3/T4, TSH, thyroglobulin, thyroid antibodies, calcitonin, calcium)
    - TSH is the only screening test needed in a patient without symptoms of hyper- or hypothyroidism
    - If concern of clinical hyper- or hypothyroidism, free T4 is preferred to total T4 as it is not affected by levels of thyroid-binding globulin

An FNA can often distinguish benign from malignant tumors and is considered to be the gold standard initial test for the evaluation of thyroid nodules.

A 38-year-old woman is found to have a benign thyroid nodule upon FNA. What is the next step in management?

Observation is appropriate in the absence of symptoms.

Benign Thyroid Nodule

- Usually represents one of the following:
  - Adenomatous or hyperplastic nodule
  - Hashimoto thyroiditis
  - Colloid cyst
- Follow with repeat imaging in 1 year
  - Repeat FNA if nodule grows >2 mm in two dimensions
  - Refer for surgery if symptomatic or if suspicion of malignancy
  - T4 replacement only given to treat hypothyroidism (do not give to euthyroid patients)

What percent of FNAs performed for thyroid lesions are malignant?

5% are malignant and 75% are benign (20% are suspicious or nondiagnostic).

Malignant Thyroid Nodule

- Cancer type can sometimes be identified on FNA
- All malignant or suspicious results should be followed up with surgery

---

> A patient with a thyroid goiter underwent thyroid function testing. What is a normal T4/T3 ratio?

A normal T4/T3 ratio is 10:1 or 20:1.

Thyroid Function Tests

- Measuring levels of thyroid-stimulating hormone (TSH) is the best test of thyroid function
- A normal T4:T3 ratio is 10:1 or 20:1 (although T3 is three times more active than T4)
- Thyroglobulin stores T3 and T4 in colloid
- Most T3 is made in the periphery by conversion from T4 (by peroxidases)
- The half-life of T3 is 1 to 3 days
- The half-life of T4 is 7 days

TSH levels provide the most sensitive indication of gland function.

> A 44-year-old woman presents with an enlarged thyroid gland and pretibial edema. Lab tests reveal an undetectable level of TSH. What is the most likely diagnosis?

Graves' disease presents with goiter and signs and symptoms of hyperthyroidism.

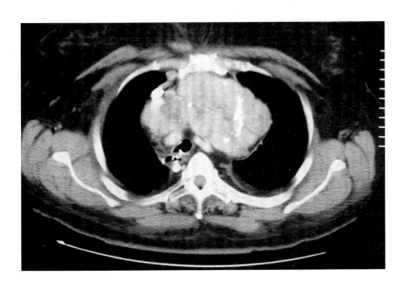

Large multinodular goiter with substernal component. (With permission from Mulholland MW, Lillemoe KD, Doherty GM, Maier RV, Upchurch GR, eds. *Greenfield's Surgery.* 4th ed. Philadelphia, PA: Lippincott Williams & Wilkins; 2005.)

Graves Disease

- The most common cause of hyperthyroidism
- Autoimmune IgG antibody to the TSH receptor
- Diagnosis
  - Signs and symptoms include tremors, hyperreflexia, tachycardia, a-fib, thyroid enlargement, palpitation, nervousness, heat intolerance, pretibial edema, weight loss, and hair loss
  - Exophthalmos is characteristic (and may not resolve with treatment)
  - Labs show decreased or undetectable TSH, elevated T3, T4, and thyroid antibodies (TRAB—TSH receptor antibody, TSI—thyroid-stimulating immunoglobulins)
  - A thyroid scan will reveal a diffuse goiter with high radiolabel uptake
  - Obtain an ultrasound to rule out focal nodules—this is essential if cold nodules are identified on the uptake scan

Graves disease is the most common cause of hyperthyroidism.

> A 33-year-old woman with Graves' disease and severe ocular involvement has failed medical therapy. What is the next step in management?

Preoperative preparation with anti-thyroid medications (until euthyroid), beta blockade if needed, and Lugol's solution, followed by thyroidectomy.

Treatment for Graves Disease

- Radioactive iodine is the most common therapy in the United States (except in children, pregnant women, and in those with Graves ocular disease)
  - Good for patients in whom medication has failed but no clear surgical indication exists
  - Pre-treat with anti-thyroid medications to establish a euthyroid state for 3 to 4 weeks if significant hyperthyroidism; discontinue medications 3 to 5 days prior to iodine treatment
  - Oral iodine-131
  - 80-90% cure rate
  - 40% to 90% become hypothyroid after treatment
- Medical therapy: Propylthiouracil (PTU) and methimazole
  - Inhibits the iodination of tyrosine residues in the thyroid
  - If unable to wean medications off by 18 months, will likely need definitive management or lifelong treatment.
  - Use PTU in the first trimester of pregnancy, otherwise utilize methimazole
  - Can be associated with hepatotoxicity and agranulocytosis
- Surgery: Total (or subtotal) thyroidectomy
  - Indications
    - Children
    - Women who want to become pregnant or are breastfeeding
    - Need for rapid control (e.g., acute control of cardiac problems)
    - Compressive symptoms
    - If unable to rule out malignancy (suspicious nodule)
    - Failure of medical management (especially in pregnancy)
    - Non-compliant patients
    - Patient preference for surgical management
  - Pre-op preparation
    - PTU or methimazole until euthyroid
    - Lugol's (iodine) solution for 10 to 15 days pre-op to decrease the friability and vascularity (Start after the patient is euthyroid!)
    - β-blocker pre-op if significant tachycardia

Radioactive iodine may worsen Graves' eye disease.

> A 49-year-old woman with a goiter has vomiting and mental status changes following an elective hernia repair. On further evaluation, she is found to have a temperature of 39.2°C, a heart rate of 165 bpm, and manic symptoms. What is the next step in treatment?

Emergent medical therapy for a thyroid storm.

Thyroid Storm

- A life-threatening condition
- Can occur following elective surgery in patients with uncontrolled or unrecognized hyperthyroidism
- Prevented by ensuring a euthyroid state before any surgery
- Treat with emergent
  - Fluid resuscitation
  - Anti-thyroid medications (PTU blocks the synthesis of thyroxine)
  - Beta blockade
  - Hypothermia
- Iodine solutions and steroids can also be used

What are the indications for operating on a benign goiter?

- Development of thyrotoxicosis
- Compressive symptoms
- Suspicion of malignancy
- Cosmetic concerns

A 40-year-old female presents with a tender and enlarged thyroid gland following a recent upper respiratory tract infection. What is the next step in management?

An ultrasound can help identify the need for urgent incision and drainage for a localized abscess. Both acute suppurative thyroiditis and subacute thyroiditis may present with unilateral tenderness following an upper respiratory tract infection.

The Tender Goiter

- Acute (suppurative) thyroiditis
  - Due to bacterial infection—most commonly staph or strep
  - Rare
  - Presents with fever, redness, fluctuance, and elevated WBC
    - Have normal thyroid function tests
  - Ultrasound can localize the abscess
  - Treatment is operative incision and drainage
- Subacute thyroiditis
  - De Quervain thyroiditis
    - Due to a viral infection
    - Have a URI prodrome and a painful, enlarged thyroid
    - Lab tests: $\uparrow$fT4, $\downarrow$TSH, and $\uparrow$ESR
    - Treatment is nonsteroidal anti-inflammatory drugs and occasionally steroids
    - Usually self-limited (2 to 3 weeks)
  - Post-partum thyroiditis
    - Autoimmune
    - Patients are usually asymptomatic

- Lab tests: ↑fT4, ↓TSH, and *normal* ESR
- Treat symptoms of hyperthyroidism
- Chronic thyroiditis
  - Hashimoto thyroiditis (see below)
  - Riedel thyroiditis
    - Autoimmune
    - Symptoms: Woody, enlarged thyroid that can cause compressive symptoms of the airway or esophagus
      - Associated with sclerosing cholangitis, retroperitoneal fibrosis, and other fibrotic diseases
    - Diagnosis: Lymphocytic infiltration of thyroid
    - Treatment
      - Tamoxifen or steroids
      - Surgery (isthmectomy or tracheostomy) for compressive symptoms

---

A 45-year-old woman with no significant medical history presents to your office complaining of excessive fatigue. Notably, 2 months ago, she had more energy than she had ever had and was having palpitations. At that time, she also lost 5 pounds. Then, over the last 2 months, she had a slow decline in her energy that was also associated with weight gain. Her mother has a history of systemic lupus erythematosus. What is the patient's most likely diagnosis?

She has Hashimoto thyroiditis.

Hashimoto Thyroiditis

- The most common cause of hypothyroidism in adults
- Autoimmune disease affecting the thyroid
- Labs
  - Anti-Tg and anti-thyroperoxidase antibodies
    - Have both humoral and cell-mediated immune disease due to microsomal and thyroglobulin antibodies
  - ↑TSH, ↓fT4; ↑ESR (early in course may present with transient period of hyperthyroidism—low TSH and elevated fT4)
  - Decreased iodine uptake on radionuclide scan
- Treatment
  - Treat hypothyroidism with thyroxine
  - Can do surgical treatment if there are compressive symptoms or concern for malignancy

---

A 55-year-old woman with a history of radiation therapy for acne presents with a 2.5-cm firm thyroid mass. It is not tender on physical exam. An FNA of an enlarged lateral neck lymph node reveals normal thyroid tissue. What is the next step in management?

Papillary thyroid cancer is the most common type of thyroid cancer and radiation exposure is the most important risk factor. Based on the size of the tumor, the history of radiation, and the patient's age, a total thyroidectomy is indicated. In addition, a lymph node dissection is indicated because a metastatic lymph node is present.

Papillary Thyroid Cancer

- It is the most common thyroid cancer (85%), but has the best prognosis (>92% 10-yr survival)
- Usually multicentric (50%)
- Papillary cancer spreads via lymphatics first, but nodal status does not predict survival
- Rarely metastasizes
  - The lung is the most common site for distant metastasis
- For a lesion <1.0 cm in a low-risk patient (unifocal, intrathyroidal, no radiation exposure, young age) lobectomy alone may be adequate
- For a lesion >1.0 cm, patients >45, or with a history of radiation, or extracapsular invasion, treatment is a total thyroidectomy
- Advantage of a total thyroidectomy: Can monitor for recurrence with thyroid scans and thyroglobulin levels
- A preoperative ultrasound to evaluate for lymphadenopathy is the standard of care and suspicious nodes should undergo preoperative FNA
- A positive regional lymph node requires an ipsilateral lymph node dissection
- Remove involved nodes en bloc with a compartment-oriented dissection
- Treat high risk patients post-operatively with radioactive iodine followed by T4 suppression

---

What are the features of papillary thyroid cancer on FNA?

- Psammoma bodies
- Intranuclear grooves and inclusions
- Prominent nucleoli
- Overlapping and optically clear nuclei ("Orphan Annie eyes")

Psammoma bodies are characteristic of papillary thyroid cancer.

What is the most important factor in the prognosis of thyroid cancer?

The most important prognostic factor is age.

What is the prognosis of thyroid cancer in children?

The prognosis is excellent. There is a 95% 10-yr survival (even though 50% to 80% have cervical lymph node metastases).

A 64-year old woman has a firm, nontender thyroid mass that is indeterminate by FNA cytology. A repeat FNA is performed and is also indeterminate. What is the next step in management of the thyroid mass?

An indeterminate FNA result should be followed up with a repeat FNA as in this case. If the FNA is indeterminate twice, then consider a thyroid lobectomy for diagnosis.

> A 44-year-old woman presents with a palpable mass in her thyroid. FNA reveals a follicular neoplasm. What is the next step in management?

Any patient with a follicular neoplasm found on FNA should undergo a diagnostic thyroid lobectomy. FNA is unable to distinguish benign from malignant lesions. Up to 20% of all follicular neoplasms are carcinomas.

Follicular Thyroid Adenoma and Cancer

- 80% are benign and 20% are malignant
- FNA is unreliable and cannot distinguish between benign and malignant
- Frozen section is also unreliable
- Surgery is often required for diagnosis—operation is a thyroid lobectomy and isthmectomy (no frozen section)
- A cancer diagnosis is made on evidence of capsular and vascular invasion
- A completion total thyroidectomy should be performed for a cancer >1 cm
- Unilateral lymph node dissection is reserved for involved nodes identified on physical exam, ultrasound, or intraoperative inspection—RARE
- Hematogenous spread is more common, especially to bone and lung
- Follicular CA should be treated with post-op radioactive iodine

Frozen section is usually unreliable with follicular thyroid cancer.

> A 4-year-old boy with a nontender thyroid mass is found to have an elevated calcitonin level upon laboratory testing. What is the most likely diagnosis?

An elevated calcitonin level in the setting of a thyroid mass is very concerning for a diagnosis of medullary thyroid cancer. Medullary thyroid cancer may be the first manifestation of MEN IIa or MEN IIb in children.

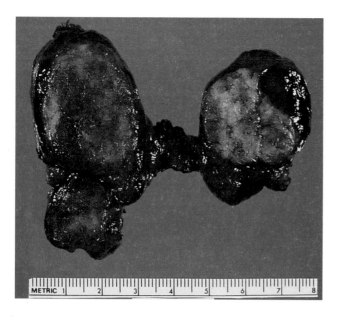

Medullary thyroid carcinoma. (With permission from Mulholland MW, Lillemoe KD, Doherty GM, Maier RV, Upchurch GR, eds. *Greenfield's Surgery*. 4th ed. Philadelphia, PA: Lippincott Williams & Wilkins; 2005.)

Medullary Thyroid Cancer

- Arise from parafollicular C cells of neural crest origin
  - C cells secrete calcitonin (can cause flushing and diarrhea)

- Amyloid found on pathology
- Treatment
  - TOTAL thyroidectomy and central lymph node dissection
  - Also perform an ipsilateral neck dissection for abnormal lateral neck nodes identified on imaging
  - T4 replacement is needed post-operatively (no role for radioactive iodine or TSH suppression)
- Operate by age 1 for MEN IIB (by age 5 for MEN IIA)
- Follow the patient postoperatively with serial calcitonin and carcinoembryonic antigen levels
- Liver, bone, or lung metastases may not be curable (unlike in papillary and follicular cancer)
- Should perform genetic testing for the RET proto-oncogene mutation
  - If positive, test family members
- Should test for MEN II associated conditions (pheochromocytoma and hyperparathyroidism) prior to surgery

It is important to rule out a pheochromocytoma prior to thyroidectomy for medullary thyroid cancer so that, if found, the pheochromocytoma can be resected first.

Medullary thyroid cancer is the most common initial manifestation of MEN II syndrome.

A 72-year-old man is found to have a Hürthle cell carcinoma with metastasis to a local lymph node. What is the operation of choice?

Total thyroidectomy with lymph node dissection.

Hürthle Cell Carcinoma

- Often considered a variant of follicular carcinoma
- Difficult to distinguish adenomas from carcinomas by FNA or frozen section
- High incidence of invasion with size >4 cm
- Treatment is total thyroidectomy plus a lymph node dissection if nodes are positive
- Radioactive iodine is used for ablation of remaining tissue
- There is only a minimal role for therapeutic radioactive iodine since most Hürthle cell cancers are not responsive

A 68-year-old man with metastatic anaplastic thyroid cancer presents with dyspnea and dysphagia secondary to his large thyroid mass. What is the next step in management?

Anaplastic thyroid cancer is a very aggressive tumor. A debulking surgery can be performed if the lesion is felt to be resectable. If the lesion is not felt to be resectable, then urgent radiation therapy can help to relieve airway obstruction.

Anaplastic Thyroid Cancer

- An FNA can be diagnostic
- Can be confused with Reidel thyroiditis
- Treat most with chemotherapy and radiation since most are at an advanced stage
- Debulking surgery is used for severe compressive symptoms or if the disease is caught early and is confined to the thyroid
- 10-year survival is <2%

A 41-year-old woman has a thyroidectomy for a well-differentiated papillary thyroid cancer with pulmonary metastasis. What is the next step in the management of her cancer?

This patient should be treated with radioactive iodine. Follow TSH levels until they peak at 3 to 6 weeks post-operatively at which point radioactive iodine treatment is best performed. Administration of (short-acting) cytomel (T3) in the interim can help prevent symptoms of hypothyroidism.

Indications for Radioiodine Therapy

- Regional, or distant metastases
- Inoperable cancer
- Residual cancer following surgery (positive margin)
- High risk for recurrence (tumor >4 cm, older age, aggressive histology, extra thyroidal extension)
- Recurrent cancer for well-differentiated papillary or follicular thyroid cancers, not amenable to surgery

Timing of Post-Operative Iodine Therapy

- An elevated TSH is needed to optimize an iodine scan. There are two ways to achieve this:
  - Thyroid hormone withdrawal—TSH peaks 3 to 6weeks post-op when off of thyroid hormone
    - An ideal TSH is >30 mIU/L prior to radioactive iodine therapy
    - Administration of cytomel (T3) in the meantime can minimize symptoms of hypothyroidism while awaiting clearance of T4 post-operatively (T3 has a shorter half-life)
    - Cytomel (T3) must be discontinued prior to initiating radioiodine therapy
  - Administration of recombinant TSH given as an injection on the 2 days prior to treatment causing the TSH to rise prior to therapy

Side Effects of Radioiodine Therapy

- Infertility
- Sialadenitis
- Pancytopenia
- GI complaints

A 48-year-old man presents to the office 1 year following a total thyroidectomy and I-131 ablation for well-differentiated thyroid cancer. What is the best test to follow for recurrent disease?

Follow-up 1 year after resection should include a neck ultrasound and a stimulated thyroglobulin level (either stimulated via thyroid hormone withdrawal or recombinant TSH administration). Serum thyroglobulin should be undetectable following total thyroidectomy and iodine ablation.

Thyroglobulin

- Glycoprotein made by normal or neoplastic thyroid tissue
- Undetectable following total thyroidectomy/thyroid remnant ablation
  - Thus it is a good tumor marker to follow patients post-operatively
- If detectable, and the neck ultrasound is negative, then do an I-131 scan:
  - If scan is positive, treat with I-131 if microscopic disease
  - If scan is negative, do CT and/or PET scan

- If macroscopic disease is found, resect
- Suppress T4 with L-thyroxine long-term

> A 29-year-old man presents with an asymptomatic thyroid mass. FNA demonstrates a thyroid lymphoma. What is the next step in management?

Appropriate staging for lymphoma and radiation ± chemo depending on the stage. Hashimoto thyroiditis increases the risk of thyroid lymphoma.

Treatment of Thyroid Lymphoma
- Radiation therapy for Stage I or II
- Radiation therapy + chemotherapy for Stage III or IV
- Surgery for palliation or obstructive symptoms in rare situations, and occasionally for treatment of localized disease

> What is the blood supply of the thyroid gland?

- Superior thyroid artery: First branch of the external carotid artery; divides into a superior and posterior branch just before entering the thyroid
- Inferior thyroid artery: Branch of the thyrocervical trunk off of the subclavian
- Thyroid ima artery: Present in 12% of people; originates from the innominate, internal mammary or the aortic arch

> Three months following a total thyroidectomy, a patient notes she is unable to sing high-pitched notes. Which nerve was most likely injured?

The external branch of the superior laryngeal nerve is responsible for high-pitched sounds via the cricothyroid muscle.

Nerves at Risk in Thyroid and Parathyroid Surgery
- Superior laryngeal nerve
  - External branch: Motor to the cricothyroid muscle
  - Lies adjacent to the vascular pedicle of the superior thyroid vessels
  - Injury to the external branch is usually minimally symptomatic (may lose vocal projection/ high pitch)
- Recurrent laryngeal nerve
  - Next to the inferior thyroid artery (nerve is posterior and medial)
  - Motor function to the vocal cord abductors
  - Unilateral injury: Hoarseness and/or swallowing difficulties
  - Bilateral injury: Cords adducted and airway occluded, causing stridor

> A 47-year-old female is found to have a calcium level of 12.1 following an episode of nephrolithiasis. What other test should she undergo?

The diagnosis of primary hyperparathyroidism is based on an elevated serum calcium and parathyroid hormone (PTH) level.

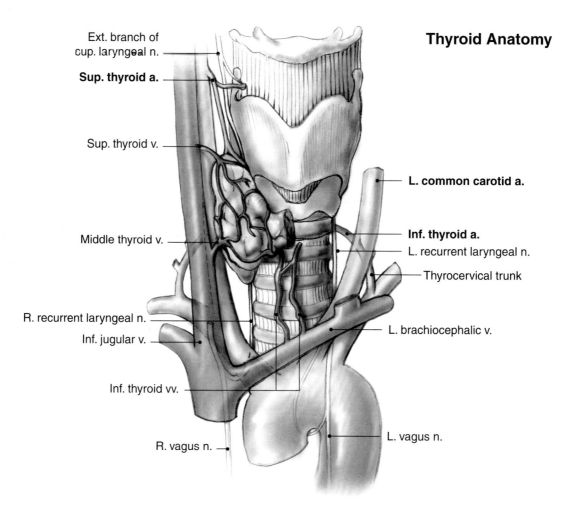

Thyroid Anatomy

Ext. branch of cup. laryngeal n.

Sup. thyroid a.

Sup. thyroid v.

Middle thyroid v.

R. recurrent laryngeal n.

Inf. jugular v.

Inf. thyroid vv.

R. vagus n.

L. common carotid a.

Inf. thyroid a.

L. recurrent laryngeal n.

Thyrocervical trunk

L. brachiocephalic v.

L. vagus n.

Anatomy of the thyroid region demonstrating the arterial and venous drainage of the thyroid gland.

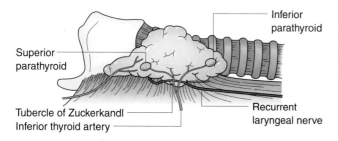

Superior parathyroid

Inferior parathyroid

Tubercle of Zuckerkandl

Inferior thyroid artery

Recurrent laryngeal nerve

Relationship of recurrent laryngeal nerve to thyroid. (With permission from Mulholland MW, Lillemoe KD, Doherty GM, Maier RV, Upchurch GR, eds. *Greenfield's Surgery*. 4th ed. Philadelphia, PA: Lippincott Williams & Wilkins; 2005.)

Primary Hyperparathyroidism

- More common in older women
- The PRAD-1 oncogene is associated with large adenomas
- Caused by an adenoma (80%), multiple adenomas (5%), or hyperplasia (15%)
- Hyperplasia associated with MEN I and IIA
- Symptoms of stones, bones, moans, and groans
  - Due to bone resorption
  - Increased: Calcium, chloride, and renal cAMP
  - Decreased: Phosphorous
  - Osteitis fibrosa cystica (brown tumor)

- Indications for surgery
  - Symptoms (bone involvement, peptic ulcers, nephrolithiasis, etc.)
  - Age <50 years
  - Calcium >1.0 mg/dL above the upper limit of normal
  - Cr clearance <30% of age matched controls
  - Bone marrow density T-score of <−2.5 at hip, lumbar spine, or distal radius
  - Inability to perform follow-up
- For an adenoma, resect the tumor and inspect the other three glands or utilize intraoperative PTH testing to confirm cure
- For hyperplasia, perform a 3½ gland parathyroidectomy, or total parathyroidectomy with autotransplantation
- A localizing study is needed only if planning a minimally invasive approach
  - First-line test for localization is a sestamibi scan
- Minimally invasive surgery can be performed if positive localization and intraoperative PTH testing is available

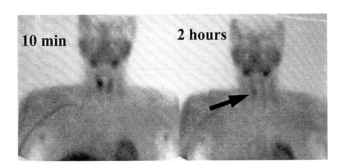

Sestamibi scan for localization of parathyroid gland. (With permission from Mulholland MW, Lillemoe KD, Doherty GM, Maier RV, Upchurch GR, eds. *Greenfield's Surgery*. 4th ed. Philadelphia, PA: Lippincott Williams & Wilkins; 2005.)

A patient with primary hyperparathyroidism is noted to have a markedly increased serum calcium and chloride. What is the most likely acid–base disorder?

Hyperchloremic metabolic acidosis can occur in patients with primary hyperparathyroidism.

What are the expected electrolyte abnormalities in patients with chronic renal failure?

- Decreased calcium (which can stimulate PTH in secondary hyperparathyroidism)
- Decreased magnesium
- Decreased sodium
- Increased potassium
- Increased phosphorous

A 66-year-old man with chronic renal failure has a decreased serum calcium and a markedly elevated PTH. What is the next step in management?

In most cases, secondary hyperparathyroidism is treated by changes in the patient's diet. Surgery is reserved for calciphylaxis (urgent and can be lifesaving), bone pain, fractures, severe pruritus, failure of medical therapy, or persistent symptoms in spite of successful renal transplantation (tertiary hyperparathyroidism).

Secondary Hyperparathyroidism

- A complication of renal failure (a.k.a., "renal osteodystrophy")
- PTH is increased in response to calcium loss
- Aluminum accumulates in bones from renal failure, contributing to osteomalacia
- Treatment is dietary (calcium and activated vitamin D supplements)
- Can also treat with a phosphorous-binding gel
- Most do not require surgery
- Surgery is indicated (and effective) for bone pain, fractures, pruritus, and calciphylaxis
- Since patients have hyperplasia, the operation used is a subtotal parathyroidectomy and bilateral thymectomy or total parathyroidectomy with/without forearm implantation

Tertiary Hyperparathyroidism

- Secondary hyperparathyroidism refractory to renal transplantation
- Surgery is often required
- Subtotal parathyroidectomy is the operation of choice, although a lesser resection may be appropriate if only one gland is clearly enlarged and the remaining glands are normal

What is the embryological origin of the parathyroid glands?

The superior parathyroid glands originate from the 4th brachial pouch. The inferior parathyroid glands originate from the 3rd brachial pouch.

What is the blood supply of the parathyroid glands?

The inferior thyroid artery supplies both the superior and inferior parathyroid glands.

An asymptomatic patient presents with a serum calcium level of 10.2, an incidental finding during routine laboratory testing. Her PTH is normal. What condition other than primary hyperparathyroidism should be in your differential diagnosis?

Familial hypercalcemic hypocalciuria (FHH) is an inherited disorder that affects the calcium sensing receptor in the kidney altering urinary calcium excretion. This condition can mimic mild primary hyperparathyroidism and should be in the differential diagnosis of any patient with mild hypercalcemia.

	PTH	Serum Ca^{2+}	Serum phosphate
Primary Hyperparathyroidism	↑	↑	↓
Secondary Hyperparathyroidism	↑	Normal/↓	↑
Tertiary Hyperparathyroidism	↑	↑	↓
Familial Hypercalcemic Hypocalciuria	Normal/↑	↑	↓

Familial Hypercalcemic Hypocalciuria

- Due to a calcium sensing receptor abnormality in the kidney resulting in calcium resorption
- The hypercalcemia is mild
- Distinguishing features from hyperparathyroidism: PTH is normal or only mildly elevated and urine calcium is very low (both are usually elevated in hyperparathyroidism)
- No treatment is required

A decreased urinary calcium and a normal serum PTH distinguishes familial hypercalcemic hypocalciuria from hyperparathyroidism.

During an exploration for a parathyroid adenoma, only three normal parathyroid glands are identified, each in their normal positions. The left lower gland is missing. Where is the most likely location of an ectopic lower parathyroid gland?

The most common location for an ectopic lower parathyroid gland is the thymus. Further exploration is warranted in this patient.

Location of an Aberrant Parathyroid

- Thymus gland
- Carotid sheath
- Retroesophageal
- Superior pharynx
- Thyroid gland
- If, after a thorough exploration, no gland is found, an intraoperative ultrasound can be performed to look for an intrathyroidal parathyroid gland
- If exploration and ultrasound do not reveal the location of the fourth gland, the patient should be closed and additional imaging obtained post-operatively

A 52-year-old man who underwent a parathyroidectomy 2 years ago presents now with a peptic ulcer. His serum calcium level is 10.8, his urinary calcium and serum PTH levels are also elevated. What is the next step in management?

The indications for surgery are the same as in primary hyperparathyroidism.

Recurrent Hyperparathyroidism

- Review operative notes and pathology reports
- Localization studies include sestamibi scan, ultrasound, CT, MRI, or venous sampling
- Two localization studies must be obtained prior to proceeding with surgery
- The most commonly missed sites for parathyroid glands:
  - Superior: Paraesophageal, thyroid parenchyma, or posterior mediastinum
  - Inferior: Tracheoesophageal groove, thymus, anterior mediastinum, or thyroid parenchyma

A 68-year-old man with squamous cell carcinoma of the lung presents with mental status changes and a serum calcium level of 14.5. What is the next step in the management of his hypercalcemia?

A multimodality treatment to increase calcium excretion and inhibit bone resorption is often required to treat a hypercalcemic crisis.

Treatment of Hypercalcemia

- Increase calcium excretion
  - Hydration with saline
  - Loop diuretics (use with caution when hydration alone is ineffective)
  - Dialysis if renally impaired
- Inhibit bone resorption
  - Bisphosphonates (3- to 6-day onset, weeks duration)
  - Calcitonin (rapid onset and short-lived)
  - Mithramycin (hepatotoxic and nephrotoxic)

Squamous cell carcinoma of the lung or metastatic cancer is the most common cause of cancer-related hypercalcemia.

If hypercalcemic crisis is related to primary hyperparathyroidism, then hydration to correct the acute hypercalcemia, followed by urgent parathyroidectomy is the best management. Avoid bisphosphonates in a patient who will be operated on for primary hyperparathyroidism as this will exacerbate their post-operative hypocalcemia.

A 55-year-old man presents with a serum Ca of 14.8 and a palpable mass in the area of the parathyroid gland. A parathyroid cancer is found at the time of surgical exploration. What is the best operation to perform?

Parathyroid cancer is treated with an en bloc resection of the tumor with the thyroid lobe and any associated lymph nodes.

Parathyroid Cancer

- A rare tumor
- Very high calcium level and a palpable mass
- Perform an en bloc resection of the tumor with the thyroid lobe and any associated lymph nodes

12 | Esophagus

Molly Sebastian and Michael R. Marohn

A 73-year-old man presents to the ED complaining of recent vomiting followed by severe, persistent chest pain. The pain is excruciating. Nothing he does mitigates the intensity of the pain. During his evaluation, the ED physician has a difficult time passing an NG tube. His extensive cardiac workup is negative. What is the most likely diagnosis?

The classic presentation of an incarcerated paraesophageal hernia is the Buchard triad: pain, history of violent retching, and difficulty passing a nasogastric (NG) tube. Because chest pain is a hallmark finding, these patients are often extensively worked up for cardiac problems before they are properly diagnosed.

Hiatal and Paraesophageal Hernias

- There are four types of gastroesophageal (GE) junction hernias
    - **Type I** "sliding" hiatal hernia: the GE junction moves up into the chest and returns to the abdomen as intra-abdominal pressure fluctuates
        - Most common type of hiatal hernia (90% of all hernias)
        - Usually asymptomatic and do not require surgery
        - When patients do have symptoms, they are most often GERD
    - **Type II** "rolling" or paraesophageal hernia: the GE junction is below the diaphragm (normal location) but the stomach herniates up beside the esophagus into the chest
    - **Type III** is a combination of both type I and type II hernias
    - **Type IV** involves at least one other organ (colon, spleen, etc.) prolapsed into the chest
- Type II, III, and IV are paraesophageal hernias for which operative repair prevents future complications of gastric volvulus or incarceration
- When a gastric volvulus occurs within a paraesophageal hernia, it is usually an organoaxial volvulus (i.e., the stomach folds on itself along its longitudinal axis)
- A paraesophageal hernia can cause difficulty in breathing because of compression on the lung (usually left)
- A Cameron ulcer is a gastric ulcer in a stomach that has herniated into the chest due to a paraesophageal hernia
    - Most commonly found on the lesser curve of the stomach
    - Can cause chronic anemia
- The goals of surgical repair are to reduce the hernia, excise the sac, and repair the defect (primarily or with mesh)

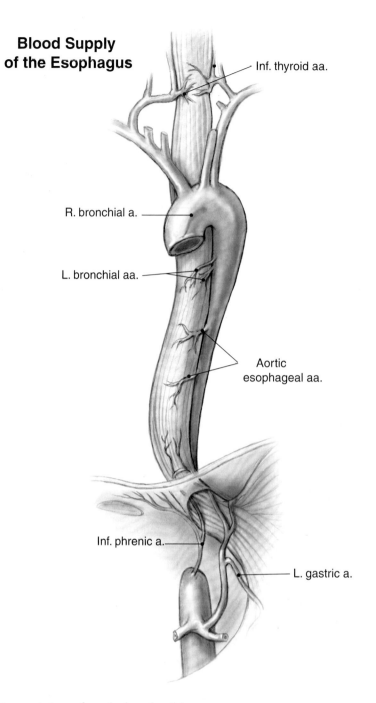

**Blood Supply
of the Esophagus**

Inf. thyroid aa.

R. bronchial a.

L. bronchial aa.

Aortic
esophageal aa.

Inf. phrenic a.

L. gastric a.

- A laparoscopic repair is preferred when feasible
- Observation (without surgery) should be considered if the patient is frail and has a short life expectancy and the paraesophageal hernia is asymptomatic

Symptomatic paraesophageal hernias require operative repair to prevent future incarceration.

An 80-year-old woman presents to clinic complaining of halitosis. She notes that periodically she regurgitates food soon after she eats. What is the next step for diagnosing her condition?

A barium swallow study is helpful for demonstrating a Zenker diverticulum.

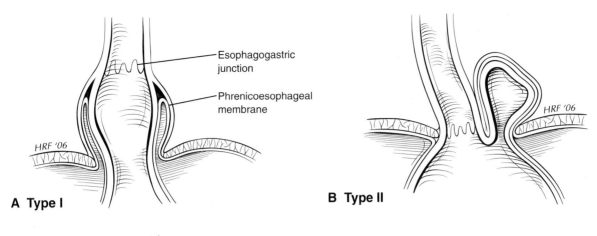

A Type I

Esophagogastric junction

Phrenicoesophageal membrane

B Type II

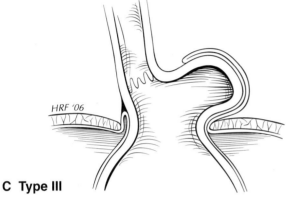

C Type III

Hernia types. (With permission from Fischer JE, Bland KI, Callery MP, et al., eds. *Mastery of Surgery.* 5th ed. Philadelphia, PA: Lippincott Williams & Wilkins; 2006.)

Esophageal Diverticula

- Pharyngoesophageal (Zenker) diverticulum is the most common type
    - Considered a false diverticulum or pseudodiverticulum—not a full-thickness defect of the esophagus
    - Protrudes posteriorly between the inferior pharyngeal constrictors and cricopharyngeus muscle (in Killian triangle)
    - Caused by pulsion forces due to cricopharyngeal dysfunction
        - There is a lack of coordination between UES relaxation and swallowing
    - Small pharyngeoesophageal diverticula can be treated with cricopharyngeal myotomy alone
    - Other options include myotomy with diverticulopexy or diverticulectomy
- Other types of esophageal diverticula include midesophageal or parabronchial diverticula
    - These are true diverticula involving all layers of the esophageal wall
    - Most commonly caused by granulomatous infections
    - Unlike the other esophageal diverticula, these are rarely symptomatic
    - Surgical excision is reserved for severe symptoms like dysphagia (pain with swallowing)
- Epiphrenic diverticulum (within 10 cm of the stomach)
    - Like Zenker diverticulum, this lesion is a pseudodiverticulum due to pulsion forces
    - It is associated with diffuse esophageal spasm, hiatal hernia, and achalasia
    - Most are asymptomatic
    - If the patient has dysphagia, the operation recommended is a diverticulectomy with contralateral long esophagomyotomy via a left thoracotomy

The most important step in the operative repair of a Zenker diverticulum is the cricopharyngeal myotomy because it is a pulsion diverticulum caused by a defect in the sphincter muscles.

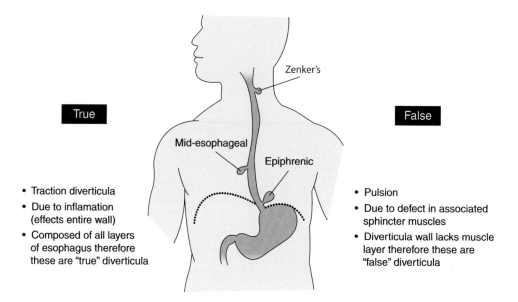

- True
  - Traction diverticula
  - Due to inflamation (effects entire wall)
  - Composed of all layers of esophagus therefore these are "true" diverticula

- False
  - Pulsion
  - Due to defect in associated sphincter muscles
  - Diverticula wall lacks muscle layer therefore these are "false" diverticula

Zenker's
Mid-esophageal
Epiphrenic

A 45-year-old woman who has been taking proton pump inhibitors for over a year has persistent heartburn and chest pain after eating. After an upper endoscopy, she is told that her biopsy showed moderate dysplasia in the lower esophagus. What is the most appropriate management for this patient?

If this patient has normal esophageal motility, a Nissen fundoplication is recommended for her persistent symptoms.

Fundoplication

- Fundoplication is generally indicated if a patient has persistent, severe, bipositional reflux symptoms despite optimal medical management for 3 to 6 months
- Other indications include ulcerative esophagitis; Barrett ulcer; presence of a large, fixed hiatal hernia; recurrent aspiration; or bile reflux esophagitis
- Contraindications include cancer, achalasia, diffuse esophageal spasms, or other causes of dysphagia
- All patients being considered for fundoplication need:
  - Esophageal manometry to rule out diffuse esophageal spasm or achalasia
  - Upper endoscopy to rule out high-grade dysplasia or cancer
  - Optional 24-hour pH monitoring to document the severity and duration of esophageal exposure to gastric acid
- Fundoplication halts the progression of Barrett esophagus but does NOT reverse it
  - If the esophagus is short (less than 2 cm of esophagus below the diaphragm), a Collis gastroplasty is used to "lengthen" the esophagus

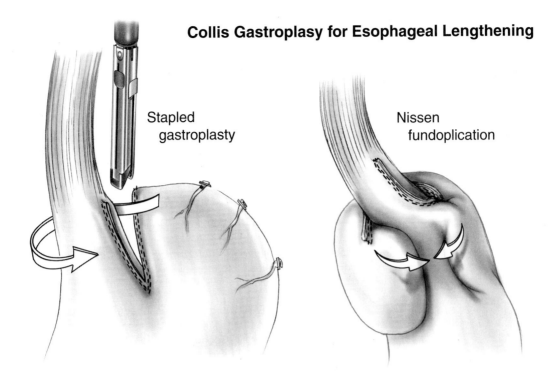

Collis Gastroplasy for Esophageal Lengthening

Stapled gastroplasty

Nissen fundoplication

- The most common intraoperative complication is a pneumothorax
  - A stable, asymptomatic pneumothorax can be managed with observation, as they usually resolve spontaneously (especially when CO_2 from laparoscopy is implicated)

Esophageal Metaplasia and Dysplasia

- Barrett esophagus (or Barrett metaplasia) is a condition in which columnar cells replace the normal squamous epithelium of the esophagus
- Goblet cells are the distinctive feature of Barrett metaplasia
- 10% to 15% of people with GERD have Barrett esophagus
- Less than 1% of people with Barrett will develop adenocarcinoma
- Although *Helicobacter pylori* is a cause of gastritis, it has NOTHING to do with esophagitis
- Patients with esophagitis but no signs of dysplasia should undergo annual screening endoscopy
- If low-grade or moderate dysplasia is present, a surveillance esophagogastroduodenoscopy (EGD) should be performed every 3 to 6 months
- High-grade dysplasia necessitates esophagectomy

High-grade dysplasia in the esophagus should be treated like cancer.

Scleroderma

- 90% of patients with scleroderma have esophageal involvement
- Have degeneration and fibrous replacement of smooth muscle
  - Striated muscle is spared
- Motility studies demonstrate:
  - Diminished peristalsis or complete aperistalsis of the esophagus
  - LOW lower esophageal sphincter (LES) pressure
  - Beware: These patients can present with reflux symptoms

Esophageal dysmotility MUST be ruled out before a fundoplication is performed. A full wrap of the distal esophagus in a patient with poor esophageal motility results in severe dysphagia postoperatively. These patients can sometimes be managed with medical management or a partial wrap.

A 76-year-old man who has a history of alcohol abuse and a 40-pack-year history of smoking is being evaluated for recent unintended weight loss (20 lbs over 2 months). He also has vague chest discomfort after eating. He first noticed difficulty swallowing solid food but now he has trouble with liquids as well. His cardiac work up is unrevealing. He is found to have a mass on a contrast study of his esophagus. Biopsy later shows adenocarcinoma. What is the best test for determining the stage of this esophageal cancer?

Endoscopic ultrasound (EUS) has become the standard of care for determining depth of invasion for esophageal tumors.

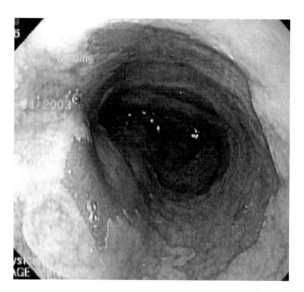

EGD showing Barrett esophagus. (With permission from Mulholland MW, Lillemoe KD, Doherty GM, Maier RV, Upchurch GR, eds. *Greenfield's Surgery.* 4th ed. Philadelphia, PA: Lippincott Williams & Wilkins; 2005.)

Esophageal Cancer

- Risk factors include alcohol abuse, smoking, poverty, and malnutrition
- Achalasia, a history of corrosive injury, and Barrett esophagus are also risk factors
- The highest incidence of this cancer is in China, Japan, Scotland, Russia, and Scandinavia
- EUS is highly sensitive for local staging
- Spreads by both lymphatic and vascular routes
- Adenocarcinoma is most common in the lower third of the esophagus
- Squamous cell cancer typically occurs in the proximal one-third of the esophagus
- If a full-thickness tumor (T3) or nodal disease is present, neoadjuvant chemoradiation followed by resection is increasingly becoming the standard of care
- With neoadjuvant therapy, up to 40% of patients can achieve pathologic complete response
- A complete pathologic response portends much better survival after surgery
- Smaller tumors can be resected without neoadjuvant therapy
- Esophagectomy can be achieved via a transhiatal or thoracic approach
  - A cervical location for the anastomosis is preferred

- If the anastomosis is in the chest, the patient is at high risk for developing mediastinitis if a leak occurs
- If the stomach is not available as a conduit, an intestinal limb or colonic interposition graft should be prepared
- The 5-year survival for advanced esophageal cancer is very low (6% to 8%)
- Patients in need of palliative procedures for obstructive symptoms might benefit from placement of an endoscopic expandable stent

The incidence of Barrett esophagus and esophageal adenocarcinoma is increasing; however, the chance of developing cancer in patients with Barrett esophagus is still less than 1%.

A 53-year-old man is being worked up for dysphagia. On upper endoscopy, the mucosa of his esophagus appears normal but the lumen seems to be narrowed from extrinsic compression. What is the most likely diagnosis in this case?

Endoscopic or barium swallow findings of an esophageal mass effect with normal mucosa are typical of a leiomyoma.

Benign Esophageal Masses

- Leiomyomas are the most common benign tumor of the esophagus
- Well circumscribed, intramural, submucosal lesions
- Confirm diagnosis with a CT showing a hypodense mass or an EUS, which will demonstrate a homogeneous hypoechoic mass
- Small risk of future malignancy
- Removed by enucleation
- Do NOT biopsy these masses!
  - Scarring after the biopsy will fix the mass to the mucosa
  - A biopsy increases the risk of perforation during subsequent attempts at enucleation

Although it is a benign lesion, an esophageal leiomyoma should be removed by enucleation due to its malignant potential.

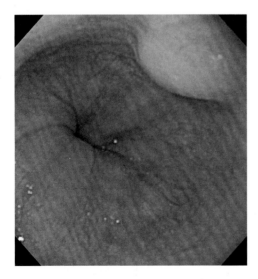

Esophageal leiomyoma. (With permission from Mulholland MW, Lillemoe KD, Doherty GM, Maier RV, Upchurch GR, eds. *Greenfield's Surgery*. 4th ed. Philadelphia, PA: Lippincott Williams & Wilkins; 2005.)

Schatzki Ring

- A constrictive ring of tissue involving the mucosa and submucosa
- Often located at the squamocolumnar junction
- Patients present with dysphagia
- The best treatment is pneumatic dilation of the constriction
- These patients rarely require surgical intervention
- Can also have a webs with iron deficiency in Plummer-Vinson syndrome

---

A 32-year-old woman has been experiencing increasing difficulty swallowing. The problem has become more pronounced over the past 2 months and it is now significantly hindering her ability to eat. She has lost 10 pounds during this period. What is the most likely diagnosis?

The most common cause of dysphagia in a young adult is achalasia, a condition marked by poor peristalsis on manometry and failure of the LES to relax during swallowing.

Achalasia

- Achalasia is a neurogenic condition caused by the absence of ganglion cells in Auerbach plexus
- In developing countries, achalasia can be a manifestation of Chagas disease, which results from infection with the parasite, *Trypanosoma cruzii*
- Manometry demonstrates:
  - Failure of the LES to relax (i.e., increased LES resting pressure)
  - Lack of coordinated peristaltic waves in the body of the esophagus
- The classic sign of achalasia on esophagram is a very dilated esophagus and "Bird's Beak" narrowing
- Nonoperative therapy includes:
  - Forced pneumatic dilatation
  - Nitrates, calcium channel blockers, and Botox injections
  - All "medical" treatments have a high recurrence rate
- A Heller myotomy is the definitive treatment for achalasia
- For patients with normal esophageal motility, a partial fundoplication can address the high incidence of reflux in these patients (30% to 40%)
  - The most common partial wrap is a Toupet (270 degree) wrap
  - Dor fundoplication folds the anterior stomach upward and is another option
- A Nissen (360 wrap) is considered to have too much resistance and should not be performed with a myotomy

Achalasia is best characterized by the failure of the LES to relax.

A 45-year-old male presents with substernal chest pain and dysphagia to both solids and liquids. A cardiac workup is negative. What should be the next diagnostic test?

A barium swallow should be performed to evaluate for diffuse esophageal spasms. The test will demonstrate a corkscrew esophagus.

Diffuse Esophageal Spasm

- Have disordered, high-amplitude contractions of the esophagus
- Symptoms: Substernal chest pain that mimics an MI, dysphagia of both solids and liquids

---

Laparoscopic Heller Myotomy for Achalasia

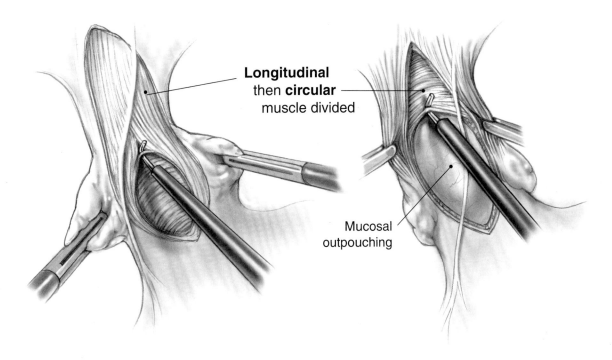

Longitudinal then **circular** muscle divided

Mucosal outpouching

- Diagnosis
  - Barium swallow: Corkscrew esophagus
  - Manometry: Frequent, high-amplitude, simultaneous contractions
- LES pressure is normal
- Treatment
  - Medical: Calcium-channel blockers, nitrates
  - Botulinum toxin injection—has a high recurrence rate
  - Forced pneumatic dilatation
  - Definitive treatment is a myotomy

After a terrible bout of violent emesis, a 67-year-old alcoholic man comes to the ED complaining of substernal chest pain. He feels slightly short of breath and notes that his pain is worse whenever he swallows. How would you evaluate him to determine a diagnosis?

An esophagram with water-soluble contrast is crucial to prove the presence of an esophageal rupture.

Esophageal Perforation (Boerhaave Syndrome)
- Patients usually remember the painful inciting event
- Commonly caused by violent episodes of emesis
- Results from a sudden increase in intraesophageal pressure
- The most common site of perforation is in the *left lateral aspect of the distal esophagus*

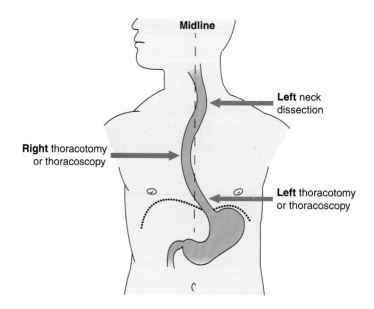

- If a surgeon is able to intervene within 12 hours of the inciting event, a primary closure of the esophageal tear with buttress to the repair (pleural flap or intercostal muscle flap) is recommended
    - If, at the time of exploration, the rupture is discovered to be due to an esophageal cancer, resection of that segment or total esophagectomy can be indicated
- The repair is at high risk for a leak given the local inflammation
- Placing a drain near the repair can facilitate early detection and control of a potential leak
- Remember that the esophagus lacks a serosa layer
    - The mucosa is the strongest layer in the esophagus
    - Therefore, buttressing with a pleural or muscle flap to cover the primary repair is important
- The dreaded complication of a failed esophageal perforation repair is mediastinitis
    - Without treatment, patients with an esophageal leak decompensate abruptly and become septic
    - There is high mortality associated with this complication
    - Any leak from the repair requires early operative intervention with irrigation, debridement, and wide drainage (chest tubes or drains)

Esophageal perforation from Boerhaave syndrome can be repaired primarily with a local flap and precautionary drain if the patient comes to surgical attention within 12 to 24 hours of the time of injury.

An 18-year-old male with an extensive history of depression and multiple suicide attempts is brought to the ED by his family after swallowing 2 pints of Draino. He is complaining of chest pain, but his vitals are stable and his abdomen is benign. What is the next step in management?

Do NOT insert an NG tube. Do a flexible esophagoscopy to determine the extent of esophageal injury.

Caustic Injury to the Esophagus

- Do NOT insert an NG tube as this can cause a perforation
- Do NOT induce vomiting

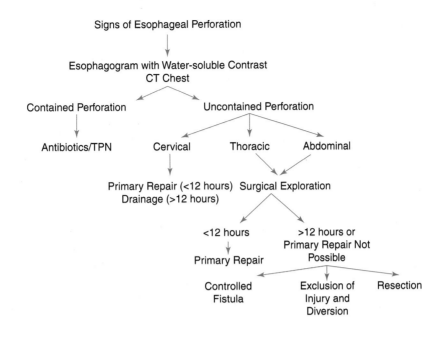

- Patient must be maintained strict NPO
- Alkali agents (e.g., draino)
  - Cause liquefactive necrosis
  - Can cause more extensive damage than acidic agents
- Acidic agents
  - Cause coagulation necrosis
- Degree of injury
  - First-degree burn
    - Hyperemia
    - Treatment: IV fluids, antibiotics, oral intake after 3 to 4 days
  - Second-degree burn
    - Ulcerations, exudates, sloughing
    - Treatment: Prolonged observation, TPN
  - Third-degree burn
    - Deep ulcers, charring
    - Treatment: Esophagectomy
- Long-term complications: Stricture, reflux, cancer

13 | Stomach

Michael G. House

After a gastrectomy, a patient overall does well, but has a persistent anemia. What is the cause?

Pernicious anemia secondary to decreased intrinsic factor post gastrectomy.

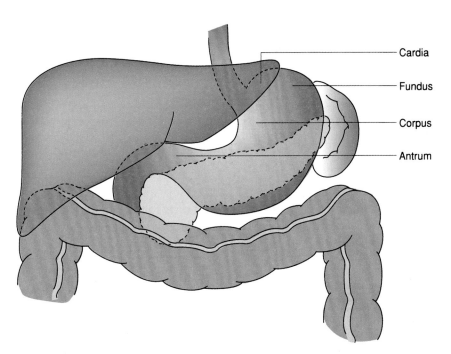

Gastric anatomy. (With permission from Mulholland MW, Lillemoe KD, Doherty GM, Maier RV, Upchurch GR, eds. *Greenfield's Surgery.* 4th ed. Philadelphia, PA: Lippincott Williams & Wilkins; 2005.)

Gastric Anatomy

- Cardia
  - Immediately distal to GE junction
  - Cell types: Surface epithelial cells, mucous cells

- Fundus
  - Most superior portion of stomach
  - Separated from stomach by the angle of His
  - Cell types: Mucous cells, some parietal and chief cells
- Corpus
  - Extends from the fundus to the antrum/pylorus
  - Cell types: Mucous cells, parietal cells, chief cells, ECL cells, D cells
- Antrum
  - Begins at the angularis incisura and goes to the pylorus
  - Cell types: Mucous cells, G cells, some D cells

Gastric Cell Types

- Chief cells (40% of gastric epithelium): Pepsinogen
  - Pepsinogen produced in response to food
  - Pepsinogen → pepsin at pH < 5
  - Pepsin breaks down protein
- Parietal cells: HCl, IF (intrinsic factor)
  - Intrinsic factor binds B12, aiding its absorption in the distal ileum
- Mucous cells: Mucous, HCO_3
- G cells: Gastrin
- D cells: Somatostatin
- ECL cells: Serotonin
- ECL-like cells: Histamine

Pernicious Anemia

- Due to autoimmune disease against the parietal cells
- Leads to B12 deficiency → megaloblastic anemia
- Diagnosis: Endoscopy with biopsy; have ulcers in the fundus
- Treatment: Vitamin B12 injection

A 67-year-old man develops overt gastric bleeding 3 days following an open surgical debridement for infected pancreatic necrosis. Gastroscopy reveals diffuse bleeding from the fundus and body of the stomach. What measure could have prevented this condition?

Early prophylaxis with an H2 receptor antagonist or a proton pump inhibitor is often effective in treating bleeding secondary to stress gastritis.

Stress Gastritis

- Mucosal ischemia that typically occurs 3 to 10 days after a stress event (e.g., operation, shock, and sepsis).
- Cushing ulcer occurs with severe head trauma
  - Due to increased gastrin and HCl hypersecretion
- Curling ulcer occurs with severe burns
  - Due to mucosal ischemia
- Develops in only 10% of critically ill patients receiving prophylactic therapy
- Treatment options include endoscopic injection or coagulation, angiographic embolization, vasopressin infusion, subtotal/total gastrectomy, or a gastric devascularization procedure

Blood Supply of the Stomach

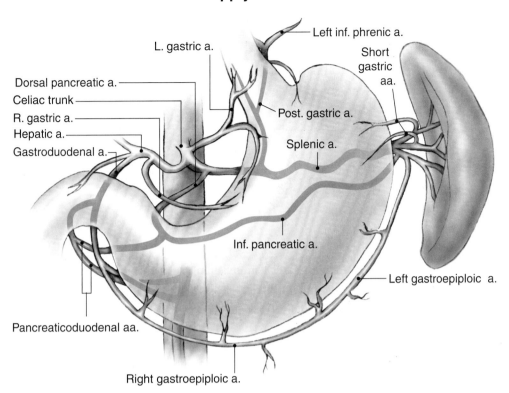

The major supply of the stomach arises from five sources: left gastric artery arising from the celiac axis, right gastric artery typically arising from the hepatic artery proper, the right gastroepiploic artery sourced from the gastroduodenal artery, the short gastric arteries and left gastroepiploic artery sourced from the splenic artery.

Alkaline Reflux Gastritis

- Due to bile reflux into the stomach
  - Most commonly seen after pyloroplasty or Billroth II reconstruction
- Symptoms: Postprandial abdominal pain
- Diagnosis: Endoscopy
- Treatment: Roux-en-Y reconstruction

Histamine induces acid production by binding to adenylate kinase to increase cAMP and protein kinase A.

A 41-year-old woman presents with recurrent epigastric pain and new onset gastric bleeding. She is hemodynamically stable and has an endoscopy, which reveals an actively bleeding vessel within an ulcer base in the pre-pyloric region. What is the most appropriate initial intervention?

This is a Dieulafoy lesion, which is seen with a submucosal artery at the base of an ulcer. Endoscopic injection therapy and coagulation are effective in treating most bleeding gastric ulcers. Remember that all gastric ulcers should be biopsied.

Gastric Ulcer

- Causes
  - *Helicobacter pylori* infection—60% to 90%
  - Nonsteroidal anti-inflammatory drug (NSAID) overuse

- Zollinger-Ellison syndrome
- Gastric cancer
- Types of gastric ulcer
  - Type I—distal lesser curvature
    - Normal to decreased acid secretion
  - Type II—distal lesser curvature and duodenal ulcer
    - Acid hypersecretion
  - Type III—prepyloric or pyloric
    - Acid hypersecretion
  - Type IV—proximal lesser curvature
    - Normal to decreased acid secretion
  - Type V—anywhere
    - Medication induced
- Treatment
  - *H. pylori*: proton pump inhibitor (PPI) + amoxicillin + clarithromycin or metronidazole
  - Infusional PPI therapy is used for active ulcer disease
  - Indications for surgical management after failed medical/endoscopic therapy include bleeding, perforation, or obstruction
  - Surgical options (depending on location of the ulcer) include
    - Omental plication for perforated ulcers in unstable patients (but remember to biopsy gastric ulcers)
    - Simple ulcer excision
    - Gastrotomy with ulcer oversewing, vagotomy, and pyloroplasty
    - Antrectomy and vagotomy
    - Subtotal gastrectomy
    - Highly selective vagotomy
    - The right vagus nerve travels posterior to the stomach and gives off the Criminal nerve of Grassi (if undivided during vagotomy, can have recurrent ulcers)
  - Unlike a highly selective vagotomy, a standard vagotomy must be done in conjunction with a pyloroplasty or at least an antral resection (in order to prevent an unopposed absence of vagal tone)
  - ALWAYS send tissue from a gastric ulcer to pathology, given the increased risk of malignancy compared to duodenal ulcers.

Ulcers with active pulsatile bleeding or a visible vessel are at highest risk for re-bleeding following endoscopic intervention.

A 53-year-old man experiences severe lightheadedness and diaphoresis after meals ever since he had a partial gastrectomy several months ago. What is the best treatment?

The dumping syndrome is often treated with fiber and avoidance of hyperosmolar liquids. Conversion to a Roux-en-Y gastroenterostomy may ultimately be required.

Post-gastrectomy Problems
- Dumping
  - Can occur early (15 to 30 minutes after meal) or late (2 to 3 hours after meal)
    - Early dumping: Due to rapid passage of high osmolarity food from the stomach to the small intestine → water shift into the lumen of the small intestine

---

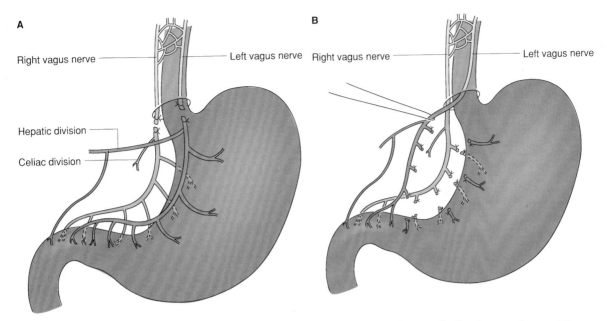

Truncal vagotomy (A) and highly selective vagotomy (B). (With permission from Mulholland MW, Lillemoe KD, Doherty GM, Maier RV, Upchurch GR, eds. *Greenfield's Surgery.* 4th ed. Philadelphia, PA: Lippincott Williams & Wilkins; 2005.)

- Late dumping: Due to hyperactive insulin release
- Treatment includes avoidance of hyperosmolar liquids, addition of fiber to the diet, and octreotide
- If symptoms persist, convert to a Roux-en-Y gastroenterostomy
- Diarrhea
  - 10% of post-gastrectomy patients
  - Mechanisms include accelerated intestinal transit, bile malabsorption, rapid gastric emptying, and bacterial overgrowth
  - Treatment includes anti-motility agents, antibiotics (for bacterial overgrowth), and surgical reversed intestinal interposition
- Bile reflux gastritis
  - Typically develops several months following pylorus resection
  - Presents with nausea, epigastric pain, and bilious vomiting
  - Diagnosed with endoscopy (or bile reflux scintigraphy)
  - Treatment includes conversion of Billroth I/II to Roux-en-Y gastroenterostomy, duodenal switch, and addition of Braun enteroenterostomy to a Billroth II
    - Billroth I procedure = partial gastrectomy and gastro*duoden*ostomy
    - Billroth II procedure = partial gastrectomy and gastro*jejun*ostomy
- Gastroparesis
  - A complication associated with a Roux-en-Y procedure
  - Consider abnormal gastric motility only after excluding mechanical obstruction downstream
  - Work-up includes esophagogastroduodenoscopy (EGD), upper GI series, gastric emptying study, and gastric manometry
  - Treatment includes metoclopramide, domperidone, erythromycin (motilin agonist), and subtotal or near total gastrectomy

- Marginal and recurrent ulcers
  - A marginal ulcer is a jejunal ulcer distal to the gastrojejunostomy anastomosis
  - Recurrent ulcers can occur in the duodenum, jejunum, or stomach
  - Work-up should consider the possibility of a gastrinoma, incomplete vagotomy, and retained antrum
  - Treatment includes discontinuation of NSAIDs, *H. pylori* eradication, and subtotal gastrectomy to remove a retained antrum, total gastrectomy, or truncal vagotomy
- Malabsorption
  - Decreased absorption of iron, vitamin B12, folate, Ca, and vitamins A, D, E, K (fat soluble), especially with bacterial overgrowth
- Gastric remnant cancer
  - Can arise several years after gastric surgery, especially after a Billroth II operation, but typically occurs 15 years or more after a gastric resection
  - Usually advanced at the time of detection and carries a poor prognosis

Metoclopramide is an effective treatment of gastroparesis, even in patients with diabetic gastroparesis.

A 21-year-old college student presents with hematemesis after binge alcohol use. Upper endoscopy reveals a mucosal tear at the GE junction with active bleeding. What is the most appropriate intervention?

Endoscopic injection therapy is the treatment of choice.

Mallory-Weiss Syndrome
- Typically presents with hematemesis following an episode of vomiting/retching
- Appears as a single linear tear or multiple tears along the lesser curvature, gastric cardia, or GE junction
- Diagnosed by EGD (or angiography)
- 90% of tears are self-limited
- The highest risk for re-bleeding occurs in patients with portal hypertension, coagulopathy, or when there is a visible vessel within the tear
- Treatment options include endoscopic injection, electrocoagulation, hemoclipping/banding, left gastric artery embolization, arterial-directed vasopressin infusion, or Blakemore tube placement

---

A 40-year-old woman presents with early satiety and epigastric pain. A CT scan reveals an isolated 8 cm epigastric mass that appears to arise from the left lobe of the liver. Upper endoscopy is normal, and there is no history of liver disease. At the time of exploration, the mass proves to arise from the stomach. What histological features would be expected from this tumor?

This is clearly a submucosal tumor consistent with a normal endoscopy, most likely a gastrointestinal stromal tumor (GIST). Characteristics of a mesenchymal tumor with positive immunohistochemistry for c-kit protein are consistent with a GIST.

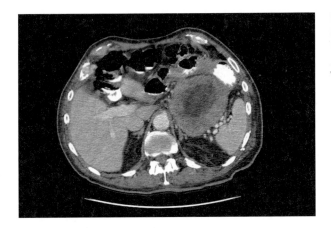

Large gastric GIST. (With permission from Mulholland MW, Lillemoe KD, Doherty GM, Maier RV, Upchurch GR, eds. *Greenfield's Surgery*. 4th ed. Philadelphia, PA: Lippincott Williams & Wilkins; 2005.)

Gastrointestinal Stromal Tumor

- Most common sarcoma associated with the GI tract
- 65% arise from the stomach
- Present with vague abdominal symptoms, early satiety, or are discovered incidentally
  - Less commonly may present with bleeding (intra- or extra-luminal) or perforation as a result of tumor necrosis, or obstruction
- Putative cell of origin is the interstitial cell of Cajal (gastrointestinal pacemaker cells)
- Rarely associated with lymphatic spread
- Primary tumor features associated with early recurrence and metastatic spread
  - Size >10 cm
  - Mitotic rate >5/50 hpf
  - Location (small intestine)
- Treatment for GIST without metastatic disease
  - En-bloc resection with 1 to 2 cm free margins of primary site
  - Avoid simple enucleation and/or capsular disruption
  - Lymphadenectomy is not necessary
  - Adjuvant therapy with Gleevec (a tyrosine kinase inhibitor) if tumor size is > 5 cm or mitotic rate > 5/50 hpf
- Treatment for GIST with metastatic or recurrent disease
  - Gleevec (imatinib) therapy
  - Resect only if all gross disease can be removed
  - Systemic chemotherapy if disease progresses
- Outcomes
  - With complete resection, 5-year survival is 55%
  - Survival is influenced by negative prognostic indicators
  - Monitor with CT every 6 months for 2 years then yearly thereafter to detect early recurrences

Mutation of the c-kit proto-oncogene (transmembrane tyrosine kinase receptor) underlies abnormal cell growth and differentiation in GIST.

A 21-year-old college student presents two hours after ingesting 250 mL of drain cleaner in an apparent suicidal gesture. She is hypotensive, actively drooling, and is found to have a rigid abdomen. What is the most appropriate course of action?

The most appropriate treatment is to secure her airway, resuscitate her with IV fluids, and plan an emergent laparotomy for presumed gastric necrosis or perforation.

Caustic Gastric Injury

- Usually associated with esophageal injuries
- Most severe with liquid alkalis (liquefactive necrosis)
- Gastric necrosis and perforation may present immediately or several days post-ingestion
- Gastric necrosis requires subtotal/total gastrectomy or esophagogastrectomy as indicated
- In the absence of shock or perforation, upper endoscopy can delineate the extent of esophageal and/or gastric injury
- Late sequelae include gastric outlet obstruction as a result of antral/pyloric stricture

Caustic injuries in the setting of shock often require surgical resection of the perforated or necrotic area involved.

What are the four subtypes of gastric adenocarcinoma that can be identified on gastroscopy?

Ulcerative (most common), polypoid, scirrhous, and superficial.

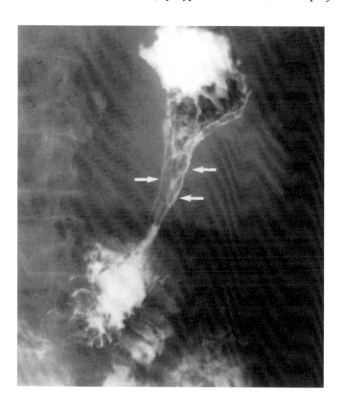

Linitis plastica. (With permission from Mulholland MW, Lillemoe KD, Doherty GM, Maier RV, Upchurch GR, eds. *Greenfield's Surgery.* 4th ed. Philadelphia, PA: Lippincott Williams & Wilkins; 2005.)

Gastric Adenocarcinoma

- Risk factors include diet (especially nitrosamines), chronic *H. pylori*/ulcer disease, pernicious anemia, atrophic gastritis, smoking, and hereditary non-polyposis colon cancer (HNPCC)
- The two histologic subtypes are intestinal and diffuse
- The majority arise along the lesser curvature, 40% to 50% involve cardia, and 10% involve entire stomach (linitis plastica)
- The most common presenting symptoms are abdominal pain and weight loss
- Use EGD for diagnosis, CT and laparoscopy for disease staging
- Surgery is indicated in the absence of disseminated disease

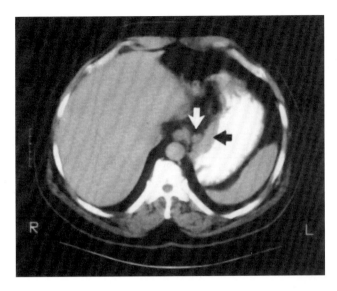

Mass along lesser curvature (*black arrow*) and enlarged lymph node (*white arrow*). (With permission from Mulholland MW, Lillemoe KD, Doherty GM, Maier RV, Upchurch GR, eds. *Greenfield's Surgery.* 4th ed. Philadelphia, PA: Lippincott Williams & Wilkins; 2005.)

- Treatment includes resection with negative margins with en bloc removal of the greater omentum, lymph nodes, and adherent organs
- Depending on the site of disease, treatment may include total gastrectomy, subtotal gastrectomy, or esophagogastrectomy
- Extent of lymphadenectomy
  - D1 resection includes perigastric lymph nodes
  - D2 includes perigastric + celiac + hepatic + splenic lymph nodes
    - D2 resections are rarely performed in the United States
- Perioperative chemotherapy (before and after surgery) including epirubicin, cisplatin, and 5-FU is indicated for advanced stage cancers, i.e., node-positive, T3 or T4 primary tumors
- Adjuvant therapy includes chemotherapy (5-FU) and radiation
- Survival 5-year: Stage 1 = 60% to 80%, Stage 4 = 5%

A 60-year-old man is diagnosed with a MALToma after undergoing endoscopic biopsy of the antral portion of his stomach. What is the most appropriate initial therapy?

Eradication therapy against H. pylori (PPI and antibiotics).

Gastric Lymphoma

- Second most common gastric cancer
- The most common symptoms at presentation are pain, weight loss, and fatigue/anemia
- Work-up involves a physical exam, serum lactate dehydrogenase (LDH) and microglobulin levels, and a CT scan of the chest, abdomen, and pelvis
- Non-Hodgkin lymphoma is the most common type (B cell, diffuse histiocytic)
  - First-line treatment is with chemotherapy (doxorubicin + cyclophosphamide)
  - Surgery ± radiation is reserved for non-responders, those with recurrent disease, or those having complications associated with chemotherapy treatment (i.e., hemorrhage or perforation)
- MALToma
  - A non-Hodgkin lymphoma that is associated with *H. pylori*
  - Treatment
    - Early stage: *H. pylori* eradication—many will resolve with this alone
    - Late stage: As for other non-Hodgkin lymphoma

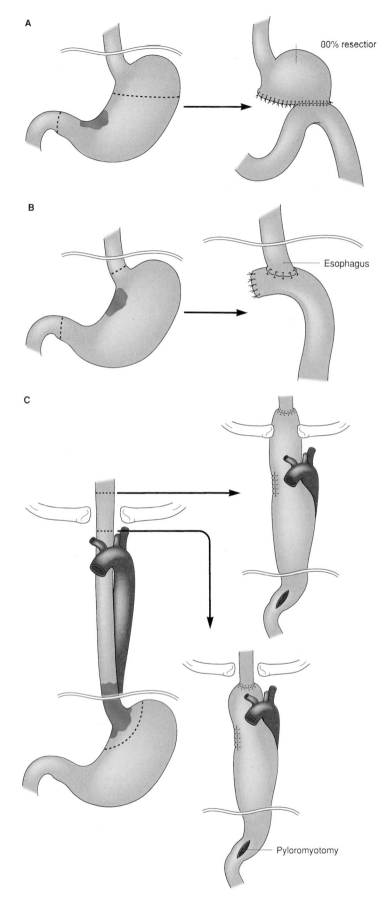

Surgical options for gastrectomy for gastric cancer: (A) distal gastrectomy and (B) total gastrectomy. (With permission from Mulholland MW, Lillemoe KD, Doherty GM, Maier RV, Upchurch GR, eds. *Greenfield's Surgery.* 4th ed. Philadelphia, PA: Lippincott Williams & Wilkins; 2005.)

Surgical intervention is rarely indicated for gastric lymphoma.

What are the three types of bezoars found in the stomach, and how are they treated?

Trichobezoars, composed of hair, are the most common type and typically require surgical removal unless they can be broken up endoscopically. Phytobezoars, which are composed of vegetable matter, can be managed with chemical dissolution with papain and acetylcysteine combined with endoscopic fragmentation. Lactobezoars result from milk precipitates and respond to endoscopic rehydration.

Gastric Foreign Bodies

- Ingested foreign objects most common among children and patients with a psychiatric history
- If the object passes through the esophagus into the stomach, then it will usually transit through the intestines
- Objects unlikely to pass through the pylorus are larger than 2 cm in diameter or 5 cm in length
- Endoscopic retrieval is appropriate for objects that remain in the stomach for >4 weeks and those with sharp ends
- Batteries, which can produce alkaline mucosal injury, should be removed from the esophagus immediately and from the stomach if they fail to pass within 48 hours

14 Obesity Surgery

Kashif A. Zuberi, Kimberley Eden Steele, and Thomas H. Magnuson

> A healthy, 37-year-old woman comes to your office requesting a gastric bypass operation. She is 5'6" tall and weighs 215 lbs. Does she meet criteria to qualify for the operation?

Obesity now affects 31% of Americans, with 5% classified as morbidly obese (BMI of 40 kg/m², weight 100 lbs above ideal body weight, or weight that is twice the ideal body weight). A patient must have a BMI > 40, or a BMI > 35 with multiple comorbidities to undergo obesity surgery. This patient has a BMI of 34.7 but is otherwise healthy; therefore, she does not meet the standard criteria.

Body Mass Index (BMI)	Class	BMI
• BMI = weight (kg)/square of the height (m²)	I	>30
• A BMI > 25 is considered overweight	II	>35
• There are three classes of obesity which are defined according to BMI thresholds	III	>40

National Institute of Health Criteria for Obesity Surgery

- BMI > 40
- BMI > 35 with one or more obesity-related comorbidities
  - Comorbidities include a history of diabetes, hypertension, or degenerative joint disease
- Failed previous attempts at non-surgical weight reduction
- No active alcohol or substance abuse
- Realistic expectations of outcomes
- Commitment to long-term vitamin supplementation and follow-up
- Acceptable risk for surgery

> A 37-year-old woman comes to your office requesting a gastric bypass operation. She has a BMI of 36. Her past medical history consists of diabetes mellitus, hypertension, and depression. She has attempted various diets and exercise programs only to regain her weight and more. Does she qualify for surgery?

The patient qualifies for obesity surgery because her patient's BMI is >35 and she has multiple comorbidities. However, be mindful of patients with depression or an endocrine etiology for weight gain. Guidelines established by the American Society of Bariatric Surgeons (ASBS) include preoperative psychological evaluation. This helps identify those who have unrealistic expectations or are unable to give informed consent. Weight gain caused by an endocrine disorder, though rare, must be identified and dealt with prior to considering surgical intervention. Examples include patients with a history of MEN I (hyperparathyroidism, insulinoma, or pituitary adenoma). Most bariatric centers emphasize the importance of a multidisciplinary approach to patient screening and education. This includes evaluation by a dietician, psychologist, and internist (for preoperative risk assessment), and a sleep study if sleep apnea is suspected.

> A 32-year-old obese but otherwise healthy male (BMI = 42) has undergone comprehensive preoperative testing for obesity surgery. His insurance company has approved the procedure. He comes today to discuss his surgical options. The dietician noted that this patient is a sweet eater and consumes milkshakes as his main source of protein. What are the different surgical options and which would you recommend for this patient?

A variety of surgical procedures have been developed to achieve weight loss, either by mechanical restriction of caloric intake through the creation of a small gastric reservoir, or the induction of malabsorption by bypassing variable lengths of small bowel. Surgical options include laparoscopic adjustable gastric band, vertical sleeve gastrectomy, Roux-en Y gastric bypass, and biliopancreatic diversion/duodenal switch. This patient would benefit most from a gastric bypass. (In fact, 80% of bariatric (obesity) procedures in the United States are Roux-en Y gastric bypass procedures, though the vertical sleeve gastrectomy is becoming more popular.)

Bariatric surgical procedures can be classified as:

Restrictive	Restrictive + Malabsorptive	Malabsorptive
LAGB	Roux-en-Y GB	Jejuno-ileal bypass
VSG	BPD/DS	
VBG		

LAGB, laparoscopic adjustable gastric band; VSG, vertical sleeve gastrectomy; VBG, vertical banded gastroplasty; Roux-en-Y GB, Roux-en-Y gastric bypass; BPD/DS, biliopancreatic diversion/duodenal switch.

Roux-en-Y Gastric Bypass

- Operation of choice for obesity at most centers
- Produces both restriction and malabsorption (bypasses duodenum and proximal jejunum)
- Creates a small gastric pouch (20 to 30 mL) along the lesser curvature
- Includes a gastrojejunostomy utilizing a Roux-en-Y limb to empty the gastric pouch
- Average weight loss is 60% to 70% of excess body weight
- Maximal weight loss occurs in the first 2 years
- Obesity-related diseases (diabetes, hypertension, and sleep apnea) are dramatically reversed within the first year of surgery
- A laparoscopic approach is associated with a shorter length of stay and fewer complications (wound, infection, hernia, etc.)
- Complications
  - Anastomotic leak—most commonly secondary to ischemia
  - Small bowel obstruction
  - Stenosis—responds to serial dilation
  - Internal hernia
    - Mesenteric defects should be closed to prevent this

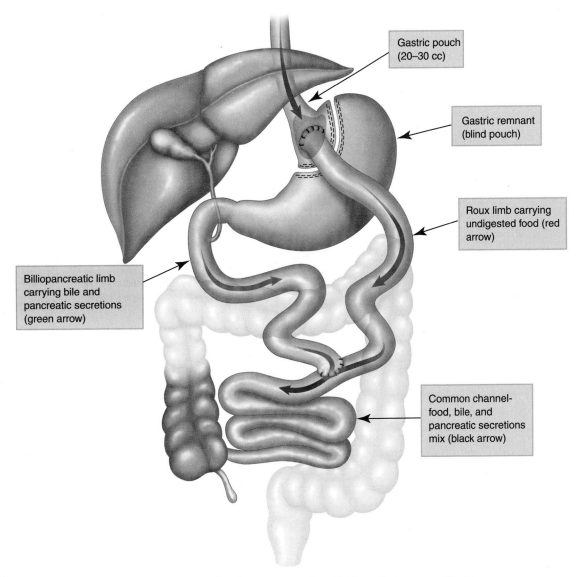

Gastric pouch
(20–30 cc)

Gastric remnant
(blind pouch)

Roux limb carrying
undigested food (red
arrow)

Billiopancreatic limb
carrying bile and
pancreatic secretions
(green arrow)

Common channel-
food, bile, and
pancreatic secretions
mix (black arrow)

Roux-en-Y gastric bypass. (Reproduced with permission from Ethicon Endosurgery 2011.)

- Marginal ulcer near stomach anastomosis
- B12 deficiency
    - Because IF needs an acidic environment to bind B12
- Iron deficiency
    - Iron is absorbed in the duodenum, which is bypassed
- Gallstones—secondary to rapid weight loss

Laparoscopic Adjustable Band

- Only a restrictive procedure (not malabsorptive)
- A silastic collar or band is placed around the proximal stomach, creating a 15 mL pouch and a narrow adjustable outlet
- The outlet is adjusted by changing the volume of saline in a surgically placed subcutaneous reservoir to tighten or loosen the band
- Average weight loss approaches 45% to 50% of excess body weight
- Complications include band migration or erosion and malfunction of the subcutaneous port

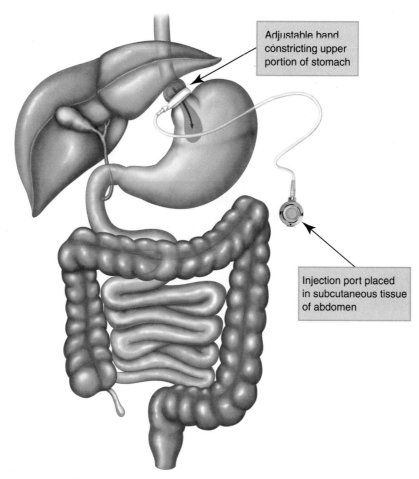

Adjustable band constricting upper portion of stomach

Injection port placed in subcutaneous tissue of abdomen

Laparoscopic adjustable gastric band. (Reproduced with permission from Ethicon Endosurgery 2011.)

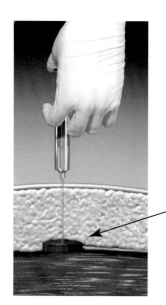

Injection port in subcutaneous fat

Laparoscopic adjustable gastric band adjustment. Adjustments are done by accessing the port which lies in the subcutaneous fat and is secured to the abdominal wall fascia. A Huber needle attached to a syringe is used to access the port. Sterile saline solution is used to fill the band. Fluid is removed from the band via the same technique. (Reproduced with permission from Ethicon Endosurgery 2011.)

Biliopancreatic Diversion/Duodenal Switch

- Achieves weight loss primarily through malabsorption
- A distal gastrectomy (80%) along the greater curvature is performed to create some restriction
- The distal small bowel is divided 250 cm proximal to the ileocecal valve
  - The proximal end is rejoined to the ileum 50 cm proximal to the ileocecal valve
  - The distal end is brought up and anastomosed to the duodenum
- Causes weight loss of up to 80% excess body weight
- The duodenal switch operation is a modification of the BPD
- The pylorus is preserved and the anastomosis is made to the duodenum instead of the stomach
- Appropriate candidates include the super-obese (BMI > 60) and those who have failed to lose weight with other obesity procedures

Vertical Banded Gastroplasty

- Entirely restrictive in nature
- Creates a small gastric reservoir or pouch measuring 15 to 20 mL in volume, which then empties into the residual stomach via a banded outlet
- The primary advantages of VBG are the avoidance of a gastrointestinal anastomosis and the preservation of normal gastroduodenal continuity
- Patients lose, on average, 40% to 50% of their excess body weight over 2 years
- Rarely performed in the 21st century
- Complications include pouch expansion, Marlex band migration or obstruction, and breakdown of the staple line that partitions the stomach

---

A 60-year-old male with DM, HTN, CAD s/p drug eluting stent placement in the LAD, and obstructive sleep apnea, has a BMI of 62. He has been referred to your clinic for evaluation. He is motivated and willing to go through the preoperative process for insurance approval. You find on inspection that most of his weight appears to be concentrated within his abdomen (central obesity). What operation would be the safest and easily performed in this type of patient?

A laparoscopic Roux-en-Y gastric bypass procedure could be offered to this patient. However with a BMI of 62 and central obesity, a laparoscopic approach would be more challenging. Additionally, he may not tolerate the operative time required for laparoscopic Roux-en Y gastric bypass. Therefore, he would be an ideal candidate for a laparoscopic vertical sleeve gastrectomy. Another option would be to offer a two-stage procedure: (1) the vertical sleeve gastrectomy and (2) revision to a Roux-en-Y gastric bypass in the future when his weight loss plateaus.

The Super-obese Patient

- Super-obese patients (BMI > 60) present both a technical and functional challenges
- Functional challenges
  - Poor cardiopulmonary reserve
  - Exercise intolerance
  - Restrictive and obstructive lung disorders (anesthesia tolerance)
  - Inability to ambulate
- Technical challenges
  - Difficult access to abdominal cavity—higher pneumoperitoneum pressures
  - Exercise intolerance

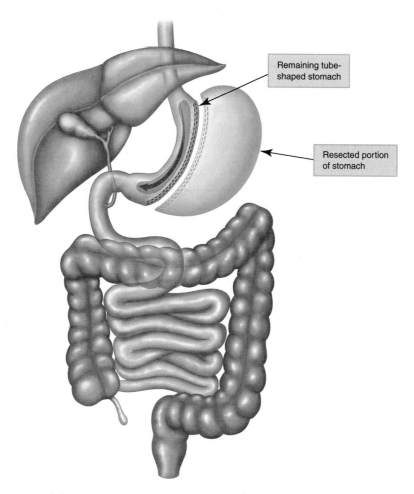

Remaining tube-shaped stomach

Resected portion of stomach

Vertical sleeve gastrectomy. (Reproduced with permission from Ethicon Endosurgery 2011.)

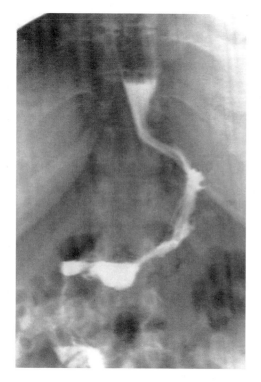

Normal upper GI study showing the restrictive properties of a sleeve gastrectomy.

- Large and stiff abdominal wall—limited port maneuverability
- Large vulnerable left liver lobe—difficult retraction and visualization of GE junction
- Thick and foreshortened small bowel mesentery—difficult Roux limb mobilization and increased risk of tension on gastro-jejunostomy

Laparoscopic Vertical Sleeve Gastrectomy

- Is a purely restrictive operation
- There are currently no long-term results of sleeve gastrectomy outcomes
- In the short term, there has been improved diabetic control, management of hypertension and obstructive sleep apnea
- There are fewer bowel obstructions or internal hernias than with Roux-en-Y gastric bypass procedures

On postoperative day #1 after laparoscopic gastric bypass, a 52-year-old man begins a clear liquid diet. Eight hours later, he complains of epigastric discomfort. The nurse notices that he is somewhat short of breath. Vital signs show a temperature of 38.5, HR 122, BP 152/80, RR 20, and pulse oximetry of 94% on 4L. Name two common and life-threatening complications that must be ruled out in this patient. What diagnostic procedures should be carried out?

Two serious complications for which bariatric patients are at high risk are pulmonary embolism and anastomotic leak. A CT scan and gastrografin swallow study can help in the diagnosis of these complications.

A postoperative gastrografin swallow study shows the following. What is the next step in management?

Extravasation of oral contrast is visualized. An emergent exploratory laparotomy to drain and repair the anastomotic leak is indicated.

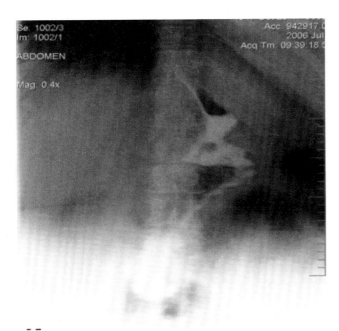

Gastrografin swallow study.

On postoperative day #2 after an open gastric bypass, the patient complains of abdominal bloating, LUQ abdominal pain, and nausea. The patient's WBC is 14,000. A swallow study completed on POD#1 showed no evidence of a leak. A CT scan is ordered, revealing the following. What is the next step in management?

This is an example of an afferent limb syndrome caused by obstruction at the jejunojejunostomy site. Insertion of a gastrostomy tube and drainage of the stomach remnant can help decompress the biliopancreatic limb until the inflammation subsides and the anastomosis opens up.

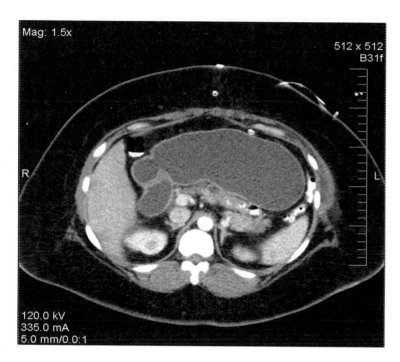

CT showing SBO due to afferent limb syndrome.

Obesity Surgery Complications

Afferent Limb Syndrome

- Partial obstruction of the afferent limb
- Symptoms
  - RUQ postprandial pain and fullness
  - Projectile bilious vomiting
- Caused by increased afferent loop pressure secondary to mechanical obstruction with increased GI secretions
- Treatment
  - Balloon dilatation
  - Revision of JJ anastomosis

Efferent Loop Syndrome

- Partial obstruction of efferent limb
- Symptoms
  - Abdominal pain
  - Bilious vomiting

- Treatment
    - Exploration
    - Reduction of internal hernia and closure of mesenteric defect

Roux Syndrome

- Have stasis of chyme in Roux limb and abnormal gastric emptying
- Symptoms
    - Epigastric pain
    - Vomiting
    - Weight loss
- Due to abnormal motility of the jejunum
- Treatment
    - Promotility agents
    - Gastrectomy to decrease gastric remnant size
    - Shortening of Roux limb

Blind Loop Syndrome

- Seen with Billroth II and Roux-en-Y
- Symptoms
    - Diarrhea
    - Malabsorption
    - Abdominal pain
    - B12 deficiency—secondary to bacteria using it up
    - Steatorrhea—due to bacterial deconjugation of bile
- Caused by bacterial (*Escherichia coli*, GNRs) overgrowth and stasis in afferent limb
- Treatment
    - Antibiotics: Tetracycline, flagyl
    - Promotility agents: Metoclopramide

Dumping

- Early dumping
    - Symptoms
        - Explosive diarrhea
        - Abdominal pain
        - Diaphoresis
        - All symptoms within 20 to 30 minutes of eating
    - Caused by rapid passage of high osmolarity food from stomach to small intestine → water shift into the lumen of the small intestine
    - Treatment
        - Small meals with high protein and low simple carbohydrates
        - Octreotide
- Late dumping
    - Symptoms: Same as early dumping, but 2 to 3 hours post-prandial
    - Due to hyperactive insulin release → hypoglycemia after glucose load
    - Treatment: Same as for early dumping

Overweight patients can mask an intra-abdominal catastrophe. Persistent tachycardia may be the only manifestation of a problem and should be taken seriously.

A 35-year-old woman presents to clinic for her 6-month follow-up after having undergone a laparoscopic band procedure. The band has been filled to its maximum. She complains that she no longer feels any restriction and is unable to lose weight despite following a strict diet and a vigorous exercise plan. A barium swallow study reveals no obvious slippage. What is the next step?

Diagnostic upper endoscopy should be performed to rule out gastric band erosion. Such a condition would require removal of the band.

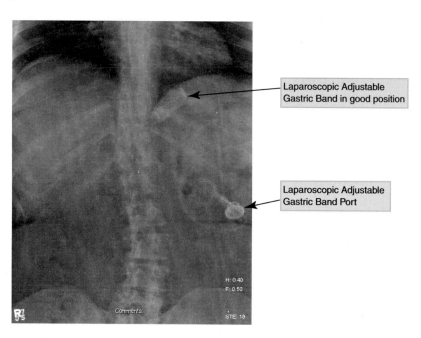

AXR showing an adjustable gastric band in good position.

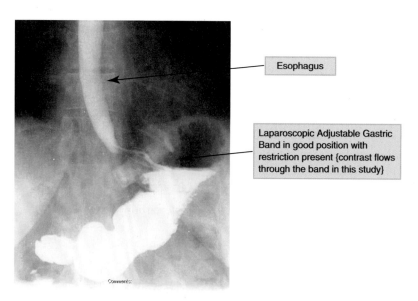

Upper GI showing an adjustable gastric band in good position with no erosion and with restriction present.

Complications of Laparoscopic Adjustable Gastric Banding

- Port site infection
- Breakage of the band itself, the band balloon, and/or the band tubing
- The port flipping its orientation
- Overfill of bands leading to persistent vomiting, inability to tolerate liquids or swallow saliva, nocturnal reflux or persistent reflux and heartburn
- Gastric band erosion
  - Symptoms: No weight loss despite being compliant with diet, the ability to eat anything without a feeling of restriction
  - Presentation: Low grade or recurrent fevers
  - Upper GI is diagnostic test of choice and may also be therapeutic
  - Treatment: Most will require re-operation for removal

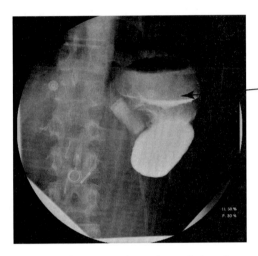

Laparoscopic Adjustable Gastric Band in poor position with stomach incarcerated above the band (A band slip)

Upper GI showing a slipped gastric band.

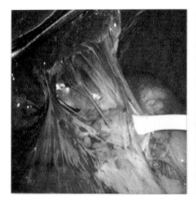 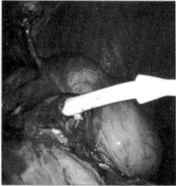

Intraoperative view of slipped gastric band.

- Gastric prolapse or "band slippage"
  - A cephalad herniation of gastric fundus through the band
  - Occurs in up to 5% of LAGB
  - Symptoms: Persistent vomiting, nocturnal reflux, regurgitation, or an inability to swallow liquids and one's own saliva
  - Pain in the left upper quadrant or left chest is an ominous sign that requires urgent re-operation as the prolapsed portion of the stomach can become ischemic or necrotic
  - Upper GI is diagnostic test of choice

- Treatment: Operative reduction and band repositioning or replacement with plication of the fundus to prevent recurrence
- Hiatal hernia
  - Hiatal hernias should be evaluated preoperatively and treated at the time of band placement
  - If a hiatal hernia recurs or occurs after band placement, it can present with recurrent or persistent heartburn and reflux
  - Symptoms are improved with removing fluid from the band
  - Ultimately may require revision of band with surgical correction of the hernia
- Pouch dilation
  - Tends to be concentric and can be asymmetric
  - Symptoms: Persistent heartburn and reflux
  - Diagnosis: Upper GI
    - Can differentiate from gastric prolapse or band overfill
    - If there is no overhang of stomach over the band and no change in the band axis then the diagnosis is usually pouch dilation
  - Treatment usually requires removal of fluid from the band and liquid diet for 2 to 4 weeks with re-evaluation
  - Recurrent symptoms can be treated with band repositioning

An upper GI is the most common test of choice to evaluate obesity surgery complications.

A 43-year-old man presents to the ER for acute onset abdominal pain. He underwent laparoscopic Roux-en Y gastric bypass 2 years ago and has done well until this admission. He now weighs 104 kg, down from 192 kg preoperatively. He is otherwise healthy with no other medical issues. On physical exam his abdomen is soft and nondistended with positive bowel sounds. No groin hernias are identified. His WBC is normal. The ER orders an abdominal X-ray, which is negative for bowel obstruction, and a RUQ ultrasound, which is negative for gallbladder disease. What is the most likely diagnosis?

An internal hernia through a mesenteric defect can be life-threatening in any bariatric patient.

Internal Hernia
- Herniation of bowel through a defect in the mesentery
- Difficult to diagnose
  - May require surgical exploration to diagnose
- Should be suspected when a patient complains of persistent abdominal pain, yet diagnostic tests are negative
- The incidence is 2.5% to 5%
- The most common location depends on the original operative technique
  - Peterson defect (located where the small bowel mesentery drapes up over the transverse colon) with antecolic approach
  - Transverse mesocolon with retrocolic approach
- The greatest risk is immediately postoperatively, and during the initial few years of weight loss
- Treatment includes laparoscopic or open exploration, reduction of the hernia, and repair of the mesenteric defect

Anastomotic Stricture
- Occurs most commonly during the initial 6 months
- Incidence is 5% to 12%

- Patients present with nausea, vomiting, or retching, and become dehydrated
- Diagnosis is made by upper endoscopy
- Treatment is with balloon dilatation

Marginal Ulcers

- An ulcer at the gastrojejunostomy
- May present as abdominal pain with upper GI bleeding, nausea, and vomiting
- Diagnosis requires upper endoscopy
- Conservative treatment includes proton pump inhibitors
- A revision gastrojejunostomy is indicated for bleeding or perforation

---

A 28-year-old woman underwent a laparoscopic gastric bypass operation for morbid obesity 2 years ago. She presents to the emergency department with vomiting and significant mental status changes. What is the most likely diagnosis?

Thiamine deficiency can cause Wernicke encephalopathy and may not be reversible with thiamine administration. It commonly presents with episodes of vomiting and is due to non-compliance with maintenance vitamins.

Micronutrient Deficiencies after Obesity Surgery

- Following a malabsorptive procedure, the distal stomach, duodenum and proximal jejunum are bypassed and micronutrient deficiencies can result
  - Intrinsic factor is produced in the distal stomach and is needed to bind *Vitamin B12* for absorption at the terminal ileum
  - *Folate* is best absorbed at the jejunum
  - Absorption of *iron* and *calcium* occur maximally in the duodenum and thus gastric bypass patients are at high risk for deficiency (>50%); as a result, anemia is common in these patients
- Gastric bypass and duodenal switch patients are counseled to monitor their protein intake (increased by protein powder supplementation) and to take a multivitamin and vitamin B-12 supplement for life
- Fat-soluble vitamins (Vitamin A, D, E, and K) are absorbed in the terminal ileum and are at low risk for deficiency following gastric bypass surgery

---

A 42-year-old woman underwent a laparoscopic gastric bypass 2 months ago. She presents to the emergency room with a chief complaint of epigastric pain radiating to her right upper quadrant. She is a febrile, with HR 89, RR 12, and BP 135/72. She is nauseated but has not vomited. What is the next step in the workup of this patient?

A right upper quadrant ultrasound is needed to rule out gallstones and/or acute cholecystitis.

What medication is given postoperatively to bariatric patients to decrease the risk of future gallstone formation?

After gastric bypass, there is an increased risk of gallstone formation because of rapid weight loss and biliary stasis. Ursodeoxycholic acid (ursodiol) has been shown to limit the formation of gallstones in gastric bypass patients. It works by both inhibiting the formation of cholesterol within the liver and decreasing its intestinal absorption. Patients are routinely discharged to home on daily ursodiol for 6 months postoperatively.

15 | Gallbladder and Biliary System

Nicole E. Lopez and Jason K. Sicklick

During a laparoscopic cholecystectomy, a bile duct variation is suspected. What is the most common variation in bile duct anatomy?

Right sectoral duct joins directly to the common bile duct (CBD).

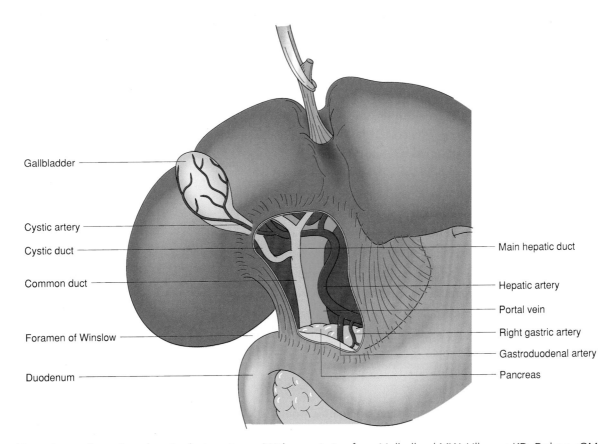

Gallbladder	
Cystic artery	Main hepatic duct
Cystic duct	Hepatic artery
Common duct	Portal vein
	Right gastric artery
Foramen of Winslow	Gastroduodenal artery
Duodenum	Pancreas

Normal porta hepatis and cystic duct anatomy. (With permission from Mulholland MW, Lillemoe KD, Doherty GM, Maier RV, Upchurch GR, eds. *Greenfield's Surgery*. 4th ed. Philadelphia, PA: Lippincott Williams & Wilkins; 2005.)

Bile Duct Anatomy

- The most common hepatic ductal anomaly is either of the right sectoral ducts (i.e., anterior or posterior) draining directly into the CBD (16% to 20%)
- The cystic duct usually joins the common hepatic duct approximately 2 to 4 cm distal to the bifurcation of the right and left hepatic ducts. Common variants include:
    - Joins the middle 1/3 of the hepatic duct at an angle (75%)
    - Fused to the hepatic duct along a parallel course (20%)
    - Spiral course to enter at the left side (5%)
    - Most rarely, the cystic duct can empty in the proximal hepatic duct or directly into the right hepatic duct (0.3%)

Porta Hepatis Anatomy

- The portal triad
    - Portal vein—posterior
    - CBD—lateral
    - Common hepatic artery—medial and anterior
- Portal venous anatomy is relatively constant and has much less variation than the biliary ductal and hepatic arterial systems

---

What is the most common hepatic artery anomaly?

A replaced right hepatic artery occurs in 15% to 20% of the population and originates from the superior mesenteric artery (SMA).

Hepatic Artery Anomalies

- Definitions
    - Replaced artery: A substitute for the normal/usual hepatic artery, which is absent
    - Accessory artery: Appears in addition to one that is normally/usually present
- Normal anatomy present in 51% to 76%
- Replaced right hepatic artery originating from the SMA
    - The most common anomaly
    - 10.6% to 21% of people
    - Runs behind the head and uncinate process of the pancreas
    - Courses posterolateral to the CBD
    - If in question, can aspirate with 25G needle
- Replaced left hepatic artery originating from the celiac trunk
    - 4.6% to 18% of people
- Accessory left hepatic artery originating from left gastric artery
    - 8% to 18% of people
- Accessory right hepatic artery
    - 7% of people
- Replaced common hepatic artery originating from the SMA
    - 1.4% to 5% of people
- Anterior location of right hepatic artery
    - The artery originates from the proper hepatic artery and courses anterior to the common hepatic duct

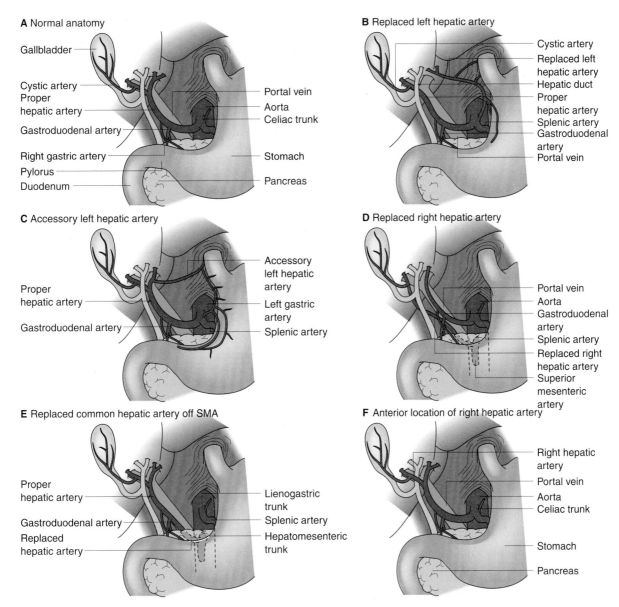

A Normal anatomy

Gallbladder

Cystic artery
Proper hepatic artery
Gastroduodenal artery

Right gastric artery
Pylorus
Duodenum

Portal vein
Aorta
Celiac trunk

Stomach

Pancreas

B Replaced left hepatic artery

Cystic artery
Replaced left hepatic artery
Hepatic duct
Proper hepatic artery
Splenic artery
Gastroduodenal artery
Portal vein

C Accessory left hepatic artery

Proper hepatic artery

Gastroduodenal artery

Accessory left hepatic artery
Left gastric artery
Splenic artery

D Replaced right hepatic artery

Portal vein
Aorta
Gastroduodenal artery
Splenic artery
Replaced right hepatic artery
Superior mesenteric artery

E Replaced common hepatic artery off SMA

Proper hepatic artery

Gastroduodenal artery
Replaced hepatic artery

Lienogastric trunk
Splenic artery
Hepatomesenteric trunk

F Anterior location of right hepatic artery

Right hepatic artery
Portal vein
Aorta
Celiac trunk

Stomach

Pancreas

Variations in hepatic artery anatomy. (A) Normal anatomy. (B) Replaced left hepatic artery originating from the left gastric artery. (C) Accessory left hepatic artery originating from the left gastric artery in addition to the normal arterial supply. (D) Replaced right hepatic artery originating from the SMA. (E) Replaced common hepatic artery originating from the SMA. (F) Anterior location of the right hepatic artery (courses anterior to the common hepatic duct). (With permission from Mulholland MW, Lillemoe KD, Doherty GM, Maier RV, Upchurch GR, eds. *Greenfield's Surgery*. 4th ed. Philadelphia, PA: Lippincott Williams & Wilkins; 2005.)

A replaced left hepatic artery is a potential pitfall during a Nissen fundoplication and a replaced right hepatic artery is a potential pitfall during a pancreaticoduodenectomy.

What layers of the bowel are not present in the gallbladder (GB) wall?

The GB lacks a submucosa and muscularis mucosa.

Layers of the Gallbladder

- The GB has a mucosa, a muscularis propria, a perimuscular subserosal connective tissue, and a serosa

- It lacks the submucosa and muscularis mucosa layers
  - The lack of submucosa makes the GB wall weaker than the intestinal wall
- Rokitansky-Aschoff sinuses—form from the invagination of the epithelium through the fibromuscular layer as a result of inflammation and increased pressure in the GB (e.g., during cholecystitis)
- During cholecystectomy, the plane of dissection is the subserosal plane and therefore, all T2 and higher GB cancers require additional resection if a cancer is incidentally identified following a cholecystectomy

---

What is the blood supply of the CBD?

The CBD has a segmental blood supply.

Blood Supply of the Common Bile Duct

- Derived inferiorly from the gastroduodenal artery—the main blood supply
- Derived superiorly from the right hepatic artery
- Supply blood vessels on the CBD are located at the cross-sectional 3 and 9 o'clock positions
  - Occasionally, these may need to be oversewn when performing a bile duct resection or pancreaticoduodenectomy

---

Upon an ultrasound examination for cholelithiasis, a 5-mm CBD is noted. What is the normal diameter of the CBD?

A normal CBD is 4 to 6 mm in diameter, with a couple of exceptions.

Common Bile Duct Size

- A normal CBD is up to 4 to 6 mm
- Add 1 mm per decade over 50 to the normal CBD size
- The CBD is normally enlarged status post cholecystectomy
  - The size of the CBD accommodates for the removed GB
- Ultrasound is the best method for determining CBD size

When performing a manual Pringle maneuver, what structure is located directly posterior to the surgeon's finger in the foramen of Winslow?

The inferior vena cava is directly posterior to the porta hepatis.

What is the average volume of daily bile production per day?

Approximately 600 to 1,000 mL of bile is produced each day.

What is the source of routine bilirubin formation?

80% of bilirubin is derived from hemoglobin.

20% of bilirubin is derived from hemoproteins and a small pool of free heme.

What is the most common element in bile?

Bile is 90% water.

Composition of Bile

- Iso-osmotic (about 300 mOsm)
- pH 7.8
- Water 90%
- Electrolytes 10%
- Bile is high in: Na, K, HCO_3
- Bile is low in: Cl, Ca, Mg
- At higher flow rates, stimulated by secretin and vasoactive intestinal peptide, $[HCO_3]$ increases and [Cl] decreases
- Organic solutes
- Primary and secondary bile acids > phospholipids [lecithin] > cholesterol > proteins > bilirubin
  - Bile acid pool: Approximately 5 g
  - Recirculate in enterohepatic circulation approximately every 4 hours
  - 0.5 g (10%) of bile acids lost in stool each day

What are the primary bile acids? What are the secondary bile acids?

The primary bile acids are cholic acid and chenodeoxycholic acid.

The secondary bile acids are deoxycholic, lithocholic, and ursodeoxycholic acid.

Where are secondary bile acids synthesized?

Small intestine.

Primary Bile Acids

- Cholic acid and chenodeoxycholic acid
- Synthesized from cholesterol in the liver
  - The rate-limiting enzyme in bile acid production is cholesterol 7α-hydroxylase
- Each of these comprise approximately 40% of bile acids
- Conjugated with either glycine or taurine in the liver to render them more useful for fat digestion and absorption

Secondary Bile Acids

- Deoxycholic acid, lithocholic acid, and ursodeoxycholic acid
- Synthesized in the small intestine from primary bile acids via intestinal bacterial enzymes
- Conjugated with either glycine or taurine in the liver for fat emulsification
- Note that lithocholic acid is insoluble and lost in stool
- Bile is reabsorbed in the terminal ileum/colon in order to enter the enterohepatic circulation
  - Bile acids are resorbed via an Na-dependent bile salt transporter
  - They are then returned to the liver via portal venous flow

How is hemoglobin degraded?

Hemoglobin Degradation

- Hgb → heme → biliverdin → bilirubin
- Free, unconjugated bilirubin undergoes glucuronidation (glucuronyl transferase) to the conjugated, water soluble form that is excreted
- Conjugated bilirubin is actively secreted in bile
- Urobilinogen
  - Breakdown of bilirubin by bacteria in the terminal ileum → resorption of bilirubin into blood → release of bilirubin in urine

What is the main type of bile pigment?

Bilirubin glucuronide (via conjugation of bilirubin to glucuronic acid by glucuronic transferase).

What are the main functions of bile?

- Fat emulsification
- Aids with absorption of lipid-soluble vitamins A, D, E, and K
- Excretion of bilirubin derived from senescent erythrocytes
- Cholesterol excretion via transport in biliary lecithin vesicles

What is the principal hormone involved in GB contraction?

Cholecystokinin (CCK) is the main hormone involved in GB contraction. 80% of the GB empties within 2 hours post-prandially.

The Gallbladder and Pregnancy

- GB contraction is decreased in the second half of the menstrual cycle and the third trimester of pregnancy
- There are more gallstones, sludge, and cholesterol content in bile, derived from estrogen, during pregnancy
- Optimal timing for the operation is during the second trimester

What happens to the enterohepatic circulation following a cholecystectomy?

The enterohepatic circulation increases to accommodate increased bile flow into the small bowel.

Changes Status Post-cholecystectomy

- CBD dilatation
- Decreased bile acid pool

- More continuous flow of bile into the intestine
  - Cholesterol solubility in the bile increases
  - Bile acid secretion increases
  - Enterohepatic recycling increases

A 25-year-old male with no past medical history presents after a football injury with a ulnar fracture. He undergoes reduction of the fracture, but postoperatively is noted to have an elevated bilirubin of 4.0; his other LFTs are normal. You fractionate the bilirubin and the conjugated portion is 0.5 and the unconjugated portion is 3.5. Does this need further workup?

This patient has Gilbert syndrome, which results in elevation of unconjugated (indirect) bilirubin, particularly after stress. No further workup is needed.

Unconjugated Hyperbilirubinemia
- Causes: Hemolysis, hepatic deficiency of uptake or conjugation
- Gilbert disease
  - Abnormal bilirubin uptake in the liver
  - Hyperbilirubinemia, particularly during stress
  - Usually asymptomatic; no treatment needed
- Crigler-Najjar disease
  - Inability to conjugate bilirubin secondary to a glucuronyl transferase deficiency
  - Have high unconjugated bilirubin
  - A life-threatening disease
- Physiologic jaundice of a newborn
  - Due to immature glucuronyl transferase

Conjugated Hyperbilirubinemia
- Causes: Secretion defects into bile ducts, excretion defects into GI tract (stones, stricture, tumor)
- Rotor syndrome
  - Deficiency in storage ability
- Dubin-Johnson syndrome
  - Deficiency in secretion ability

A 41-year-old obese Native American woman underwent resection of her terminal ileum for Crohn's disease and was maintained on TPN for 6 weeks. What is her predisposition to have cholelithiasis?

She has multiple risk factors for cholelithiasis.

Risk Factors for Cholelithiasis
- Middle age
- Female
- Obesity
- Rapid weight loss (secondary to GB sludge)
- Exogenous estrogen

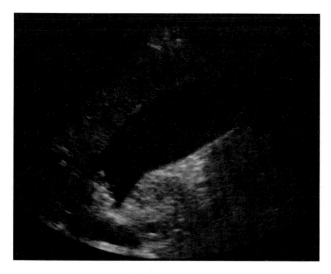

Gallstones on ultrasound.

- Pregnancy
- Terminal ileum resection
- Total parenteral nutrition (cholestasis leads to increased pigmented stone formation)
- Truncal or hepatic branch vagotomy (loss of cholinergic stimulation for GB contraction leads to stasis)
- Genetic susceptibility to cholesterol stone formation (e.g., Native Americans)
- Cirrhosis
- Crohn's disease
- Hereditary spherocytosis
- Hemolytic anemia
- Gallstones in obese people with no other risk factors. Usually secondary to overactive HMG Co-A reductase
- Gallstones in thin people with no other risk factors: Due to underactive 7α-hydroxylase

What types of gallstones are most common following a terminal ileum resection?

Pigmented stones.

Gallstones

- Cholesterol stones (most common)
  - Yellow stones
  - Recurrent stones are usually cholesterol stones
  - Due to a failure of cholesterol and calcium salts to remain in solution as a result of an imbalance of cholesterol, lecithin, and bile acids (relatively increased cholesterol)
  - Pure cholesterol stones
    - Nearly 100% cholesterol
    - Typically multiple with bumpy, spheroid, or faceted shape
  - Mixed cholesterol stones
    - ≥70% cholesterol
    - Typically single, ovoid, spherical

- Pigmented stones
    - Dark stones due to calcium bilirubinate, i.e., a precipitation of unconjugated bilirubin with Ca
    - Most contain <20% cholesterol
    - Causes
        - Congenital or acquired hemolytic anemia (i.e., sickle cell disease or thalassemia)
        - Higher incidence after terminal ileum resection
        - Crohn's disease (secondary to bile salt malabsorption)
    - Black pigment stones
        - Jet black, brittle, and spiculated shape
        - Generally form in the GB
        - May contain polymerized bile pigments
        - Found with cirrhosis, hemolysis, Crohn's disease, long-term TPN administration
    - Brown pigment stones
        - Brown or brownish-yellow with a soft or malleable consistency
        - Pliable due to a higher percent composition of cholesterol and calcium palmitate (bacterial derived)
        - Associated with infected bile and are largely composed of bacterial cell bodies and precipitated calcium bilirubinate
        - Also associated with parasitic infections (*Opisthorchis viverrini*, *Clonorchis sinensis*, and *Ascaris lumbricoides*)
        - Generally form in the bile ducts and result in CBD stones

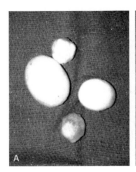 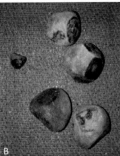 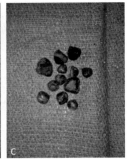

(A) Cholesterol gallstones. (B) Brown pigment gallstone. (C) Black pigment gallstones.

What is the best laboratory test for biliary obstruction?

Alkaline phosphatase. It can also be elevated during childhood, pregnancy, and due to primary/metastatic bone malignancies.

Differential Diagnosis of Conjugated Hyperbilirubinemia
- Choledocholithiasis
- Intrinsic or extrinsic periampullary, biliary, or hepatic tumors
- Primary sclerosing cholangitis (PSC)
- Parasitic infections (adult *A. lumbricoides* or eggs of *C. sinensis* or *Fasciola hepatica*)
- AIDS cholangiopathy (*Cryptosporidium*, CMV, or HIV)
- Biliary stricture
- Sepsis

What is the imaging method of choice for the initial workup of right upper quadrant pain?

RUQ ultrasound is the imaging study of choice for patients with RUQ pain. It is useful in diagnosing cholelithiasis, cholecystitis, liver masses, and pyelonephritis.

Imaging Studies for Gallstones

Imaging Study	Sensitivity
Endoscopic ultrasound (EUS)	95% (choledocholithiasis)
Ultrasound	>97%
MRCP	85–100%
CT scan	75%
X-rays	15–20%

A 43-year-old obese woman presents to the emergency department with right upper quadrant pain. Her pain is colicky in nature, has been intermittent for several months, and is worse after consuming fatty foods. She has no fever or leukocytosis. An abdominal ultrasound confirms gallstones in the GB. What is the next step in her management?

Discharge the patient with dietary instructions to avoid fatty foods and to take analgesics as needed. An elective cholecystectomy should be planned for symptomatic cholelithiasis. Admission to the hospital is generally reserved for patients who cannot tolerate a regular diet or have severe pain.

Cholelithiasis

- Defined as the presence of gallstones within the GB
- Typically asymptomatic (8% to 15% prevalence in the general population)
- Approximately 1% to 2% of those with asymptomatic gallstones may develop symptoms annually
- Biliary colic is often the presenting symptom, although nausea and vomiting may be present in severe cases
- Approximately 70% of patients will have one or more recurrent episodes of pain within a year of onset of symptoms
- Laparoscopic cholecystectomy should be performed for patients with symptoms

Biliary Colic

- The symptom of biliary pain
- It is caused by GB contraction in response to a fatty meal, which leads to pressing of a gallstone against the cystic duct opening
- This closed system leads to increased intra-GB pressure and pain
- It may be mistaken for irritable bowel syndrome, acute myocardial infarction, or peptic ulcer disease

A 40-year-old woman presents with a 5-mm GB wall and pericholecystic fluid on ultrasound. What is the most likely diagnosis?

Acute cholecystitis is the most likely diagnosis. 90% to 95% of cases are associated with cholelithiasis.

Acute Cholecystitis

- Prolonged or recurrent cystic duct blockage by a gallstone or biliary stasis can progress to total obstruction
- If untreated, acute cholecystitis can progress into gangrenous cholecystitis or lead to GB perforation
- Patients typically complain of RUQ or epigastric abdominal pain with possible radiation to the right shoulder or back
- Ultrasound is the most commonly used test for diagnosis
- HIDA is the most sensitive test for acute cholecystitis

Ultrasound

- Findings consistent with acute cholecystitis
  - GB wall thickening (>3 mm)
  - Pericholecystic fluid
  - Distended GB
  - Positive sonographic Murphy sign
  - Gallstones (supportive)

HIDA Scan

- A functional test using technetium-99m pertechnetate iminodiacetic acid to evaluate the biliary system
  - Technetium is taken up by the liver and concentrated in the biliary tract
  - If GB cannot be seen, it is secondary to cystic duct obstruction by a stone → need cholecystectomy
  - If <25% of the GB volume is excreted after CCK over 20 minutes, have biliary dyskinesia
- 50% of these patients will benefit from cholecystectomy
- Highly sensitive for cholecystitis, although it is more invasive than an ultrasound and is usually reserved for cases when the diagnosis is in question
- HIDA specificity is confounded by high false positive rates when patients are NPO for prolonged periods (>3 days)

Definitive therapy for cholecystitis includes broad-spectrum antibiotic coverage followed by laparoscopic cholecystectomy within 48 hours.

A 30-year-old female presents to the emergency department with right upper quadrant pain for the last 5 days, an ultrasound is consistent with cholecystitis. What is the next step in management?

Classically, IV antibiotics and plan for interval cholecystectomy have been advocated for patients presenting more than 72 hours after the onset of symptoms. Newer studies would suggest that laparoscopic cholecystectomy can be performed in selected patients.

You have just performed a laparoscopic cholecystectomy on a 32-year-old otherwise healthy female and the post-anesthesia care unit (PACU) calls you to inform you that she is becoming progressively more hypotensive and tachycardic. What are you concerned about and what is your next step in management?

This is concerning for the clip falling off of the cystic artery and the patient should be taken back to the OR immediately for exploration.

Shock after Laparoscopic Cholecystectomy

- Early (first 24 hours): Hemorrhagic from a clip that fell off the cystic artery
- Late (after first 24 hours): Septic shock from accidental clip on CBD with subsequent cholangitis

Persistent Nausea/Vomiting after Laparoscopic Cholecystectomy

- Do ultrasound to look for fluid collection
- If there is a fluid collection
    - Drain collection
    - If bilious then perform endoscopic retrograde cholangiopancreatography (ERCP) and sphincterotomy to create a "path of least resistance" by which the bile can flow out through the CBD as opposed to the cystic duct remnant
        - If bilious fluid collection persists, may need to do hepaticojejunostomy
- If no fluid collection and hepatic ducts are dilated, likely have a transected CBD with stricture

A 65-year-old woman has been on TPN for 12 weeks following a prolonged ICU course. She reports new right upper quadrant pain at the time of a new-onset fever and leukocytosis. An ultrasound demonstrates no gallstones, but significant GB wall thickening and pericholecystic fluid. What is the next step in management?

The patient likely has acalculous cholecystitis. A laparoscopic cholecystectomy and a cholecystostomy tube are the only ways to relieve the infection.

Acalculous Cholecystitis

- Bile stasis leads to GB distention and ischemia
- Risk factors include prolonged fasting, dehydration, narcotic use, and hyperalimentation
- Overall, a rare condition, but more commonly seen in critically ill patients who have been on TPN for an extended period
    - Multiple trauma, prolonged critical illness, or sepsis
    - Consider in any postoperative or acutely ill patient with upper abdominal pain and fever or with unexplained fever and leukocytosis
- Ultrasound is first test of choice; HIDA scan is sensitive but not specific (especially when patients have been NPO for a significant period of time)
- Treatment
    - Laparoscopic cholecystectomy for stable patients
    - Cholecystostomy tube placement for unstable or high-risk patients

Emphysematous Gallbladder Disease

- Gas in GB wall that can be seen on plain film
- Usually secondary to *Clostridium perfringens*
- Increased incidence in diabetics
- Symptoms: Severe, rapid onset abdominal pain, nausea/vomiting, and sepsis
- Treatment: Same as for acalculous cholecystitis

A 29-year-old woman is evaluated in the office for right upper quadrant pain. Her symptoms are consistent with biliary colic and have been intermittent for 2 years.
An ultrasound is normal without evidence of gallstones. Following dietary instruction, her symptoms improve slightly but persist. What is the next step in management?

Obtain a HIDA scan with ejection fraction to determine if the patient has biliary dyskinesia.

Biliary Dyskinesia

- Classically associated with RUQ pain, fatty food intolerance, nausea, and a normal ultrasound
- Abdominal CT and EGD are often necessary to rule out other causes of symptoms
- A HIDA ejection fraction of less than 20% at 20 minutes is considered abnormal
- Treatment is laparoscopic cholecystectomy

Which noninvasive study may be utilized to evaluate the biliary tree?

Magnetic resonance cholangiopancreatography (MRCP) is a non invasive method of imaging the biliary tree that improves upon the ability of CT and ultrasound to exclude CBD stones or stenosis.

A 62-year-old man with biliary obstruction from a CBD stone seen on MRCP is febrile and has an increased WBC. What is the most likely organism causing his cholangitis?

This patient most likely has an ascending cholangitis secondary to biliary obstruction. Escherichia coli is the most common organism.

Acute (Ascending) Cholangitis

- Occurs when a bile duct obstruction, most commonly from an impacted stone, causes dilation of the obstructed duct, stasis, and bacterial superinfection
- Can result from instrumentation including ERCP or PTC (percutaneous transhepatic biliary catheter)
- Characterized by Charcot triad (fever, jaundice, and abdominal pain), which occurs in only 50% to 75% of cases
- Occasionally can progress to biliary sepsis characterized by Reynold pentad—Charcot triad plus hypotension and mental status changes
- Organisms: *Escherichia coli* >> *Enterococcus* > *Klebsiella* > *Proteus* > *Pseudomonas* > *Enterobacter*
- Treatment consists of emergent biliary decompression by ERCP with sphincterotomy or percutaneous transhepatic biliary drainage

During a laparoscopic cholecystectomy and cholangiogram, CBD stones were seen. What is the next step in management?

After administering glucagon, flush the CBD with saline.

Common Bile Duct Stones

- If found during MRCP:
  - Perform an ERCP with stone retrieval and sphincterotomy
  - If ERCP is unsuccessful, perform a laparoscopic CBD exploration to remove the stones
- If discovered by intra-operative cholangiography:
  - Administer glucagon and then flush the CBD with saline
  - CBD exploration can be performed
    - Saline irrigation with repeated flushes of the CBD
    - Fogarty balloon technique
    - Gentle pushing of CBD stones with coronary dilators
    - Basket retrieval system
    - Choledochoscopy—be sure to examine both antegrade and retrograde
  - Alternatively, a postoperative ERCP can be performed
    - Ideal for small stones
- In cases in which the patient is septic or hemodynamically unstable, ERCP, percutaneous biliary drainage, or cholecystostomy should be performed to decompress the obstruction and treat the cholangitis
- Conversion from a laparoscopic to an open CBD exploration
  - A more invasive option for cases where multiple preoperative ERCP procedures fail or the cholangitis is life threatening
  - Transduodenal sphincteroplasty is a last resort for CBD stones refractory to ERCP and CBD exploration

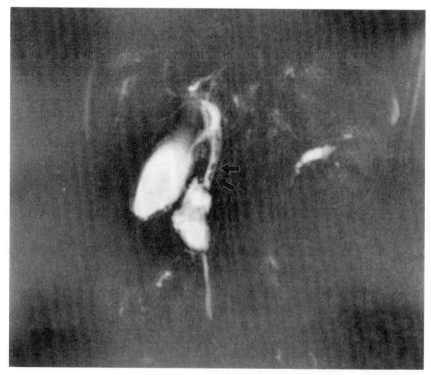

MRCP demonstrating CBD stones. (With permission from Mulholland MW, Lillemoe KD, Doherty GM, Maier RV, Upchurch GR, eds. *Greenfield's Surgery.* 4th ed. Philadelphia, PA: Lippincott Williams & Wilkins; 2005.)

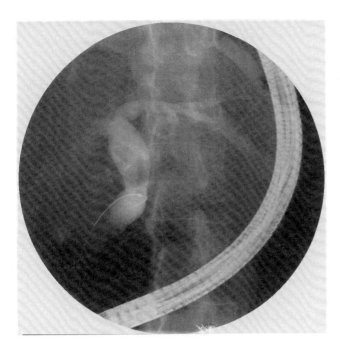

ERCP with CBD stones. (With permission from Mulholland MW, Lillemoe KD, Doherty GM, Maier RV, Upchurch GR, eds. *Greenfield's Surgery*. 4th ed. Philadelphia, PA: Lippincott Williams & Wilkins; 2005.)

If preoperative ERCP and other less invasive techniques are unsuccessful in relieving a CBD obstruction in the setting of cholangitis, an open CBD exploration should be performed.

What is the minimum level of bilirubin needed to have clinically apparent jaundice?

A bilirubin level of 2.5 to 3.0 mg/dL or greater usually results in clinically apparent jaundice.

- Sublingual jaundice occurs before scleral icterus. This is followed by jaundice of the skin.

A 48-year-old man with a history of gallstones presents with a bilirubin level of 25 mg/dL. What is the most likely cause of his hyperbilirubinemia?

Complete biliary obstruction is one of the few conditions that can cause a markedly elevated bilirubin. Liver failure, hemolytic anemia, and viral hepatitis should also be considered.

A 45-year-old man has persistent jaundice 3 weeks following resection of a chronically obstructing bile duct cancer. What is the most likely cause of his persistent hyperbilirubinemia following biliary decompression?

Increased delta bilirubin.

Delta Bilirubin
- Defined as bilirubin bound to albumin (half-life = 3 weeks)
- Occurs with prolonged hyperbilirubinemia
- Not cleared by hepatic or renal metabolism
- Persistent hyperbilirubinemia can also lead to skin deposition of bilirubin, resulting in a prolonged appearance of jaundice

> What is the Mirizzi syndrome?

Mirizzi syndrome describes an impacted cystic duct stone that leads to compression of the extrahepatic bile ducts leading to elevated LFTs with no CBD obstruction.

> During a laparoscopic cholecystectomy, the GB is noted to have a strawberry appearance. What is the most likely etiology?

A strawberry appearance of the GB may result from the deposition of triglycerides, cholesterol precursors, and cholesterol esters into macrophages of the lamina propria. The lipid accumulation creates yellow deposits that, on a background of hyperemic mucosa, lead to this appearance.

> A 43-year-old female with a history of a car accident 1 year ago complicated by a hepatic laceration that was managed conservatively, but with no other significant medical history, presents with an upper GI bleed, jaundice, and RUQ pain. What is the next step in management?

An angiogram to evaluate for a fistula between the biliary and hepatic arterial system.

Hemobilia

- Most commonly presents with an upper GI bleed, jaundice, and RUQ pain
- Most commonly have a fistula between the biliary and hepatic arterial system
- Most commonly occurs with trauma
- Diagnosis: Angiogram
- Treatment: Angiogram with embolization first—if that fails, surgical exploration

Bilhemia

- Bile in the venous system
- Bilhemia is a rare complication after liver injury that is associated with a high mortality
- Occurs due to an intrahepatic fistula between the biliary and venous system
- Clinical signs are a rapid increase in the direct and total bilirubin up to extreme values with an increase in the serum bile acids

> A 65-year-old woman with a history of diabetes presents with right upper quadrant pain. A CT scan reveals a porcelain GB. What is the significance of this finding?

A porcelain GB may be associated with GB cancer, or more commonly, simple thickening and calcification of the GB wall.

Porcelain Gallbladder

- An uncommon manifestation of chronic cholecystitis characterized by intramural calcification of the GB wall
- GB develops a bluish hue and brittle consistency
- Associated with cholelithiasis in >95% of patients
- More common in diabetics

- Associated with a 0% to 7% risk of GB cancer
  - Higher incidence of GB cancer with selective calcification over diffuse calcification
- A porcelain GB is an indication for cholecystectomy

> During a laparoscopic cholecystectomy, the GB is perforated and a white secretion is noted to extrude from the GB. What does this white fluid indicate?

The white bile results from long-term complete obstruction of the cystic duct and is referred to as biliary hydrops. This obstruction leads to increased intraluminal pressure and cessation of biliary secretion.

- Indications for needle decompression of hydrops during laparoscopic cholecystectomy:
  - GB is overdistended and taught, increasing the risk of rupture or tear with retraction
  - Insufficient visualization of the triangle of Calot due to GB distention

> A 27-year-old woman is found to have an incidental 0.5 cm polyp. What is the next step in management?

For an asymptomatic GB polyp measuring less than 1 cm, there is no evidence that surgery is warranted. A follow-up ultrasound in 1 year is a reasonable management strategy.

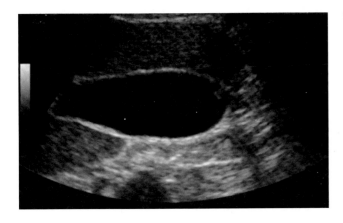

Ultrasound showing GB polyp.

Gallbladder Polyps

- Majority are benign, but imaging studies are insufficient to exclude the possibility of GB carcinoma or premalignant adenomas
- Operate for symptoms, size >1 cm, increasing size, family history of GB cancer, or in the setting of PSC
- Underlying pathologies
  - Cholesterolosis (most common)
  - Adenomyomatosis
  - Inflammatory process
  - Adenoma
  - Leiomyoma
  - Lipoma
  - Adenocarcinoma

- To distinguish a polyp from gallstone, an ultrasonographer may have the patient roll during the ultrasound—with rolling, a stone should be mobile whereas a polyp will be stationary

---

A 4-year-old Asian girl presents with right upper quadrant pain and jaundice. An ultrasound demonstrates a cystic dilation of the CBD. What is the next step in management?

An ERCP or CT scan can confirm the presence of a Type I choledochal cyst. The treatment is a cyst excision and Roux-en-Y choledochojejunostomy or hepaticojejunostomy.

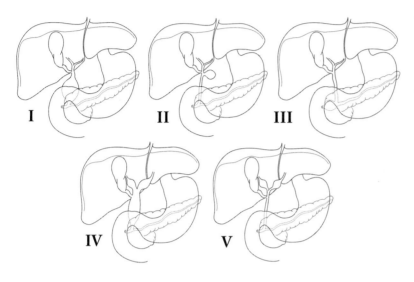

Types of choledochal cysts. (With permission from Fischer JE, Bland KI, Callery MP, et al., eds. *Mastery of Surgery*. 5th ed. Philadelphia, PA: Lippincott Williams & Wilkins; 2006:1183.)

Choledochal Cyst
- More common in females and Asians
- Predispose to cholangiocarcinoma
- Type I is the most common (approximately 90%)
    - Solitary extrahepatic fusiform or cystic dilation of the CBD that spares the intrahepatic bile ducts
    - Treatment: Cyst excision with a Roux-en-Y hepaticojejunostomy
- Types II–IV describe variations of intra- and extrahepatic involvement
    - Type II: Extrahepatic supraduodenal diverticulum
        - Treatment: Cyst excision with primary choledochorrhaphy including T-tube placement, or cyst excision with a Roux-en-Y hepaticojejunostomy
    - Type III: Intraduodenal diverticulum, choledochocele
        - Treatment: Transduodenal cyst excision with reimplantation of the CBD and pancreatic ducts
    - Type IV: Two types
        - Type IVa: Fusiform extrahepatic and intrahepatic cysts
            - Treatment: Cyst excision with a Roux-en-Y hepaticojejunostomy; hepatic lobectomy if cysts are localized to one lobe; or liver transplantation
        - Type IVb: Multiple extrahepatic cysts
            - Treatment: Cyst excision with a Roux-en-Y hepaticojejunostomy
    - Type V: Caroli disease—involves only intrahepatic ducts
        - Treatment: Liver transplantation

- Neonates often present only with jaundice
- Children present with pain, but sometimes a mass may be palpated
- Pancreatitis and cholangitis can be early manifestations
- Overall, there is a 2.5% to 30% risk of malignant transformation
- Liver transplantation is reserved for Caroli (intrahepatic only) disease with liver failure

Surgical resection of a choledochal cyst is indicated due to increased risk of malignancy.

A 37-year-old woman presents 5 years after a hepaticojejunostomy performed for a CBD injury. She complains of right upper quadrant pain and is febrile.
Her laboratory tests demonstrate a WBC of 19,000 and a total bilirubin of 7.2. What is the most likely etiology of her illness?

Following hepaticojejunostomy or any biliary surgery, an anastomotic stricture can result, leading to increased susceptibility to episodes of cholangitis.

Biliary Stricture
- Differential diagnosis of presentation
  - Cholangiocarcinoma
  - Ampullary tumor
  - Pancreatic head or uncinate tumor
  - Duodenal tumor
  - CBD injury
  - CBD stones
  - Sclerosing cholangitis
  - Pancreatitis
  - Ascending cholangitis
  - Recurrent pyogenic cholangiohepatitis
  - Intraductal papillary neoplasm of the bile duct
- Biliary anastomotic stricture
  - May present years after biliary surgery
  - Treatment is balloon dilatation by ERCP or PTC if thought to be benign (i.e., anastomotic stricture)
- Extrahepatic bile duct resection may be indicated for lesions suspicious for malignancy
- For more distal lesions, pancreaticoduodenectomy may be considered
- Malignant masquerade (Pseudo-Klatskin tumor)
  - Benign idiopathic fibroinflammatory causing stricture of the common hepatic duct confluence that is clinically and radiologically indistinguishable from hilar cholangiocarcinoma
  - Causes include:
    - Lymphoplasmacytic sclerosing pancreatitis and cholangitis
    - PSC
    - Granulomatous disease
    - Nonspecific fibrosis and inflammation
    - Occult choledocholithiasis
  - Recognition of this pseudotumor emphasizes the importance of offering surgery to all patients with resectable hilar cholangiocarcinoma

Now biliary strictures may represent malignancy and must be evaluated. This is especially the case if there is a history of malignancy, or if there is no history of prior biliary surgery, pancreatitis, cholangitis, or other process to explain the presence of a benign stricture.

Common Bile Duct Injury

- A common cause of lawsuits in general surgery
- Most commonly secondary to incorrect identification of the CBD as the cystic duct
- Present with bile leak/biloma, jaundice, cholangitis, vague abdominal pain, inappropriately high level of pain following a routine laparoscopic cholecystectomy, and sepsis
- Workup includes an RUQ ultrasound, HIDA scan, CT, and/or ERCP
- Treatment when recognized immediately
  - If the injury is <50% of CBD circumference, perform an end-to-end repair
  - If >50% of CBD circumference, or involves the right or left bile duct, perform a hepaticojejunostomy
  - If an experienced hepatobiliary surgeon is not available, simply place drains and transfer the patient
- Treatment if the injury is recognized postoperatively
  - If the injury is <50% of CBD circumference, insert an ERCP-placed bile stent or percutaneous transhepatic biliary drain
    - Many patients will heal with this and will not need subsequent reconstructive surgery
  - If >50% of CBD circumference, or involves the right or left bile duct, perform an hepaticojejunostomy before POD #7 or after 6 weeks
    - Can place drains as a temporizing measure until surgery if injury is recognized after POD 7

The ideal time to repair a major bile duct injury is in the initial few days postoperatively or about 6 weeks later once the inflammation has resolved. An ERCP or PTC drain can temporize and sometimes resolve the situation in the interim.

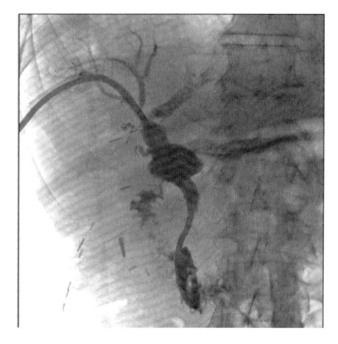

Percutaneous transhepatic biliary drain after a CBD injury.

A 79-year-old woman with a known history of cholelithiasis presents with a 6-day history of intermittent nausea, vomiting, obstipation, and crampy abdominal pain. A CT scan demonstrates pneumobilia. What is the best way to treat her illness?

A bowel obstruction with pneumobilia is highly suspicious for "gallstone ileus." An exploratory laparotomy is indicated to search for obstructing gallstones in the small bowel.

Gallstone Ileus

- Most common in elderly women
- The inciting event is a fistula between the GB and bowel, most commonly the duodenum
- Large stones are often caught at the narrow area of the terminal ileum/ileocecal valve
- Symptoms of bowel obstruction with gallstone ileus are often intermittent, with brief periods of relief when the stone moves into a non-obstructing position
- Pneumobilia is present in 50% of cases
- Often associated with cholecystitis
- Treatment is laparotomy with removal of the obstructing stone, exploration of the entire bowel, cholecystectomy, and possible CBD exploration
  - Always inspect the GI tract from the stomach to the colon for a second or third stone
  - Stones in the duodenum should be milked into the stomach where a gastrostomy can be safely performed
  - Perform a cholecystectomy and fistula repair only if the patient is stable and can tolerate the procedure; otherwise, this procedure can be deferred

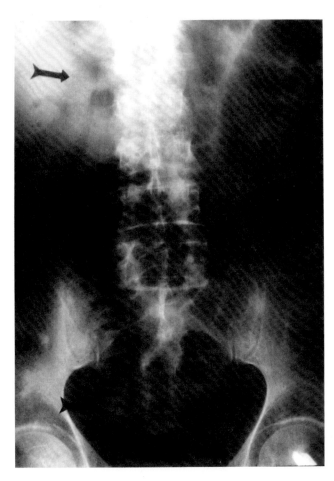

Gallstone ileus. Air in the biliary tree (*superior arrow*). Stone in the terminal ileum causing bowel obstruction (*inferior arrow*). (With permission from Mulholland MW, Lillemoe KD, Doherty GM, Maier RV, Upchurch GR, eds. *Greenfield's Surgery.* 4th ed. Philadelphia, PA: Lippincott Williams & Wilkins; 2005.)

A 41-year-old man presents with pruritus and fatigue. Laboratory tests demonstrate a mildly elevated alkaline phosphatase and gamma-glutamyl transferase (GGT). An ERCP reveals multifocal intrahepatic and extrahepatic bile duct strictures. What is the next step in management?

A liver biopsy is indicated for patients with suspected PSC to determine the stage of the disease.

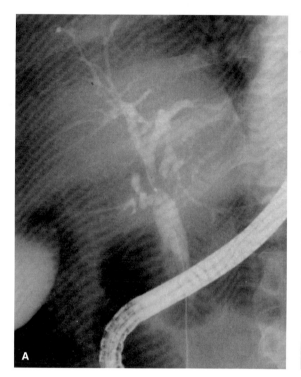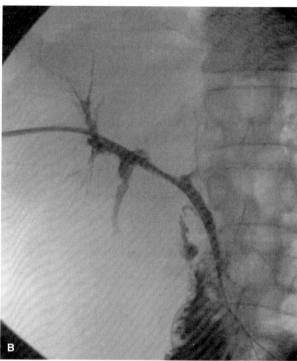

Typical ERCP findings with PSC. (With permission from Fischer JE, Bland KI, Callery MP, et al., eds. *Mastery of Surgery*. 5th ed. Philadelphia, PA: Lippincott Williams & Wilkins; 2006.)

Primary Sclerosing Cholangitis

+ Probable autoimmune disorder
+ More common in young men
+ Other associated diseases: Ulcerative colitis, Crohn's disease, pancreatitis, diabetes mellitus, retroperitoneal fibrosis, Riedel thyroiditis, and multiple other autoimmune disorders
+ Typical presentation includes RUQ pain, jaundice, pruritus, weight loss, and fatigue
+ ERCP often reveals multifocal intrahepatic and extrahepatic bile duct strictures
+ Increased risk of cholangiocarcinoma
+ Pruritus can be controlled with cholestyramine
+ Treatment is liver transplantation
+ A Roux-en-Y hepaticojejunostomy can serve as a bridge to transplant in select cases

Primary Biliary Cirrhosis

+ Women with medium-sized hepatic ducts
+ Cholestasis → cirrhosis → portal hypertension
+ Symptoms: Pruritus, fatigue, jaundice, xanthomas

- Diagnosis: Anti-mitochondrial antibodies
- Treatment: Transplant
    - There is NO increased cancer risk with PBC

PSC is associated with ulcerative colitis in 50% to 75% of cases and therefore aggressive colon cancer screening is necessary.

Two weeks following a laparoscopic cholecystectomy for symptomatic cholelithiasis, the GB specimen of a 68-year-old woman is found to have a 2-cm adenocarcinoma invading to the subserosa. What is the next best step in management?

The patient should undergo a metastatic cancer workup including tumor markers (CEA and CA 19-9) as well as thoracic and abdominal CT scans followed by surgery as appropriate.

Gallbladder Cancer
- RUQ pain is the most common symptom
- More common in elderly women
- Gallstones occur in 80% of cases
- Because GB cancer often presents with pain, it can be easily confused with symptomatic cholelithiasis
    - CEA >4 ng/mL: Highly specific and moderately (50%) sensitive
    - Serum CA19-9 >20 units/mL: Highly specific and sensitive
- 80% are adenocarcinomas
- Similar to pancreatic cancer, needle biopsies are NOT indicated
    - The only exception is if the tumor is clearly unresectable and a diagnosis is needed for chemotherapy
- 10% of cases are incidental diagnoses following laparoscopic cholecystectomy; cancer is found incidentally in 1% of cholecystectomies performed for benign disease

Staging and Treatment—Based upon AJCC TNM System
- Stage 0: Tis, N0, M0: Small cancer in the epithelial layer only
- Stage I: T1, N0, M0: Tumor invades mucosa (*T1a*) or muscularis (*T1b*).
- Stage II: T2, N0, M0: Tumor invades perimuscular connective tissue and does not extend beyond serosa
- Stage IIIA: T3, N0, M0: Tumor perforates the serosa and/or directly invades the liver and/or one other adjacent organ or structure
- Stage IIIB: T1-3, N1, M0: Metastases to nodes along the cystic duct, CBD, hepatic artery, and/or portal vein
- Stage IVA: T4, N0-1, M0: Tumor invades main portal vein or hepatic artery or invades at least two extrahepatic organs or structures
- Stage IVB: Any T, N2, M0 or any T, any N, M1: Metastases to distant nodes, including periaortic, pericaval, SMA, and celiac artery lymph nodes

Surgery for Gallbladder Cancer
- Surgical resection is the only potentially curative treatment; however, this is only possible in 25% to 50% of patients at presentation
- 5-year survival is very poor (<5%)
- Resectable

- Simple cholecystectomy: Tis, T1a
- Radical or extended cholecystectomy: For T1b and more advanced tumors
  - Radical cholecystectomy: Cholecystectomy, partial hepatectomy (IVB/V), and regional lymph node dissection
  - Extended hepatectomy if hepatic artery of portal vein is involved
  - Bile duct resection if cystic duct margin is positive or if extensive dissection of the porta hepatis puts the bile duct at risk for ischemia
- Radical cholecystectomy with segmental or lobar hepatic resection: T3-4 tumors may require a major hepatectomy and/or bile duct resection/reconstruction
- Unresectable: Advanced in the porta hepatis, local invasion into critical structures or metastasis beyond locoregional confines
  - Endoscopic or percutaneous stents for biliary drainage
  - Recent trials suggest that chemotherapy with cisplatin plus gemcitabine offers improved survival in patients with advanced biliary cancer

Incidental GB cancer discovered in a specimen following laparoscopic cholecystectomy does not warrant further surgery if the cancer is limited to the mucosa. Tumors limited to the mucosa layer may only require a careful inspection of the margins and a cancer workup.

Following laparoscopic cholecystectomy for symptomatic cholelithiasis, the GB specimen of a 52-year-old man is found to have a 0.75-cm GB adenocarcinoma invading to the muscularis layer. All margins are negative except the cystic duct margin, which is positive for malignancy. What is the next step?

Following a cancer work-up, a resection of the CBD and hepaticojejunostomy with regional lymphadenectomy should be performed. It remains a topic of debate whether laparoscopic port sites should be excised full thickness.

During an exploration to resect a GB adenocarcinoma, a suspicious para-aortic lymph node is identified and biopsied. Frozen section is consistent with adenocarcinoma of the GB. What is the next step?

No further surgery—stop the operation and close. Positive retropancreatic, paraduodenal, celiac, superior mesenteric, or para-aortic nodes contraindicate surgical resection since there is no proven improvement in survival with resection of these lymph nodes.

Absolute Contraindications to Resection of Gallbladder Cancer

- Non-contiguous liver metastases
- Carcinomatosis
- N2 disease
- Contraindications to major abdominal surgery such as cirrhosis, ascites, insufficient remnant liver

Relative Contraindications to Resection of Gallbladder Cancer

Stage IV A: Hepatic artery or portal vein invasion (this finding may manifest as atrophy of a liver segment) or invasion into two adjacent organs

GB cancer with limited spread to local/regional lymph nodes of the hepatoduodenal ligament and most superior pancreatic nodes should be resected along with a partial liver resection.

> During an exploration to resect a GB adenocarcinoma, a regional lymphadenectomy is performed, which shows no evidence of lymphadenopathy. Upon further exploration, no evidence of metastases to peripancreatic, periduodenal, periportal, or other distant lymph nodes is found. The GB is diffusely hard, but not invading adjacent structures. What is the next step in management?

Following regional lymphadenectomy and an inspection of other lymph nodes in the area, an en bloc GB and liver resection should be performed (laparoscopic or open), to anatomically resect of liver adjacent to the GB (segments IVB and V). If criteria are met, localized invasive GB cancer is surgically managed with cholecystectomy and an en bloc non-anatomic liver resection 1 to 4 cm deep.

> A 58-year-old Asian woman with history of *C. sinensis* infection and PSC presents with painless jaundice and weight loss. What is the next step in management?

Bile duct cancer usually presents with painless jaundice and is evaluated by ERCP or PTC.

Bile Duct Cancer (Cholangiocarcinoma)
 - Risk factors include
   - Liver flukes (*C. sinensis*)
   - Typhoid fever (*Salmonella typhi*)
   - Choledochal cysts
   - Sclerosing cholangitis
   - Ulcerative colitis
   - Nitrosamines
   - Methyldopa
   - Oral contraceptive pills
   - Thorium dioxide
   - Chronic inflammatory states (i.e., pancreatic reflux whereby there is anomalous pancreatic ductal drainage in which the pancreatic duct drains into the CBD)
 - Hilar cholangiocarcinomas are referred to as Klatskin tumors
 - Preoperative studies can include cytologic brushing at ERCP or PTC, endoscopic ultrasound, and CT
 - However, if there is a suspicion of cancer, only a localization imaging study is needed to evaluate whether tumor is present in the left or right bile duct or both
 - Resection of bile duct cancers varies by the location of the tumor (Bismuth classification system)
   - Excision of the extra-hepatic biliary tree including the bifurcation followed by Roux-en-Y hepaticojejunostomy is reserved for hilar tumors
   - Right versus left hepatic lobectomy is reserved for unilobar tumors or involvement of the right or left secondary/tertiary bile ducts, respectively
   - Distal bile duct tumors are treated with a pancreaticoduodenectomy
 - Unresectable tumors are treated with a palliative stent or biliary bypass

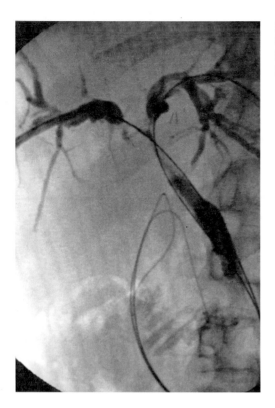

ERCP appearance of a Klatskin tumor. (With permission from Mulholland MW, Lillemoe KD, Doherty GM, Maier RV, Upchurch GR, eds. *Greenfield's Surgery*. 4th ed. Philadelphia, PA: Lippincott Williams & Wilkins; 2005.)

Similarities of Bile Duct Cancer to Gallbladder Cancer

- Tumor type is usually adenocarcinoma and invades locally
- Can present as painless jaundice with elevations of alkaline phosphatase and GGT
- Cholangitis is an infrequent presentation
- Surgical resection is the only potential cure; however, it is only possible in <40% of patients
- There is no proven benefit from chemotherapy or radiation therapy
- 5-year survival very poor (<10%)

SUGGESTED READINGS

Edge SB, Byrd DR, Compton CC, et al. *American Joint Committee on Cancer Staging Manual*. 7th ed. New York, NY: Springer; 2010.

Banz V, Gsponer T, Candinas D, et al. Population-based analysis of 4113 patients with acute cholecystitis: defining the optimal time-point for laparoscopic cholecystectomy. *Ann Surg* 2011; 254(6):964–970.

Endo I, Gonen M, Yopp AC, et al. Intrahepatic cholangiocarcinoma: rising frequency, improved survival, and determinants of outcome after resection. *Ann Surg* 2008; 248(1):84–96.

Massarweh NN, Flum DR. Role of intraoperative cholangiography in avoiding bile duct injury. *J Am Coll Surg* 2007; 204(4):656–664.

Jayaraman S, Jarnagin WR. Management of gallbladder cancer. *Gastroenterol Clin N Am* 2010; 39(2):331–342.

Valle J, Wasan H, Palmer DH, et al. Cisplatin plus gemcitabine versus gemcitabine for biliary tract cancer. *N Engl J Med* 2010; 362 (14):1273–1281.

16 | Liver

Ana L. Gleisner and Nestor F. Esnaola

What are the two main classification systems for the macroscopic anatomy of the liver?

The segmental (French-Couinaud) and lobar (American) systems.

Segmental Classification

- Liver is divided into eight segments
- Segments correspond mostly to venous drainage

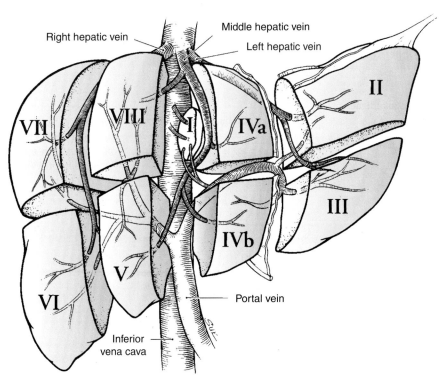

Segmental classification of the liver. (With permission from Mulholland MW, Lillemoe KD, Doherty GM, Maier RV, Upchurch GR, eds. *Greenfield's Surgery*. 4th ed. Philadelphia, PA: Lippincott Williams & Wilkins; 2005.)

Lobar Classification

- Liver is divided into the right and left lobes
- Lobes are separated by Cantlie line, which runs from the gallbladder fossa to the inferior vena cava (IVC)
- The caudate lobe is distinct from the right and left lobes because its venous drainage is directly into the IVC

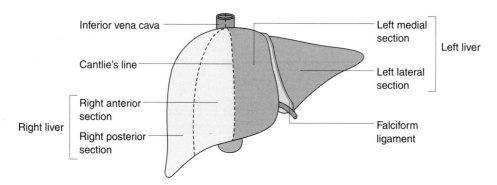

Lobar classification of the liver. (With permission from Mulholland MW, Lillemoe KD, Doherty GM, Maier RV, Upchurch GR, eds. *Greenfield's Surgery*. 4th ed. Philadelphia, PA: Lippincott Williams & Wilkins; 2005.)

Other Perihepatic Structures

- Falciform ligament
  - Separates the medial and lateral segments of the left lobe
  - Attaches the liver to the abdominal wall
- Ligamentum teres
  - Carries the obliterated umbilical vein
- Triangular ligaments
  - Lateral and medial extensions of the coronary ligaments on the posterior surface of the liver
  - Made of peritoneum

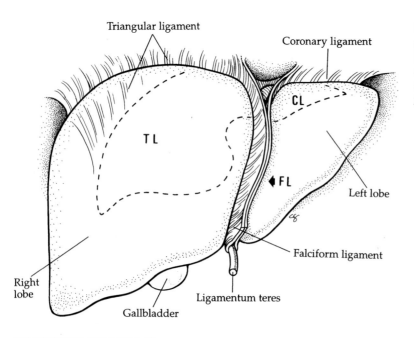

Perihepatic ligaments. (With permission from Fischer JE, Bland KI, Callery MP, et al., eds. *Mastery of Surgery*. 5th ed. Philadelphia, PA: Lippincott Williams & Wilkins; 2006.)

- Hepatoduodenal ligament
  - Where the bile duct, portal vein, and hepatic artery meet (the portal triad)
- Foramen of Winslow
  - Anterior—portal triad
  - Posterior—IVC
  - Inferior—duodenum
  - Superior—liver

What cells in the liver are most susceptible to ischemic insult and what cells are most susceptible to toxic or chemical injury?

The hepatocytes are the most susceptible to ischemic injury, and the biliary ductule is the most susceptible to toxic or chemical injury.

Microscopic Anatomy of the Liver

- Acinar unit
  - The functional unit of the liver
  - Includes the biliary ductule, the hepatic arteriole, and the portal venule
  - Zones are defined relative to oxygen and solute concentration gradients
  - Zone 1
    - Closest to portal triad
    - Most susceptible to toxic injury, least susceptible to ischemia
  - Zone 3
    - Contains hepatocytes
    - Adjacent to the terminal hepatic vein
    - Most susceptible to ischemic injury
- Alkaline phosphatase is in the canalicular system
- Nutrient uptake occurs in the sinusoidal membrane

During a routine cholecystectomy, the gallbladder is very inflamed and due to poor visualization, the common hepatic artery is mistaken for the cystic artery and is ligated. What will be the remaining blood flow and oxygen supply to the liver?

The liver will still have 75% of its original blood flow, but only 50% of its original oxygen delivery.

Blood Supply of the Liver

- Portal vein
  - Supplies 75% of the blood flow to the liver and 50% of the oxygen supply
  - Formed by the superior mesenteric vein (SMV) and splenic veins
    - Inferior mesenteric vein drains into the splenic veins (or occasionally, into the SMV)
- Hepatic artery
  - Supplies 25% of the blood flow to the liver and 50% of the oxygen supply
  - Becomes the proper hepatic artery after the gastroduodenal artery branches off, and then branches into the right and left hepatic arteries
    - Approximately 10% of patients will have

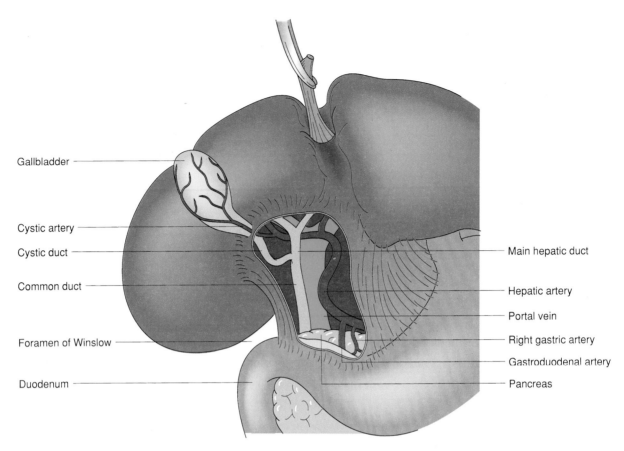

Gallbladder

Cystic artery

Cystic duct

Common duct

Foramen of Winslow

Duodenum

Main hepatic duct

Hepatic artery

Portal vein

Right gastric artery

Gastroduodenal artery

Pancreas

Periportal anatomy. (With permission from Mulholland MW, Lillemoe KD, Doherty GM, Maier RV, Upchurch GR, eds. *Greenfield's Surgery*. 4th ed. Philadelphia, PA: Lippincott Williams & Wilkins; 2005.)

- *A replaced*/accessory right hepatic artery arising from the superior mesenteric artery that travels posterolateral to the common bile duct (CBD) in the porta hepatis
- A replaced/accessory left hepatic artery arising from the left gastric artery that travels through the gastrohepatic ligament into the falciform ligament
- Hepatic vein (HV)
  - 3 venous branches
    - Left HV: Drains segments II, III, and IVA
    - Right HV: Drains segments VI, VII, and VIII
    - Middle HV: Drains segments IV and V
  - Caudate lobe (segment I) drains directly into the IVC

What is the lymphatic drainage of the liver?

Lymphatic Drainage of the Liver
- Lymphatic drainage starts in perisinusoidal spaces of Disse and clefts of Mall
- These drain into the porta hepatis
- Porta hepatis drains to cisterna chili
- Cisterna chili drains into thoracic duct
- Lymphatics are on the right side of the CBD
- Pathophysiology of ascites
  - Decreased permeability of sinusoidal epithelial cells → altered lymphatic drainage→ ascites

> In addition to bile production and hemoglobin degradation, what are the physiologic functions of the liver?

The liver also does detoxification, nutrient storage, glucose, lipid and protein metabolism, and protein synthesis.

Detoxification

- Cytochrome P450 system
  - Conversion of hydrophobic to hydrophilic compounds to improve solubility for secretion
  - Reactions include reduction, hydroxylation, and hydrolysis to expose functional groups
- Phase II reactions
  - Conjugation to alter solubility

Nutrient Storage

- Glycogen
- Triglycerides
- Vitamin B12
- Copper
- Fat-soluble vitamins

Protein Synthesis

- Coagulation factors: I, II, V, VII, IX, X, and XI, antithrombin III, protein C/S
  - Factor VIII is made primarily by endothelial cells, but a small proportion is made in the liver
- Complement factors
- Acute phase proteins: Transferrin, CRP, fibrinogen, haptoglobin, albumin, ceruloplasmin

Protein, Lipid, and Glucose Metabolisms

- Glycogenesis and glycogenolysis + gluconeogenesis, depending on the body's state of metabolism
- Lipogenesis (from amino acids and glucose)
- Deamination and transamination of amino acids
- Urea cycle—conversion of ammonia to urea
- Production of non-essential amino acids

> A 63-year-old woman with a history of unresectable bile duct cancer (cholangiocarcinoma) status post biliary stenting presents with a 1-week history of fevers, chills, and jaundice. An abdominal CT reveals multiple rim-enhancing fluid collections in the liver. What is the most likely diagnosis?

A hepatic abscess usually presents following episodes of intra-abdominal infection or bacteremia and is characterized by a rim-enhancing fluid collection on CT scan. Common organisms include Escherichia coli, Klebsiella, Proteus, Staphylococcus, and Streptococcus. Fungus may be found in immunocompromised patients or in patients with multi-organism hepatobiliary infection. Amebic abscesses are caused by Entamoeba histolytica.

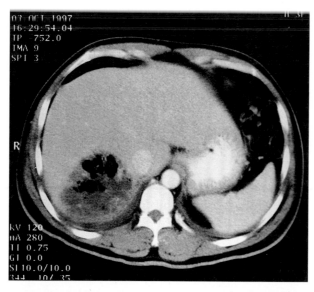

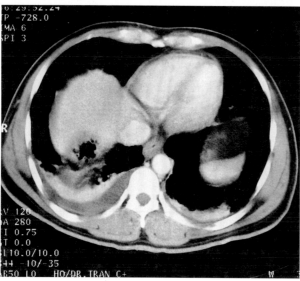

Pyogenic liver abscess. (With permission from Fischer JE, Bland KI, Callery MP, et al., eds. *Mastery of Surgery*. 5th ed. Philadelphia, PA: Lippincott Williams & Wilkins; 2006.)

Pyogenic Liver Abscess

- Causes
  - Biliary instrumentation (most common)
  - Biliary obstruction from stones, strictures, and tumors
  - Portal vein spread of gastrointestinal infections such as diverticulitis, appendicitis, or perforated ulcers
  - Hematogenous spread via hepatic artery in the setting of systemic bacteremia
  - Unknown etiology in up to 20% of patients
- Diagnosis
  - Most common type of liver abscess in the United States
  - Patients present with fever, chills, and right upper quadrant abdominal pain
  - Jaundice, weight loss, nausea, and vomiting can also be seen
  - Up to one-quarter of patients will be septic
  - Lab tests show leukocytosis, elevated bilirubin, and alkaline phosphatase
  - Plain abdominal films or abdominal CT may show gas in the abscess cavity and elevation of the right hemidiaphragm

- CT can also demonstrate contrast-enhancing, well-defined round masses with low internal density
- Ultrasound demonstrates hypoechoic lesions
  - Treatment
    - Percutaneous drainage is the treatment of choice
    - Laparoscopic or open surgical drainage is used when percutaneous drainage is not possible or the source of infection is surgically correctable
    - Microabscesses in patients in good condition can be treated with antibiotics alone
    - Broad-spectrum antibiotics should be substituted with culture-guided antibiotics as soon as the organisms are identified

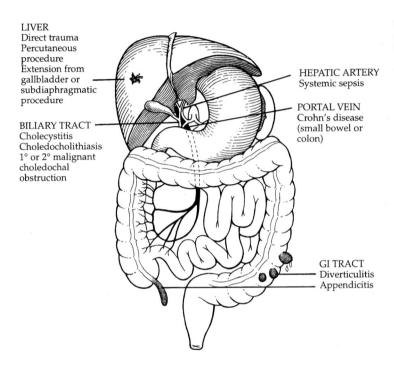

LIVER
Direct trauma
Percutaneous procedure
Extension from gallbladder or subdiaphragmatic procedure

BILIARY TRACT
Cholecystitis
Choledocholithiasis
1° or 2° malignant choledochal obstruction

HEPATIC ARTERY
Systemic sepsis

PORTAL VEIN
Crohn's disease (small bowel or colon)

GI TRACT
Diverticulitis
Appendicitis

Causes of pyogenic liver abscess. (With permission from Fischer JE, Bland KI, Callery MP, et al., eds. *Mastery of Surgery*. 5th ed. Philadelphia, PA: Lippincott Williams & Wilkins; 2006.)

When choosing a method of drainage, factors that should be considered include the anesthetic risk and underlying clinical condition of the patient, as well as the local expertise in and availability of each drainage method.

Amebic Liver Abscess

- Most common cause of liver abscess worldwide
- Complication of intestinal amebiasis (*E. histolytica*) in 3% to 10% of cases; spreads to the liver via the portal vein
- Symptoms/history
  - History of travel to a tropical climate
  - Fever
  - Abdominal pain and hepatomegaly
  - Diarrhea is present in only 20% to 30% of the cases
  - Often patients do NOT have jaundice
  - The abscess can rupture into pleura, pericardium, or peritoneum
- Diagnosis
  - Often a solitary lesion in the right lobe of the liver
    - CT scan shows low internal density and smooth margins

- Serology (*indirect hemagglutination* and gel diffusion precipitation) is the most accurate test for diagnosis
- Stool testing for the cyst of the protozoan is negative in most cases
- Treatment
  - *Metronidazole* is effective in most cases
  - Aspiration may be required for larger abscesses
  - Surgical drainage is reserved for patients with secondary infection, perforation with peritoneal irritation, or failure of metronidazole therapy

History of travel to a tropical area in a young patient with a solitary liver cavity should prompt serology investigation for an amebic abscess.

A 38-year-old man who recently emigrated from Sudan presents to the emergency department with nausea, vomiting, and jaundice. A CT scan reveals a large, solitary, calcified cyst in the right lobe of the liver. Serologic tests confirm infection with *Echinococcus*. What is the next step in the management of this cyst?

The cyst should be excised completely, including sterilization of the cyst and excision of the germinal layer.

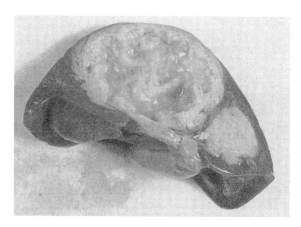

Echinococcal cyst. (With permission from Mulholland MW, Lillemoe KD, Doherty GM, Maier RV, Upchurch GR, eds. *Greenfield's Surgery*. 4th ed. Philadelphia, PA: Lippincott Williams & Wilkins; 2005.)

Echinococcal Cyst

- Caused by the larval stage of the tapeworm Echinococcus
- Infection occurs through ingestion of parasite eggs
  - Eggs are released in the feces of the definitive host (carnivores and rodents)
  - Eggs hatch and migrate across the intestinal wall of the intermediate host, spreading to the liver (most commonly), brain, lungs, and bones
- Patients are often from endemic areas such as the Mediterranean and Baltic areas, Middle and Far East, South America and South Africa
- There is an asymptomatic phase of variable duration
- Clinical manifestations include fever, abdominal pain, jaundice, and weight loss
- Serology (indirect hemagglutination) has good sensitivity
  - Can also have a positive Casoni skin test (intradermal injection of sterilized fluid from hydatid cysts that results in wheal response; high false positive rate limits its utility)
- Imaging with ultrasound or CT scan usually shows a unilocular or complex lesion with daughter cysts
- Thick calcified rims are seen in dead cysts

- Rupture, most commonly to the biliary tree, is a serious complication
- Rupture can result in dissemination and hypersensitivity or anaphylactic shock
- Cure is achieved with surgical removal of all living parasites
  - Options include simple cystectomy with *deroofing and evacuation* of contents or partial hepatectomy
  - Spillage of cyst contents should be prevented; the cyst may be aspirated and injected with scolicidal agents (70% to 90% ethanol, 15% to 20% hypertonic saline, 0.5% silver nitrate or hydrogen peroxide)
  - The operative cyst can be packed with 20% saline-moistened gauze or povidone iodine-soaked gauze to kill parasites
- Surgery may also be indicated for symptomatic dead cysts
- *Albendazole* is used in preparation for surgery and to reduce recurrence after surgical removal
  - May be effective when used in lieu of surgery in up to 30% of the cases but recurrence is common

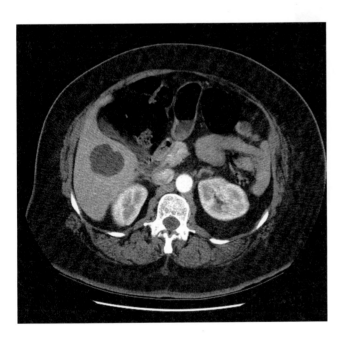

Simple hepatic cyst. (With permission from Mulholland MW, Lillemoe KD, Doherty GM, Maier RV, Upchurch GR, eds. *Greenfield's Surgery.* 4th ed. Philadelphia, PA: Lippincott Williams & Wilkins; 2005.)

Simple Liver Cyst

- Simple cysts may be congenital in origin and have no malignant potential
- True simple cysts have a secretory epithelium
- Pseudocysts are trauma-related
- Small cysts are usually asymptomatic and are often incidentally discovered
- Larger cysts can cause abdominal pain and, rarely, obstructive jaundice
- Imaging shows a thin-walled cyst and a water-dense content
- Symptomatic cysts are treated with laparoscopic or open marsupialization
- However, evidence of ovarian stroma on pathology is diagnostic of cystadenoma for which resection is indicated

Asymptomatic simple liver cysts are common and can be found in up to 5% of the population.

A 41-year-old woman presents to her primary care physician complaining of early satiety and persistent right upper quadrant discomfort. An ultrasound reveals a large, distinct, hyperechoic mass. A CT scan with IV contrast shows central filling of the lesion on delayed films. What is the most sensitive and specific diagnostic study for this type of lesion?

A dynamic-contrast MRI is the study of choice in the diagnosis of hemangiomas that are not obvious on CT with arterial and venous imaging. Hemangiomas constitute greater than 50% of incidental solid liver masses.

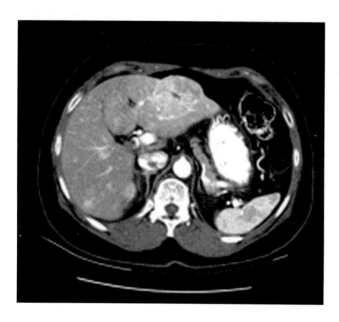

Hepatic hemangioma. (With permission from Mulholland MW, Lillemoe KD, Doherty GM, Maier RV, Upchurch GR, eds. *Greenfield's Surgery*. 4th ed. Philadelphia, PA: Lippincott Williams &Wilkins; 2005.)

Overview of Solid Lesions in the Liver

- Benign
    - Hemangioma
    - Adenoma
    - Focal nodular hyperplasia (FNH)
- Primary malignant tumors
- Metastatic tumors (most common)

Benign Solid Liver Lesions

- *Hemangiomas* are thought to represent progressive growth of congenital lesions
    - Most common benign solid tumor of the liver (2% to 7% liver autopsies)
    - When manifested in infants, they may be associated with the Kasabach-Merritt syndrome (congestive heart failure and risk of disseminated intravascular coagulation from bleeding)
- *Adenomas* are associated with oral contraceptive pill use
    - These lesions are usually asymptomatic and incidentally discovered
    - Symptoms are related to distension of Glisson capsule or infarction within the mass
    - Extrinsic compression of the mass can cause increased abdominal girth or early satiety
- *FNH* and adenomas are usually diagnosed in women of child-bearing age
- All lesions are more common in women

- Tumor markers should always be checked (AFP, CEA, CA 19-9) to rule out malignancy
- Biopsy has largely been replaced by imaging studies
- Imaging characteristics
  - *Hemangioma*
    - US: Hyperechoic, well-demarcated, increased vascular flow
    - CT: Rim-enhancement with central filling on delayed images during the arterial phase
    - MRI: Isodense on T1, hyperdense on T2, peripheral enhancement with Gadolinium
    - Tc 99 RBC scan: Highly sensitive and specific
  - **Adenoma**
    - US: Non-specific
    - CT: Hypodense; heterogeneous on contrast injection
    - MRI: Hypodense
    - Tc 99 sulfur colloid: No enhancement
    - Angiography: Multiple vessels penetrating the tumor from the peripheral parenchyma; occasionally, areas of necrosis and hemorrhage
  - **FNH**
    - US: Non-specific
    - CT: May demarcate on contrast with a central, stellate scar on portal venous phase
    - MRI: Isodense in T1 and T2, early hyperdensity with gadolinium
    - Tc 99 sulfur colloid: Enhancement due to bile proliferation

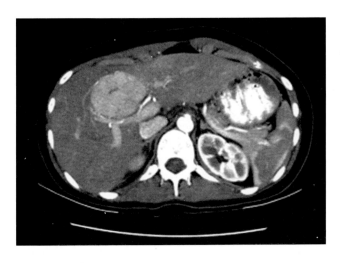

FNH. (With permission from Mulholland MW, Lillemoe KD, Doherty GM, Maier RV, Upchurch GR, eds. *Greenfield's Surgery.* 4th ed. Philadelphia, PA: Lippincott Williams & Wilkins; 2005.)

Hepatic Adenoma

- Hepatic adenomas have a risk of rupture (common) and malignant transformation
  - Risk increases with size >5 cm
  - Pregnancy increases the risk of adenoma rupture and hemorrhage
- Serial imaging (every 6 months) should be performed to observe for change in size, which is suggestive of malignancy
- If hepatic adenoma is suspected, oral contraceptive pills (OCPs) should be discontinued
  - Adenomas usually regress completely after OCP cessation
- Surgical resection is reserved for patients with large/superficial lesions, severe symptoms, or when malignancy cannot be ruled out

- Hepatic resection is usually effective in symptom relief
- Ruptured adenomas may be treated with emergent embolization

Hemangiomas and FNHs have a negligible risk of rupture and no risk of malignant transformation and do not need to be resected unless they are symptomatic.

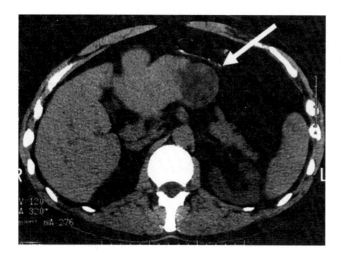

Hepatic adenoma. (With permission from Fischer JE, Bland KI, Callery MP, et al., eds. *Mastery of Surgery*. 5th ed. Philadelphia, PA: Lippincott Williams & Wilkins; 2006.)

Primary Malignant Tumors

Hepatocellular Carcinoma

- Most common type of primary tumor
  - Associated with hepatitis B virus (HBV) chronic infection and carrier states
  - Associated with liver cirrhosis due to any cause, but especially hepatitis C virus (HCV)
  - Patients with alpha-1-antitrypsin deficiency, tyrosinemia, and type 1 glycogen storage disease are also at increased risk
  - Aflatoxin-rich diet is also associated with an increased risk of hepatocellular carcinoma (HCC)
- Clinical manifestations include rapid clinical deterioration, painful hepatomegaly, weight loss, anorexia, and weakness
  - Signs and symptoms of cirrhosis may also be evident
  - Non-cirrhotic HCC is mainly associated with hepatitis B infection
- An elevated AFP is present in 85% of patients and correlates with tumor size
  - AFP levels greater than 400 μg/L is generally diagnostic of HCC
- Patients with cirrhosis should have periodic imaging and AFP evaluation
  - Ultrasound is a sensitive (60% to 78%) screening tool for patients with cirrhosis
- The fibrolamellar variant of HCC is usually diagnosed in younger patients
  - Not associated with cirrhosis nor hepatitis
  - Often no increase in AFP levels
  - Has a more favorable prognosis
- In endemic areas, HCC is a common cause of hemoperitoneum; spontaneous rupture may approach 8%

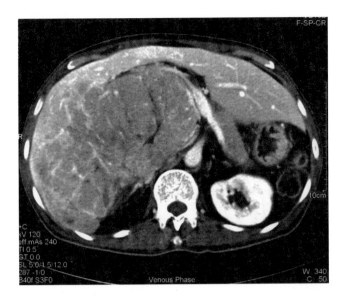

Hepatocellular carcinoma. (With permission from Fischer JE, Bland KI, Callery MP, et al., eds. *Mastery of Surgery.* 5th ed. Philadelphia, PA: Lippincott Williams & Wilkins; 2006.)

Treatment Options for Hepatocellular Carcinoma

- **Tumor ablation**
  - May be curative for small tumors or serve as a bridge to transplantation
  - Options include percutaneous treatment (ethanol injection or radiofrequency ablation [RFA]) or surgical (laparoscopic or open) RFA
  - Associated with a low complication rate
  - Causes some surrounding tissue burn injury, so should not be used near large vascular or biliary structures
- **Transcatheter arterial chemoembolization**
  - Effective in larger tumors as a palliative procedure or as a bridge to transplantation
  - May be contraindicated in patients with portal vein thrombosis
- **Surgical resection**
  - Usually limited to patients with good hepatic reserve (non-cirrhotic or Child A patients, no portal hypertension)
  - High recurrence rate (up to 70% at 5 years) in patients with underlying liver fibrosis/cirrhosis
- **Liver transplantation**
  - Good long-term results in patients who meet the Milan criteria (solitary lesion up to 5 cm, or a maximum of three lesions, none greater than 3 cm in size; no involvement of portal vein or IVC)
  - Best option for patients with Child B or C cirrhosis
  - Limited by donor availability
  - Patients are conferred higher priority on the transplant waiting list when HCC is diagnosed

The best long-term results for HCC are achieved with surgical resection or transplantation.

Other Primary Liver Tumors

- Include angiosarcoma, cholangiocarcinoma, and hepatoblastoma
- Angiosarcoma
  - Associated with exposure to chemical carcinogens (arsenic, vinyl chloride)
  - Often unresectable at diagnosis; prognosis is dismal

- Cholangiocarcinoma
  - Classified as intrahepatic (arising at/above the second order biliary radicals) or extrahepatic (includes hilar, or Klatskin tumors)
  - Associated with chronic cholestasis, primary sclerosing cholangitis, *Clonorchis sinensis*, ulcerative colitis, choledochal cysts, chronic bile duct infection, cirrhosis, hemochromatosis, and congenital cystic disease of the liver
  - Signs/symptoms
    - More common in older males
    - Present with painless jaundice, pruritus
    - ↑ alkaline phosphatase, bilirubin, GGT, and *normal* AST/ALT
  - Treatment
  - Proximal 1/3 of biliary tree (including Klatskin tumors)
    - Usually unresectable, but can attempt resection of bile duct (often with associated liver lobe) and portal lymphadenectomy
    - Reconstruction with hepaticojejunostomy
  - Middle 1/3 of biliary tree
    - Resection of bile duct and portal lymphadenectomy
    - Reconstruction with choledocho- versus hepaticojejunostomy
  - Distal 1/3 of biliary tree
    - Whipple procedure
  - Consider palliative stenting (endoscopic or via percutaneous transhepatic cholangiography) for unresectable disease
  - Chemoradiation may be used for attempted cure (definitive chemoradiation) or palliation.

While HCC is the most common cause of liver cancer worldwide and is endemic in Asia, metastatic lesions are the most common liver malignancy in the United States.

Tumors Metastatic to the Liver
- Virtually any malignant tumor can metastasize to the liver
- Elevated tumor markers can help distinguish a primary malignancy from metastatic disease (e.g., carcinoembryonic antigen [CEA] in CEA-producing colorectal tumors)
- On imaging, metastatic tumors are generally less vascular than primary liver tumors
  - Exception: Metastatic neuroendocrine tumors (NETs), which are highly vascular/visible on arterial phase CT images
- CT, MRI, or intraoperative ultrasound detects 90% to 95% of lesions
- The best potential curative treatment is surgical resection
  - Limitations to surgery include inability to achieve negative margins with sufficient remnant liver parenchyma
  - Contraindications to attempted curative hepatic resection include central (celiac) or periaortic lymph node involvement, carcinomatosis, or unresectable extrahepatic disease
  - Exceptions to contraindications include rare tumors where debulking has an accepted benefit in survival (e.g., symptomatic NETs)

Colorectal Cancer Metastases to the Liver
- Most common cause of liver metastases
  - Synchronous presentation (i.e., at the same time as the primary tumor) in up to 15% of patients
  - Up to 2/3 of patients with colorectal tumors will develop metastatic disease
    - Approximately half of these patients will present with liver-only disease

- Prognosis is based on the ability to achieve an R0 (microscopically negative margins) resection and/or combined R0 resection/complete ablation of the primary tumor (if still present) and *all* the metastases
- When combined with chemotherapeutic agents, 5-year survival after complete resection (± ablation) approaches 30% to 50%
- Percutaneous or surgical RFA can be used in unresectable colorectal metastasis measuring up to 5 cm, either alone or in combination with surgical resection of other lesions
- Selective internal radiation therapy (with Yttrium 90) can also provide a palliative benefit

Metastatic tumors are as common as FNH and adenomas among patients with an incidental solid liver mass and no other apparent cancers.

A 55-year-old man who underwent a total colectomy has progressive deterioration of his mental status, and develops ascites and jaundice. After an extended stay in the ICU, he is diagnosed with severe liver failure. What will be the most likely cause of the patient's ultimate demise?

Uncal herniation due to cerebral edema is the most common cause of death in patients with severe liver failure.

Acute Liver Failure

- Most commonly caused by hepatitis, liver toxins, and drug hepatotoxicity
- Unknown etiology in 20% to 40% of the cases
- Predictable with acetaminophen toxicity; idiosyncratic for other drugs
- Rare causes include Budd-Chiari syndrome, Wilson disease, and malignancy
- Patients present with rapid hepatocellular dysfunction, jaundice, coagulopathy, and encephalopathy
- Encephalopathy may develop within 2 weeks of the onset of jaundice (fulminant hepatic failure) or between 2 weeks and 3 months (sub-fulminant hepatic failure)
- Severe encephalopathy can result in diminished sensorial awareness/coma and is often associated with infectious complications (e.g., pneumonia)
- Fulminant failure is usually complicated by cerebral edema and uncal herniation
- Sub-fulminant failure is associated with the development of portal hypertension
- Infectious complications may develop in up to 80% of patients
- Clinical parameters of acute liver failure are similar to sepsis
- Patients with irreversible liver failure need urgent liver transplantation
- Kings College criteria for liver transplantation in cases of acetaminophen toxicity are as follows:
  - pH less than 7.3 (irrespective of grade of encephalopathy)
  - Prothrombin time (PT) greater than 100 seconds or INR >7.7
  - Serum creatinine level greater than 3.4 mg/dL in patients with grade III or IV encephalopathy
- Measurement of lactate levels at 4 and 12 hours after acetaminophen ingestion also helps in early identification of patients who require liver transplantation
- Kings College criteria for liver transplantation in other cases are as follows:
  - PT greater than 100 seconds (irrespective of grade of encephalopathy) or
  - Any three of the following criteria:
    - Age younger than 10 years or older than 40 years
    - Non-A/non-B hepatitis, halothane hepatitis, or idiosyncratic drug reactions as etiology of acute hepatic failure

- Duration of jaundice of more than 7 days before onset of encephalopathy
- PT greater than 50 seconds
- Serum bilirubin level greater than 17 mg/dL
- Supportive treatment (prophylaxis for GI bleeding, correction of hypoglycemia, intracranial pressure monitoring and control with osmotherapy and barbiturates, hemodynamic support) until organ availability
- With liver transplantation, 5 years survival is about 70%

Chronic Liver Failure

- Chronic liver injury is caused by infection (HBV, HCV—most common cause worldwide), toxins (e.g., alcohol—most common cause in the United States), as well as autoimmune and inherited diseases (e.g., cystic fibrosis)
    - Hepatitis A
        - Picornavirus
        - Fecal–oral transmission
        - Do not develop post-transplant infection

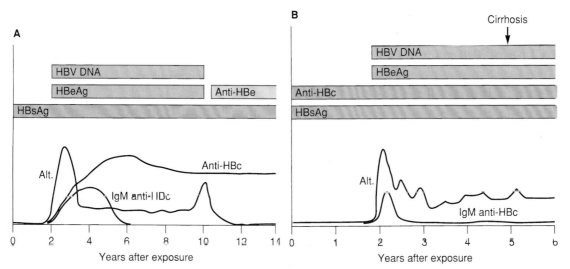

Hepatitis B Ag and Ab. (With permission from Mulholland MW, Lillemoe KD, Doherty GM, Maier RV, Upchurch GR, eds. *Greenfield's Surgery*. 4th ed. Philadelphia, PA: Lippincott Williams &Wilkins; 2005.)

- Hepatitis B
    - Hepadnavirus
    - Venereal transmission
    - Tests
        - With vaccination should have anti-HBs Ab only
        - Increased anti-HBc and anti-HBs Abs with no hepatitis B antigens → patient had infection, but has cleared it and is immune
        - Increased anti-HBc and anti-HBs Abs with hepatitis B antigens → patient has active disease
        - If has a liver transplant, new liver will become infected
- Hepatitis C
    - Flavivirus (RNA virus)
    - Transmitted through blood
    - If has a liver transplant, new liver will become infected

- Hepatitis D
  - Co-factor for hepatitis B
- Hepatitis E
  - RNA virus
  - Fecal–oral transmission
  - Can cause fulminant hepatic failure in pregnancy, most commonly in the third trimester
    - Non-alcoholic steatohepatitis can progress to cirrhosis
    - Chronic inflammation leads to hepatocyte destruction and regeneration as well as fibrosis; fibrosis leads to portal hypertension
    - Characterized by
      - Impaired synthesis of clotting factors
      - Coagulopathy (increase in the PT time)
      - Decrease in liver excretory capacity: Jaundice and encephalopathy
      - Liver failure → inability to metabolize → buildup of ammonia, methane thiols, and false neurotransmitters → encephalopathy
    - Portal hypertension: Splenomegaly/thrombocytopenia, esophageal varices
  - Portal hypertension can lead to bleeding from esophageal varices
  - Hypoalbuminemia results in decreased effective intravascular volume and causes sodium and water retention via the renin-angiotensin-aldosterone pathway and ADH secretion
  - Ascites develops in the setting of sodium and water retention, portal hypertension, and dilated hepatic hilar lymphatics
  - The presence of ascites increases the risk of spontaneous bacterial peritonitis (SBP)

Worsening encephalopathy may be associated with infectious complications, excessive diuretic treatment, or SBP. Ascites fluid can be aspirated to rule out SBP (diagnosed if fluid contains >250 PMNs/L).

Management of Complications of Liver Failure

- Endoscopic variceal obliteration (i.e., banding, sclerotherapy) to treat and prevent bleeding, along with beta blockers
- Diuretics and sodium restriction for ascites control
  - Frequent paracentesis may be necessary to treat refractory ascites
- Transjugular intrahepatic portosystemic shunts (TIPS) and (rarely) surgical shunts can be used to treat acute and recurrent variceal bleeding refractory to medical treatment, refractory ascites, hydrothorax due to cirrhosis, and Budd-Chiari syndrome
  - TIPS should not be performed in patients with severe liver failure, primary pulmonary hypertension, or severe encephalopathy
  - The procedure may be associated with new-onset or worsening encephalopathy as blood is diverted from the liver
  - Portocaval or mesocaval interpositions (10 to 12 mm in width) are the most commonly performed surgical shunts
- Antibiotics to prevent SBP
- Hepatic encephalopathy
  - May need to embolize previous therapeutic shunts or embolize other collaterals
  - Lactulose: A cathartic that clears bacteria in the gut and prevents NH_3 uptake by converting it to ammonium
  - Limit protein intake
    - Can feed branched chain amino acids, which are metabolized by skeletal muscle

- Dopamine receptor agonists (ı-DOPA and bromocriptine) may help
  - Perform gastric lavage (via an NG tube) and guaiac stools and to rule out GI bleed
- Hepatorenal syndrome
  - Same appearance as pre-renal azotemia
  - Treatment: Stop diuretics and give volume
- Periodic liver imaging and AFP evaluation for early detection of HCC
- Liver transplantation is the mainstay of treatment and is indicated in patients with poor hepatic reserve (Child B or C) and/or a history of serious/recurring complications

Liver Scoring Systems

- The prognosis of patients with chronic liver disease can be determined by the Child-Pugh classification

Child-Pugh Classification

PTT (seconds)	Total bilirubin (mg/dL)	Albumin (mg/dL)	Ascites	Encephalopathy (grade)	Points
<4	<2	>3.5	None	None	1
4–6	2–3	2.8–3.5	Controlled	I–II	2
>6	>3	<2.8	Refractory	III–IV	3

Class	Points	Operative mortality (%)	1-year survival rate after TIPS (%)
A	5–6	1	75
B	7–9	3–10	68
C	10–15	30–50	50

- *The MELD score* has been shown to have excellent predictive power for 3-month mortality in patients with chronic liver disease
  - Used to determine organ allocation priorities
  - Calculated using only laboratory values (INR, total bilirubin, and creatinine) and no subjective criteria

MELD Score Formula

$3.8 \times \ln [\text{total bilirubin (mg/dL)}] + 11.2 \times \ln [\text{INR}] + 9.6 \times \ln [\text{creatinine (mg/dL)}] + 6.4$

A 35-year-old female with a history of factor V Leiden deficiency presents with hematemesis, jaundice, and altered mental status. She is also noted to have ascites and hepatomegaly. What is the next step in treatment?

The patient has Budd-Chiari syndrome and should be initially treated with anticoagulation.

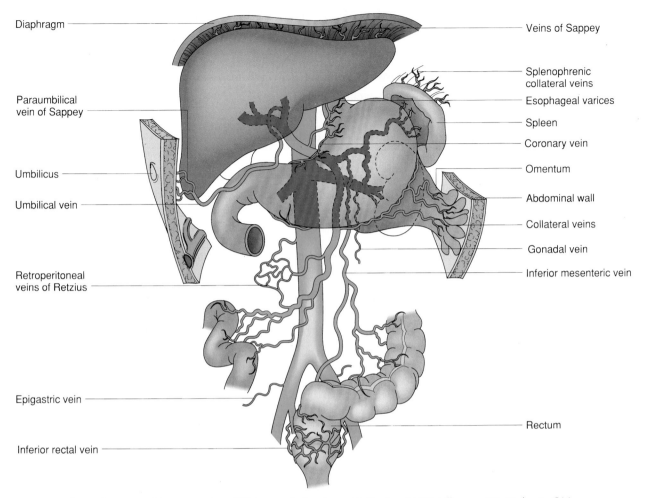

Venous collaterals in portal hypertension. (With permission from Mulholland MW, Lillemoe KD, Doherty GM, Maier RV, Upchurch GR, eds. *Greenfield's Surgery*. 4th ed. Philadelphia, PA: Lippincott Williams & Wilkins; 2005.)

Portal Hypertension

- Portal pressure gradient >12 mmHg
- Obstruction → portal venous hypertension → vasodilatation and increased splanchnic inflow → development of collateral flow between portal and systemic circulation
- Varices
  - Coronary vein → esophageal varices (lower esophagus)
  - Superior hemorrhoidal vein → hemorrhoids
  - Paraumbilical veins → peri-umbilical varices (caput medusae)
  - Veins of Retzius → in retroperitoneum and shunt portal vein blood from the bowel and other organs to the vena cava
  - Treatment
    - Banding/sclerotherapy for esophageal varices—90% effective
    - Vasopressin—splanchnic artery constriction
      - *Patients with CAD should* be on nitroglycerin while on vasopressin
    - Octreotide—decreases portal pressure by decreasing portal flow
    - Propranolol can help to prevent re-bleeding—no role acutely
    - TIPS should be considered for refractory variceal bleeding

Extrahepatic Causes of Portal Hypertension

- Portal vein thrombosis
  - Congenital
    - In childhood, often caused by umbilical vein catheterization
    - Liver function is generally well preserved
  - Sepsis
    - Secondary to hypercoagulable state or dehydration
  - Infection
    - Schistosomiasis
  - Trauma
  - Treatment
    - Long-term anticoagulation
    - Clot lysis via transhepatic infusions through the portal vein
- Malignant occlusion
  - HCC

Intrahepatic Causes of Portal Hypertension

- Schistosomiasis
- Congenital hepatic fibrosis
- Cirrhosis

Hepatic Venous Causes of Portal Hypertension

- Budd-Chiari syndrome
  - Causes occlusion of major hepatic veins → postsinusoidal portal hypertension
  - More common in women, particularly those with hypercoagulable states
  - Symptoms: RUQ pain, jaundice, ascites, complications of portal HTN
    - Caudate lobe is spared in most cases
  - Treatment: Anticoagulation, portacaval shunting (TIPS *not* effective)
- Veno-occlusive disease
- Constrictive pericarditis
- CHF

17 | Pancreas

Martin A. Makary and Vicente Valero

Which artery can provide blood supply to the liver in the event that the common hepatic artery is occluded?

The portal vein (PV) provides 60% to 75% of the blood flow and 50% of the oxygen to the liver. The gastroduodenal artery (GDA), with its origin from the superior mesenteric artery (SMA), also supplies the liver via retrograde flow in the event of a common hepatic artery occlusion.

Blood Supply of the Pancreas

- The head of the pancreas is supplied primarily by the SMA and the GDA, which give rise to the pancreaticoduodenal arteries
- The body is supplied by branches from the splenic artery
- The tail is supplied by branches from the splenic, gastroepiploic, and dorsal pancreatic arteries
  - Islet cells have a large blood supply relative to their size, and thus islet cell tumors tend to be hypervascular

The SMA is the main artery supplying the head of the pancreas.

Blood Supply of the Pancreas

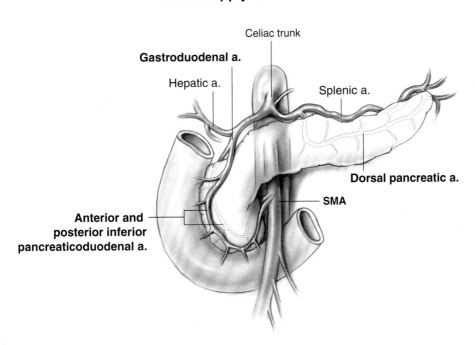

> What is the normal pressure within the bile duct compared to the pancreatic duct?

The pancreatic duct has a higher resting pressure compared to the bile duct, which prevents bile reflux into the pancreatic duct. The pressure in both ductal systems increases following meals.

> What are the pancreatic enzymes and hormones?

Exocrine Pancreas

- **Amylase**
  - Responsible for the digestion of dietary carbohydrates consisting primarily of starch, sucrose, and lactose
  - Secreted by the salivary glands (S-type amylase) and by the pancreas (P-type amylase)
  - Digestion begins in the mouth where 30% to 40% of starch is converted to maltose, isomaltose, and dextrins before S-amylase is inactivated by gastric juice
  - Pancreatic amylase completes the hydrolysis of the remaining starch in the jejunum
- **Lipase**
  - Most sensitive marker of pancreatitis
  - *Amylase and lipase are secreted in their active forms, unlike trypsinogen and phospholipase A2, which are activated by duodenal enzymes*
- **Endocrine Pancreas**
  - **Cells**
    - Alpha cells $\Rightarrow$ Glucagon
    - Beta cells $\Rightarrow$ Insulin
    - Delta cells $\Rightarrow$ VIP
    - G-Cells $\Rightarrow$ Gastrin
  - **GI hormones that increase pancreatic activity**
    - Secretin (released in response to a low duodenal pH)
    - Cholecystokinin
    - Acetylcholine (vagal stimulation) secretions
    - Gastrin
    - Serotonin (less important)
  - **GI hormones that decrease pancreatic activity**
    - Somatostatin
    - Glucagon

Somatostatin (or its long-acting analogue octreotide) has many therapeutic applications including the treatment of diarrhea and flushing in carcinoid syndrome and the treatment of intestinal fistulas and variceal bleeding.

Secretin is the primary stimulant of pancreatic water and electrolyte secretion. The bicarbonate concentration in pancreatic secretions is increased when the pancreas is maximally stimulated due to carbonic anhydrase activity in the pancreatic duct.

> A 6-month-old boy with Down syndrome presents with a gastric outlet obstruction. An annular pancreas is suspected. What is the best test to establish the diagnosis?

An upper GI contrast study is the diagnostic test of choice for an annular pancreas.

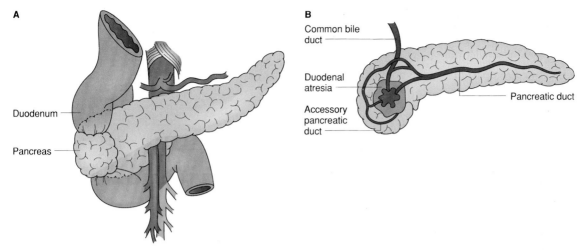

Annular pancreas. (With permission from Mulholland MW, Lillemoe KD, Doherty GM, Maier RV, Upchurch GR, eds. *Greenfield's Surgery*. 4th ed. Philadelphia, PA: Lippincott Williams & Wilkins; 2005.)

Annular Pancreas

- Pancreas encircling the second part of the duodenum
  - Due to incomplete rotation of the ventral pancreatic bud
- Associated with trisomy 21
- An UGI is diagnostic
- Most patients are asymptomatic
- The treatment is a duodenojejunostomy and should be reserved for symptomatic patients
  - The pancreas is NOT resected as the band around the duodenum frequently carries a pancreatic duct remnant

The treatment of symptomatic annular pancreas is bypass rather than resection.

A 31-year-old woman presents with recurrent epigastric pain radiating to her back and a history of pancreas divisum. What is the most likely cause of her symptoms?

In pancreas divisum, two separate ductal systems drain bile and pancreatic juice into the duodenum via a major and minor papilla. It is associated with recurrent episodes of acute pancreatitis.

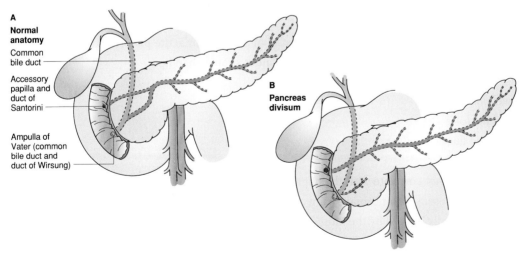

Pancreas divisum. (With permission from Mulholland MW, Lillemoe KD, Doherty GM, Maier RV, Upchurch GR, eds. *Greenfield's Surgery*. 4th ed. Philadelphia, PA: Lippincott Williams & Wilkins; 2005.)

Pancreas Divisum

- Failure of pancreatic duct fusion at the time of developmental rotation
  - The smaller duct (duct of Santorini) often drains the majority of the pancreas in this condition
- Found in up to 11% of the population and often asymptomatic
- ERCP is the gold standard for diagnosis
  - Demonstrates two non-communicating ductal systems
- Main treatment option is endoscopic sphincterotomy

Pancreas divisum is associated with recurrent episodes of acute pancreatitis and can lead to chronic pancreatitis, a condition in which the pancreatic gland is hardened and the ductal system is often dilated.

> What is the most sensitive test for pancreatitis?

A CT scan with IV contrast is the best radiographic study for pancreatitis. Serum lipase is the most sensitive and specific lab test.

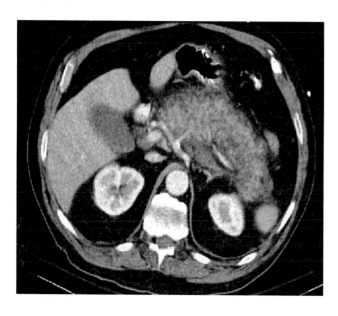

Acute pancreatitis on CT scan. (With permission from Mulholland MW, Lillemoe KD, Doherty GM, Maier RV, Upchurch GR, eds. *Greenfield's Surgery*. 4th ed. Philadelphia, PA: Lippincott Williams & Wilkins; 2005.)

Acute Pancreatitis

- Serum lipase is a more sensitive and specific test than amylase for acute pancreatitis
- Amylase is often elevated but returns to baseline values sooner than lipase
- Amylase levels can be elevated from other conditions
  - Bowel obstruction
  - Bowel necrosis
  - Perforated duodenal ulcer
  - Salivary tumors
- Amylase level may not correlate with the degree of the pancreatitis
- Pancreatitis can present with normal serum amylase levels for the following reasons:
  - Amylase is rapidly cleared by the kidneys
  - Pancreatic parenchyma can be destroyed in chronic pancreatitis (i.e., the pancreas has exhausted its enzymatic production capacity)
  - Hyperlipidemia interferes with amylase determination

- ERCP is a poor test for pancreatitis and can induce or worsen pancreatitis 5% to 15% of the time
- Ranson criteria are not clinically useful for the following reasons:
  - Ranson criteria only predict outcomes based on initial presentation: age, WBC, glucose, LDH, AST, BUN, PaO_2, Ca, Hct, base deficit, and fluid sequestration
  - It is limited by the 48-hour waiting period and the inability to recalculate the score throughout the patient's clinical course
  - Even low-grade pancreatitis can spontaneously lead to infected pancreatic necrosis and death

Elderly patients with new-onset pancreatitis have pancreatic cancer until proven otherwise.

A 35-year-old morbidly obese woman presents with pancreatitis. What is the most likely etiology?

Gallstones are the most common cause of acute pancreatitis in the United States.

Causes of Acute Pancreatitis
- Gallstones (35% to 45% of cases)
- Alcoholic pancreatitis (30% to 40%)
- Idiopathic/other (30% to 35%)
  - ERCP, viruses, medications (antiretrovirals, azathioprine, and others)
  - Trauma is a common cause of pancreatitis in children

A 41-year-old woman presents with new-onset epigastric and right upper quadrant pain. Her total bilirubin is 4.1, amylase 2500, and lipase 2800. Magnetic resonance cholangiopancreatography (MRCP) demonstrates common bile duct stones and pancreatitis. When should a cholecystectomy be performed?

The management of gallstone pancreatitis is conservative (supportive) until symptoms improve. Once the pancreatitis resolves, a laparoscopic cholecystectomy should be performed prior to discharge.

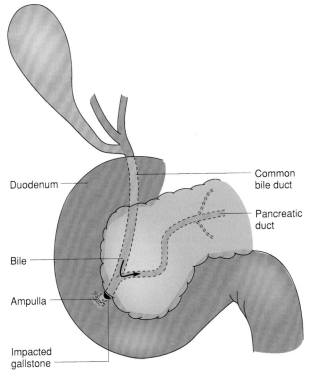

Gallstone in common bile duct leading to gallstone pancreatitis. (With permission from Mulholland MW, Lillemoe KD, Doherty GM, Maier RV, Upchurch GR, eds. *Greenfield's Surgery.* 4th ed. Philadelphia, PA: Lippincott Williams & Wilkins; 2005.)

Duodenum

Common bile duct

Pancreatic duct

Bile

Ampulla

Impacted gallstone

Gallstone Pancreatitis

- Pancreatitis caused by a stone passing through the common bile duct (CBD)
- Associated with increased liver function tests (LFTs), amylase, and lipase
- Following LFTs and clinically distinguishing biliary "colic" from pancreatitis symptoms can be useful in determining whether or not a stone has passed
- Transabdominal ultrasound is poor for looking at stones in the common bile duct, but it does identify CBD dilatation, a finding consistent with CBD stones
- A normal CBD diameter is 4 to 6 mm, with an increased normal limit for older patients (1 mm larger per decade over 50)
- The CBD is normally dilated post cholecystectomy (because the CBD accommodates for a missing gallbladder)
- MRCP is the screening test of choice for common bile duct stones

Laparoscopic cholecystectomy for gallstone pancreatitis should be performed during the same admission. Interval laparoscopic cholecystectomy should be avoided because of the high risk of recurrent gallstone pancreatitis.

A 47-year-old alcoholic presents with severe pancreatitis and signs of early sepsis. He is febrile and has a markedly increased white blood cell count, but is hemodynamically stable. What is the next diagnostic step in management?

A CT scan is critical for making the important diagnosis of necrotizing pancreatitis. Ascending cholangitis should also be considered with the above clinical picture. The total bilirubin is classically elevated in cholangitis.

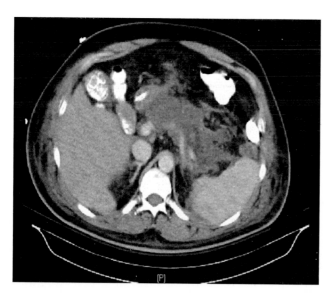

Necrotizing pancreatitis on CT scan. (With permission from Mulholland MW, Lillemoe KD, Doherty GM, Maier RV, Upchurch GR, eds. *Greenfield's Surgery*. 4th ed. Philadelphia, PA: Lippincott Williams & Wilkins; 2005.)

Necrotizing Pancreatitis

- Hypoperfusion of the pancreas results in necrosis which can be sterile or infected
- Distinguishing sterile versus infected necrosis can be difficult
- Subtle or overt signs of sepsis often accompany infected necrosis
- Gas in the pancreas is pathognomonic for infected necrosis
- Infected necrosis requires operative necrosectomy or percutaneous drainage
- Sterile necrosis with clinical improvement should be managed nonoperatively

- Percutaneous drainage should not be performed as it can introduce bacteria and convert the sterile necrosis into infected necrosis
- A necrosectomy can be performed with several variations in management: Open packing, closed packing, repeat second-look laparotomies, and continuous lavage
- Treat infected necrosis with broad spectrum antibiotics (carbapenems)

A 61-year-old woman develops a high-output pancreatic fistula following a Whipple procedure. What acid–base disturbance is likely?

A metabolic acidosis can develop from a high-output pancreatic fistula secondary to high bicarbonate losses.

Pancreatic Fistula
- Results from disruption of the pancreatic duct
- Sodium and bicarbonate losses in the pancreatic fluid result in an electrolyte and acid–base imbalance
- The treatment is controlled drainage via operatively placed drains or percutaneous drains
- Insert a chest tube for pancreatic-pleural fistulas
- Patients should be kept NPO and receive TPN for high-output fistulas
- ERCP can be useful for diagnosing ductal disruption and provides the option of possible stenting

A 45-year-old male presents with mild abdominal pain and a new 7-cm pancreatic pseudocyst on CT scan. What is the most appropriate next step in management?

A repeat CT scan should be performed in at least 6 weeks since most pseudocysts resolve over time.

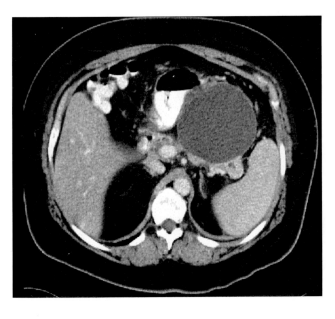

Pancreatic pseudocyst on CT scan. (With permission from Mulholland MW, Lillemoe KD, Doherty GM, Maier RV, Upchurch GR, eds. *Greenfield's Surgery.* 4th ed. Philadelphia: Lippincott Williams & Wilkins; 2005.)

Pancreatic Pseudocyst
- Often presents with persistent epigastric discomfort, hyperamylasemia, early satiety, or nausea and vomiting
- Presents following an episode of acute pancreatitis

- The vast majority resolve spontaneously
- Complications include infection, rupture, small bowel obstruction, and bleeding
- General indications for intervention
  - Symptomatic AND
  - >6 weeks duration (to allow for wall maturation) AND
  - >6 cm in size (larger pseudocysts tend to be more symptomatic)
- Treatment options are endoscopic, laparoscopic, or open cystogastrostomy, or cystojejunostomy
  - These are all ways to "internally" drain the pseudocyst cavity into the GI tract
  - If you operate, remember to biopsy the wall of the pseudocyst
- For an infected pseudocyst, percutaneous "external" drainage may be required to treat sepsis
- It is important to distinguish a pseudocyst from a cystic neoplasm. History and clinical course are the most important factors in differentiating the two.
  - Pseudocysts follow episodes of pancreatitis and aspirates contain inflammatory cells and lack epithelial cells
  - Cystic neoplasms are low in amylase, may contain mucin, and can have high levels of tumor markers

---

A large simple pancreatic abscess is identified on CT during an evaluation for fever in the setting of pancreatitis. What is the next step in management?

Immediate percutaneous drainage and broad-spectrum antibiotics is indicated for any abdominal abscess. Surgical intervention is reserved for cases where percutaneous drainage is not possible or the patient has severe worsening sepsis following percutaneous drainage.

A 51-year-old man is noted to have a "chain of lakes" appearance of his pancreatic duct on ERCP. What is the most likely diagnosis?

A chain of lakes is a characteristic appearance of chronic pancreatitis on ERCP.

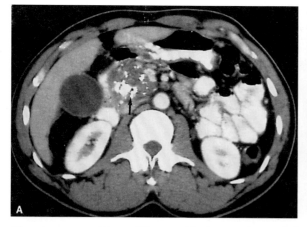 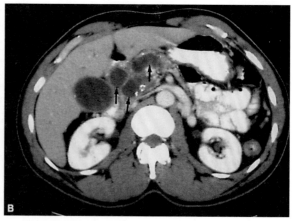

Chronic pancreatitis on CT scan with characteristic calcifications. (With permission from Mulholland MW, Lillemoe KD, Doherty GM, Maier RV, Upchurch GR, eds. *Greenfield's Surgery*. 4th ed. Philadelphia, PA: Lippincott Williams & Wilkins; 2005.)

Chronic Pancreatitis

- Intermittent epigastric pain that can result in constant, chronic pain after a period of years
- 85% to 90% of cases of chronic pancreatitis are due to recurrent episodes of alcoholic pancreatitis, with most of the remaining cases of unknown etiology
- Amylase and lipase are usually normal (the pancreas is "burnt-out" of enzymes)
- It is common to see calcifications of the pancreas and impacted stones in the pancreatic duct on CT scan
- Treatment for chronic pancreatitis with a small pancreatic duct is celiac nerve splanchnicectomy for pain relief
  - Surgery is rarely indicated
  - In select patients, total pancreatectomy with autoislet transplant can be successful for symptom relief
- For chronic pancreatitis with a large pancreatic duct (AT LEAST >8 mm), the surgical goals are to relieve high ductal pressures with a drainage procedure and resect diseased pancreatic tissue. Different surgical options include:
  - Lateral pancreaticojejunostomy (Puestow procedure)
  - Duodenal-preserving pancreatic head resection and lateral pancreaticojejunostomy (Frey or Beger procedure)
  - Whipple (pancreaticoduodenectomy) resection or distal pancreatectomy
- In general the majority get complete pain relief, and most others have an improvement in pain control
- An isolated duct stricture from pancreatitis can occasionally be managed with an endoscopic stent; however, it is important to rule out malignancy when not clearly associated with alcoholic or gallstone pancreatitis

---

A 62-year-old man presents with new-onset painless jaundice and a 30-lb weight loss. What is the next step in management?

This patient most likely has a periampullary cancer. Painless jaundice occurs in over 60% to 75% of patients with periampullary cancers. A high-resolution CT should be performed to evaluate the pancreas for a mass (including resectability) and to evaluate the liver and abdomen for metastatic lesions.

Periampullary Cancers

- Pancreatic cancer (worst prognosis)
- Distal bile duct cancer
- Ampullary cancer
- Duodenal cancer (best prognosis)

During dissection of the ligament of Treitz for a tumor in the fourth portion of the duodenum, a large vein is noted immediately to the left of the ligament of Treitz. What vessel is this?

The inferior mesenteric vein joins the splenic vein left of the ligament of Treitz. The ligament of Treitz is not a true ligament; it is the peritoneal reflection at the exit of the 4th portion of the duodenum as it arises out of the mesentery.

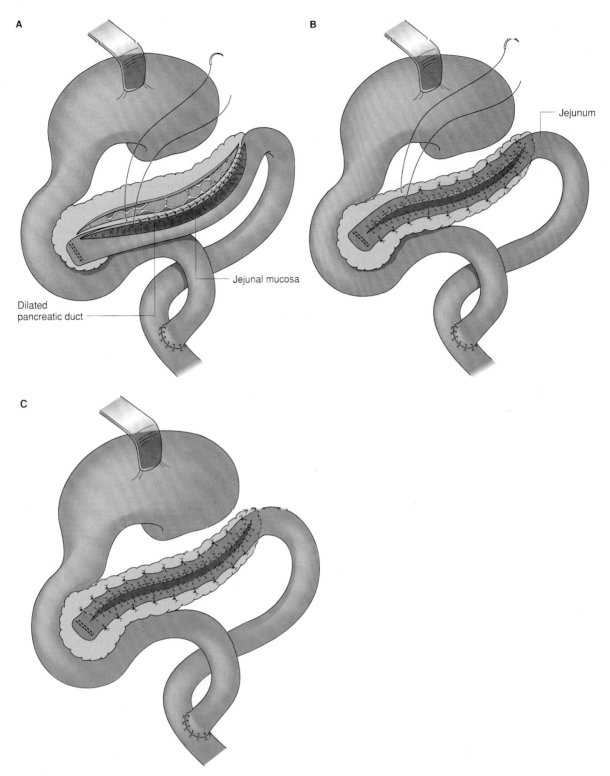

A

B

Jejunum

Jejunal mucosa

Dilated
pancreatic duct

C

Puestow procedure. (With permission from Mulholland MW, Lillemoe KD, Doherty GM, Maier RV, Upchurch GR, eds. *Greenfield's Surgery*. 4th ed. Philadelphia, PA: Lippincott Williams & Wilkins; 2005.)

Relationship of IMV to Ligament of Treitz

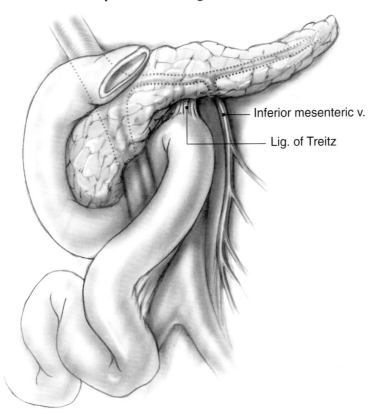

Inferior mesenteric v.

Lig. of Treitz

A 63-year-old man with a 3-cm incidentally discovered pancreas head mass presents for evaluation. What is the most common clinical tumor marker used in evaluating pancreas masses?

CA 19-9 is the most common tumor marker. Although it is only moderately specific (also elevated in pancreatitis and in some patients with normal glands), it can be helpful, especially when markedly elevated (to the thousands). It can also be used postoperatively to assess recurrence. A high-resolution CT scan with an experienced reader will predict resectability >90% of the time.

Candidacy for Surgical Resection

- Candidacy for surgical resection is based on:
  - The absence of distant metastases
  - The absence of local vascular invasion into life-critical veins
  - The patient's age and operative risk/comorbid conditions
  - The patient's motivation to proceed with a major operation associated with a 1% to 3% mortality rate
  - Vascular invasion to the superior mesenteric vein (SMV) and PV is the most common reason patients are not good surgical candidates
    - Vascular invasion to the PV/SMV can only be definitively determined by looking at the venous phase of the CT (the delayed phase in which IV contract lights up the vein)
    - In rare cases where invasion is limited to a small area of the PV/SMV, a Whipple with vein resection can be performed

Dissection of the Pancreatic Neck off the SMV/Portal Vein

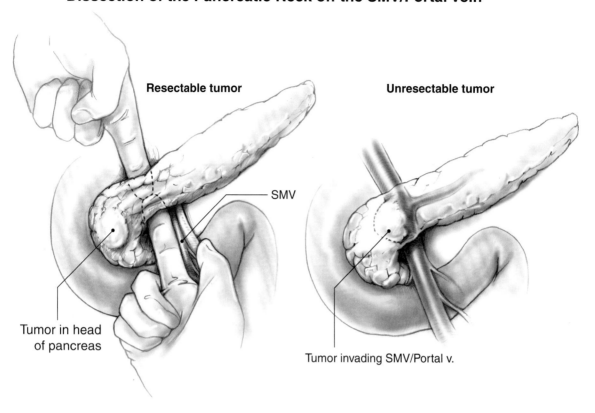

Resectable tumor

Unresectable tumor

SMV

Tumor in head
of pancreas

Tumor invading SMV/Portal v.

Pancreatic Cancer

- 90% are ductal adenocarcinoma
- Associated with the K-ras mutation
- 70% in the pancreatic head
- A markedly increased CA 19-9 can be diagnostic
- Biopsies are not necessary in the preoperative evaluation
- Lymphatic spread is common
- 80% of patients present with advanced disease that is not resectable
- The liver is the most common site of distant metastases
- A *Whipple procedure* (pancreaticoduodenectomy) is the standard operation to treat tumors of the pancreatic head
- The Whipple procedure is also the surgical treatment for other tumors in the area:
  - Distal bile duct cancer (cholangiocarcinoma)
  - Ampullary cancer
  - Duodenal cancer
  - Cysts >3 cm in size that are not believed to be pseudocysts or benign by appearance
- The main complication of a Whipple procedure is a pancreatic anastomotic leak/fistula
  - Often successfully treated with controlled drainage using drains placed prophylactically at the time of operation or with percutaneously inserted drains
- 5-year survival after a Whipple resection for cancer is poor (10% to 20%)
- Improved surgical outcomes have been observed at high-volume centers

Kocher Maneuver

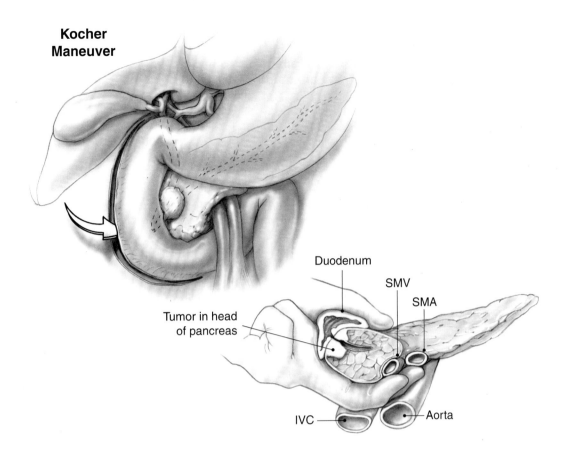

Duodenum

SMV

SMA

Tumor in head
of pancreas

IVC

Aorta

Pancreaticoduodenectomy (Whipple Procedure)

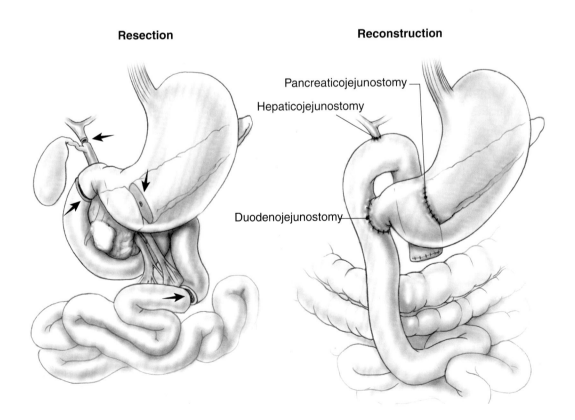

Resection

Reconstruction

Pancreaticojejunostomy

Hepaticojejunostomy

Duodenojejunostomy

If a patient has a mass that is clearly resectable on CT, routine biopsy of the pancreas should not be performed. The only exception is if a tissue diagnosis is needed to begin chemotherapy (assuming that the patient is amenable to having chemotherapy if a cancer diagnosis if made, and that there are no other distant lesions that can be more readily biopsied).

> Following a Whipple for pancreatic cancer, what adjuvant therapy is recommended?

Folfirinox or gemcitabine is routinely given, although the survival advantage is small and occurs in a minority of patients who are chemosensitive. Radiation therapy is added at some centers although there is no level one data to support a survival benefit. Some centers routinely give neoadjuvant chemotherapy prior to surgical resection.

> A 52-year-old-man is explored for pancreatic cancer and gastric outlet obstruction. At the time of operation, he is found to have an unresectable tumor, metastatic disease in the liver, and a dilated stomach due to tumor compression on the duodenum. What is the next step in operative management?

Perform a gastrojejunostomy to palliate the patient's gastric outlet obstruction. A liver biopsy to confirm metastatic disease and a celiac plexus alcohol block for pain control should also be performed at the time of surgery. While some surgeons may also perform a hepaticojejunostomy for a bile duct obstruction, many would simply have the obstruction managed by a subsequent endoscopic or transhepatic percutaneous bile duct stent once biliary symptoms present.

Palliative Surgery for Pancreatic Cancer
- Any gastric outlet obstruction noted at the time of surgery must be addressed
  - A gastrojejunostomy is preferred over a gastrostomy tube
- Endoscopically placed duodenal stents have also been used to manage gastric outlet obstructions
- Any suspicious liver or other distant lesion should be biopsied to accurately stage the cancer
- An alcohol block of the celiac plexus for pain relief in symptomatic patients can be performed surgically or percutaneously (at a later date)
- Concomitant biliary obstruction can be addressed with either a hepaticojejunostomy, or a wallstent placed subsequently by upper endoscopy or percutaneously by interventional radiology
- Administer postoperative chemotherapy (5-FU or gemcitabine)

A celiac plexus block with alcohol is an effective treatment of pancreatic pain in patients with unresectable disease.

> A 72-year-old man underwent an endoscopic evaluation of a pancreatic head cyst. During the duodenoscopy, mucin is found to be oozing from the papilla. What is the most likely diagnosis?

Mucin fluid arising from the ampulla is pathognomonic for an intraductal papillary mucinous neoplasm (IPMN).

Intraductal Papillary Mucinous Neoplasm
- Male predominance (60%)
- More common in the elderly (age 60s to 80s)

- Communicates with the pancreatic duct (i.e., mucin can drain out of the ampulla)
- High levels of amylase in the cyst
- Considered premalignant (90% of patients are cured with definitive surgery)
- Commonly occurs in the head which necessitates treatment with a Whipple procedure
  - The uncinate is the most common location.

A 45-year-old woman underwent a distal pancreatectomy for a cystic lesion in the pancreatic tail. Histologic analysis demonstrates an ovarian-like stroma and no communication with the pancreatic ductal system. What is the most likely diagnosis?

The above case is a typical presentation for a mucinous cystic neoplasm.

Mucinous Cystic Neoplasm

- Female predominance
- More common in younger patients (age 40 to 50s)
- More common in the pancreatic tail (unlike IPMNs)
- No communication with pancreatic duct
- Ovarian-like stroma
- Considered premalignant (100% are cured with definitive surgery)
- The usual treatment is a distal pancreatectomy

A 32-year-old man presents with abdominal pain, severe esophagitis, and multiple distal duodenal ulcers. What is the most likely diagnosis?

A gastrinoma, or Zollinger-Ellison syndrome, presents with multiple ulcers in atypical locations which fail to respond to or recur following conventional therapy.

Gastrinoma

- 70% malignant
- 70% male
- 70% mutation-associated (sporadic)
- 30% MEN-associated (better prognosis)
  - Test for other MEN I tumors—pituitary adenoma and parathyroid hyperplasia
  - If MEN I syndrome and patient also has a pituitary adenoma, the pituitary adenoma should be removed first

What is the best test to diagnose a gastrinoma?

An octreotide scan detects 85% of lesions. Lab tests can also be helpful in establishing a diagnosis.

Diagnosis of Gastrinoma

- A gastric pH < 2.5 and a gastrin level >500 can be diagnostic
  - Hold PPI for at least 1 week or H_2 blocker for at least 2 days prior to measuring gastrin level
- If gastrin levels are between 200 and 500, injecting 4 mg of calcium will increase the gastrin level by 400 in the presence of a gastrinoma

- Increase in gastrin with injection of secretin can also be used for diagnosis (usually secretin causes a decrease in gastrin)
  - Give 2 U/kg secretin
  - Take gastrin levels at 2, 5, 10, 15, and 30 minutes
  - If gastrin >200 is diagnostic for ZES
- The serum secretin level can be elevated

Localizing a Gastrinoma

- Octreotide scan (85% sensitive)
- CT (65%)
- EUS (65%)
- Angiography (65%)
- Although fractionated venous sampling is 90% accurate, it is also invasive and therefore NOT the best test

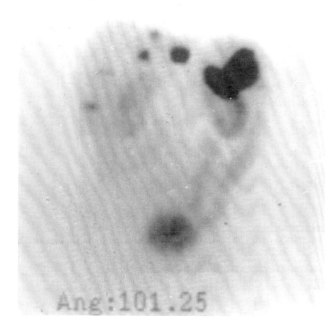

Octreotide scan in a patient with large endocrine tumor in the tail of the pancreas with several hepatic metastases. (With permission from Mulholland MW, Lillemoe KD, Doherty GM, Maier RV, Upchurch GR, eds. *Greenfield's Surgery.* 4th ed. Philadelphia, PA: Lippincott Williams & Wilkins; 2005.)

What is the most common anatomical location for a gastrinoma?

The duodenum is the most common location. 70% to 90% of tumors are found in the gastrinoma triangle.

The Gastrinoma Triangle

- Confluence of the cystic duct and common bile duct
- Junction of the second and third portions of the duodenum
- Junction of the neck and body of the pancreas

During an operative exploration for a gastrinoma, the tumor is not found in the pancreas after an extensive Kocher maneuver. Preoperative endoscopy intraoperative ultrasound is performed, but neither reveals a mass. What is the next intraoperative step?

Perform a duodenotomy. Duodenal gastrinomas are submucosal and sometimes can be identified with palpation.

> During an operative exploration for a gastrinoma, the tumor is not found in the pancreas or the duodenum. What is the next step?

A distal pancreatectomy may be performed if all localization techniques fail to identify the tumor. A highly-selective vagotomy should also be performed if the tumor is not seen, if there is evidence of metastatic disease, or if the patient has the familial type.

Treatment of Gastrinoma

- Enucleation
- Whipple or distal pancreatectomy procedures may be required for tumors involving the pancreatic duct
- Sandostatin, streptozotocin, and debulking may be indicated for metastatic disease

> A 34-year-old woman presents with visual disturbances, bizarre behavior, and memory lapses. What is the most likely pancreatic etiology?

Hypoglycemia from an insulinoma can induce hunger, irritability, coma, or even psychosis.

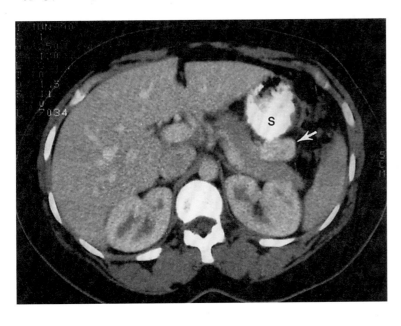

CT of a patient with an insulinoma. (With permission from Mulholland MW, Lillemoe KD, Doherty GM, Maier RV, Upchurch GR, eds. *Greenfield's Surgery.* 4th ed. Philadelphia, PA: Lippincott Williams & Wilkins; 2005.)

Insulinoma

- Can present with hypoglycemia
- 90% are benign
- 75% are solitary
- Symptoms: Whipple's triad—symptoms of hypoglycemia, hypoglycemia (<50 mg/dL) with symptoms, relief with glucose
- The best test is an intraoperative ultrasound
- Elevated C-peptide distinguishes a true insulinoma from the surreptitious administration of insulin
- Does NOT light up on a nuclear medicine scan (other endocrine tumors often do)
- Treatment is enucleation for head/body insulinomas and distal pancreatectomy for tail insulinomas
- Debulking is appropriate for metastatic disease.

Do not perform a blind resection if unable to localize an insulinoma.

What is the nonoperative management of symptomatic insulinomas?

- *Small meals*
- *Administer a calcium channel blocker (calcium may stimulate the tumor).*
- *Follow radiographically every 6 months.*

A 48-year-old female presents with a 6-month history of watery diarrhea with intermittent flushing and swelling of the face and neck. During this time period she has been experiencing episodes of abdominal cramping. On physical exam, she appears to be lethargic with poor skin turgor and dry mucous membranes. Laboratory studies demonstrate hypokalemia. A CT scan of the abdomen and pelvis reveals a tumor in the pancreas. What is the most likely diagnosis?

She most likely is suffering from dehydration secondary to a VIPoma.

VIPoma (Watery Diarrhea, Hypokalemia, Achlorhydria Syndrome)

- Symptoms: Watery diarrhea, hypokalemia, achlorhydria
- Characterized by elevated VIP and calcium levels
- Associated with severe diarrhea, often with asymptomatic periods between bouts
- The distal pancreas is a common site
- Sandostatin can be used for symptomatic relief

A 48-year-old man presents with a rash and a pancreatic mass. What is the most likely diagnosis?

Glucagonomas are classically associated with dermatitis and can present as a red skin patch with a healing center.

Glucagonoma

- Cutaneous rash (migratory necrolytic erythema)
- Mild diabetes
- Cachexia
- Venous thrombosis

Glucagonomas are common in the pancreatic tail and can be blindly resected with a distal pancreatectomy if localization studies and operative exploration fail to identify the tumor.

A 44-year-old man has neurofibromatosis and a peripancreatic mass. What is the most likely diagnosis?

Duodenal somatostatinomas can be associated with neurofibromatosis (this is a classic test question).

Somatostatinoma

- Consists of type II diabetes, cholelithiasis, and steatorrhea
- 90% are malignant

- 25% are located in the small bowel
- Sandostatin levels can be diagnostic
- The pancreatic head is a common site

> What islet cell tumor is the least malignant?

Insulinomas are least likely to be malignant. Little data exists on some of the other types of islet cell tumors since many are rare (e.g., there have been fewer than 60 reported cases of somatostatinoma).

Malignant Potential of Islet Cell Tumors

- Somatostatinomas (90%) > glucagonoma (80%) > gastrinoma (70%) > VIPoma (50%) > insulinoma (10%)

> Excluding pancreatic adenocarcinoma, which pancreatic tumors are common in the pancreatic head versus the tail?

Location of Pancreatic Tumors

- Pancreatic tumors commonly found in the head
  - IPMN
  - Distal bile duct cancer
  - Periampullary and duodenal tumors
  - Gastrinoma
  - Somatostatinoma
- Pancreatic tumors commonly found in the tail
  - Mucinous cystic neoplasm
  - VIPoma
  - Glucagonoma
- Insulinomas are distributed evenly between the head and the tail.

18 | Spleen

Joseph E. Chebli and Joseph J. Ricotta

In searching for an accessory spleen during an exploratory operation, which area should be inspected first?

The splenic hilum is the most common site for an accessory spleen.

Accessory Spleen

- Occurs in 15% to 35% of the population
- Location (in decreasing order of frequency)
  - Splenic hilum
  - Gastrosplenic, splenocolic, gastrocolic, and splenorenal ligament
  - Other sites include the greater omentum, mesentery, pelvis (left ureter), and left gonad

What are the three components of the splenic microanatomy and their functions?

Red pulp serves a phagocytic function. White pulp has an immunologic function. A marginal zone filters material from the white pulp.

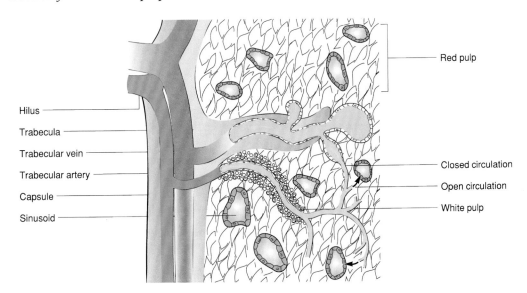

Red and white pulp. (With permission from Mulholland MW, Lillemoe KD, Doherty GM, Maier RV, Upchurch GR, eds. *Greenfield's Surgery.* 4th ed. Philadelphia, PA: Lippincott Williams & Wilkins; 2005.)

Red Pulp

- Comprises 85% of the spleen
- Cell types: Mononuclear phagocytes
- Functions
  - Clears nucleated remnants from immature RBCs
  - Clears dead or damaged RBCs
- Without spleen—have Howell-Jolly bodies (nuclear remnants)

White Pulp

- Comprises 15% of the spleen
- Cell types: Lymphoid, mostly B cells
- Functions
  - Clears bacteria without preexisting antibodies
  - Clears poorly opsonized bacteria
  - Clears foreign particles
  - Clears cellular debris

What are the two types of arterial supply of the spleen?

Magistral and distributed (most common).

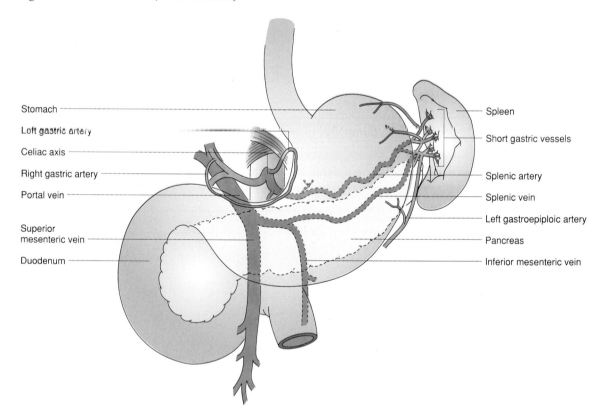

Arterial supply of the spleen. (With permission from Mulholland MW, Lillemoe KD, Doherty GM, Maier RV, Upchurch GR, eds. *Greenfield's Surgery*. 4th ed. Philadelphia, PA: Lippincott Williams & Wilkins; 2005.)

Arterial Supply of the Spleen

- Magistral: A single arterial pedicle
- Distributed: Multiple branches enter the spleen arising from main trunks 2 to 3 cm from the hilum

> A 32-year-old man who underwent a splenectomy does not have any Howell-Jolly bodies on a peripheral smear. What does this finding indicate?

The lack of Howell-Jolly bodies suggests that the patient may have unresected accessory splenic tissue or splenosis. Splenosis refers to the auto transplantation of splenic fragments.

Products Removed by the Spleen

- Howell-Jolly bodies (nuclear remnants)
- Pappenheimer bodies (iron granules)
- Heinz bodies (denatured hemoglobin)
- Target cells (deformed cells)
- Stippling (inclusions)
- Acanthocytes (spurred cells)

> After splenectomy, a patient has persistent thrombocytopenia. What should you look for?

Perform imaging evaluation to see if the patient has an accessory spleen.

> During a splenectomy, the tail of the pancreas was inadvertently resected with the specimen. What is the next step?

Place a surgical drain or multiple drains at the cut end of the pancreas (the pancreatic stump).

> A 55-year-old male presents with a mass in the tail of the pancreas on CT scan that appears to be arising from the spleen. What is another test to evaluate the possibility an accessory spleen?

A sulfur colloid ("liver-spleen") scan can help determine if the mass has the same consistency of the spleen.

> What is the difference between splenomegaly and hypersplenism?

Splenomegaly is an enlarged spleen. Hypersplenism refers to any combination of neutropenia, anemia, or thrombocytopenia due to splenic sequestration.

> A 48-year-old man with a history of cirrhosis presents with severe portal hypertension and a massive spleen. What is the best management of the splenomegaly?

Do NOT perform a splenectomy for portal-venous hypertension. Any operation in this setting carries an extremely high operative mortality. The best management is treatment of the underlying portal hypertension.

The most accepted contraindication to a splenectomy is portal hypertension.

> A 59-year-old man with a history of IV drug abuse presents with a partial splenic infarction. What volume of normal splenic volume is required for full function?

Approximately 30% to 50% of the spleen's mass can achieve most of the function of the entire spleen.

Splenic Infarction

- Rarely requires surgery
- Most resolve spontaneously
- Pain may persist for weeks
- There is no correlation between spleen infarctions and abscess formation

> A 34-year-old man has a splenectomy performed for trauma. What is the most common trend in platelet count postoperatively?

The spleen normally stores approximately one-third of the body's platelets, resulting in decreased sequestration and increased circulating platelets following a splenectomy.

Post-splenectomy Changes

- RBC increases
- WBC increases
- Platelet count increases
- Decreased antibody response to antigens (the opsonins, tuftsin, and properdin are produced in the spleen)

> Against which organisms should one be vaccinated prior to splenectomy?

Encapsulated organisms: Streptococcus pneumoniae, Haemophilus influenzae, and Neisseria meningitidis.

> When should the splenectomy patient be immunized?

At least 2 weeks prior to surgery is ideal so that fevers associated with the vaccine are not confused with postoperative sepsis. If the surgery is unplanned, vaccination should be delayed until the patient has regained immunocompetence. Vaccination is given prior to discharge for a poorly compliant patient.

> A 48-year-old man presents with refractory bleeding varices and a long-standing history of pancreatitis. What intervention may be indicated?

Bleeding gastric varices in the setting of splenic vein thrombosis are effectively treated with splenectomy.

Splenic Vein Thrombosis

- Associated with pancreatitis because of the proximity of the vessel to the pancreas
- Can result in gastroesophageal varices
- Splenectomy is the definitive treatment for bleeding
- Prophylactic splenectomy is not indicated (less than 10% of splenic vein thromboses result in bleeding)

> A 28-year-old woman presents with a new diagnosis of idiopathic thrombocytopenic purpura (ITP) by her hematologist. What is the next step in her management?

Steroids are the mainstay treatment for ITP. Surgery is reserved for refractory ITP.

Adult Immune or Idiopathic Thrombocytopenic Purpura

- Antiplatelet IgG directed at the fibrinogen receptor (IIb/IIIa) that triggers platelet destruction in the spleen
- More common in young women
- Medical treatment
  - Successful in 15% of adults
  - Steroids or IV gamma globulin
- Surgery
  - Indicated for ITP refractory to the medical treatment above
  - Successful in 85% of adults
  - Transfuse platelets if necessary after the splenic artery is ligated

> What is the size of a typical spleen in ITP?

Normal size; therefore, many patients are good candidates for laparoscopic splenectomy.

> A 5-year-old girl presents with a new diagnosis of ITP following an upper respiratory infection. What is the likelihood that the disease will resolve without surgery?

Surgery is rarely indicated for childhood ITP. Approximately 70% of children with ITP will have complete resolution regardless of therapy.

Childhood Idiopathic Thrombocytopenic Purpura

- Occurs after viral illness
- Self-limited in most cases: Usually lasts 6 to 12 months
- Treatment
  - Avoid contact sports
  - Pulse high-dose steroids may help
  - Surgery is rarely indicated and is reserved for cases when there is no remission within 12 months and severe thrombocytopenia persists despite medical therapy

When indicated, a platelet transfusion is best given at the time of the skin incision.

> A 14-year-old woman presents with a new-onset fever, purple rash, jaundice, paresthesia, and renal failure. What is the best initial step in treatment?

Steroids and plasmapheresis are the standard treatments for thrombotic thrombocytopenic purpura (TTP).

Thrombotic Thrombocytopenic Purpura

- Histology shows occlusion of arterioles and capillaries by deposits of hyaline
- Morbidity and mortality can result from deposition of platelet thrombi in end organs

- Pentad of TTP
  - Fever
  - Purpura
  - Hemolytic anemia
  - Neurologic symptoms
  - Renal failure
- Treatment
  - Plasmapheresis (80% respond)—the most appropriate initial treatment
  - High-dose steroids
  - Surgery is rarely indicated and reserved for failed medical therapy
  - Success of surgery: 65%
  - The most common causes of mortality are intracerebral hemorrhage or acute renal failure

Platelet transfusions should be avoided in patients with TTP.

A 55-year-old woman presents with severe rheumatoid arthritis, splenomegaly, and neutropenia. What is the best treatment?

Splenectomy prevents further antibody production and reduces inflammation.

Felty Syndrome
- Antibodies directed against granulocytes
- Triad of rheumatoid arthritis, splenomegaly, and neutropenia
- Treatment is splenectomy for symptomatic splenomegaly

A 16-year-old woman presents with mild jaundice, splenomegaly, and a strong family history of splenectomy. What is the most likely treatment required?

Hereditary spherocytosis is the most common hemolytic anemia treated by splenectomy. Because of the high incidence of concomitant gallstones, a cholecystectomy is indicated for the presence of gallstones.

Hereditary Spherocytosis
- Autosomal dominant
- Membrane defect in the RBC membrane (spectrin)
- Jaundice, splenomegaly, and cholelithiasis (55%) are common
- There is an increased risk of gallstone formation from recurrent hemolysis
- Splenectomy leads to resolution of anemia
  - The need for splenectomy is based on the severity of disease, which is based on the degree of hemolysis
  - If the patient carries the trait or has mild disease, splenectomy is generally not indicated
- Partial splenectomy is also a possible treatment
  - You can have splenic regrowth, but this is not necessarily associated with increased hemolysis
  - If a partial splenectomy is performed, it is important to watch closely for signs of post-operative bleeding as it is more likely after partial splenectomy

Hereditary Elliptocytosis
- Membrane defect in spectrin chain association and protein 4.1
- Mild anemia
- Most patients are asymptomatic

Hereditary Pyropoikilocytosis

- Severe alterations of RBC structure
- Primarily in African Americans
- Splenectomy reduces hemolysis

If a child under the age of 4 requires a splenectomy, every effort should be made to wait until after age 4 to minimize the risk of post-splenectomy sepsis.

A 25-year-old male presents with a history of sickle cell disease, mild left upper quadrant pain, and a normal spleen on abdominal CT. Is a splenectomy indicated?

A splenectomy is rarely indicated for sickle cell disease.

Sickle Cell Disease

- Normal hemoglobin A is replaced by hemoglobin S
- Caused by valine for glycine substitution
- Decreased oxygen tension leads to Hg S crystallization and sickling
- Splenic infarcts, transient hypersplenism with chronic hyposplenism from scarring, and splenic abscesses are common
- A splenectomy is indicated only for acute sequestration, symptomatic hypersplenism, or abscess

Which hemolytic disease is considered to be a contraindication to splenectomy?

Glucose 6 phosphate dehydrogenase deficiency (G6PDD) is considered to be a contraindication to splenectomy.

Glucose 6 Phosphate Dehydrogenase Deficiency

- X-linked
- Causes anemia after drug or chemical exposure
- African, Middle Eastern, Mediterranean races
- No indication for splenectomy

Pyruvate Kinase Deficiency

- Autosomal recessive
- Abnormality of Embden-Meyerhof pathway of anaerobic glycolysis: RBC energy needs exceed production
- Splenomegaly
- Splenectomy can be helpful (but hemolysis and anemia persist)

Thalassemia Major

- Autosomal dominant
- Can present with anemia in the first year of life
- Signs and symptoms include pallor, retarded body growth, and head enlargement
- Marked by persistence of hemoglobin F and decreased hemoglobin A
- Splenectomy reduces hemolysis
- Most patients do not survive to second decade because of hemosiderosis (iron deposition)

Thalassemia Minor
- Slightly reduced level of hemoglobin A

> When is splenectomy indicated for Gaucher disease?

Gaucher disease with symptomatic splenomegaly can be an indication for partial splenectomy.

Gaucher Disease
- Autosomal recessive disorder characterized by deficiency in beta-glucosidase
- Symptomatic splenomegaly can develop
- Splenectomy exacerbates bone involvement
- Current treatment: Enzyme replacement therapy using recombinant glucocerebrosidase

> A 16-year-old boy presents with severe left upper quadrant pain and anemia following an episode of infectious mononucleosis. What is the most likely etiology?

Infectious mononucleosis can lead to splenic rupture 2 to 4 weeks after symptoms of the infection. Malaria is also known to cause spontaneous splenic rupture.

> What is the most common primary malignant tumor of the spleen?

Non-Hodgkin lymphoma.

Primary Tumors of the Spleen
- Hemangioma (most common benign tumor and overall)
- Non-Hodgkin lymphoma (most common malignant tumor)
- Hodgkin lymphoma
- Angiosarcoma (most common non-lymphoid malignant tumor)

> What is the role of splenectomy in Hodgkin disease?

In general, splenectomy is rarely indicated in Hodgkin disease.

Hodgkin Disease
- Malignant lymphoma
- Ann Arbor classification
  - Stage I: Disease in one area or two contiguous areas of lymph node involvement
  - Stage II: Disease in two noncontiguous areas on the same side of the diaphragm
  - Stage III: Disease on both sides of the diaphragm
  - Stage IV: Disease disseminated to the liver, bone marrow, or lung
- Symptoms
  - A: Asymptomatic
  - B: Night sweats, fever, weight loss
- Histology types

- Lymphocyte predominant (best type)
- Nodular sclerosing (most common)
- Mixed cellularity
- Lymphocyte depleted
- Staging laparotomy has mostly been replaced by CT scanning

The only surgical indications for Hodgkin lymphoma are Stage I or II disease with nodular sclerosing type and no symptoms.

A 67-year-old man with chronic lymphocytic leukemia (CLL) has persistent cytopenia and mild left upper quadrant pain. A CT scan demonstrates splenomegaly. What is the next step in management?

Splenectomy can be an effective treatment for CLL.

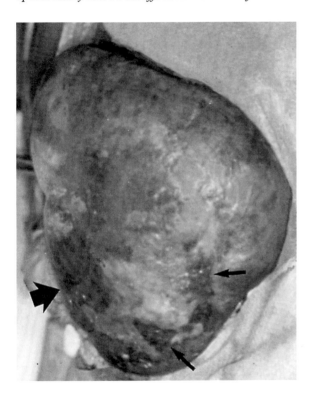

A massively enlarged spleen in a patient with CLL. (With permission from Mulholland MW, Lillemoe KD, Doherty GM, Maier RV, Upchurch GR, eds. *Greenfield's Surgery.* 4th ed. Philadelphia, PA: Lippincott Williams & Wilkins; 2005.)

Chronic Lymphocytic Leukemia
- Splenomegaly is common
- Chemotherapy is the best initial treatment for the disease
- Splenectomy is effective in improving cytopenia in most cases
- Splenectomy resolves the symptoms of splenomegaly

An 84-year-old woman with hairy cell leukemia (HCL) and severe left upper quadrant and left shoulder pain is found to have a massively enlarged spleen on ultrasound. What is the next step in management?

Splenectomy can be an effective treatment for HCL.

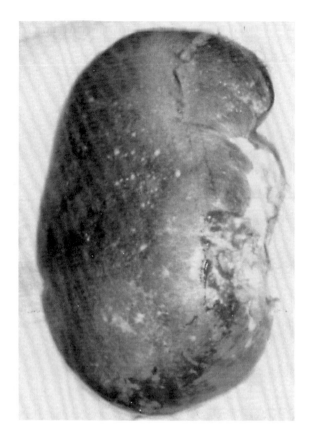

Spleen from a patient with HCL. (With permission from Mulholland MW, Lillemoe KD, Doherty GM, Maier RV, Upchurch GR, eds. *Greenfield's Surgery*. 4th ed. Philadelphia, PA: Lippincott Williams & Wilkins; 2005.)

Hairy Cell Leukemia

- "Ruffled" B-cell membranes give cells a "hairy" appearance
- Splenomegaly is very common
- Chemotherapy (Cladribine) is the best initial treatment for the disease
- Splenectomy is effective in improving cytopenia in most cases
- Splenectomy is indicated for symptomatic splenomegaly

CLL with anemia and HCL are the two types of leukemia most amenable to splenectomy.

What is the role for splenectomy in acquired immune hemolytic anemia?

Only the warm antibody type may respond.

Acquired Immune Hemolytic Anemia

- Warm antibody type
  - IgG binds to RBC cell membranes and the RBCs are removed by the spleen
  - Usually does not involve complement fixation or direct hemolysis
  - The medical treatment is steroids (30% to 40% do not respond or relapse)
  - 80% respond to splenectomy
- Cold antibody type
  - IgM mediated
  - Complement fixation and direct intravascular cell lysis
  - Splenectomy NOT indicated

> A 6-year-old boy presents with a large, unilocular splenic cyst and a recent history of parasitic infection. What is the most likely organism?

Echinococcus granulosus is the most common cause of parasitic splenic cysts.

Splenic Cyst

- Parasitic (5%)
  - Echinococcus granulosus (unilocular)
    - Associated with echinococcal liver cysts
    - Most splenic manifestations are asymptomatic
  - *Echinococcus multilocularis* and *Echinococcus vogeli* (multiloculated)
    - Calcifications
    - Internal cysts or scoleces
- Non-parasitic true cyst (20%)
  - Epithelial lined
  - Rarely symptomatic if <8 cm
  - Remove if >10 cm
- Pseudocyst (80%)
  - Occurs after pancreatitis or trauma
- Symptomatic cysts >4 cm in size should be removed

> What is the most appropriate treatment for a nonparasitic splenic cyst that is symptomatic?

Splenectomy.

> A 44-year-old man with a history of IV drug abuse presents with generalized abdominal pain, fever, and evidence of bacterial endocarditis. A CT scan reveals a low density mass in the spleen with no enhancement upon administration of IV contrast. What is the most likely diagnosis?

Splenic abscesses are rare but typically result from the hematogenous spread of bacteria from a primary source.

Splenic Abscess

- *Staphylococcus* and *Streptococcus* are the most common organisms
- Sources typically include IV drug injections, pyelonephritis, osteomyelitis, or an intra-abdominal source
- Splenomegaly and generalized abdominal symptoms are common
- Administer broad-spectrum antibiotics
- Treatment is splenectomy for a multiloculated abscess
- Treatment is CT-guided drainage for a unilocular abscess

> A 24-year-old man presents 3 months status post splenectomy with a temperature of 39.5°C, chills, and tachycardia. What is the next step in management?

The immediate recognition of post splenectomy sepsis is critical. The rapid initiation of IV antibiotics can be life-saving. Do NOT waste time with an H&P, lab tests, cultures, or culture results before administration of IV antibiotics.

Overwhelming Post-splenectomy Infection

- Affects 0.1% to 0.3% of adults following splenectomy
- Affects 0.6% to 4.0% of children following splenectomy
- Results from a lack of IgM
- Caused by encapsulated bacteria (*Strep. pneumoniae* 50%)
- Mortality is greater in children (50%) than in adults (30%)
- Most episodes occur within 2 years of splenectomy
- If possible, a splenectomy should be delayed until age 4 in children to minimize the risk of post-splenectomy sepsis

Overwhelming post-splenectomy infection requires emergent antibiotics and may result in disseminated intravascular coagulation (DIC) if not treated early.

19 | Adrenal Gland

Alan P.B. Dackiw and Kimberley Eden Steele

> What is the relationship of the adrenal glands to the peritoneal cavity?

Also known as the suprarenal glands, the adrenal glands are located in the retroperitoneum on the superomedial border of the kidneys. The right adrenal is crescentic in shape and the left is pyramidal in shape.

> How much does a normal adrenal gland weigh?

The normal adrenal gland weighs 4 to 6 g.

> What is the main artery supplying the adrenal gland?

The main artery is the inferior phrenic artery.

Arterial Supply of the Adrenal Gland
- Three sources
  - Inferior phrenic artery (superior adrenal artery)
  - Unnamed branches from the aorta (middle adrenal artery)
  - Branches from the renal artery (inferior adrenal artery)
- The arteries penetrate the gland in a circumferential stellate fashion, leaving both anterior and posterior surfaces avascular

Venous Drainage
- Left adrenal vein
  - Also receives the left phrenic vein
  - Drains from the lower pole of the gland
  - Drains into the left renal vein
- Right adrenal vein
  - Drains from the anterior surface of the gland
  - Drains into the posterolateral IVC
  - Short
- Surgically control venous drainage first

The right adrenal vein is shorter in length (and larger in diameter) than the left adrenal vein and thus it may be more difficult to control surgically.

How is the adrenal gland innervated?

There is no innervation to the adrenal cortex. The medulla is innervated by the splanchnic nervous system.

What is the embryonic origin of the adrenal cortex?

The adrenal cortex originates from the mesoderm. During the fifth week of gestation, the adrenal cortex arises from the adrenocortical ridge, which lies near the gonads.

What are some common sites where extra-adrenal cortical tissue might be found?

Adrenal nests may be found in the ovaries, testes, or kidneys.

Adrenal Cortex

- Originates from mesoderm
- Consists of 3 zones (which correspond to 3 classes of steroid hormones)

3 Zones of the Adrenal Gland

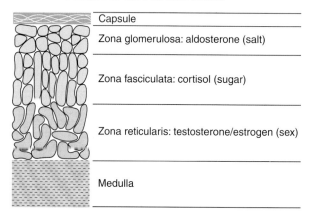

What is the embryonic origin of the adrenal medulla?

The adrenal medulla arises from ectoderm derived from the neural crest.

Adrenal Medulla

- Originates from ectoderm
- Produces epinephrine (20%) and norepinephrine (80%)

What are the only two locations where epinephrine is produced in the human body, and why is this?

The enzyme responsible for converting norepinephrine to epinephrine is phenylethanolamine-N-methyltransferase. This particular enzyme is located in only two areas of the human body: The adrenal medulla and the Organ of Zuckerkandl (sympathetic paraganglia near the aortic bifurcation).

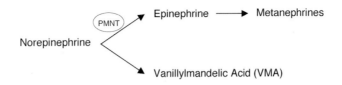

A 38-year-old female has an abdominal CT scan to evaluate her pelvic and lower abdominal pain. The CT demonstrates an ovarian cyst and a 2.5-cm left adrenal mass. What is the next step in management?

The adrenal mass is an adrenal incidentaloma. Given its small size, it does not account for the patient's symptoms and it can be further evaluated on an elective basis. Furthermore, any evaluation of an adrenal mass requires a work-up to answer the following three important questions:

1. Is it functioning or non-functioning?

2. Is it benign or malignant?

3. Is it primary or secondary?

Considerations in Evaluating an Adrenal Mass

1. **Functioning (Metabolically Active) vs. Non-functioning**
   - The vast majority of adrenal masses are non-functioning
   - Hyperfunctioning lesions should generally be resected, regardless of size
   - A diagnosis of a hyperfunctioning gland is made by history, physical exam, and blood and urine levels of primary and secondary metabolites (catecholamines, metanephrines, vanillylmandelic acid [VMA])
   - The degree of autonomous function can be measured and can aid in diagnosis (adrenal hyperplasia vs. adrenal adenoma vs. adrenal carcinoma)
     - *Hyperplasia* is sensitive to negative feedback with inhibition of secretion
     - *Adenoma* is intermediately sensitive to negative feedback
     - *Carcinoma* is usually autonomous

2. **Benign vs. Malignant**
   - The vast majority of adrenal masses are benign
     - Hyperplastic mass
     - Adenoma
     - Benign cyst
   - Carcinomas are rare and approximately 50% have metastases at the time of diagnosis
   - CT assists in diagnosis

3. **Primary vs. Secondary**
   - Secondary (metastatic) lesions originate from lung, breast, renal cell, melanoma, prostate, and colon cancers
   - In fact, metastasis to the adrenal gland is the most common cause of an adrenal mass if the patient has a history of malignancy

A colonoscopy, as well as a breast and pelvic or prostate exam should be performed in all patients with a suspicious adrenal, hepatic, or atypical intra-abdominal mass.

Adrenal Incidentalomas

- Defined as an adrenal mass discovered during abdominal imaging performed for an unrelated reason

- Most are small, benign, non-functioning cortical adenomas (and have no clinical significance)
- The prevalence of "serendipitous" masses is reported to be 1% to 2% of CT scans (similar to autopsy studies)
- The differential diagnosis includes cortical adenoma (most common), adrenocortical carcinoma (rare), pheochromocytoma, ganglioneuroma, cyst, organized hemorrhage or fibrosis, and metastasis

An incidentaloma is most commonly an adrenal adenoma.

Studies to Evaluate an Adrenal Mass

- Serum electrolytes (hypercortisolism may present as hypokalemia and hypernatremia)
- 24-hour urine cortisol
- Plasma cortisol, estradiol, testosterone, dehydroepiandrosterone, and androstenedione
- A low-dose (1 mg) dexamethasone cortisol suppression test
    - Normally, this should suppress pituitary ACTH resulting in a decrease in measured urinary cortisol levels
        - If there is no suppression, suspect Cushing disease
        - Then follow-up with a high-dose dexamethasone suppression test to diagnose an autonomously functioning adrenal tumor
- Serum renin-to-aldosterone ratio
- Urinary catecholamines, metanephrines, VMA
- Serum 17-OH steroids and 17-ketosteroids

The best diagnostic screening test for Cushing syndrome is a low-dose overnight dexamethasone suppression test.

CT Scan Characteristics of Adrenal Masses

- Benign tumors are usually round/oval, smooth, and homogenous
- Adenomas contain increased fat content and thus have a low density
- Malignant tumors are irregular and non-homogeneous from focal hemorrhage and necrosis
- A cyst can be identified and further evaluation may include aspiration with cytology
- Positive (malignant) cytology, evidence of hormonal activity, and recurrence after needle aspiration are indications for surgical resection
- Homogeneous fatty lesions (myelolipoma and lipomas) may be diagnosed by CT scan and generally require no further investigation or treatment regardless of size

Resect adrenal masses that are hyperfunctioning, large (>4 to 6 cm), growing, or have suspicious characteristics on CT scan (irregular borders/heterogeneity).

Magnetic Resonance Imaging Characteristics

T2-weighted density ratio of adrenal mass to liver	Tumor type
0.7–1.4	Adenoma
1.4–3.0	Malignancy (primary or secondary)
>3.0	Pheochromocytoma

Percutaneous Needle Biopsy

- Contraindicated if there is an indication for surgery—a general surgical principle true to many types of suspicious masses in the body
- May be performed when multiple masses are present and a primary diagnosis is unknown based on other tests
- May be of particular value in a patient with a known extra-adrenal malignancy
- It is not helpful in differentiating adrenal adenoma from adrenal cortical carcinoma (as with most neuroendocrine tumors in the body)
- Not appropriate for a hormonally active tumor, larger tumors, or if pheochromocytoma is even remotely suspected—all of which are surgical indications

Do not perform percutaneous needle biopsy on an adrenal mass until it is confirmed that the lesion is non-functional.

A 64-year-old man is found to have a 3.5-cm adrenal mass and hypertension. His urinary catecholamines are noted to be markedly elevated. Is surgical resection indicated?

While this patient does not meet criteria for resection based on adrenal size alone, the presence of biologic activity (i.e., hyperfunction) is an indication for surgical resection. Other criteria for surgical resection include malignancy and size.

Indications for Surgery

- Hyperfunction
    - Increased aldosterone (Conn syndrome)
    - Increased cortisol (Cushing syndrome)
    - Increased catecholamines (pheochromocytoma)
- Malignancy
    - CT findings may indicate the presence of a malignancy
- Size >4 to 6 cm
    - For non-functioning masses <4 cm, DO NOT OPERATE
        - Follow size and character with CT at regular intervals (e.g., 3, 6, 12 months, and yearly)
        - Resect if there is an increase in size or if it becomes metabolically active (i.e., hyperfunctioning)
    - For non-functioning masses 4 to 6 cm, INDIVIDUALIZE
        - May resect or observe (consider Magnetic resonance imaging [MRI])
        - In younger patients (<40 years), in whom adenomas are less common, consider surgery
        - In elderly patients with significant comorbidity and operative risk, consider not operating, since the natural history of such intermediate size incidentalomas is still poorly understood
        - Resect if the mass becomes metabolically active
    - For non-functioning masses >6 cm, OPERATE
        - Resect because of increased risk of malignancy
        - Begin a metastatic work-up for cancer
        - The only contraindications to resection are
            - Adrenal metastasis
            - Other metastatic disease
            - An asymptomatic, well-characterized lipoma or myelolipoma

A 47-year-old woman with refractory hypertension on three antihypertensive medications is noted on routine blood-work to be hypokalemic. A CT scan is obtained. What is the most likely diagnosis?

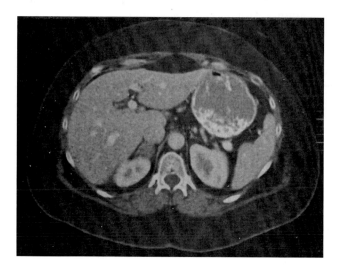

CT demonstrates a low-density, 1.5 cm *right* adrenal mass, anteromedial to the right kidney.

Refractory hypertension and hypokalemia are signs of hyperaldosteronism (Conn syndrome). Aldosterone causes sodium and water resorption with potassium and hydrogen wasting. Hyperaldosteronism should be suspected in any patient with refractory hypertension accompanied by unexplained hypokalemia or an adrenal mass.

Primary Hyperaldosteronism (Conn Syndrome)
- May present with hypertension, hypokalemia, polyuria, polydipsia, alkalosis, and muscle weakness
- Caused by adrenal adenomas (60%) or bilateral adrenal hyperplasia (40%)
- Plasma aldosterone is elevated and plasma renin is low (i.e., high aldosterone:renin ratio)
- Urinary aldosterone (following salt loading) is elevated

Distinguishing Adenoma versus Hyperplasia
- After hyperaldosteronism is diagnosed, the next step is to determine whether the cause is an adenoma or hyperplasia
- Image with CT scan or MRI
- Adrenal vein sampling for aldosterone may be used to confirm the diagnosis
- 18-hydroxycorticosterone levels are elevated with adenoma (>100 μg/dL) and low with hyperplasia
- Hyperfunctioning (or large) adenomas are treated with unilateral adrenalectomy
- Carcinomas and bilateral adenomas are exceedingly rare
- When adrenalectomy is indicated, pre-op treatment with spironolactone helps normalize potassium levels
- Hyperplasia is treated medically
- Medical treatment includes spironolactone, calcium channel blockers, and potassium

Hyperaldosteronism due to an adrenal adenoma is treated surgically, while hyperaldosteronism due to hyperplasia is treated medically.

Secondary Hyperaldosteronism

- High plasma aldosterone, high plasma renin
- Secondary to renovascular hypertension
- Results from diuretic use

Tertiary Hyperaldosteronism

> A 25-year-old woman presents with mild symptoms of emotional lability, weight gain, and hirsutism. A 2.5-cm left adrenal mass is seen on CT. What is the next step in management?

A low-dose dexamethasone test is the best way to distinguish an incidental, non-functional adrenal tumor from a Cushing adenoma.

Hypercortisolism (Cushing Syndrome)

- Presents with weight gain (most common), hypertension, diabetes, centripetal obesity, buffalo hump, hirsutism, acne, purple striae, and mental status changes
- 24-hour urinary and serum cortisol levels can distinguish hypercortisolism from the normal diurnal variation of cortisol levels
- **Cushing "Syndrome"**
    - Refers to excess circulating glucocorticoids
    - Can be due to adrenal hyperplasia, adenoma, or carcinoma
    - Also caused by ectopic ACTH or corticotropin releasing factor secretion (small cell carcinoma/paraneoplastic syndrome)
    - Occurs with exogenous steroid use
- **Cushing Disease**
    - Refers to ACTH hypersecretion from the pituitary causing a secondary increase in cortisol from the adrenal gland
    - A pituitary adenoma may be treated medically (with bromocriptine) or surgically (transsphenoidal or transcranial hypophysectomy)
    - Other (less desired) options include pituitary radiation, or bilateral adrenalectomy with steroid replacement
        - Reserved for rare cases of recurrent disease after pituitary surgery

The Low-dose Dexamethasone Suppression Test

- The best test for hypercortisolism/Cushing syndrome
- A low-dose dexamethasone bolus (1 mg) is given
- ACTH level is used to distinguish the level of dysfunction along the pituitary-adrenal axis (primary versus secondary hypercortisolism)
    - Low plasma ACTH = primary hypercortisolism
        - An adrenal adenoma, hyperplasia, or (rarely) carcinoma
    - High plasma ACTH = secondary hypercortisolism
        - A pituitary adenoma with increased ACTH or an ectopic ACTH-secreting tumor

The High-dose Dexamethasone Suppression Test

- Identifies if secondary hypercortisolism is from the pituitary or an ectopic source
- A high dose of dexamethasone is given (2 mg every 6 hours, for 48 hours)
    - Ectopic ACTH production will not be suppressed by a high dose test
    - Pituitary ACTH will be suppressed (by at least 50%) by a high dose test

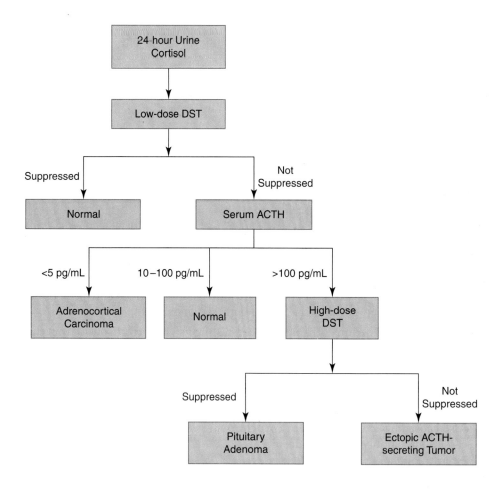

Adrenalectomy in Cushing Syndrome

- Indications
  - Adrenal adenoma or carcinoma
  - Adrenal hyperplasia (requires bilateral adrenalectomy)
  - Selected cases of secondary hypercortisolism in which the primary tumor cannot be identified in the sella turcica or elsewhere (requires bilateral adrenalectomy)
- Following unilateral adrenalectomy, patients must be given perioperative steroid coverage until they regain contralateral adrenal cortical function
- Mineralocorticoid replacement is generally not necessary unless a bilateral adrenalectomy is performed

The most common cause of a Cushingoid appearance is exogenous steroid administration.

A 43-year-old woman presents with left-sided abdominal pain, weight gain, and abnormal hair growth. A CT scan demonstrates a 10-cm left adrenal mass and enlarged periaortic and vena caval lymph nodes. What is the most likely diagnosis?

Adrenal cortical carcinoma often presents with vague abdominal symptoms and a large retroperitoneal adrenal mass in a middle-aged woman. It is a very aggressive tumor with a poor prognosis.

Adrenal Cortical Carcinoma

- Usually occurs in women age 40 to 50 years
- Usually large (90% are >6 cm)

- Left-sided tumors more common
- CT scan shows irregular features, sometimes necrosis, calcifications, and invasion into adjacent organs
- Can present with liver metastases
- Most are functional tumors
  - Cushing syndrome present in up to 50%
  - Virilizing in some women
  - Feminization in some men
  - Hyperaldosteronism (rare) with cancer
- Treatment
  - Adrenalectomy (may require a thoraco-abdominal approach, especially on the right side)
  - Adjacent involved organs may need to be resected en bloc
  - Although 50% are localized to the adrenal gland, most eventually develop metastases (85%)
  - Overall 5-year survival is poor (~20%)
  - Chemotherapy and radiation therapy are not beneficial

A definitive margin-negative resection is the most important prognostic factor for adrenal cortical carcinoma.

A 37-year-old woman with refractory hypertension and worsening headaches describes having frequent palpitations and episodes of diaphoresis. What is the next step in management?

Headache, palpitations, and diaphoresis are the three classic hallmark findings of a pheochromocytoma. Serum and urine catecholamine and metabolites should be tested.

Pheochromocytoma
- A rare tumor of the adrenal medulla (neuroectodermal origin)
- Involves the chromaffin cell of the adrenergic system
- May originate in extra-adrenal adrenergic tissue
  - Organ of Zuckerkandl (at the base of the IMA or aortic bifurcation)
  - Scattered along the midline retroperitoneum (para-aortic, bladder, etc.)
- Presents as paroxysmal hypertension (most common) or sustained hypertension
- Screen for multiple endocrine neoplasia (MEN) syndrome
- The majority are sporadic
- Rule of "10s"
  - 10% are familial
  - 10% are extra-adrenal
  - 10% are multiple
  - 10% are bilateral
  - 10% are pediatric
  - 10% are malignant
- Diagnostic test: 24-hour urine collection
  - Quantitate urinary catecholamines (dopamine, epinephrine, norepinephrine) and their metabolites (VMA, metanephrines)
  - 80% of patients will have at least one urinary metabolite greater than twice the normal level
- May also find elevated plasma catecholamines/metanephrines
- **MRI** reveals characteristically bright areas on T2 weighted images

- A "Pheo Scan" uses **MIBG I131**, a norepinephrine analogue, which concentrates in adrenergic vesicles
  - Good for identifying extra-adrenal pheochromocytomas
  - False negative rate = 5%
  - False positive rate = 1% to 2%

Evaluate for MEN in all patients with a pheochromocytoma prior to surgical resection.

A 22-year-old woman undergoing a laparoscopic adrenalectomy for a pheochromocytoma develops sudden arrhythmias and hypertension at the time of operation during surgical manipulation of the adrenal gland. What is the next step in management?

Sudden arrhythmias and hypertension may indicate incomplete adrenergic blockade. Treat hypertension with nipride. Occasionally arrhythmias require propranolol or lidocaine. Surgical manipulation of the gland can result in a dangerous release of catecholamines and thus should be minimized.

A 43-year-old man is about to undergo a laparoscopic adrenalectomy for pheochromocytoma. What preoperative considerations are important?

Patients with a pheochromocytoma are classically hypertensive and volume depleted. Preoperative preparation must consider these potential issues.

Preoperative Preparation for a Pheochromocytoma
- Alpha blockade first!
  - Phenoxybenzamine for 7 to 10 days prior to operation
  - Prazosin can also be used
- Next, beta blockade (if needed) to treat reflex tachycardia
  - Propranolol for 48 hours prior to operation
- Hydration for 1 to 2 days prior to surgery

The Case for Alpha Blockade First
- Administration of a beta blocker in the presence of high circulating levels of catecholamine can cause a hypertensive crisis
- Beta blockers abolish beta-2-mediated vasodilation, leaving alpha-1-mediated vasoconstriction unopposed
- Preoperative volume expansion with saline is important to minimize blood pressure lability at the time of operation
- Surgical manipulation of the adrenal gland should be minimized to prevent release of catecholamines
- Early ligation of the adrenal vein is desirable
- The patient should be monitored postoperatively for arrhythmias and unstable blood pressure

Preparation for an adrenalectomy for pheochromocytoma is alpha blockade followed by hydration and beta blockade.

A 6-year-old boy is brought to the pediatrician for an annual check-up. His mother has a history of medullary thyroid cancer. The pediatrician orders a series of labs including calcium and urine catecholamines, which are normal. However, the serum calcitonin is slightly elevated. What should be the next step?

MEN IIA includes pheochromocytoma, hyperparathyroidism, and medullary thyroid cancer. The patient should be tested for the RET proto-oncogene (associated with medullary thyroid carcinoma in both MEN IIA and MEN IIB). If the patient tests positive for the RET gene, then a prophylactic total thyroidectomy should be performed.

The reasons for total thyroidectomy are that medullary thyroid cancer in MEN II is a bilateral disease, and there is a greater than 30% incidence of lymph node involvement at the time of the diagnosis.

Surveillance of MEN IIA and IIB family members is done by yearly lab tests including calcium, catecholamines, and calcitonin levels. Children with a diagnosis of MEN IIA or found to have elevated serum calcitonin should have their thyroids removed before the age of 5 years.

Medullary thyroid cancer tends to be more aggressive in MEN IIB and therefore a child with positive MEN IIB genetic markers should have a prophylactic total thyroidectomy by 2 years of age.

MEN I

- The 3 Ps: Pituitary, Parathyroid, Pancreas
  - But note there is no pheochromocytoma in MEN I
- Autosomal dominant trait (chromosome 11)
- **Pit**uitary tumors
  - Most common = Prolactinoma
  - Treatment begins with bromocriptine
  - Then (rarely) surgical transsphenoidal hypophysectomy
- Hyper**para**thyroidism
  - Four gland hyperplasia
  - Requires bilateral exploration/resection
  - Most common manifestation of MEN I
- Neuroendocrine **Pan**creatic tumors
  - Most common are non-functional tumors of pancreatic polypeptide production

The 3 Ps of MEN I

Tumor location	Common manifestation	Treatment
Pituitary	Prolactinoma	Bromocriptine
Hyperparathyroid	four gland hyperplasia	three gland resection
Pancreas	Non-functional	None in most cases

The parathyroid is the most commonly affected organ in MEN I.

MEN IIA

- Also an autosomal dominant trait (chromosome 10)
- Medullary thyroid cancer (in 100% of patients)
- Pheochromocytoma
- Hyperparathyroidism

MEN IIB

- Also autosomal dominant but can occur sporadically
- Medullary thyroid carcinoma (in 100% of patients)
- Pheochromocytoma
- Mucosal neuromas/marfanoid habitus

Medullary thyroid cancer is present in nearly 100% of patients with MEN II (A and B).

A 32-year-old woman just underwent an uncomplicated ileocecectomy for active Crohn's disease. While in the recovery room, the patient's blood pressure dropped to 72/36 and did not improve with aggressive fluid administration. Her hematocrit was stable. What cause of hypotension should be considered?

Patients with Crohn's disease are often on chronic corticosteroids—a special consideration in surgical patients. This patient is most likely having symptoms of acute adrenal insufficiency, referred to as an Addisonian crisis. Prior steroid use can result in suppression of the hypothalamic–pituitary–adrenal axis. Thus "stress dose" steroids should be given to treat severe, unexplained, or refractory hypotension in any patient with a history of corticosteroid use during the past year, and especially in patients with a long-standing history of corticosteroid use.

Adrenal Insufficiency (Addison Disease)

- Iatrogenic
  - Commonly due to exogenous corticosteroids
    - Transplant patients
    - Inflammatory bowel disease patients
    - Young athletes (taking steroids undisclosed)
  - Most common type of adrenal insufficiency
  - Exogenous corticosteroids suppress ACTH secretion
  - Also known as secondary adrenal insufficiency
- Primary adrenal insufficiency
  - Most common cause is autoimmune destruction of adrenal cortex
  - Can also be caused by infection
    - Histoplasmosis
    - Tuberculosis
    - Meningococcus (with bilateral adrenal hemorrhage = Waterhouse-Friderichsen syndrome)
- Lab findings
  - Hyperkalemia, hyponatremia, hypochloremia
  - Hypoglycemia
  - Acidosis
  - Elevated blood urea nitrogen
- Cosyntropin stimulation test
  - Synthetic ACTH is administered (250 μg IV)
  - Plasma cortisol levels are measured 30 and 60 minutes later
    - Plasma cortisol <20 μg/dL is suggestive of insufficiency
  - Primary versus secondary can be diagnosed by measuring ACTH levels
    - Elevated ACTH levels are suggestive of primary disease

- Treatment of adrenal insufficiency
  - Acute adrenal insufficiency: Give glucocorticoids and IV hydration (normal saline)
  - Chronic adrenal insufficiency: Chronic daily administration of oral glucocorticoids and fludrocortisone

A lack of endogenous steroids following an IV administration of synthetic ACTH (cosyntropin stimulation test) is diagnostic for adrenal insufficiency.

When in doubt, give IV steroids to any patient with a history of steroid use and sudden intraoperative or postoperative unexplained hypotension that is refractory to fluid resuscitation. These patients need immediate steroid administration (hydrocortisone 100 mg IV) rather than pressors.

SUGGESTED READINGS

Brunt LM. The positive impact of laparoscopic adrenalectomy on complications of adrenal surgery. *Surg Endosc.* 2002;16:1432-2218.

NIH Consensus Statement on Adrenal Incidentaloma.

http://consensus.nih.gov/2002/2002AdrenalIncidentalomasos021html.htm.

20 | Small Bowel

Genevieve Melton-Meaux and Anne O. Lidor

> What is the function of the migrating motor complex (MMC)? What is the primary hormone associated with MMC initiation?

The MMC, which is mediated by the hormone motilin, provides a basic motility pattern resulting in the propagation of cellular debris, bacteria, and chyme through the stomach and small bowl. It is composed of 4 phases that cycle approximately every 2 hours and stop with meals.

Layers of the Bowel Wall

- Mucosa: Villi and crypts, responsible for absorption
- Submucosa: Contains muscularis mucosa, blood vessels, lymphatics, and nerves (Meissner nerve plexus)
- Muscularis: Inner circular, outer longitudinal, and the Myenteric plexus of Auerbach
- Serosa: Single layer of mesoepithelial cells lining the exterior of the small intestine

The submucosa is the strongest layer of the small bowel wall.

Cell Types in the Small Intestine

- Enterocytes
  - Arise from pluripotential cells in the crypts of Lieberkuhn
  - Migrate to the tips of the villi
  - Specialized for digestion and absorption
  - Glutamine is the key energy source for enterocytes
    - Decreased uptake of glutamine → decreased enterocyte integrity → bacterial translocation → sepsis
- Enteroendocrine cells
  - I cells—secrete CCK
    - Stimulates gallbladder contraction and pancreatic enzyme secretion
    - Stimulates sphincter of Oddi relaxation
  - S cells—secretin
    - Stimulates HCO_2, pancreatic enzyme, and intestinal secretion
    - Stimulated by duodenal acidification (pH <3)
  - D cells—somatostatin
    - Inhibits release of all GI hormones

- K cells—gastric inhibitory peptide
  - Stimulates insulin secretion
  - Inhibits gastric acid secretion
- Paneth cells
  - In the bases of the crypts of Lieberkuhn
  - Aid in phagocytosis and mucosal defense
- M cells
  - Ag presenting cells in Peyer patches
- Brunner glands
  - In the duodenum
  - Produce alkaline solution to protect against gastric acid

Portions of the Small Intestine

- Duodenum
  - Bulb (first portion)—90% of ulcers occur here
  - Descending (second portion)—contains ampulla of Vater
  - Transverse (third portion)
  - Ascending (fourth portion)
  - Descending and transverse portions are retroperitoneal
  - third and fourth portions are the transition point at the acute angle between the aorta (posterior) and the superior mesenteric artery (SMA) (anterior)
    - With a narrowing of this angle, can have SMA syndrome
- Jejunum
  - Starts at the ligament of Treitz and is about 100 cm long
  - Long vasa recta and circular muscle folds
  - Maximum site of all absorption except for
    - B12—terminal ileum
    - Folate—terminal ileum
    - Bile acids—terminal ileum
    - Iron—Duodenum
  - 95% of NaCl and 90% of water absorbed in jejunum
- Ileum
  - 150 cm long
  - Short vasa recta
- Blood supply to duodenum is celiac and SMA
- Blood supply to jejunum and ileum is SMA

Nutrient Absorption

- Water and electrolytes
  - Sodium transport creates an osmotic gradient that drives water absorption
  - Na, Cl, K, Ca, Mg, and Fe are absorbed in the small bowel
- Carbohydrate digestion
  - Begins in the mouth with salivary amylase

- Continues with pancreatic amylase and disaccharidases
- Intestinal brush border has maltase, sucrase, dextrinase, and lactase
- Carbohydrates are broken down into glucose, galactose, and fructose
- Glucose and galactose
    - Absorbed at brush border by secondary active transport via sodium co-transporter SGLUT1
- Fructose
    - Absorbed at brush border by facilitated diffusion by GLUT5
- All then enter the bloodstream via GLUT-2 facilitated diffusion at the basolateral surface of the enterocytes

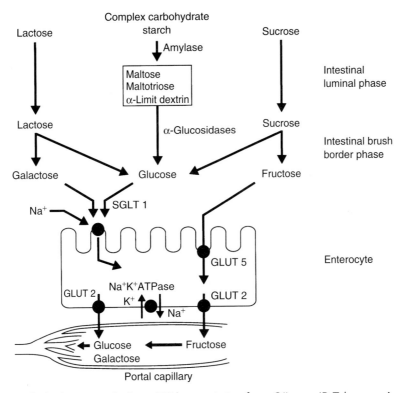

Carbohydrate metabolism. (With permission from O'Leary JP, Tabuenca A, eds. *Physiologic Basis of Surgery*. 4th ed. Philadelphia, PA: Wolters Kluwer Health/Lippincott Williams & Wilkins; 2007.)

- Protein digestion
    - Begins in stomach with pepsin
    - Continues in small intestine with trypsin, chymotrypsin, and carboxypeptidase where proteins are broken down into amino acids and di- and tripeptides
    - Amino acids are absorbed at the brush border by secondary active transport with Na
    - Di- and tripeptides are absorbed at the brush border by secondary active transport with H
    - They then enter the bloodstream via diffusion at the basolateral surface

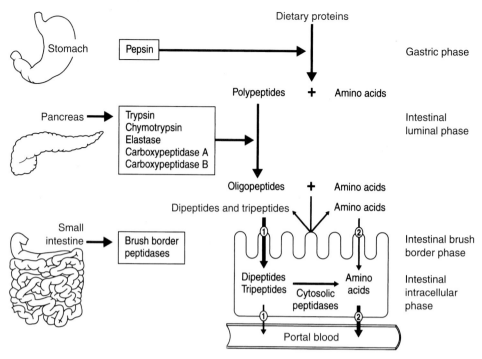

Protein metabolism. (With permission from O'Leary JP, Tabuenca A, eds. *Physiologic Basis of Surgery.* 4th ed. Philadelphia, PA: Wolters Kluwer Health/Lippincott Williams & Wilkins; 2007.)

- Lipid digestion
  - Triglycerides (TGs) are digested by lipases at the brush border to form monoglycerides and free fatty acids (FFAs)
  - Micelles are then formed with the monoglycerides, FFAs, bile salts, phospholipids, and cholesterol
    - Bile salts increase absorption area for fats, helping for micelles
    - Fat soluble vitamins A, D, E, and K are also absorbed in micelles
  - Micelles then enter the enterocyte by fusing with the membrane
  - In the enterocytes, TGs reform
  - TGs and cholesterol then form chylomicrons, which are transported to lymphatics (lacteals) via basolateral exocytosis
    - Chylomicrons are 90% TGs, 10% phospholipid, cholesterol, and protein
  - Long chain fatty acids are also released into lymphatics
  - Medium and short chain fatty acids are released into portal vein (as with amino acids and carbohydrates)
  - Lipoprotein lipase
    - On the liver endothelium
    - Clears chylomicrons and TAGs from blood and breaks them down into fatty acids and glycerol
    - Fatty acids and glycerol are then are taken up by hepatocytes
  - FFA-binding protein
    - On liver endothelium
    - Binds short and medium chain fatty acids

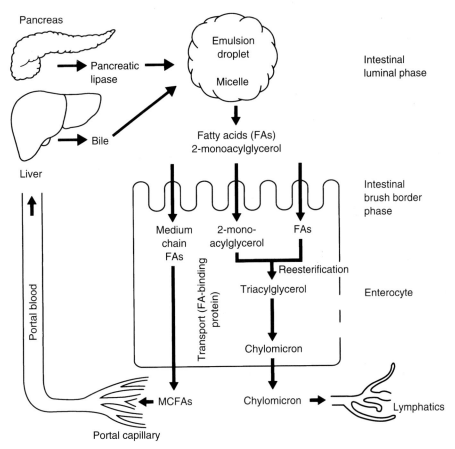

Lipid metabolism. (With permission from O'Leary JP, Tabuenca A, eds. *Physiologic Basis of Surgery*. 4th ed. Philadelphia, PA: Wolters Kluwer Health/Lippincott Williams & Wilkins; 2007.)

Small Bowel Motility

- MMC
  - Basic motility pattern resulting in the propagation of cellular debris, bacteria, and chyme
  - Starts in the stomach and progresses through the small intestine over approximately 2 hours
    - Phase I: Period of inactivity (60 to 75 minutes)
    - Phase II: Period of increasing irregular bowel contractions (up to 60 minutes)
    - Phase III: Period of maximal contractions, rapid spikes, and muscular contraction (5 to 10 minutes)
    - Phase IV: Slowing of activity
  - Motilin is the hormone that mediates the MMC
  - Erythromycin acts as a motilin analogue and induces the MMC in the fasted state in humans
  - Cyclic activity continues until interrupted by a meal
    - After a meal, the MMC is replaced by 3 to 4 hours of rapid spiking activity, similar to Phase II
    - Contractions occur throughout the intestine with a caudal spread

Small Bowel Immunity

- Largest immune organ in the body
- Gut-associated lymphoid tissue is composed of aggregated tissue (Peyer patches, lymph nodes, and lymphoid follicles) and free leukocytes
- B lymphocytes produce secretory IgA

The small bowel is the largest immune organ of the body, with a large role in antigen presentation. Secretory IgA is a key mediator of gut immune defenses.

A 50-year-old woman with a history of multiple previous pelvic operations presents to the emergency department with a 2-day history of abdominal pain, distention, nausea, vomiting, and reports no bowel movements for 36 hours. What is the first diagnostic test of choice?

An abdominal X-ray series (flat and upright) is the initial study for a suspected small bowel obstruction. A hernia is the most common cause of a small bowel obstruction in a patient without a history of previous abdominal operations.

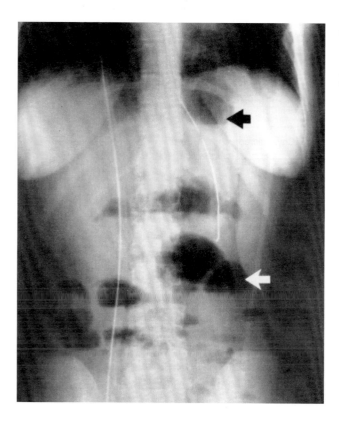

AXR showing an SBO. (With permission from Mulholland MW, Lillemoe KD, Doherty GM, Maier RV, Upchurch GR, eds. *Greenfield's Surgery.* 4th ed. Philadelphia, PA: Lippincott Williams & Wilkins; 2005.)

Small Bowel Obstruction

- Caused by adhesions (most common cause), hernias, and tumors
- Other causes include volvulus, intussusception, Crohn's disease, and radiation enteritis
- The most common cause in patients with a virgin abdomen is an incarcerated hernia
  - It is important to check the groin for both inguinal and femoral hernias
- History of recent bowel movements
  - Diarrhea can be a finding with obstruction
  - No bowel movements for >3 days indicates obstruction or constipation
- Typical findings on an abdominal X-ray with flat and upright (or decubitus) views include air fluid levels and dilated small bowel
  - The absence of gas in the colon or rectum can indicate a complete obstruction
- A CT scan is 90% sensitive and specific for diagnosing a small bowel obstruction and can isolate the obstruction site (transition point)

- Conservative management includes bowel rest and possible decompression using an NG tube
- Indications for surgery include signs of strangulation or perforation (progressive pain, peritoneal signs, fever, increasing white cell count) or a lack of improvement with conservative management

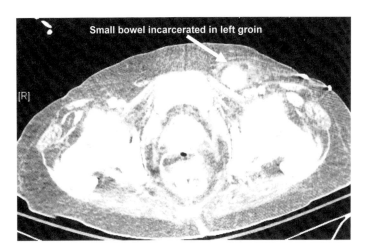

Incarcerated hernia. (With permission from Mulholland MW, Lillemoe KD, Doherty GM, Maier RV, Upchurch GR, eds. *Greenfield's Surgery*. 4th ed. Philadelphia, PA: Lippincott Williams & Wilkins; 2005.)

Bowel rest with an NG tube and IV fluids cures 80% of partial small bowel obstructions and 20% of complete small bowel obstructions.

A 67-year-old male who presented to the hospital with RUQ pain and jaundice and was found to have a common bile duct stone undergoes an endoscopic retrograde cholangiopancreatography (ERCP) and sphincterotomy. That evening, he develops worsening abdominal pain and peritonitis. A CT scan is performed and he is found to have retroperitoneal air. What is the next step in management?

Duodenal perforation occurs in 1% of ERCPs. If the patient is stable, they can be managed conservatively with NGT, IV antibiotics, serial abdominal exams, and bowel rest. If they become unstable or develop peritonitis, they should undergo an exploratory laparoscopy or laparotomy. In the majority of cases, the exact area of perforation is not visible at the time of exploration and wide drainage of the duodenum is usually sufficient to control the leak.

A 60-year-old man is recovering on postoperative day 6 following a low anterior colon resection. He develops nausea and emesis and has had no passage of flatus or stool since the operation. On CT scan, his bowel is diffusely dilated with no transition point. What possible factors may have contributed to his condition?

Postoperative ileus usually occurs in the first few hours after surgery and can persist for days to weeks. It is characterized by the lack of an abrupt transition point on imaging studies. It is caused by increased catecholamines, opiates, inhaled anesthetics, inflammation, surgical manipulation, electrolyte imbalance, and intra-abdominal infection. Patients with a history of prior surgery are more likely to develop a postoperative ileus because more bowel manipulation is often required. Laparoscopy is associated with lower rates of postoperative ileus.

Ileus

- Defined as a temporary inhibition of coordinated gastrointestinal motor function
- Common causes include major abdominal surgery, spinal surgery, spinal trauma, and opiates

- Treatment is with bowel rest and supportive therapy
- Postoperative ileus generally resolves 4 to 5 days following a laparotomy
- Laparoscopic surgery is associated with a shorter period of postoperative ileus
- Consider a mechanical obstruction in the differential diagnosis if the ileus does not resolve
- Parenteral nutrition may be indicated if the patient is NPO for >1 week

Return of function occurs in the small bowel first (usually within 1 to 2 days), followed by the stomach (usually within 2 to 3 days), then the colon (usually within 3 to 4 days).

A 79-year-old woman with symptoms of small bowel obstruction is found on an abdominal X-ray series (flat and upright) to have dilated small bowel loops, air in the biliary tree, and a large radiolucent round object in the right lower quadrant. What is the most likely diagnosis?

This patient has a gallstone ileus, which can occasionally be diagnosed on plain films and is caused by a fistula between the gallbladder and the bowel (typically the duodenum). Treatment is to surgically remove the impacted gallstone and, if the patient is stable, cholecystectomy and closure of the fistula.

Gallstone Ileus

- Bowel obstruction caused by a gallstone
- Classically occurs in elderly patients
- Caused by a fistula between the gallbladder and second portion of the duodenum
- Inflammation from cholecystitis causes erosion into the duodenum
    - Can erode into the transverse colon, stomach, or jejunum, but this is rare
- Bouveret syndrome refers to gastric outlet obstruction due to a gallstone impacted in the duodenal bulb
- Treatment is removal of the stone from the terminal ileum and a cholecystectomy with duodenal closure
    - A cholecystectomy and fistula closure in the setting of gallstone ileus with obstruction should only be undertaken if the patient is stable
    - The cholecystectomy can be delayed if the patient is not stable

Up to 40% of patients with gallstone ileus will have a second stone. Always search for a second stone when exploring these patients.

A 45-year-old woman with Crohn's disease and multiple bowel resections has intractable diarrhea, weight loss, and frequent admission to the hospital for dehydration and electrolyte abnormalities. What is the most likely diagnosis?

This patient most likely has short bowel (or short gut) syndrome, which typically occurs in adults with less than 150 cm of small bowel, or in those with greater than 150 cm of small bowel but with a disease causing malabsorption.

Short Bowel Syndrome

- Characterized by diarrhea, steatorrhea, weight loss, dehydration, malabsorption, and malnutrition
- The diagnosis is made based on symptoms, not length of bowel
- The Schilling test checks for enteral B12 absorption
- The Sudan red stain checks for fecal fat
- In children, short bowel syndrome occurs with <30% of the normal length for age of jejunum and ileum

- Treatment is TPN (Total or Complete Parenteral Nutrition) and enteral feeding
- Consider small bowel transplantation for patients with severe short bowel syndrome (50% 5-year graft success rate)
- TPN complications (liver failure, recurrent line sepsis, and venous thrombosis) are often the ultimate cause of death in these patients
- Preservation of the ileocecal valve and colon enhances nutrient support and can lead to increased absorptive surface area
- Loss of the ileocecal valve can lead to bacterial overgrowth which decreases the functional absorptive surface area

With bowel adaptation, many patients with short bowel syndrome can regain nutritional autonomy. For adults, the minimum length of small bowel needed to achieve nutritional autonomy is 100 to 150 cm without the ileocecal valve and as little as 50 to 70 cm of small bowel with the entire colon in continuity.

What are some of the complications associated with terminal ileum resection?

Diarrhea, steatorrhea, anemia, and renal stones may occur following resection of the terminal ileum.

Terminal Ileum Resection
- Common symptoms following resection include diarrhea, steatorrhea, anemia, and renal stones
- Diarrhea/steatorrhea is caused by decreased bile salt absorption
- Bile salts are not well tolerated in the colon
  - Treated with cholestyramine
- Macrocytic anemia is due to decreased B12/intrinsic factor absorption
- Oxalate renal stones can result from increased colonic oxalate absorption

A 26-year-old Jewish woman presents to her primary care physician with intermittent crampy abdominal pain, diarrhea, and episodic symptoms of partial small bowel obstruction. What is the next test to establish a diagnosis? How is the definitive diagnosis typically obtained?

This patient likely has Crohn's disease. A small bowel series is the next test to obtain, as it can delineate the pattern and distribution of affected bowel in Crohn's disease. Ultimately, the definitive diagnosis is made using tissue samples, often obtained via endoscopy. These can demonstrate transmural inflammation with granulomas, segmental disease ("skip lesions"), and "cobblestoning."

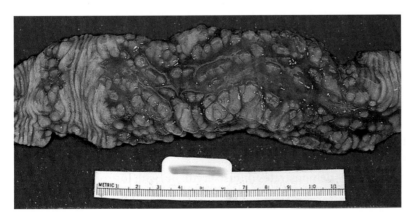

Ulceration in Crohn's disease. (With permission from Mulholland MW, Lillemoe KD, Doherty GM, Maier RV, Upchurch GR, eds. *Greenfield's Surgery.* 4th ed. Philadelphia, PA: Lippincott Williams & Wilkins; 2005.)

Crohn's Disease

- Presentation
  - Symptoms of intermittent abdominal pain, diarrhea, and weight loss
  - Bimodal distribution with the first presentation occurring between 15 to 35 years of age and a smaller number presenting in the 6th decade
  - More common in urban areas
  - Increased in Ashkenazi Jews
  - Rare in Asia and South America
  - Smokers have double the risk of nonsmokers
  - Increased risk in first degree relatives
- The diagnosis is made using endoscopic tissue samples, along with barium studies or CT scan
- Pathology shows transmural inflammation with granulomas, segmental disease ("skip lesions"), cobblestoning, creeping fat, and fistulas
- Can involve any portion of the gastrointestinal tract from mouth to anus
  - The terminal ileum is most commonly involved initially—can have signs of B12 deficiency
  - Perianal disease is characteristic of the first presentation in 10% of patients
- The initial treatment is medical: Aminosalicylates, corticosteroids, immunosuppressive drugs (azathioprine, methotrexate), antibiotics, and biologics (Remicade = infliximab, Humira = adalimumab, Cimzia = certolizamab)
  - Infliximab, adalimumab, certolizamab: Anti-TNF-α agents improve closure of refractory fistulas and can improve the natural history of Crohn's disease including maintaining remission
    - Toxicity increases with increased number of infusions with Infliximab
    - Important to check a PPD prior to starting any Anti-TNF-α agent since these can reactive *M tuberculosis*
    - Increased risk of lymphoma and other malignancies with Anti-TNF-α agents
  - Steroids can bring about remission but do not maintain remission
  - Azathioprine and the biologics are the most helpful drug for maintaining remission
    - Metabolized to 6-MP, which blocks lymphocyte proliferation and function
    - Effects are first seen 3 to 4 months after starting treatment (should be started immediately during flare)
    - The relapse rate with azathioprine is 30% (without is 75%)
- Surgery is eventually required in the majority of patients with Crohn's disease
  - The most common surgical indications are failure of medical management, obstruction, inflammatory mass or abscess, fistula, toxic megacolon, or perianal disease
  - Small bowel stricturoplasty should be performed whenever possible to maintain bowel length
  - Limited small bowel resection is reserved for perforation or lesions not amenable to stricturoplasty
  - Margins should only be grossly free of disease, not wide (to preserve bowel length when possible)
    - Loss of bowel length may lead to short bowel syndrome
  - Laparoscopy reduces adhesions which can increase the risk of future operations and thus should be performed whenever possible
- Long-standing Crohn's disease is associated with the same risk of cancer as ulcerative colitis
  - In contrast to Crohn's disease, ulcerative colitis first affects the rectum and distal colon in a continuous fashion with anal sparing
  - The pathology with ulcerative colitis demonstrates diffuse erythema with loss of goblet cells and basal plasmacytosis

- Distinguishing early ulcerative colitis from Crohn's disease can be difficult as ulcerative colitis can affect the ileum (backwash ileitis) with some spared areas

A 24-year-old male presents with a 12-hour history of right lower quadrant pain, fever to 101.5°F, leukocytosis, and two loose stools. The patient is taken to the operating room for presumed appendicitis. Intraoperatively, the appendix appears normal. The terminal ileum appears inflamed. What is the next step in management?

When acute ileitis is discovered intraoperatively with a normal appendix, an appendectomy should still be performed. An appendectomy helps to avoid difficulty or confusion with the future evaluation of right lower quadrant pain.

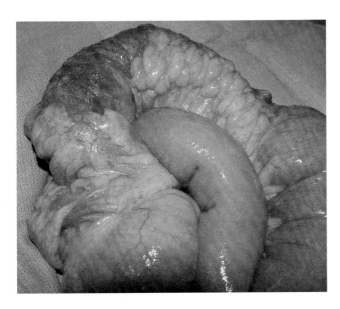

Crohn's ileitis. (With permission from Mulholland MW, Lillemoe KD, Doherty GM, Maier RV, Upchurch GR, eds. *Greenfield's Surgery.* 4th ed. Philadelphia, PA: Lippincott Williams & Wilkins; 2005.)

Acute Ileitis
- Most often caused by acute bacterial infections with *Campylobacter* or *Yersinia*
- Also found with Crohn's disease
- In the case of acute ileitis discovered intraoperatively, an appendectomy should be performed

A 55-year-old female with no previous operations presents with abdominal pain and weight loss from obstructive symptoms. A small bowel series with follow-through demonstrates an ulcerated lesion in the proximal ileum. What is the most likely type of tumor?

Most small bowel tumors are metastatic, with melanoma being the most common malignancy to metastasize to the small bowel. Among primary tumors, most are likely to be malignant. Malignant tumors of the small bowel include adenocarcinoma (30% to 50%), carcinoid, lymphoma, and gastrointestinal stromal tumor (GIST). Common presentations include obstruction, pain, bleeding, or perforation.

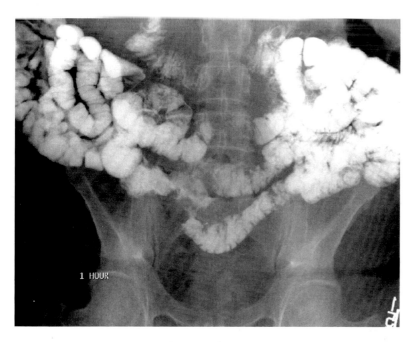

Partial SBO secondary to metastatic melanoma. (With permission from Mulholland MW, Lillemoe KD, Doherty GM, Maier RV, Upchurch GR, eds. *Greenfield's Surgery*. 4th ed. Philadelphia, PA: Lippincott Williams & Wilkins; 2005.)

A 62-year-old male presents with intermittent symptoms consistent with partial small bowel obstruction despite having no previous history of abdominal surgery. A CT scan demonstrates a small bowel mass with a partial obstruction. At laparotomy, a 6-cm lesion involving the small bowel wall is discovered. A frozen section performed by the pathologist on call reveals spindle cells. Where does this tumor commonly recur?

Spindle cells are characteristic of GISTs. GIST tumors are common in the stomach or small bowel and spread by hematogenous means (i.e., lymph nodes are rarely involved). The most common recurrence is in the liver, although occasionally it can present with diffuse intra-abdominal spread. Overall, GIST tumors have a good prognosis. Features associated with malignant behavior include larger tumors and high mitotic activity (>5 mitoses per high power field).

Small Bowel Tumors

- Most malignant lesions of the small bowel are metastatic neoplasms
- Melanoma is the most common tumor to metastasize to small bowel
- Primary small bowel tumors represent only 5% of GI tumors (1% to 2% of all neoplasms)
- The most common benign tumors are adenoma (25% to 35%), lipoma, hamartoma, and hemangioma
- The most common malignant tumors are adenocarcinoma (30% to 50%), carcinoid (20% to 30%), lymphoma (15%), and GISTs
- Small bowel tumors present with obstruction, pain, bleeding, or perforation
- Resect all tumors, even if they are asymptomatic

Malignant Small Bowel Tumors

- Adenocarcinoma (50%)
  - Increased risk with Crohn's disease, FAP, HNPCC, Gardner's syndrome, and von Recklinghausen disease
  - The duodenum is the most common location

- Only 50% of patients have resectable lesions
- Resect with at least 5 cm margins
- 5-year survival is poor (10% to 15%)
- Carcinoid (25%)
  - Most are asymptomatic and discovered incidentally
  - Can present with obstructive symptoms from intermittent intussusception
  - "Carcinoid syndrome"
    - Not seen without metastases as the liver usually clears the 5-HT
    - Develops in approximately 10% of patients with carcinoid tumor with liver metastases
    - Signs and symptoms include flushing, sweating, diarrhea, wheezing, abdominal pain, dermatosis, and fibrosis of the cardiac tricuspid or pulmonary valve
      - GI symptoms are from vasoconstriction and fibrosis (desmoplastic reaction)
  - Carcinoids can metabolize the majority of the body's tryptophan for making serotonin, which depletes niacin
    - This can lead to niacin deficiency/pellagra
    - Symptoms include the 3Ds: Dermatitis, dementia, diarrhea
  - Common locations for gastrointestinal carcinoids include the appendix (85%), ileum, rectum, and stomach
  - Use chromagranin A for diagnosis
  - Small bowel carcinoid (ileal most common)
    - Most are found within 2 feet of the ileocecal valve
    - Inspect the entire small bowel since approximately 30% of small bowel carcinoids have another synchronous lesion
    - Small bowel carcinoid has a poorer prognosis than appendiceal carcinoid
    - Arise from Kulchitsky cells in the small intestinal crypts of Lieberkuhn
    - Stain Argyrophil-positive on histology
    - The gold-standard test is electron microscopy for neurosecretory granules
    - Make and release serotonin (5-HIAA is metabolite of serotonin)
    - Elevated urinary 5-HIAA is seen *only if* the tumor drains directly into the systemic circulation (extensive liver metastases, non-gastrointestinal carcinoid)
    - Scintigraphy with ^{111}In-pentetreotide can assess the extent and locality of the lesions
    - 5-year survival: Localized disease (65%), metastatic disease (35%)
- Lymphoma (20%)
  - Most commonly non-Hodgkin B-cell lymphoma in adults and Burkitt lymphoma in children
  - Risk factors include malabsorptive and inflammatory conditions and immunosuppression (e.g., celiac sprue, Wegener's disease, SLE, AIDS, Crohn's disease)
  - Typically have no associated systemic symptoms (unlike most lymphomas)
  - Mediterranean variant in young males
  - Treated with chemotherapy
- GIST (2%)
  - Less common than stomach GISTs (65%)
  - Arise from interstitial cells of Cajal
    - Mesodermal origin
    - Function as pacemaker cells for the GI tract
    - Characteristics of both smooth muscle and neural cells
    - Express c-Kit protein (CD117)

- Located in bowel submucosa
- Can be associated with neurofibromatosis type I (rare)
- Can develop central necrosis and bleeding
- Treat with segmental resection achieving grossly negative margins (wide margins not necessary)
- Up to 30% will demonstrate malignant behavior and recurrence is common
- Pathologic features associated with malignant behavior include high mitotic activity (>5 mitoses per 50 high-powered fields) and large tumor size (>5 cm)
- Mesenteric margins are important because tumors spread hematogenously, not via the lymphatics
- The most common site of metastasis is the liver
- Tumors in difficult-to-resect locations and multiple tumors are treated with the c-Kit kinase competitive inhibitor, imatinib mesylate (a.k.a., STI571 or Gleevec)

A wide margin of resection and associated lymph node resection is not important for GISTs since they spread via the bloodstream.

Benign Small Bowel Tumors
- May present as a lead point of an intussusception ("target lesion" on CT)
  - Unlike pediatric intussusceptions, all adult cases must be managed operatively
- Small bowel hemangiomas can involve the entire GI tract (Osler-Weber-Rendu disease)
- Peutz-Jeghers syndrome present with hamartomas mainly in the jejunum and ileum
  - Hamartomas may undergo malignant transformation
  - Patients also have melanotic pigmentation of the face, palms and soles, and buccal mucosa
  - Increased risk of cancer of breast, ovaries, and pancreas
  - Need surveillance with an EGD and colonoscopy every other year

Benign small bowel tumors may present as a lead point of an intussusception, which may be diagnosed as a "target lesion" on CT scan.

Which duodenal adenomas require surgical resection versus local endoscopic resection?

All tubulovillous and villous adenomas of the duodenum require definitive surgical resection due to their high degree of malignant potential. The type of resection is dependent upon the location and size of the lesion. Both Brunner gland adenomas and simple pedunculated adenomas can be managed with endoscopic/local resection alone due to their low malignant potential.

Duodenal Adenomas
- Duodenal tubulovillous and villous adenomas
  - Frequently located at the major papilla (ampulla of Vater)
  - Associated with inherited colonic polyposis syndromes (e.g., FAP, Gardner's, von Recklinghausen's)
  - High malignant potential
  - The best treatment is surgical resection
  - If the tumor is near the papilla or large in size, treat with a pancreaticoduodenectomy
- Brunner's gland adenoma
  - Arise from Brunner glands located throughout duodenal submucosa
  - Negligible malignant potential

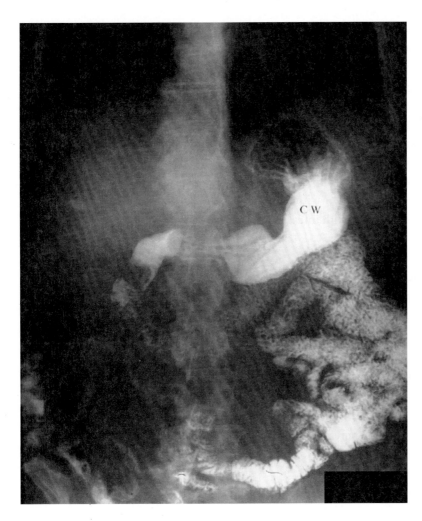

Duodenal adenoma. (With permission from Mulholland MW, Lillemoe KD, Doherty GM, Maier RV, Upchurch GR, eds. *Greenfield's Surgery*. 4th ed. Philadelphia, PA: Lippincott Williams & Wilkins; 2005.)

- Always managed with a local resection (surgical or endoscopic)
- Simple tubular pedunculated adenoma
  - Minimal malignant potential
  - Managed endoscopically unless complicated by obstruction or bleeding

Tubulovillous and villous adenomas of the duodenum that are either large or located in the second portion of the duodenumare typically treated surgically with a transduodenal resection or pancreaticoduodenectomy.

A 60-year-old female with two previous admissions for pancreatitis was admitted with nonspecific abdominal pain. The patient has no history of alcohol abuse or gallstones. An ERCP demonstrates a small duodenal diverticulum 1 cm away from the ampulla. How should this lesion be managed?

Conservative management is recommended for most duodenal diverticula.

Diverticula of the Small Bowel

- Caused by propulsion forces
- Few are symptomatic (10%)

- Most common locations: Duodenum > Jejunum > Ileum
- Indications for surgery include severe pain, perforation, obstruction, infection, and hemorrhage
- Duodenal diverticulum
  - Often on the mesenteric border of the second portion of the duodenum
  - Congenital diverticula (wind-sock diverticula) are associated with duodenal atresia or other intestinal malformations
  - Large diverticula which involve the papilla can cause sphincter dysfunction, cholangitis, pancreatitis, obstruction, hemorrhage, or perforation
  - Most cases are successfully managed without an operation
  - Occasionally, duodenal excision with or without a choledochojejunostomy is required
- Jejunoileal diverticulum are associated with intestinal dyskinesia
- Meckel diverticulum
  - Rule of 2s
    - Found in 2% of the population
    - Usually presents in the second year of life
    - Two times more common in males
    - Symptomatic in 2% of patients
    - Located 2 feet from the ileocecal valve
    - Approximately 2 inches in length
  - Congenital failure to obliterate the Vitelline duct (also called omphalomesenteric duct) in utero
  - If there is heterotopic mucosa, pancreatic tissue is the most common type, but it is usually asymptomatic
  - Can cause gastrointestinal bleeding
  - Diagnosis can be made with a Meckel scan (^{99}Tc)
  - The most common presentation in adults is volvulus with concomitant obstruction in those with a persistent fibrous band from the tip of the Meckel diverticulum to the umbilicus
  - If found incidentally, resection is indicated for any of the following criteria:
    - Patient <40 years of age
    - Meckel diverticulum longer than 2 cm
    - Presence of a fibrous band
    - Evidence of heterotopic mucosa

While pancreatic tissue is the most common tissue found in a Meckel diverticulum, gastric tissue is the most common type of tissue found in patients with symptomatic Meckel, as these lesions will present with gastrointestinal bleeding.

A 52-year-old woman with a history of rheumatoid arthritis and chronic back pain presents to the emergency department with intense abdominal pain diffusely. An upright abdominal X-ray reveals free air under the right hemi-diaphragm. She has a fever and a white blood cell count of 46,000. What is the next step in management?

This patient should be adequately resuscitated and taken to the operating room urgently for surgical exploration for a presumed perforated duodenal ulcer. A patient with a history of a chronic pain condition such as arthritis or back pain should increase the surgeon's level of suspicion for an ulcer since these conditions are often associated with long-term NSAID use.

Perforated Duodenal Ulcer

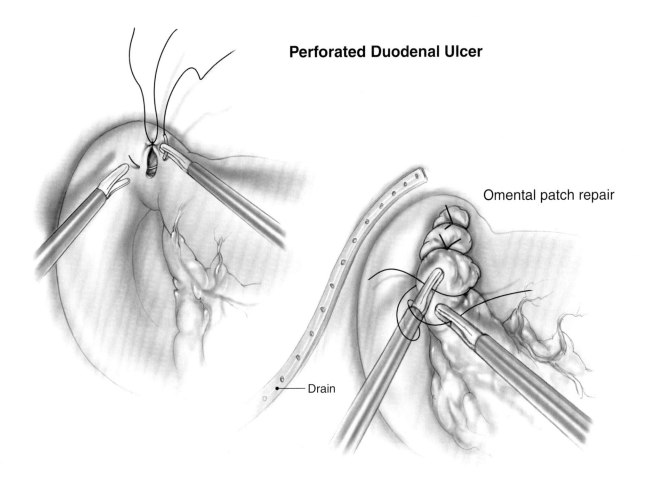

Omental patch repair

Drain

Duodenal Ulcer

- 95% are in the first part of the duodenum
- Most are associated with *Helicobactor pylori*
- Long-term NSAID use is a major risk factor
- Anterior ulcers perforate
- Posterior ulcers bleed (i.e., they erode into vessels, namely the gastroduodenal artery)
- Anterior ulcers warrant surgical exploration
  - Exceptions include patients with minimal symptoms and no systemic findings
  - Beware of the patient on steroids or with immunosuppression: Symptoms may be masked in these patients and physical exam is not always reliable. A water-soluble contrast study may be helpful to decide if surgical exploration is necessary.
- Posterior (bleeding) ulcers can be approached by
  - Endoscopic injection and/or cauterization (risk of re-bleeding)
  - Angiographic embolization (ideal when possible)
  - Surgically opening the duodenum (longitudinal duodenotomy) and oversewing the bleeding ulcer

Bleeding Duodenal Ulcer

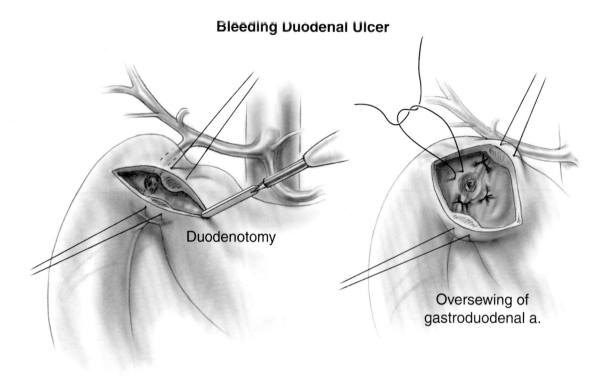

Duodenotomy

Oversewing of
gastroduodenal a.

An 82-year-old woman with new-onset atrial fibrillation presents to the emergency room with sudden, severe abdominal pain, fever, and blood in her stool. What is the most likely diagnosis?

Acute mesenteric ischemia. Most emboli lodge at the SMA origin or in the first branch of the SMA (middle colic). The gold standard for diagnosis is contrast visceral angiography, but CT angiography and magnetic resonance angiography can be equally effective in establishing the diagnosis.

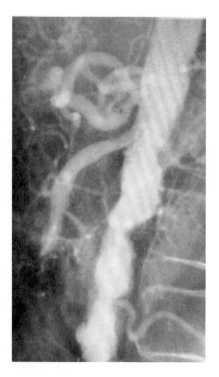

SMA embolus. (With permission from Mulholland MW, Lillemoe KD, Doherty GM, Maier RV, Upchurch GR, eds. *Greenfield's Surgery*. 4th ed. Philadelphia, PA: Lippincott Williams & Wilkins; 2005.)

> Intraoperatively, there is some question about bowel viability for several intestinal segments. What are some methods that can be used to assess bowel viability?

Acceptable techniques that can be used alone or in combination to assess bowel viability include manual palpation/Doppler examination of the arterial pulse in the mesentery, visualization of intravenous fluorescein with a Wood's lamp, and a second look laparotomy.

Mesenteric Ischemia

- The classic presentation is pain out of proportion to the physical examination
- Embolic ischemia is seen in the setting of a recent myocardial infarction, atrial fibrillation, or vascular mural thrombus
    - Most emboli lodge in the SMA at its origin or its first branch (middle colic artery)
    - Treatment is emergent surgical exploration with the goal of restoring blood flow (embolectomy or bypass) and resection of any nonviable bowel
- Thrombotic ischemia is seen in the setting of diffuse atherosclerotic disease or a hypercoagulable state
    - Treatment is surgical thrombectomy and resection of any nonviable bowel
- Non-occlusive ischemia is seen in the setting of low blood flow states (i.e., critically ill patients on vasopressors)
    - Acute ischemia requires surgical exploration with the resection of nonviable bowel
- Chronic mesenteric ischemia
    - Most often caused by atherosclerosis
    - Symptoms include abdominal pain with eating, which results in weight loss, malnutrition, and "food fear"
    - Chronic intestinal angina (pain with eating) may be managed non-operatively or with an elective arterial bypass

> A 55-year-old woman with rectal cancer is treated with radiation therapy and develops mild nausea following each treatment. What is the most likely diagnosis?

Radiation enteritis can cause nausea, and in rare cases, stricture or perforation.

Radiation Enteritis

- Acute enteritis
    - The degree of acute enteritis is a function of the rate and duration of the radiation dose
    - Can be subclinical or present with nausea, abdominal pain, and anorexia
    - The process is generally self-limited (resolves within 2 to 6 weeks after treatment)
- Chronic enteritis
    - The degree of enteritis is a function of the total dose of radiation (>4000 CGY)
    - Results from obliterative vasculitis with ischemia and full-thickness bowel wall fibrosis
    - Typical onset is 2 to 3 years after radiation exposure
    - The symptoms are related to abnormal intestinal transit
    - Can present with intermittent diarrhea, constipation, abdominal pain, perforation, bowel obstruction, or intestinal fistula

The typical onset of chronic enteritis symptoms from radiation therapy is between 2 and 3 years after exposure.

A 60 year old woman with a remote history of pelvic radiation for cervical cancer undergoes emergent laparotomy for a perforated cecal carcinoma. One week after surgery, she develops feculent drainage from her midline wound. What are some of the possible risk factors for this complication?

The patient has an enterocutaneous fistula. Risk factors include inflammatory bowel disease, cancer, steroid use, a history of radiation therapy, contaminated surgery, and preoperative malnutrition.

Enterocutaneous Fistula

- Most common fistulas are iatrogenic
- The more proximal the fistula is in the bowel, the higher the output
- Rule out distal bowel obstruction initially
- Most heal with conservative measures (bowel rest $\pm$ TPN)
- Surgery is indicated if the fistula fails to close after several weeks/months or if the patient develops sepsis from the source
- Resect the affected bowel segment and fistula tract

Fistula healing is impaired by FRIENDS (foreign body, radiation, inflammatory bowel disease/infection, epithelialization, neoplasm, distal obstruction, steroids/sepsis).

A 35-year-old woman with AIDS presents with acute right lower quadrant pain, a normal white cell count, normal hematocrit, and normal electrolytes. What are some of the major opportunistic disease entities which must be considered in the differential?

Patients who are immunocompromised due to AIDS, chemotherapy, or medications for organ transplant are at increased risk for opportunistic infectious diseases, including CMV enteritis, mycobacterial diseases, Shigella, and Salmonella.

Bowel Disease in Immunocompromised Patients

- Immunocompromised patients infected with opportunistic pathogens can present with an acute abdomen
- CMV enteritis
    - Most frequently affects the distal ileum and right colon
    - Endoscopy shows hemorrhagic ulcerated lesions
    - Nuclear inclusions ("owl's eyes") are seen on cytology
    - Treat with gancyclovir or foscarnet (viridostatic drugs)
- Gastrointestinal mycobacterial disease
    - *Mycobacterium avium* complex (MAC) and *Mycobacterium tuberculosis*
    - Affects the ileum and cecum
    - Can cause fistulas, obstructions, and free perforation
    - Diagnosed by demonstrating the organism in the tissue
    - Treat *M. tuberculosis* with a multi-drug regimen
    - Treat MAC with amikacin, clarithromycin, or ciprofloxacin
- *Shigella, Salmonella, Campylobacter jejuni*
    - Presents with blood-tinged diarrhea, weight loss, fever, and crampy abdominal pain
    - Stool cultures are diagnostic
    - Can be associated with bacteremia

CMV enteritis most frequently affects the distal ileum and right colon and is diagnosed definitively by observing "owl's eye" nuclear inclusions on tissue microscopy.

21 | Appendix

Heather G. Lyu and Jeffrey M. Hardacre

In which position does the appendix most likely reside in a patient with appendicitis that presents as right flank pain?

An inflamed retrocecal appendix will often present with right flank pain.

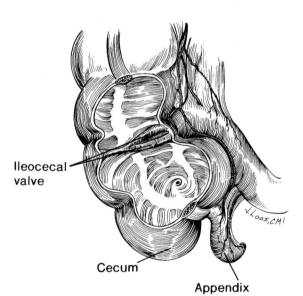

Appendix at the confluence of the three teniae. (With permission from Fischer JE, Bland KI, Callery MP, et al., eds. *Mastery of Surgery*. 5th ed. Philadelphia, PA: Lippincott Williams & Wilkins; 2006.)

Ileocecal valve

Cecum

Appendix

The Appendix

- Arises at the confluence of the three teniae
- Following the anterior tenia is a useful technique to find the appendix in a difficult operation
- Symptoms of appendicitis are related to the position of the appendix (anterior, retrocecal, pelvic, retroileal)
- The blood supply is from the appendicular artery, a branch of the ileocolic artery (from the superior mesenteric artery)
- Innervated by the autonomic nervous system
  - The early pain of appendicitis is visceral or vague periumbilical pain
  - The focused RLQ pain occurs only after the appendiceal inflammation irritates the parietal peritoneum and activates the somatic pain fibers

- Luminal obstruction is the inciting event and is most commonly due to lymphoid hyperplasia or a fecalith
- Tumors can also cause luminal obstruction (incidence of tumors is 0.1% to 1.0%)
- Obstruction leads to bacterial overgrowth and compromise of lymphatic, venous, and arterial flow, which result in ischemia, necrosis, and perforation

The most common location for a perforation is the antimesenteric border of the middle third of the appendix because it has the poorest blood supply.

A 24-year-old woman presents with a one-day history of new periumbilical pain that radiates to the right lower quadrant. A diagnosis of appendicitis is confirmed by ultrasound (US). What is the likelihood that she will also have leukocytosis?

Approximately 90% of patients with acute appendicitis have a WBC greater than 10,000.

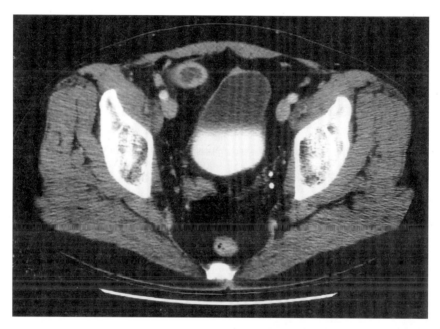

Acute appendicitis seen on computed tomography (CT) scan. (With permission from Mulholland MW, Lillemoe KD, Doherty GM, Maier RV, Upchurch GR, eds. *Greenfield's Surgery.* 4th ed. Philadelphia, PA: Lippincott Williams & Wilkins; 2005.)

Acute Appendicitis
- The "classic" presentation is periumbilical pain radiating to the right lower quadrant accompanied by:
  - Anorexia (usually first)
  - Abdominal pain (usually precedes nausea)
  - Low-grade fever and nausea are present in only 50% of patients
- Symptom duration of greater than 24 to 36 hours is uncommon in non-perforated appendicitis
- Menstrual and sexual histories as well as pelvic and rectal exams are imperative
- The most common finding on physical exam is focal abdominal tenderness with signs of peritoneal irritation
- Common signs of appendicitis include:
  - Dunphy: Increased pain with coughing
  - Rovsing: Left lower quadrant palpation induces right lower quadrant pain

- Obturator: Pain on internal rotation of the right hip
- Iliopsoas: Pain on extension of the right hip
- Urinalysis often reveals minimal white cells, red cells, and bacteria
- β-HCG must be checked in female patients to rule out an ectopic pregnancy

A WBC greater than 20,000 suggests a perforation, which is also true for the workup of many other gastrointestinal diseases.

A 32-year-old woman with suspected acute appendicitis has an abdominal CT. What findings on CT are consistent with a diagnosis of appendicitis?

CT findings consistent with appendicitis are appendiceal diameter of >6 mm, right lower quadrant fat stranding, lack of filling of the appendix with contrast, and a fecalith (non-specific).

Ultrasonography and Computed Tomography in the Evaluation of Acute Appendicitis
- A clinical diagnosis of acute appendicitis can obviate the need for any imaging workup, particularly in a male patient
- US is useful but operator-dependent
  - Sonographic criteria for appendicitis include a non-compressible tubular structure, diameter >6 mm, and presence of a fecalith or complex mass
  - US (transabdominal and transvaginal) is particularly useful in women of menstrual age to evaluate other pathologic conditions
  - Non-visualization of the appendix does not rule out appendicitis
- CT is less operator-dependent
  - Oral and/or rectal contrast can improve the yield
  - Criteria for appendicitis include a thickened appendix >6 mm in diameter, wall thickness >1.5 mm, periappendiceal inflammation, and the presence of a phlegmon, fecalith, or abscess
  - A CT scan can also suggest conditions other than appendicitis

---

A 79-year-old man presents with a recent history of right lower quadrant pain over McBurney's point, which is now generalized. He is noted to have temperature of 101.8°F and mild tachycardia. His CBC reveals a WBC of 28,000, a hematocrit of 22%, and a platelet count of 285,000. What is the most likely diagnosis?

Perforated cecal cancer can present with anemia and signs and symptoms of appendicitis.

Colon Perforation
- Signs and symptoms of appendicitis with concomitant anemia suggest colon cancer
- A history of diverticular symptoms suggests perforated diverticulitis
- Resection of the involved segment of colon is the standard management
- An ostomy may need to be created

Perforated cecal cancer should be suspected in any elderly patient with anemia and signs of appendicitis.

A 24 year old man is diagnosed in the emergency department to have acute appendicitis. What is the next step in management?

Preoperative preparation of the patient is essential. A patient with acute appendicitis should be taken to the operating room urgently, not emergently.

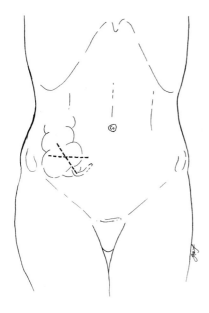

McBurney (horizontal) and Rocky-Davis (diagonal) incisions for an open appendectomy. (With permission from Fischer JE, Bland KI, Callery MP, et al., eds. *Mastery of Surgery*. 5th ed. Philadelphia: Lippincott Williams & Wilkins; 2006.)

Appendectomy

- Preoperative preparation includes fluid resuscitation based on a calculated fluid deficit
- Intravenous antibiotics that cover gram negatives should be administered
- An examination under anesthesia to search for a mass or other pathology may help determine the incision site
- Without a clear diagnosis or indication for operation, observation and serial examinations may be pursued
- An acceptable rate of finding a normal appendix is 10% to 15%
- An open appendectomy is performed via a McBurney or transverse Rockey-Davis incision with a muscle-splitting technique
- A laparoscopic appendectomy is usually performed with three ports, an ultrasonic scalpel, and a stapler

If the base of the appendix is involved or gangrenous, a limited cecectomy can be performed to utilize healthy tissue at the margin of resection.

A 23-year-old woman reports having right lower quadrant pain and relapsing fevers over the past week. She states that she had a similar episode of pain 3 weeks prior. A CT scan reveals a periappendiceal abscess. What is the next step in management?

Percutaneous drainage is often effective in treating periappendiceal abscesses.

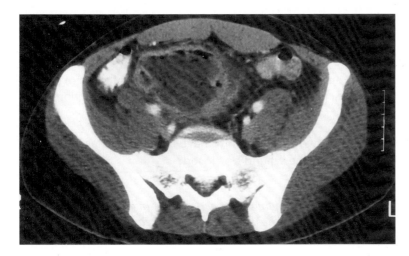

Periappendiceal abscess on CT scan. (With permission from Mulholland MW, Lillemoe KD, Doherty GM, Maier RV, Upchurch GR, eds. *Greenfield's Surgery*. 4th ed. Philadelphia, PA: Lippincott Williams & Wilkins; 2005.)

Phlegmon of the Appendix

- Generalized inflammation which obscures radiographic delineation of the appendix and cecum
- For minimal symptoms and no evidence of peritonitis, a phlegmon can be treated with intravenous antibiotics alone
- If the patient does not improve in 24 to 48 hours, then surgical exploration is indicated
- If a non-operative approach is successful and an interval appendectomy is not planned, a perforated neoplasm must be ruled out with a colonoscopy

Periappendiceal Abscess

- Often presents later in the course of disease (around 5 days)
- An abscess can often be treated with percutaneous drainage and intravenous antibiotics
- An interval appendectomy should be done in 6 weeks to 3 months
- An appropriate preoperative workup should be performed in the "interim," including a possible colonoscopy

A large and redundant sigmoid colon with pathology can cause right lower quadrant pain.

During an exploration for acute appendicitis, a normal appendix is found as well as terminal ileitis involving the cecum at the base of the appendix. What is the next step?

Close. An appendectomy should not be performed.

Exploration for Appendicitis

- If a normal appendix is found at operation, check for:
  - Acute cholecystitis
  - Drainage in the paracolic gutter suggestive of a perforated ulcer
  - Inflammatory bowel disease
  - Diverticular disease
  - Tumor
  - Meckel diverticulitis (usually within 2 feet proximal to the cecum)
  - Obstetric/gynecologic pathology
    - Ectopic pregnancy
    - Pelvic inflammatory disease

- Ruptured or torsed ovarian cyst
- Thrombosed ovarian vein
- Endometriosis
- If inflammatory bowel disease is found, an ileocecal resection is not indicated unless there is a clear indication for a bowel resection (i.e., perforation, stricture, fistula, or clear obstruction)

A 5-year-old boy is found at the time of operative exploration to have a perforated appendix. Following removal of the appendix, how should the wound be closed?

In children, the wound can be closed primarily, in spite of the finding of perforation. In adults, delayed primary closure or healing by secondary intention is usually the method of choice in cases involving perforation.

Wound Management

- Close the wound in all cases of appendicitis in children and uncomplicated appendicitis in adults
- Delayed primary closure or healing by secondary intention is appropriate for perforated appendicitis in adults
- The duration of post-operative antibiotics depends on the severity of infection but most would treat uncomplicated appendicitis for 1 day and perforated appendicitis with diffuse peritonitis for 3 to 7 days
- A post-operative intra-abdominal abscess can usually be treated by percutaneous drainage
- Complication rates vary from 5% (for uncomplicated appendicitis) to 30% (for perforated appendicitis)
- Complications of appendicitis
  - Liver abscess
  - Local abdominal or retroperitoneal abscess
  - Sepsis
  - Fistula

What are benefits of a laparoscopic appendectomy?

Earlier return to work is the main benefit in larger outcome studies. However, a laparoscopic approach can provide more diagnostic information if the appendix turns out to be normal at the time of operation.

Laparoscopic Appendectomy

- Decreased pain
- Decreased length of stay
- Increased cost
- Faster return to work/functional status

A 46-year-old man with HIV presents with right lower quadrant pain and no other symptoms. What is the next step in management?

A CT scan of the abdomen and pelvis is indicated because of the broad differential diagnosis in immunocompromised patients.

Appendicitis in the Immunocompromised Patient

- The presentation is often atypical
  - In transplant patients, concomitant steroids or other medications commonly obscure the physical exam
  - The WBC count is often confounded by HIV disease or immunosuppression
- The differential diagnosis should be expanded to include opportunistic infections, especially CMV
- Early intervention is warranted

> During an exploration for appendicitis, the appendix is identified and inspected. There are no signs of inflammation or infection, but a firm 1.5 cm mass is found at the base of the appendix. What is the next step in management?

Carcinoid tumor is the most common tumor of the appendix. A right hemicolectomy is indicated because it involves the base of the appendix.

Carcinoid of the Appendix

- Firm, yellow nodule with surrounding desmoplastic reaction
- Carcinoid is most commonly found in the small bowel > rectum > appendix
- Of those found in the appendix, 75% are located at the tip of the appendix
- Up to 15% of patients have synchronous tumors
- Size is correlated with prognosis
- Carcinoid of the appendix rarely produces serotonin
- The extent of the resection depends on tumor size, which is a surrogate for metastatic potential
- A right hemicolectomy is indicated for any one of three criteria:
  - Size >2 cm
  - Involvement of the base of the appendix
  - Palpable regional lymph nodes
- If criteria for a right hemicolectomy are not met, a simple appendectomy should be performed
- Symptoms of the carcinoid syndrome (occur only with metastasis to the liver in those tumors that produce serotonin)
  - Flushing
  - Right heart valvular disease
  - Wheezing
  - Diarrhea
- Treat diarrhea and flushing with octreotide (blocks serotonin)

> A 45-year-old man presents with a left-sided renal stone, which has passed. During his workup, a CT scan revealed a 4 cm mucocele-appearing cyst of the appendix. Upon further history taking, it appears that the mass is asymptomatic. What is the next step?

A mucocele of the appendix has a small risk of malignant transformation and thus should be removed.

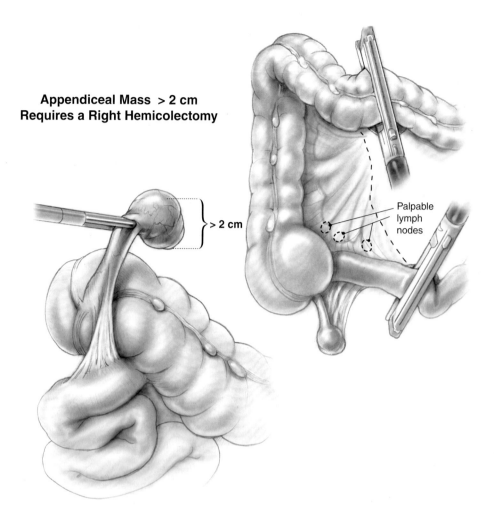

**Appendiceal Mass > 2 cm
Requires a Right Hemicolectomy**

> 2 cm

Palpable
lymph
nodes

Mucocele

- Consists of cystadenomas and cystadenocarcinomas
- Cystadenomas are adequately treated by appendectomy but are usually treated with a right hemicolectomy because they are difficult to differentiate from cystadenocarcinomas
- Do NOT biopsy
- Rupture of a cystadenocarcinoma can lead to pseudomyxoma peritonei
  - The most common complication from pseudomyxoma peritonei is small bowel obstruction

Adenocarcinoma

- Frequently presents with metastatic disease
- Treated with right hemicolectomy
- The staging and treatment is similar to that for colon cancer
- Remember to run the bowel: Up to 35% of patients have synchronous tumors

A 4-year-old girl presents with right lower quadrant pain, vomiting, fever, and an elevated WBC. An US confirms appendicitis. What is the likelihood of rupture in this patient compared to adults?

Children are more likely to have a ruptured appendix compared to adults.

Appendicitis in Children

- Often present with higher-grade fevers and more vomiting than adults
- Have higher rates of gangrene and rupture (as high as 50%), probably because of delayed diagnoses
- Periappendiceal abscess formation is less common (possibly because the omentum is less developed)

> A 22-year-old 18-week gravid woman presents with right-sided abdominal pain, fever, and an elevated WBC. What is the next step in management?

An US is a good initial test to evaluate any pregnant woman for appendicitis. A CT scan in pregnancy is also safe and can aid in making the diagnosis. A suspicion of acute appendicitis must be treated aggressively in the pregnant patient because of the increased risk of maternal and fetal mortality.

Appendicitis in Pregnancy

- Appendicitis is the most common cause of an acute abdomen in pregnancy after the first trimester
- The incidence of appendicitis in pregnancy is the same as in non-pregnant women
- 0.5% maternal mortality and 2% to 8% fetal mortality (but can be as high as 35% with perforated appendicitis)
- Anatomic alterations of intra-abdominal organs must be kept in mind
- There is a 50% incidence of inducing labor in the third trimester
- An obstetrician should be informed and ready to intervene

SUGGESTED READINGS

Guller U, Hervey S, Purves H, et al. Laparoscopic versus open appendectomy: Outcomes comparison based on a large administrative database. *Ann Surg.* 2004; 239(1):43–52.

Rao PM, Rhea JT, Rattner DW, Venus LG, Novelline RA. Introduction of appendiceal CT: Impact on negative appendectomy and appendiceal perforation rates. *Ann Surg.* 1999; 229(3):344–349.

Nguyen NT, Zainabadi K, Mavandadi S, et al. Trends in utilization and outcomes of laparoscopic versus open appendectomy. *Am J Surg.* 2004; 188(6):813–820.

22 | Colon

Danielle A. Bischof and Nita Ahuja

An 83-year-old female underwent abdominal aortic aneurysm repair 1 day ago and is now passing bloody stools. What is the next step in management?

A sigmoidoscopy or colonoscopy should be performed to rule out ischemia. Ischemic colitis should be considered in any abdominal aortic aneurysm patient with hematochezia in the postoperative period.

Ischemic Colitis

- Most cases idiopathic and not associated with recent surgery
- 1% to 7% incidence following aortic surgery
- Most commonly affects the watershed areas of the colon (splenic flexure and rectosigmoid junction)
- Gold standard for diagnosis: Flexible sigmoidoscopy and/or colonoscopy
- Treatment
  - Most cases resolve with supportive treatment
  - Surgical resection of all non-viable areas if no improvement or gangrene
  - Consider planning a second-look laparotomy in 24 to 48 hours if a borderline area of perfusion warrants re-examination

Rectal sparing is common with colon ischemia due to redundant rectal blood supply from IMA and iliac vessels.

A 62-year-old man underwent an uneventful hip surgery complicated by a *Staph aureus* infection in the postoperative period treated with a 14-day course of cefazolin. Five days after stopping treatment he developed severe watery diarrhea. What is the most likely diagnosis?

Clostridium difficile-associated colitis must be ruled out in a patient who develops diarrhea with recent antibiotic use.

Clostridium difficile

- Rising incidence, especially in immunocompromised
- Can range from asymptomatic colonization to mild diarrhea to severe disease, with high fever, abdominal pain, paralytic ileus, toxic megacolon, or even perforation
- Treatment options
  - Standard treatment: Oral metronidazole or oral vancomycin
  - If patient has ileus, can use IV metronidazole

385

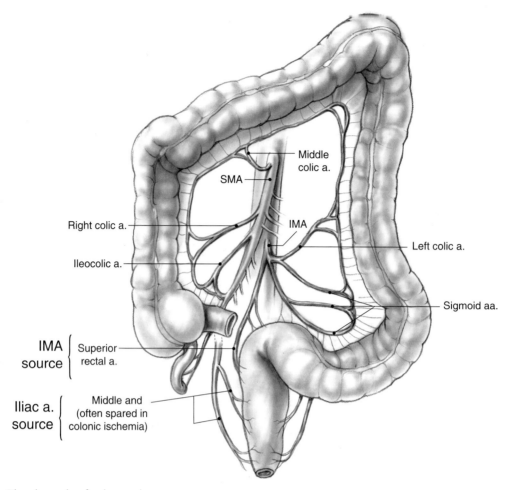

Blood supply of colon and rectum.

- Vancomycin enemas can also be used if the patient has an ileus
- Fecal enemas from a donor (fecal transplant) for patients with recurrent or drug-resistant *C. difficile*
- High relapse rate (15%) after adequate therapy
- Consider a subtotal colectomy if the patient has worsening sepsis despite adequate medical treatment
- Other surgical indications include toxic megacolon, peritonitis, and organ failure
- High surgical mortality rate

Clostridium difficile colitis is associated with the use of all antibiotics including metronidazole, clindamycin (most common), penicillins, and cephalosporins.

A 38-year-old male with AIDS presents with lower Gastrointestinal (GI) bleeding. What is the most common cause for this bleeding?

Immunocompromised patients such as HIV and transplant patients are at risk for opportunistic infections. In the GI system, the most common opportunist is cytomegalovirus (CMV), causing colitis.

Lower GI Bleeding

- Etiologies include:
    - Anatomic: Diverticulosis, Meckel diverticulum, hemorrhoids
    - Vascular: Angiodysplasia, ischemia, radiation-induced
    - Inflammatory: Inflammatory bowel disease (IBD), idiopathic

- Infections: *C. difficile* colitis, hemorrhagic *E. coli*
- Neoplastic
- Most common cause is diverticular disease (30% to 50%), yet only 15% of patients with diverticulosis will have bleeding
  - Most diverticular bleeds occur in the absence of diverticulitis and resolve spontaneously
  - Caused by disrupted vasa recta → arterial bleeding
  - The most common cause of massive LGI bleeding is diverticulosis
  - 50% to 90% of diverticular bleeds occur on the right side while most diverticular disease is on the left side
- Angiodysplasia (Arteriovenous malformation, or AVM) is the most common cause of bleeding in elderly patients
  - Most common in cecum or ascending colon
  - Usually venous source
  - Bleeding usually self-limited
  - 80% re-bleed if untreated
  - 20% to 30% patients also have aortic stenosis (Heyde syndrome).
  - Treatment of bleeding includes argon plasma coagulation, endoscopic coagulation, injection sclerotherapy, or definitive surgical resection
- While treatment should be individualized, broad indications for surgery include:
  - Transfusion of 4U PRBC within a 24-hour period
  - Persistent bleeding after 72 hours
  - Re-bleeding within 1 week of an initial episode

Remember that upper GI bleeding can cause lower GI bleeding. In fact, up to 15% of patients with lower GI bleeding have an upper GI source.

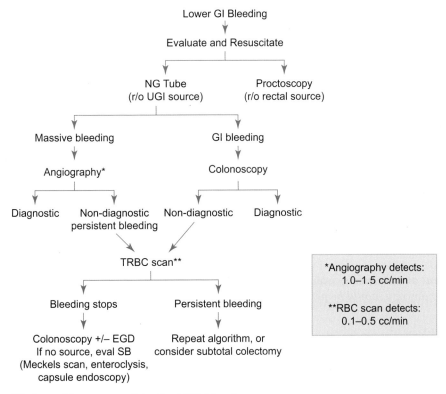

Workup of lower gastrointestinal (GI) bleeding.

An 82-year old man underwent a hip replacement 8 days ago and now has a massively distended, non-tender abdomen. An abdominal X-ray (AXR) confirms marked colonic distension with a cecum measuring 9 cm and no obstruction seen on a gastrografin enema imaging study. What is the most likely diagnosis?

While identifying a possible source of obstruction is the first thought in any patient with a massively dilated colon, elderly patients without an obstruction are known to develop colonic pseudoobstruction, also known as Ogilvie syndrome.

Ogilvie Syndrome

- Massive dilation of colon without mechanical obstruction
- Common in elderly patients who are debilitated or have had recent surgery or trauma
- Must rule out mechanical obstruction with a water-soluble contrast enema or CT with rectal contrast
- Treatment
  - Most (85%) resolve with conservative treatment
    - Bowel rest
    - Correct fluid-electrolyte imbalances
    - Avoid narcotics and anticholinergics
    - Rectal tube decompression
  - If above measures fail or cecum is >10 to 12 cm:
    - Consider a cholinesterase inhibitor (IV neostigmine)
      - *Neostigmine increases* acetylcholine activity to induce coordinated colon propulsion
      - 90% success rate but 25% will recur
      - Neostigmine is contraindicated in patients with cardiovascular disease, asthma, or on beta-blockers
      - Must administer in a monitored setting with atropine available, as patients can become profoundly bradycardiac
    - Consider colonoscopic decompression in patients who fail or have contraindications to neostigmine
    - Cecostomy is an option if the patient fails the above measures
    - Surgery is generally reserved for perforation or ischemia (rare)
      - *Procedure of choice* is subtotal colectomy with end ileostomy

A 90-year-old female from a nursing home was noted to have obstipation and a significant increase in her abdominal girth. She is brought to the hospital where an AXR demonstrated large loops of redundant colon in the left lower quadrant. She has no peritoneal signs. What is the next step in management?

Unless the patient already meets criteria for a surgical resection (worsening sepsis, perforation, etc.), a rigid or flexible sigmoidoscopy should be performed for immediate decompression of a sigmoid volvulus.

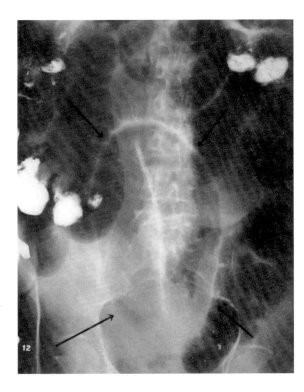

Sigmoid volvulus. (With permission from Mulholland MW, Lillemoe KD, Doherty GM, Maier RV, Upchurch GR, eds. *Greenfield's Surgery.* 4th ed. Philadelphia, PA: Lippincott Williams & Wilkins; 2005.)

Sigmoid Volvulus

- Sigmoid colon is the most common site for colonic volvulus
- Notorious in bedridden, institutionalized patients with neurologic or psychiatric conditions
- Risk factors: Redundant sigmoid colon, bedridden patients, chronic constipation
- Differential diagnosis includes obstructing colorectal cancer, cecal volvulus, and Ogilvie syndrome
- AXR shows dilated redundant colon and "bent inner tube" sign, which can extend anywhere from the pelvis to the RUQ
- Obtain a barium enema if AXR is equivocal
    - A classic "bird's beak" points to the site of obstruction
- Treatment is sigmoidoscopy to decompress and detorse the volvulus
    - Success rate 85%
- Patients with perforation, peritonitis, hematochezia, gangrene or those who fail detorsion or fail to improve should undergo rapid resuscitation and surgical resection

60% of patients will have a recurrence after endoscopic detorsion and patients should undergo elective resection (sigmoid colectomy) during the same hospitalization. These patients should be nutritionally optimized and undergo full colonoscopy in the interim.

A 55-year-old woman presents with severe abdominal pain. Physical exam reveals a distended abdomen that is tympanitic and diffusely tender. She has a marked leukocytosis. AXR shows a dilated cecum extending to the left upper quadrant. A gastrografin enema confirms the diagnosis of cecal volvulus. What is the next step?

An ileocecectomy or right colectomy to include the involved area is indicated.

Cecal Volvulus

- Less common than sigmoid volvulus
- Differential diagnosis is the same as that for sigmoid volvulus

- Treatment is resection with right hemicolectomy
- Despite higher risk of recurrence, cecopexy can be considered in:
  - Poor medical candidates with a short life expectancy, with viable bowel
  - Patients with mild symptoms caused by cecal bascule (chronic intermittent obstruction caused by a floppy cecum that folds on itself leading to obstruction)

There is no role for neostigmine in the management of volvulus.

A 78-year-old man is found to have a stricture in the sigmoid colon on contrast studies. He has a history of multiple attacks of diverticulitis. What is the next step in his management?

A stricture often recurs following endoscopic dilatation. Surgical resection of the stricture with primary colon anastomosis is the definitive treatment and will rule out neoplasia.

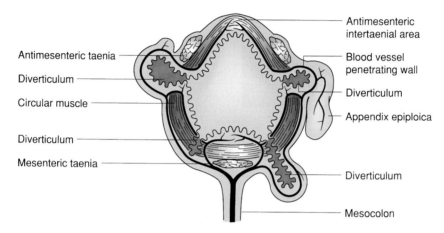

Relation of diverticula to blood vessels. (With permission from Mulholland MW, Lillemoe KD, Doherty GM, Maier RV, Upchurch GR, eds. *Greenfield's Surgery*, 4th ed. Philadelphia, PA: Lippincott Williams & Wilkins; 2005.)

Diverticular Disease

- "False" diverticula—involve herniation of the mucosa through the muscularispropria
- 90% of diverticular disease involves the sigmoid
- 35% of patients have disease outside the sigmoid
- Incidence rises with age; 30% to 50% by age 60, 80% by age 85
- Most patients are asymptomatic
  - One-third of patients present with complications (bleeding, abscess, stricture, or acute perforation)
- Surgery is only indicated for patients with diverticular complications, recurrent bleeding, or multiple hospitalizations
  - One-third of patients require an operation

A 67-year-old woman presents with a 1-day history of fever, left lower quadrant pain, and leukocytosis. AXR shows significant free air. What is the most likely diagnosis?

Perforated diverticulitis is a common cause of sudden left lower quadrant pain and free air.

Diverticulitis

- A CT scan with oral and IV contrast helps establish the diagnosis
- Right-sided (atypical) diverticulitis is more common in younger and Asian patients
- Hinchey classification
  - Stage I: Confined pericolic abscess
  - Stage II: Distant abscess (retroperitoneal or pelvic)
  - Stage III: Purulent peritonitis due to rupture of pericolonic/pelvic abscess but without communication with bowel
  - Stage IV: Fecal peritonitis due to free perforation of diverticulum with communication with bowel
- Treatment
  - Mild diverticulitis: A course of oral broad-spectrum antibiotics and a low-residue diet
    - Must cover *E. coli* and *Bacteroides fragilis*
  - Severe diverticulitis: IV antibiotics, IV fluids, bowel rest and analgesics
  - If an abscess is seen, percutaneous drainage followed by elective resection in 6 to 12 weeks
  - Patients with generalized peritonitis and fecal contamination or worsening sepsis (Stage III or IV) require immediate surgery
- All patients should undergo colonoscopy 6 weeks after episode of diverticulitis to rule out neoplasia
- High recurrence rate
  - 30% recur after first episode and 30% recur after second episode, however complications are most likely to occur with first episode
  - Elective resection recommended for patients with uncomplicated diverticulitis when the frequency and severity of episodes impact quality of life
  - Elective resection recommended after the first episode in immunosuppressed due to higher recurrence and complication rates
- Elective operation is a simple resection with primary anastomosis
- Choice of operation in an emergent situation depends on degree of inflammation and contamination
  - Anastomosis of severely inflamed/contaminated ends of bowel should be avoided given the risk of non-healing and subsequent leakage
- Emergency operation choices include:
  - Hartmann procedure (resection of involved colon with the proximal end brought out as an end colostomy)
  - Resection with primary anastomosis ± proximal diversion with a "protective" diverting loop ileostomy
  - Placement of large external drains at the site of perforation ± proximal diversion with an ostomy (useful choice when dissection is very dangerous)
- 4% to 10% can recur even after surgical resection, especially when a portion of sigmoid colon is left in place

The choice to perform a diverting ostomy depends on the bowel tissue integrity and the degree of inflammation and contamination.

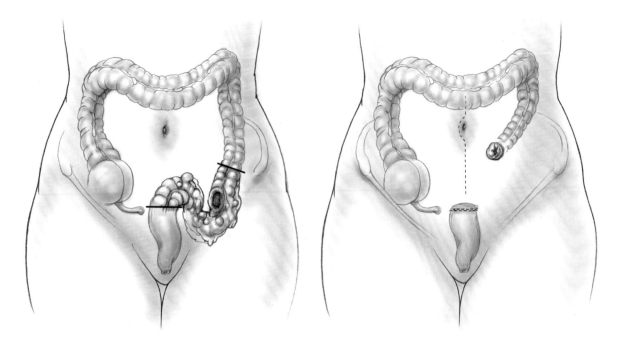

Perforated colon with local inflammatory response.

> A 55-year-old woman had a mild attack of diverticulitis treated with antibiotics 6 months ago. She now has frequent episodes of urinary tract infections and pneumaturia. What is the most likely diagnosis?

Pneumaturia (air in the urine) is a classic finding of a colovesical fistula, commonly caused by diverticular disease or a tumor.

Diverticular Fistulas

- Colovesical fistulas are the most common type of colon fistulas
  - Other types of colon fistulas include colocutaneous, colovaginal, coloenteric, and coloureteric fistulas
- Chronic and recurrent urinary tract infections are typical
- Treatment is resection of affected colon with primary anastomosis and closure of the fistula—bladder resection is not necessary
- Coloenteric fistulas are treated by resection and primary anastomosis of both small intestine and colon
- Colovaginal fistulas may present with feculent vaginal discharge
  - Most commonly occur in women with previous hysterectomy
  - Treatment is resection with primary anastomosis of diseased colon
  - Close the vaginal defect, if possible

Cystoscopy rarely identifies a fistula tract but it can show hyperemia and inflammation consistent with chronic cystitis.

> A 25-year-old man was recently diagnosed with familial adenomatous polyposis (FAP). Baseline colonoscopy shows hundreds of polyps. He is otherwise asymptomatic and referred to your clinic for surgical evaluation. What operation should you recommend?

FAP is best managed with a total proctocolectomy with ileal pouch and anal "pull-through" anastomosis.

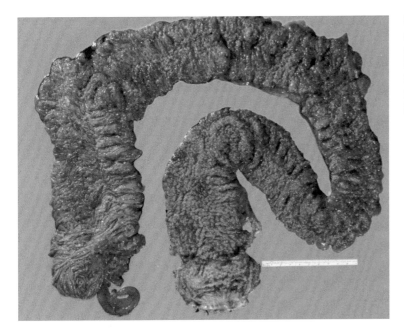

Colon of a patient with familial adenomatous polyposis (FAP). (With permission from Mulholland MW, Lillemoe KD, Doherty GM, Maier RV, Upchurch GR, eds. *Greenfield's Surgery*. 4th ed. Philadelphia, PA: Lippincott Williams & Wilkins; 2005.)

Familial Adenomatous Polyposis

- Autosomal dominant, germline mutation in **APC gene**
    - The protein truncation test identifies 80% of APC mutations
    - An attenuated form of FAP (AFAP) caused by a mutation in 5′ end of APC gene manifests with fewer polyps and later onset of cancer
    - MYH-associated polyposis is caused by an autosomal recessive mutation in the MYH gene, but patients present similarly with multiple adenomatous polyps in the colon
- Without intervention, mutation carriers develop colorectal cancer by age 40
- Mutation carriers are screened annually by sigmoidoscopy starting at age 10 to 12
    - Full colonoscopy should be performed when polyps identified
- Definitive treatment for FAP is total proctocolectomy with ileal pouch and anal anastomosis
    - Mucosectomy of the rectum is controversial—if not performed, strict surveillance of remnant rectal mucosa is required
- Prophylactic proctocolectomy is performed
    - Immediately for profuse polyposis, multiple adenomas >1 cm, or adenomas with villous histology or high-grade dysplasia
    - Patients with sparse, small (<5 mm) adenomas can be followed endoscopically with surgery to accommodate school and work schedules
    - Proctocolectomy should be performed by age 20 for all patients
- Extra-intestinal manifestations
    - Congenital hypertrophy of the retinal pigment epithelium
    - Osteomas of skull or mandible (Gardner's syndrome)
    - Supernumerary teeth
- FAP-associated tumors
    - Desmoid tumors (#1)
    - Periampullary tumors
    - Medulloblastomas (Turcot syndrome)
    - Hepatoblastoma
    - Small bowel cancer

- Thyroid cancer
- Adrenal cancer
- Concurrent duodenal polyps are common ~95% incidence
  - Endoscopic screening for polyps should be performed starting at age 25 and every 2 to 3 years thereafter
  - Surgery may be required for extensive duodenal polyps, rapid polyp growth, or a lesion demonstrating high-grade dysplasia or ulceration

---

A patient with FAP underwent prophylactic proctocolectomy 4 years ago and now has a 7 cm mass in the small bowel mesentery. Biopsies have been non-conclusive. What is the most likely diagnosis?

Desmoid tumors are common in patients with FAP and typically occur following an operation. 10% to 15% of patients with FAP develop desmoid tumors after laparotomy.

Desmoid Tumor
- Occur at surgical sites from prior surgery (e.g., mesentery and abdominal wall)
- Benign, but potentially fast-growing, mesenchymal tumor
- Can be fatal secondary to local invasion/complications
- Treatment
  - First line medical therapies
    - Cox-2 inhibitors (Sulindac)
    - Anti-estrogen therapy (Tamoxifen)
  - Cytotoxic chemotherapy can be used for intra-abdominal desmoids that are large, have rapid growth, or are symptomatic
  - Imatinib and radiotherapy are additional treatment options
  - Surgical resection with grossly negative margins is an option for abdominal wall desmoid tumors
    - Recurrence rates are high—up to 40%
  - Often, mesenteric desmoid tumors are unresectable because they involve the root of the mesentery
    - An initial non-operative approach to treatment is advised for intra-abdominal desmoids especially if they encase vessels or organs

---

A patient is diagnosed with hereditary nonpolyposis colorectal cancer (HNPCC). What is the genetic mutation involved?

HNPCC is associated with DNA repair genes hMLH1 or hMSH2.

Hereditary Nonpolyposis Colorectal Cancer (or Lynch Syndrome)
- Autosomal dominant
- Usually right-sided cancers
- Associated with endometrial, ovarian, gastric, and small bowel cancers
- Increased risk of synchronous cancers: Consider subtotal colectomy ± hysterectomy with oophorectomy

- Characterized by microsatellite instability (MSI)
- Amsterdam criteria
  - Three affected relatives (one must be a first-degree relative of one of the others)
  - Two generations affected
  - One diagnosed before age 50 years
- Revised Bethesda Guideline for testing for MSI in colorectal cancer patients
  - Diagnosis of colorectal cancer at age <50 years
  - Any patient with a synchronous or metachronous colorectal cancer or other HNPCC related cancer, regardless of age
  - Colorectal cancer with HNPCC-like histology (evidence of high MSI) at age <60 years
  - Colorectal cancer or other HNPCC-related tumors in one or more first degree relatives (cancer must be diagnosed at age <50 years or adenoma at age <40 years)
  - Colorectal cancer in two or more first or second degree relatives with HNPCC-related tumors regardless of age
- Surveillance colonoscopy is recommended every 1 to 2 years starting at age 20 to 25 years and annually after age 40 years
  - Women should also undergo an annual transvaginal ultrasound, endometrial biopsy, and CA-125 level
  - Women should consider TAHBSO after child bearing is complete
- Patients can also develop sebaceous tumors (Muir-Torre syndrome)

The name "hereditary nonpolyposis colorectal cancer" is misnomer since cancer still arises from adenomatous polyps.

A 27-year-old woman presents with a small bowel obstruction and hyperpigmented lesions on her lips and fingertips. What syndrome does she have and what is the most likely mode of inheritance of this disease?

Peutz-Jeghers syndrome is an autosomal dominant syndrome associated with multiple small bowel hamartomas.

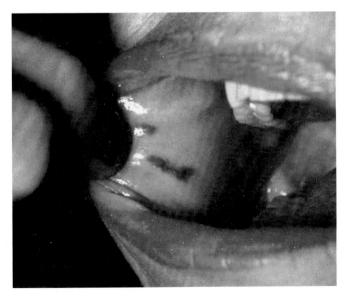

Hyperpigmented lesions seen in Peutz-Jeghers syndrome. (With permission from Mulholland MW, Lillemoe KD, Doherty GM, Maier RV, Upchurch GR, eds. *Greenfield's Surgery*. 4th ed. Philadelphia, PA: Lippincott Williams & Wilkins; 2005.)

Peutz-Jeghers Syndrome

- Autosomal dominant
- Mutation in LKB1/STK1 gene
- Multiple benign intestinal hamartomas that can involve the entire GI tract
- Characteristic mucocutaneous pigmentation of lips, buccal mucosa, hands, feet, and genitalia
- General increased risk of cancer including small bowel, gastric, pancreatic gonadal, and breast cancers
- No indication for prophylactic surgery
- Managed with close surveillance and polypectomy or surgical resection as needed

Familial Juvenile Polyposis

- Autosomal dominant
- Multiple benign hamartomas and cherry-red retention polyps filled with mucin
- Juvenile polyps are not pre-malignant but patients have an overall increased risk of colon cancer

Cowden Syndrome

- Autosomal dominant
- Germline mutation in PTEN
- Multiple gastrointestinal hamartomas
- Multiple trichilemmomas
- Increased risk of breast and thyroid cancer

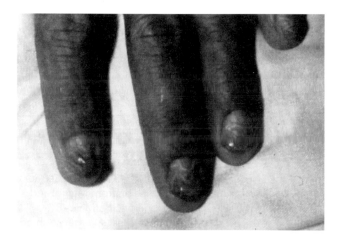

Cutaneous manifestations of Cronkhite-Canada syndrome. (With permission from Mulholland MW, Lillemoe KD, Doherty GM, Maier RV, Upchurch GR, eds. *Greenfield's Surgery.* 4th ed. Philadelphia, PA: Lippincott Williams & Wilkins; 2005.)

Cronkhite-Canada Syndrome

- Sporadic
- Characteristic cutaneous lesions (onycholysis, alopecia, and hyperpigmentation), chronic diarrhea, protein-losing enteropathy, and gastrointestinal polyps
- Diarrhea is common and often dictates therapy

A 66-year-old woman underwent a screening colonoscopy and snare polypectomy of a 1.8 cm tubular adenoma. Pathology shows invasive cancer at the margin. What is the next step in management?

This patient should be considered to have cancer at the polypectomy site. A standard en bloc colectomy with associated mesenteric lymph nodes is indicated.

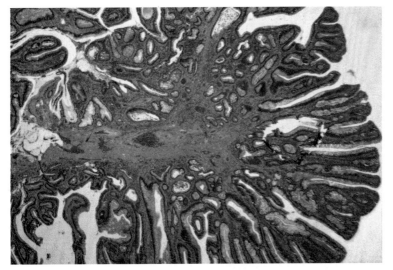

A

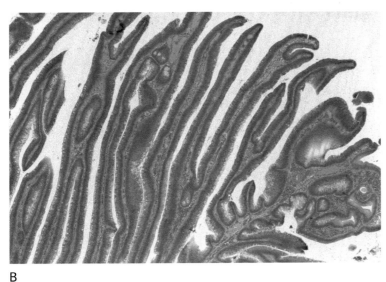

B

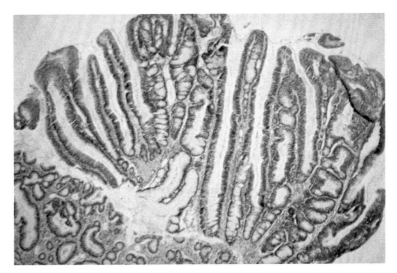

C

Histology of (A) tubular (B) villous and (C) tubulovillous adenomas. (With permission from Mulholland MW, Lillemoe KD, Doherty GM, Maier RV, Upchurch GR, eds. *Greenfield's Surgery.* 4th ed. Philadelphia, PA: Lippincott Williams & Wilkins; 2005.)

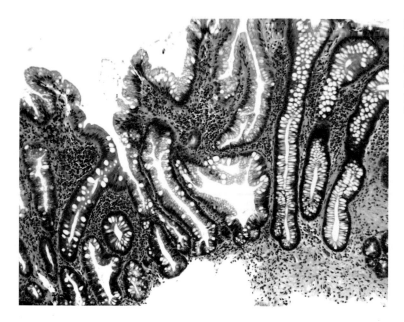

Sessile serrated adenoma. (With permission from Corman M, Nicholls MR, Fazio VW, Bergamaschi R, eds. *Corman's Colon and Rectal Surgery.* 6th ed. Philadelphia, PA: Wolters Kluwer Health/Lippincott Williams & Wilkins; 2012.)

Colorectal Polyps

- *Tubular* polyps are the most common (80%) and have a low risk of malignancy (5%)
- *Tubulovillous* polyps have an intermediate risk of malignancy (15%)
- *Villous* polyps carry a high risk of malignancy (40% to 60%)
- *Sessile serrated adenomas*
    - Typically do not have classic histologic dysplasia
    - Have significant malignant potential
    - More prevalent in the right colon
    - Are associated with development of metachronous polyps
- **Hyperplastic polyps**
    - Usually left sided and benign
    - Patients with hyperplastic polyposis (>20 large hyperplastic polyps throughout the colon in a young adult) may have an increased risk of colon cancer
- The average time for transformation from polyp to cancer is 5 to 10 years
- The risk of carcinoma in-situ within a polypectomy specimen is 6%
- Routine colon cancer screening should start at age 50 years
    - Annual fecal occult blood testing
    - Sigmoidoscopy every 5 years or colonoscopy every 10 years
    - Patients with first degree relatives with colorectal polyps/cancers should start 10 years earlier than when the affected individual was diagnosed or at age 40 years, whichever comes first
- Treatment for polyps found during endoscopy is snare polypectomy
- Indications for surgery after polypectomy
    - Positive tumor <2 mm from resection margin or deep invasion into stalk
    - Unclear margin status
    - Polyps >3 cm in size
    - Sessile polyps not amenable to endoscopic excision
    - Angiolymphatic invasion
    - Grade 3 histology

- Postpolypectomy surveillance: Colonoscopy at 3 years; then if normal, resume regular surveillance interval

Carcinoma in-situ or high-grade dysplasia should be treated like cancer—a positive margin mandates an oncologic surgical resection.

A 66-year-old female underwent a right hemicolectomy for a 6 cm tumor invading through the muscularispropria with 3 out of 16 lymph nodes positive for cancer. What should be the next step?

Adjuvant chemotherapy, 5FU/Leucovorin, or 5FU/Leucovorin/Oxaliplatin (FOLFOX) is recommended for Stage III colon cancer.

Colorectal Cancer
- Second most common cause of cancer death in the United States (lung cancer is most common)
- 95% are adenocarcinomas
- Other types include squamous cell, lymphoma, sarcoma, and carcinoid tumors
- Mutations in the APC gene (aka the "gatekeeper" gene) are found in up to 90% of all colorectal cancers
- Other common mutations: K-Ras (early event) and p53 mutation (late event)
- Must perform colonoscopy to rule out synchronous lesions
- Treatment
    - Carcinoma in-situ: Endoscopic resection
    - Invasive cancer in polyp
        - Segmental resection if lymphatic or vascular invasion, positive margin or poorly differentiated
        - Otherwise, polypectomy is sufficient
    - All other invasive cancers: Segmental resection
        - If positive lymph nodes, add post-operative chemotherapy
        - Adjuvant chemotherapy should also be considered for high risk Stage 2
            - *T4, perforation* or obstruction, <12 nodes examined, poorly differentiated histology, lymphovascular or perineural invasion
        - Need at least 12 LNs for optimal staging
    - Metastatic disease
        - Resection is indicated for isolated, resectable masses in liver and/or lung
- TNM staging: T=tumor size (T1: invades submucosa; T2: invades muscularis propria; T3: invades serosa; T4: tumor directly invades or is adherent to other organs or structures), N=lymph node status (N1: 1 to 3 nodes; N2: 4 or more nodes; Nx=any status), M=presence of metastatic disease
    - Stage 1: T1-2 N0M0
    - Stage 2: T3-4 N0M0
    - Stage 3: TxN1-2 M0
    - Stage 4: TxNxM1
- Adjuvant therapy is standard for Stage 3 and 4 cancers
- *CEA* can be useful for detecting recurrence
    - Obtain a CEA level preoperatively and a baseline level postoperatively

- Elevated preoperative CEA level is an independent poor prognostic factor
- Surveillance after colon cancer surgery
  - H&P every 3 to 6 months for 2 years then every 6 months for 3 years
  - CEA every 3 to 6 months for 2 years then every 6 months for 3 years
  - CT chest, abdomen, pelvis yearly for up to 5 years (For Stage II and III)
  - Colonoscopy at 1 year and then 3 years later, then every 5 years (assuming no polyps found)
- Metastatic disease
  - Liver (#1) and lung (#2) are the most common sites of metastasis
  - Drop metastases to ovaries (Krukenberg tumors) are found in 5%
  - Rectal cancer can metastasize to spine directly via Batson venous plexus
  - 90% of cancer recurrence occurs within 3 years
  - All patients with isolated hepatic metastases should be evaluated by a hepatic surgeon for consideration of resection
    - Resectability is dependent on an adequate future liver remnant (at least 2 segments) with intact vascular supply, venous drainage, and biliary drainage
    - The average 5-year survival for patients with resected liver metastases is 40%
    - Can repeat liver resections after recurrence
  - Isolated lung metastasis may be resectable with a 35% to 56% 5-year survival rate
  - Cytoreductive surgery with heated intraperitoneal chemotherapy is being considered in selected good biology colorectal cancers with isolated peritoneal metastases with 5-year survival approaching 35% to 40%
  - Other locoregional modalities such as liver-directed therapy or stereotactic radiation therapy for metastatic disease also shows promise

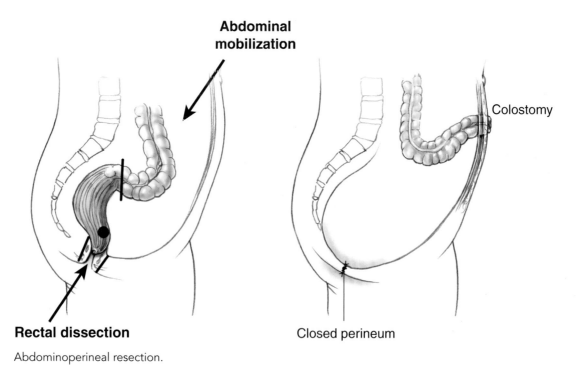

Abdominoperineal resection.

Resection

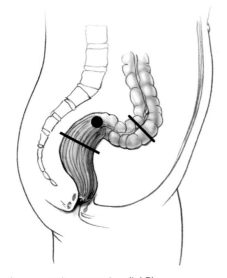

Reconstruction

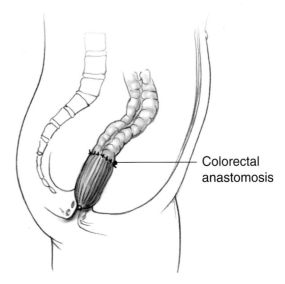

Colorectal anastomosis

Low anterior resection (LAR).

A 58-year-old woman is requesting that her right colectomy for a villous tumor be performed laparoscopically. What is the data on laparoscopic versus open colectomy?

Laparoscopic colon resection for cancer is associated with improved short-term outcomes and similar long-term survival compared to open surgery.

Laparoscopic Colectomy

- Laparoscopic colectomy is associated with decreased operative morbidity: Decreased pain, shorter hospitalization, more rapid return to work, 50% fewer wound infections, lower incidence of ventral hernia, and improved cosmesis
- COST study (Clinical Outcomes of Surgical Therapy)
  - A randomized trial comparing open versus laparoscopic colectomy for cancer
  - No difference in cancer survival
  - Local recurrence rates were the same at median follow up of 4.4 years
  - Established laparoscopic colectomy as standard of care, when technically feasible

A 45-year-old male with a 12-year history of ulcerative colitis (UC) recently underwent a screening colonoscopy. The colonoscopy revealed an area of nodularity in his descending colon. Biopsies of this region showed evidence of high-grade dysplasia. What is the next step in his management?

Proctocolectomy with ileal pouch and anal anastomosis.

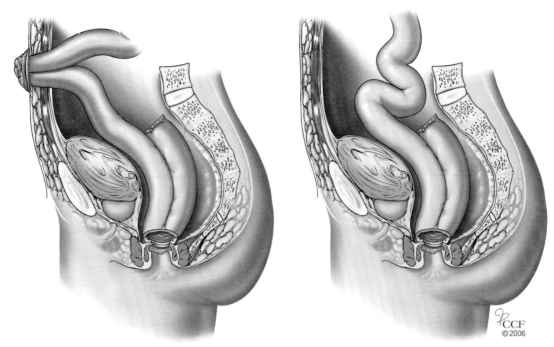

Ileoanal pouch. (With permission from Fischer JE, Bland KI, Callery MP, et al., eds. *Mastery of Surgery.* 5th ed. Philadelphia, PA: Lippincott Williams & Wilkins; 2006.)

Ulcerative Colitis

- Inflammatory condition affecting the mucosa of the colon and rectum
  - Perianal disease is rare
- Two peaks of incidence: Third and seventh decades
- Pathologic features
  - Continuous lesions
  - Crypt abscesses
  - Pseudopolyps
- Risk of malignancy is increased after 10 years of presence of disease—begin surveillance with yearly colonoscopies at that time
  - Biopsies showing reactive atypia during acute flares must be repeated when disease is in remission since atypia often resolves
- Medical therapy
  - Maintenance: 5-ASA and sulfasalazine
  - Acute attacks: Steroids, sulfasalazine and 5-ASA
  - Infliximab (Remicade)
    - A chimeric monoclonal anti-TNF antibody
    - For severe disease
    - Works well for patients with perianal fistulas
  - Cyclosporine—for fulminant, steroid-refractory disease
- Indications for surgery
  - Massive hemorrhage (4 to 6 units of blood)
  - Toxic megacolon
  - Free perforation

- Failure of medical management, inability to wean steroids
- High-grade dysplasia and/or cancer
  - Operations
    - Emergent subtotal colectomy with end-ileostomy
    - Elective proctocolectomy and ileo-anal pouch reconstruction
  - Pouch complications
    - Early: Leak (8% to 10%)
    - Late: Pouchitis (25% to 30%), adhesive SBO
    - General: Increased bowel movements, increased nocturnal incontinence

Proctocolectomy does not alter the course of primary sclerosing cholangitis.

Crohn's Disease

- Transmural inflammation of the entire GI tract
- Sites of involvement
  - Terminal ileum and cecum (ileocolic disease) 40%
  - Small bowel 30%
  - Colon and rectum 25%
  - Perianal disease is common
  - Rectal sparing in 40% of patients
- Two peaks of incidence: second and sixth decades
- Pathologic features
  - Skip lesions—ulcerations spread between normal mucosa
  - Noncaseating granulomas
  - Cobblestoning
- Diagnostic markers
  - P-ANCA (anti-neutrophil cytoplasmic antibody)
  - ASCA (anti-saccharomyces cerevisiae)
  - Both may be helpful in diagnosing IBD
- Fourfold increase in risk of colorectal cancer, but still less than the risk in UC patients
- 7% of Crohn's strictures are malignant
- Treatment
  - Medical maintenance and management of acute attacks: Similar to UC
    - Flagyl for perianal disease management
  - Surgery reserved for failed medical management, management of complications and/or worsening sepsis
    - Do not need clear microscopic margins—just need grossly negative margins

Extraintestinal manifestations of inflammatory bowel disease

- Primary sclerosing cholangitis
  - More common with UC
  - Fibrotic strictures of the intra- and extrahepatic biliary tree
  - Beaded appearance on ERCP
  - Increased risk of cholangiocarcinoma
- Erythema nodosum
- Pyoderma gangrenosum

- Uveitis
- Arthritis
- Ankylosingspodylitis

Infliximab may reactivate tuberculosis or histoplasmosis. Infliximab increases the risk of opportunistic infections and patients must avoid unpasteurized milk.

A 59-year-old male undergoing chemotherapy for lymphoma has an ANC of 200 and acute right lower quadrant pain. CT shows diffuse cecal wall thickening and pneumatosis. This finding is consistent with what condition?

Typhilitis or neutropenic enterocolitis can mimic acute ischemia, but can be treated medically.

Typhilitis
- Occurs in immunosuppressed patients
- Commonly affects the cecum
- Use GM-CSF to correct WBC
- Most episodes resolve with supportive medical management, including broad-spectrum IV antibiotics ($\pm$ antifungals), bowel rest, IV hydration, and NG decompression
- Operate for peritonitis, free perforation, persistent GI bleeding, or continued deterioration

A 45-year-old female with no significant past medical history who recently returned from a vacation in Mexico presents to the office with complaints of 3 to 4 bowel movements per day, cramping, and fever. She has also recently developed worsening RUQ pain. These findings are consistent with what condition?

Amoebic colitis due to Entamoeba histolitica.

Amoebic Colitis
- Primary infection occurs in the colon and then spreads to the liver
- Fecal-oral transmission
- Risk factors: Travel outside of the US
- Symptoms: Cramping, fevers, diarrhea
- Diagnosis
    - Antiamoebic antibodies
    - Colonoscopy: Ulcerations and trophozites
- Treatment: Flagyl

23 | Anus and Rectum

Jennifer L. Bennett, Jon D. Vogel, and Elizabeth C. Wick

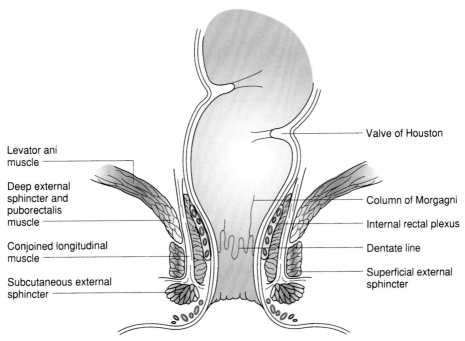

Anatomy of the anal canal. (With permission from Mulholland MW, Lillemoe KD, Doherty GM, Maier RV, Upchurch GR, eds. *Greenfield's Surgery*. 4th ed. Philadelphia, PA: Lippincott Williams & Wilkins; 2005.)

Anatomy of the Anus

- The anal canal is a muscular tube
    - Begins at the anorectal ring (the insertion of the levatorani muscles)
    - Ends at the anal verge (the junction of the anoderm and the perianal skin)
- Cell types of the anal canal and anal transition zone include squamous, cuboidal, columnar epithelial cells, endocrine, and melanin-containing cells
    - Does not have "transitional" cells
- The dentate line in the anal canal is approximately 2 cm from the anal verge
    - Separates the proximal columnar epithelium from the distal squamous epithelium lining the anal mucosa
    - At the dentate line, the anal glands drain their secretions into the anal canal

405

- Anoderm refers to the hairless squamous epithelium between the dentate line and the hair-bearing perianal skin (anal margin)
  - The anoderm and perianal skin have somatic innervation and thus are sensitive to painful stimulation
- The external anal sphincter (EAS) is composed of skeletal muscle
  - The striated skeletal muscle has three parts: Deep, superficial, and subcutaneous
  - All layers are innervated by somatic sensory fibers from the pudendal nerve
  - Is under voluntary control
- The internal anal sphincter is a continuation of the circular smooth muscle layer of the rectum
  - Innervated with visceral sympathetic and parasympathetic fibers from presacral nerves
  - Is constitutively contracted

A 54-year-old man has a complaint of daily bright red blood per rectum and protrusion from the anus after defecation that requires manual reduction. He uses fiber supplements but still strains with defecation. What is the diagnosis and treatment for this problem?

Hemorrhoidal disease manifests with the passage of bright red blood per rectum, protrusions from the anus, mucus drainage, pruritus, and/or anal discomfort.

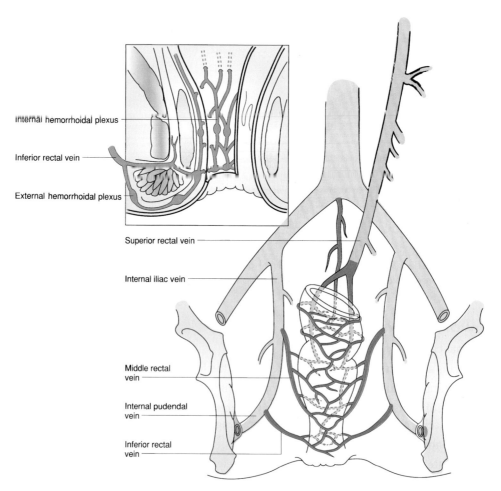

Venous drainage of the rectum and anal canal. (With permission from Mulholland MW, Lillemoe KD, Doherty GM, Maier RV, Upchurch GR, eds. *Greenfield's Surgery.* 4th ed. Philadelphia, PA: Lippincott Williams & Wilkins; 2005.)

Hemorrhoids

- Hemorrhoids are tufts of vascular and connective tissue (vascular cushions) that are normally present in the anal canal
- There are two types of hemorrhoids: Internal and external
- Internal hemorrhoids are located proximal to the dentate line and have visceral innervation, therefore rarely cause anal pain
- Internal hemorrhoid disease is graded in the following manner:
  - Grade 1: Bleeding without prolapse
  - Grade 2: Prolapse with spontaneous reduction ± bleeding
  - Grade 3: Prolapse requiring manual reduction ± bleeding
  - Grade 4: Prolapse that is not reducible
  - Grading is done by interpretation of the patients symptoms
- Treatment of internal hemorrhoid disease is directed by the grade of the disease
  - Grade 1: Dietary fiber supplementation (e.g., psyllium, methylcellulose) and avoidance of straining; rubber-band ligation (RBL)
  - Grade 2: As with Grade 1 but RBL required more frequently
  - Grade 3/4: Hemorrhoidectomy (stapled or excisional)—resect down to the internal sphincter
- External hemorrhoids (skin tags)
  - Located distal to the dentate line
  - Are innervated with somatic fibers, thus usually cause pain if thrombosed

A

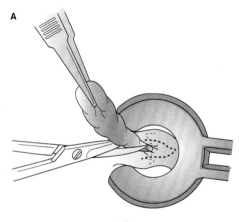

Excisional hemorrhoidectomy. (With permission from Mulholland MW, Lillemoe KD, Doherty GM, Maier RV, Upchurch GR, eds. *Greenfield's Surgery.* 4th ed. Philadelphia, PA: Lippincott Williams & Wilkins; 2005.)

B

Internal sphincter exposed

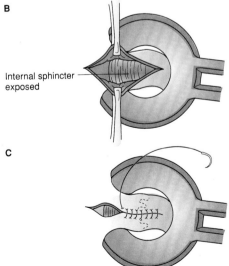

C

- The vast majority of patients with grade 1 to 3 hemorrhoids do not seek treatment
- Excisional and stapled hemorrhoidectomy procedures(for prolapsing hemorrhoids or PPH) have similar long-term efficacy
  - The stapled technique is associated with decreased post-operative pain but can be complicated by, in rare incidences, severe persistent anal pain

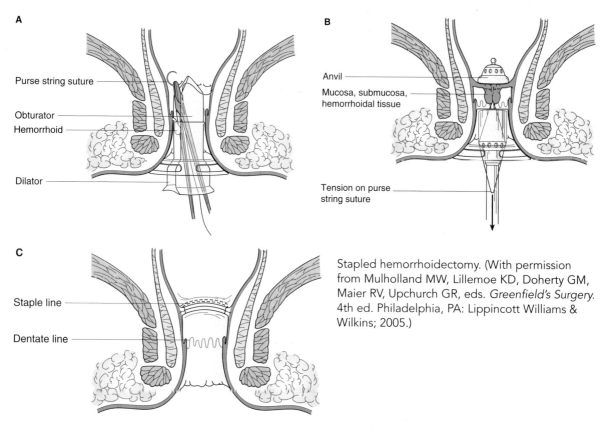

Stapled hemorrhoidectomy. (With permission from Mulholland MW, Lillemoe KD, Doherty GM, Maier RV, Upchurch GR, eds. *Greenfield's Surgery.* 4th ed. Philadelphia, PA: Lippincott Williams & Wilkins; 2005.)

Internal hemorrhoids usually present as painless bright red blood on the toilet tissue, and rarely are the cause of anal pain

Thrombosed Hemorrhoid

- A blood clot in an external hemorrhoid causing acute pain
- If diagnosed within 1 to 2 days of pain onset, treat with incision and evacuation of the thrombus, or excision of the entire thrombosed skin tag
- When diagnosis is delayed 2 to 4 days after pain onset, treatment with warm soaks ("sitz baths") and pain medications alone are effective
  - In this case, the pain caused by excising the clot is generally greater than the pain from the resolving hemorrhoid so intervention should be avoided

---

A 49-year-old man has a complaint of 2 months of severe anal pain that occurs during a bowel movement and after wiping he notices bright red blood on the toilet tissue. What is the diagnosis and treatment for this problem?

An anal fissure is most likely the result of the passage of hard stool that tears the lining of the anal canal as it passes. The treatment is based on decreasing muscle tension.

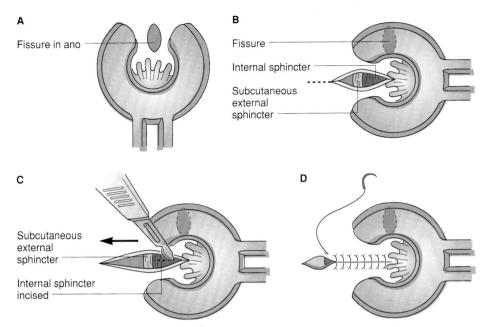

Lateral internal sphincterotomy. (With permission from Mulholland MW, Lillemoe KD, Doherty GM, Maier RV, Upchurch GR, eds. *Greenfield's Surgery.* 4th ed. Philadelphia, PA: Lippincott Williams & Wilkins; 2005.)

Anal Fissure

- A painful ulceration in the anoderm from local trauma in the anal canal below the dentate line
- 90% occur along the posterior midline
  - With lateral or recurrent fissures, IBD should be considered
- Treatment begins with warm soaks (sitz bath), stool bulking agents (e.g., methylcellulose), nifedipine ointment (to relax increased sphincter tone), and topical anesthetics (e.g., lidocaine jelly)
- The next treatment option is topical nitroglycerine or nifedipine ointment
  - Goal is to relax the sphincter muscle to increase blood supply to the mucosa to improve healing
  - Nitroglycerine treatment is more likely to be successful with an acute fissure (<2 months) rather than a chronic fissure
- Botulinum toxin injection is an option for treating chronic anal fissures
- Lateral internal sphincterotomy is the surgical treatment of choice for anal fissures refractory to "conservative" management
  - To decrease the risk of incontinence, the fistulotomy should be tailored to the size of the fissure
  - Fissures secondary to IBD should NOT undergo surgical treatment. In general this type of fissure is not as painful as a non-IBD related fissure.
- If a fissure fails to heal or looks atypical, biopsy should be considered to rule out malignancy

The most common reason for persistent anal pain following a left internal sphincterotomy is that the sphincterotomy was inadequate.

A 34-year-old man presents with 3 days of perianal pain and swelling. Examination reveals a tender, cellulitic lesion involving the skin adjacent to the anus. What is the diagnosis and treatment?

An anoperineal abscess occurs when anal gland drainage is occluded, resulting in an infection of the gland and abscess formation. Antibiotics are reserved for those patients with an increased risk for an infectious complication.

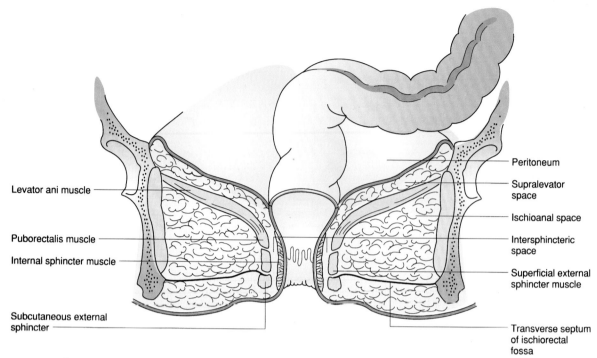

Anatomy of perianorectal spaces. (With permission from Mulholland MW, Lillemoe KD, Doherty GM, Maier RV, Upchurch GR, eds. *Greenfield's Surgery*. 4th ed. Philadelphia, PA: Lippincott Williams & Wilkins; 2005.)

Anoperineal Abscess

- The abscess is labeled according to its location around the anus or rectum
  - Perianal abscess: In the soft tissue overlying the sphincter complex
  - Intersphincteric abscess: Between the internal and external sphincters
  - Ischioanal abscess: In the ischioanal space
  - Supralevator abscess: Between the levators and the overlying peritoneum
- Treatment is incision and drainage (I&D) of the abscess. Patients should NOT be treated with antibiotics alone.
  - Adequate drainage can be achieved via a small "stab" incision and insertion of a mushroom-type drain into the abscess cavity
  - The incision should be made as close to the anal verge as possible to prevent formation of a long-track fistula-in-ano (FIA)
  - The drain is left for 7 to 10 days
  - Large or deep abscesses may require I&D under general anesthesia
- Antibiotics are indicated for individuals with immunosuppression, diabetes, prosthetic implants, as well as valvular or developmental cardiac defects
- Patients should be counseled that they could develop a subsequent perianal fistula

A FIA and a recurrent abscess are the main complications following an I&D procedure.

A 34-year-old man presents 3 months after incision and drainage of an ischioanal abscess complaining of discharge from a fleshy lump near his anus. What is his diagnosis and how is this treated?

A FIA is often managed with seton placement or a fistulotomy procedure.

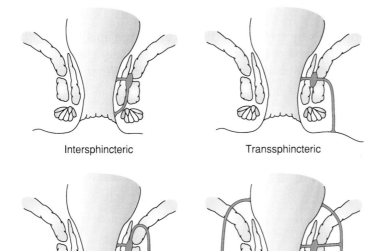

Types of fistula-in-ano. (With permission from Mulholland MW, Lillemoe KD, Doherty GM, Maier RV, Upchurch GR, eds. *Greenfield's Surgery.* 4th ed. Philadelphia, PA: Lippincott Williams & Wilkins; 2005.)

Intersphincteric   Transsphincteric

Suprasphincteric   Extrasphincteric

Fistula-in-ano

- An abnormal connection between the lumen of the anus (or rectum) and the perianal skin
- Most often, the internal opening of the FIA is at the dentate line
- Presents with drainage of mucus or flatus from a skin opening (external opening)
- The external opening often corresponds with the drainage site of a previous abscess
- May be associated with an abscess, prior anal surgery, Crohn's disease, radiation, or cancer
- An examination under anesthesia (EUA) may be necessary to identify the anatomy
- The "Parks classification" defines FIA by their relationship to the anal sphincters
  - Intersphincteric FIA: Tracks between the internal anal sphincter (IAS) and EAS
  - Transsphincteric FIA: Tracks through both the IAS and EAS
  - Suprasphincteric FIA: Tracks up and over the EAS
  - Extrasphincteric FIA: The internal opening is in the rectum, not at the dentate line
- Goodsall rule is a general guide to the trajectory and location of the fistula tract
  - Anterior or anterolateral external openings usually track directly radially into the anal canal (i.e., a straight path)
  - Posterior or posterolateral external openings typically track curvilinearly in the anal canal
- Draining setons (e.g., silastic vessel loops)
  - Used to prevent recurrent abscess formation
  - Can be used for extended periods (years) in patients with Crohn's disease
- Cutting setons (e.g., silk sutures)
  - Allow for the gradual eradication of the fistula while aiming to preserve sphincter integrity
- Fistulotomies (opening and curettage of the fistula tract) are performed for "simple fistulas" involving less than 30% to 50% of the EAS
- Fibrin glue and collagen "fistula plugs" have been used with moderate success
- More recently, the ligation of intersphincteric fistula tract (LIFT) procedure has gained popularity. This requires closing the internal opening and debriding the tract.

FIA is considered the "chronic phase" of an anoperineal abscess and may occur in up to 50% of patients following incision and drainage of anoperineal abscesses.

A 22-year-old woman underwent a vaginal delivery and suffered a fourth degree anal sphincter injury. The injury was repaired at the time of delivery. Several weeks later she presents to you with the complaint of stool and flatus passage from her vagina. What is the diagnosis and treatment?

Fourth degree anal sphincter lacerations involve the entire anal sphincter complex and the anal canal mucosa. Episiotomies with third and fourth degree anal sphincter laceration injuries occur in 5% of deliveries. With immediately repaired lacerations, a rectovaginal fistula (RVF) complicates about 10% of cases. Most RVFs require operative repair.

Rectovaginal Fistula

- Obstetric injury is the leading cause of RVFs
  - Also associated with Crohn's disease, prior anorectal surgery, radiation, and infection
- Small RVF from obstetrical trauma will spontaneously heal in about 50% of patients; therefore, if tolerable to the patient, intervention should be delayed for 6 months
- Repair should be delayed until resolution of any infection and acute inflammation
- Antibiotics, sitz baths, and fecal diversion may be required in treatment
- Simple fistulotomy is not appropriate for RVF, unless the fistulotomy will avoid muscle division
- Options for repair are:
  - Full-thickness fistulotomy (episioproctotomy) with layered closure of the defect (anorectal mucosa, anal sphincters, vaginal mucosa)
  - Rectal mucosa advancement flap ± sphincteroplasty
  - In some cases, anterior resection with colorectal or coloanal anastomosis
- Repair in patients with Crohn's disease is challenging and only should be considered in patients with no rectal inflammation
- In complex patients, optimizing bowel function (preventing diarrhea or loose stools) may significantly improve symptoms and obviate the need for surgery

For the above patient, the initial treatment is aimed at resolving her infection first. Sitz baths and antibiotics may be needed.

A 45-year-old homeless man presents with a complaint of "itching and lumps near my anus." Your examination reveals an anal condyloma. How is this condition treated?

Topical treatments are often successful when patients are compliant and monitored closely. Surgery is necessary in select cases.

Condyloma Acuminatum (Anal Condyloma, Anal Warts)

- Caused by human papillomavirus infection
- Pink or white papillary lesions ranging in size from millimeters to several centimeters in diameter
- May be located in the perianal skin, anal canal, or rectal mucosa
- Risk factors for infection include anal receptive intercourse, a partner with cervical dysplasia, immunosuppression, and immunocompromise (HIV)
- Condyloma acuminatum is strongly associated with the development of anal intraepithelial neoplasia (AIN) and anal squamous cell carcinoma

- Eradication of the condyloma is required to avoid transmission to sexual partners and prevent malignant transformation
- Topical application of podophyllin, bichloroacetic acid, and imiquimod have all been tried as treatment options
- Extended treatment periods and high recurrence rates limit the utility of these treatments
- Surgical excision and fulguration at the base of the lesion is a fast and effective treatment
- A verrucous carcinoma (Buschke-Lowenstein tumor) shares many similar features with condyloma acuminatum, but is a locally invasive, non-metastasizing squamous cell carcinoma. Treatment is complete excision.
- In some cases, patients with HPV infection develop AIN, which can be a precursor to anal cancer
- High resolution anoscopy can be used to identify areas of AIN and apply local treatment (either chemical or cautery)

All patients with condyloma acuminatum must be evaluated every 4 to 8 weeks, repeating therapy for recurrent lesions as needed. Yearly surveillance should be performed after complete eradication.

A 56-year-old female has a complaint of anal pain. Examination reveals an ulcerated lesion in the anal canal. The biopsy result shows squamous cell carcinoma of the anus (SCCA). How is this treated?

Chemotherapy with 5-FU/mitomycin and radiation therapy (Nigro protocol).

Squamous Cell Carcinoma of the Anus

- Comprise 80% of all anal cancers
- Five-times more common than anal margin (perianal) SCCA
- Risk factors for anal SCCA include immunocompromise, chronic inflammation, radiation, and HPV
- Combination chemoradiation therapy (Nigro protocol)
  - External beam irradiation (30 to 50 Gy) of the tumor/nodal drainage basin
  - 5-flourouracil and mitomycin
  - Cures 75% to 90% of patients with anal SCCA
- Abdominoperineal resection (APR) is indicated when chemoradiation therapy fails, resulting in long-term survival in 60% to 90% of patients
- PET-CT is used to stage anal cancer
- The most common site of metastatis is the inguinal lymph nodes, so it is important to evaluate these as part of the physical exam

Other Malignancies of the Anal Canal and Anoderm

- Adenocarcinoma of the anal canal is treated surgically as with low rectal cancer
- Melanoma of the anal canal
  - 40% to 70% are amelanotic
  - Resistant to radiation and chemotherapy
  - Treatment is a wide local excision or an APR
  - Prognosis is very poor
- Basal cell cancer
  - Need 3 mm resection margins
  - Wide local excision is typically sufficient

- Rarely, an APR may be needed if the sphincter is involved
- Anal margin cancers are generally managed with wide local excision

The World Health Organization and the American Joint Committee on Cancer define anal canal cancers as those that are located between the upper and lower borders of the internal sphincter muscle, i.e., from the anorectal ring to the anal verge. Anal margin cancers involve the perianal skin within 5 cm of the anal verge.

> An 85-year-old woman complains that her "rectum falls out" during defecation. You diagnose her with full-thickness rectal prolapse. How is this treated?

The operative approach to rectal prolapse depends on the etiology.

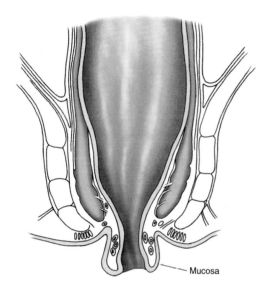

Rectal prolapse. (With permission from Fischer JE, Bland KI, Callery MP, et al., eds. *Mastery of Surgery.* 5th ed. Philadelphia, PA: Lippincott Williams & Wilkins; 2006.)

MUCOSAL PROLAPSE

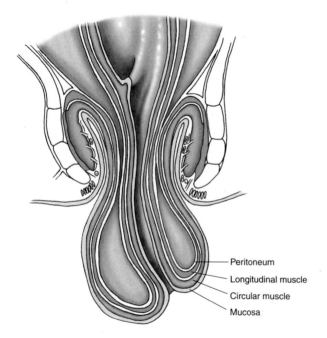

COMPLETE RECTAL PROLAPSE

Rectal Prolapse

- Full-thickness intussusception of a part of the rectum
- Most common in women (90%)
- Often associated with constipation
- Rectal prolapse is distinguished from prolapsing internal hemorrhoids by the circular mucosal folds visualized with rectal prolapse compared to the radial creases seen with prolapsed hemorrhoids
- Examining the patient while straining on the toilet can reproduce the prolapse
- Internal prolapse can be diagnosed via defecography or dynamic MRI
- Impaired fecal continence is often associated with prolapse, but improves for many patients after repair of the prolapse
- Common surgical techniques to repair rectal prolapse include:
  - Open or laparoscopic or robotic rectopexy
  - Rectopexy plus sigmoid colectomy—for prolapse associated with constipation
  - Transabdominal proctopexy (the Ripstein procedure)—for massive rectal prolapse
  - The Delorme (rectal mucosectomy) or Altemeier (perineal proctosigmoidectomy) procedures may be used for patients when trying to avoid an abdominal operation

Colonoscopy should be performed in all patients with rectal prolapse to determine if mucosal pathology is associated with the prolapse.

A 65-year-old woman complains of fecal incontinence. How is this condition evaluated?

A thorough "history of present illness" is one of the most important steps in the evaluation of fecal incontinence. Medication use, childbirth history, and prior anal surgery should also be investigated.

Fecal Incontinence

- A shorter anal canal and childbirth-related injuries put women at an increased risk
- Incontinence may be caused by traumatic injury to the anal sphincters (vaginal delivery, anal surgery), rectal prolapse, central nervous system deficits, connective tissue disorders, or medications
- Examine the anoperineum for scars, lesions, and prolapse
- Evaluate the sphincter tone assessing both the resting pressure (internal anal sphincter) and the squeeze pressure (EAS) while considering that patulous anus (lack of anal muscle tone) is a possibility
- Diagnostic studies include:
  - Endoluminal ultrasound—evaluates sphincter defects
  - Sphincter manometry—evaluates sphincter contraction deficits
  - Physiology studies—evaluates rectal sensation deficits
  - Pudendal nerve studies—evaluates external sphincter innervation deficits
- The underlying abnormality drives the treatment approach
- Direct or overlapping sphincter repair is indicated when there is a sphincter defect
- Biofeedback training is effectively used in patients with incontinence and intact sphincters
- A bowel management regime (fiber supplements, scheduled trips to the toilet, enemas after a bowel movement), the Secca procedure (radiofrequency treatment of the anal sphincter), artificial bowel sphincter, and colostomy construction are additional treatment choices

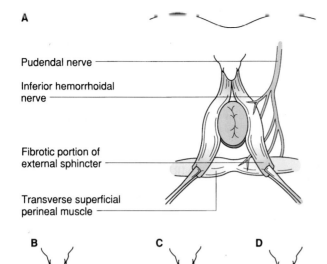

A

Pudendal nerve

Inferior hemorrhoidal nerve

Fibrotic portion of external sphincter

Transverse superficial perineal muscle

B C D

Overlapping anal sphincteroplasty. (With permission from Mulholland MW, Lillemoe KD, Doherty GM, Maier RV, Upchurch GR, eds. *Greenfield's Surgery*. 4th ed. Philadelphia, PA: Lippincott Williams & Wilkins; 2005.)

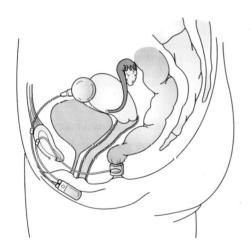

A

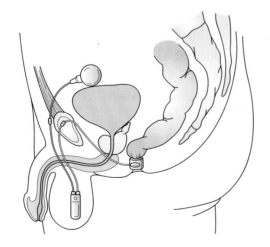

B

Artificial sphincter. (With permission from Mulholland MW, Lillemoe KD, Doherty GM, Maier RV, Upchurch GR, eds. *Greenfield's Surgery*. 4th ed. Philadelphia, PA: Lippincott Williams & Wilkins; 2005.)

> A 55-year-old man is referred to you with a "low rectal adenocarcinoma." What studies are required to determine the precise location and stage of the cancer?

A complete colonoscopy or contrast enema must be performed to exclude a synchronous neoplasm before initiating treatment for the rectal cancer.

Rectal Adenocarcinoma

- Depth of invasion of the primary tumor (T), lymph node involvement (N), and presence of metastasis (M) define the staging for colon and rectal cancer
- T stages
  - T1: Limited to the submucosa
  - T2: Invades the muscularis propria
  - T3: Invades through the muscularis propria into the subserosa
  - T4: Invades into adjacent structures (e.g., prostate)
- Rectal cancer staging
  - Stage1 = T1 or T2 N0 M0
  - Stage 2 = T3 or T4 N0 M0
  - Stage 3 = N1 or N2
  - Stage 4 = M1
- Preoperative pelvic irradiation and chemotherapy
  - Indicated for both Stage 2 and 3 rectal cancers in the lower two-thirds of the rectum (within 10 cm of the anorectal ring)
- Transanal full-thickness excision
  - Appropriate for well-differentiated or moderately differentiated T1N0 cancers without lymphovascular invasion
  - Benefits of transanal excision, a low risk surgery, must be carefully weighed against the 10% to 15% risk of missing lymph node involvement
- APR
  - Performed for low rectal cancers with anal sphincter invasion or tumors within 1 to 2 cm of the sphincter where complete resection would result in excision of the sphincter
- Total mesorectal excision
  - Involves excision of the rectum and its surrounding "mesorectum" via sharp dissection in the avascular plane between the presacral fascia and the fascia propria of the rectum
  - The anterior dissection is performed anterior to Denonvilliers fascia for anterior cancers and posterior to Denonvilliers fascia for posterior cancers
- Palliative interventions for metastatic rectal cancer include a range of therapies including fulguration of the tumor, endostent placement for obstructing cancers, colostomy, or palliative APR

Total mesorectal excision has been shown to decrease the rate of local recurrence from about 30% to less than 10% after radical resection of the rectum for cancer.

> A 35-year-old woman with Crohn's disease has a complaint of diarrhea and anal pain. Examination reveals large external skin tags, internal hemorrhoids, and a posterior midline anal fissure. How are these conditions treated?

The goals in treating anoperineal Crohn's disease are to relieve symptoms, prevent harm to the sphincters, and avoid creating wounds that are unable to heal.

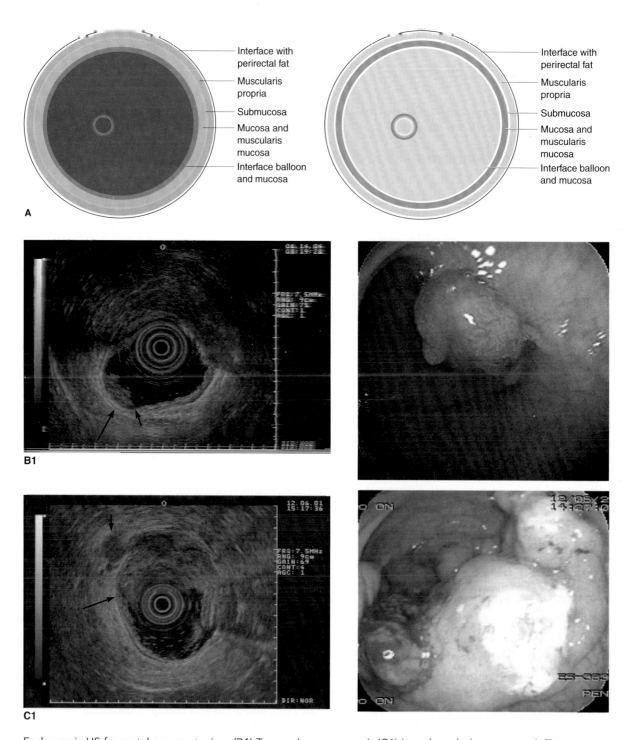

Endoscopic US for rectal cancer staging. (B1) Tumors (*upper arrows*). (C1) Lymph node (*upper arrow*), Tumor (*bottom arrow*). (With permission from Mulholland MW, Lillemoe KD, Doherty GM, Maier RV, Upchurch GR, eds. *Greenfield's Surgery*. 4th ed. Philadelphia, PA: Lippincott Williams & Wilkins; 2005.)

Perianal Crohn's Disease

- May present as an anal fissure, fistula, pain, bleeding, abscess, or a complaint of "hemorrhoids"
- Skin tags (external hemorrhoids) in Crohn's disease are often large, edematous, and pink in color with an appearance resembling "elephant ears"
  - These do not typically cause problems and should NOT be excised

- In Crohn's disease, an anal fissure may occur anywhere around the anus with or without associated pain
  - A fissure lateral to the midline should be investigated further for the possibility of Crohn's disease, cancer, or an infectious etiology
  - A painful fissure in a patient with Crohn's disease and normal rectal mucosa is treated with the same approach as an idiopathic fissure
- The initial treatment for a fissure in the setting of active rectal Crohn's disease is systemic medical therapy directed at the underlying disease (steroids, infliximab, metronidazole). Eventually radical surgery (proctectomy) may be necessary.
- A perianal abscess is treated with incision and drainage
- A fistula is typically treated by placing a draining seton

A 24-year-old woman has a complaint of rectal fullness and a sensation of incomplete passage of stool. Digital rectal examination (DRE) reveals an extramucosal lesion posterior to the rectum. What is your diagnosis and how is this problem treated?

You will never diagnose a presacral tumor unless you include it in the differential diagnosis for every patient with anorectal symptoms.

Retrorectal "Presacral" Tumors

- May be cystic or solid,
- Most often are benign, congenital, cystic lesions
  - Can occasionally be malignant
  - Most common malignant tumor is a chordoma
- Are more common in females
- The tumors can be classified as congenital, neoplastic, inflammatory, or metastatic
- DRE is useful in describing the extent of the lesion, its fixation to the sacrum or sphincters, and whether it is solid or cystic
- MRI and/or CT are useful for gaining more information about these lesions
- Complete excision both diagnoses and treats the tumor
  - Percutaneous and transrectal biopsies should be avoided due to the risk of lesion infection, destruction of the tissue planes, and seeding of tumor cells along the needle track
  - Low lesions (below S3) can be excised via a posterior (Kraske) incision
  - Lesions above S3 typically require a combined anterior-posterior approach with laparotomy and mobilization of the rectum off the presacral fascia

A 52-year-old man underwent colonoscopy with complete endoscopic removal of a 1.5 cm mid-rectal carcinoid tumor. He is referred to you for further management. How is this treated?

Rectal carcinoid tumors larger than 1 cm require surgical resection (anterior proctosigmoidectomy or APR).

Rectal Carcinoid

- Rectal carcinoid tumors up to 1 cm in diameter are treated by excisional biopsy without any further treatment
- Rectal carcinoid tumors 2 cm or larger require a radical resection (anterior proctosigmoidectomy or APR)
- In rectal carcinoid tumors 1 to 2 cm in size, up to 11% of cases have lymph node spread

- Muscle and lymphovascular invasion are risk factors for lymph node involvement
- Metastatic evaluation includes CT scan of the abdomen and pelvis, and octreotide scintigraphy (octreoscan)

Carcinoid syndrome is not associated with rectal carcinoid tumors.

> A 25-year-old man presents to the emergency room with a bullet wound through his buttocks and bright red blood per rectum. How is this treated?

The patient needs to go to the operating room. At the very least, a thorough rectal exam under anesthesia (EUA) and rigid sigmoidoscopy should be performed. Bleeding injury sites can be oversewn transanally. A colostomy may be required for fecal diversion to allow the injury to heal.

Traumatic Injury to the Rectum

- Extra-peritoneal injuries to the rectum are treated with colostomy construction
  - Exploration of the extra-peritoneal rectum is indicated with non-rectal injuries in the pelvis requiring assessment and/or repair
  - Presacral drainage and irrigation of the rectum may be useful for destructive lesions of the extra-peritoneal rectum
- Intra-peritoneal rectal injuries are treated like colon injuries
  - Minimally destructive lacerations are repaired primarily without the creation of a colostomy
  - Destructive lesions (>50% circumference, extensive necrosis) are safely treated by resection of the damaged segment and colostomy formation

Most rectal injuries are identified by bright red blood per rectum and an obvious mucosal injury on rigid proctoscopy.

> A 32-year-old man is referred to you for treatment of a low back abscess. You examine him and find a pilonidal sinus. How is this condition treated?

Pilonidal means "nest of hair." Treatment depends on whether it is in the acute or chronic phase. All infected fluid collections require drainage. Once the infection has cleared, a definitive resection of the pilonidal sinus may be necessary to prevent recurrence.

Pilonidal Sinus

- A pilonidal sinus is the chronic phase of pilonidal disease
- Treat with unroofing of the sinus, curettage of the contained debris, and serial dressing changes to allow healing by secondary intention
- An infected sinus (abscess) is treated with incision and drainage
  - In about 40% of patients, this is the only treatment required
- If the sinus recurs, excision of the tract maybe required—it is essential that the entire tract be removed during this procedure

> A 52-year-old woman complains of difficulty evacuating stool from the rectum and needs to insert a finger into her vagina to allow passage of stool. You suspect a rectocele. How is this treated?

Rectoceles are commonly present but rarely problematic, and should be repaired only when symptomatic.

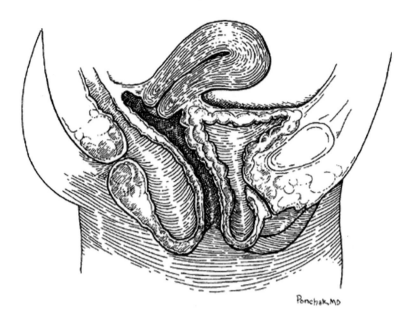

Cystocele and rectocele. (With permission from Fischer JE, Bland KI, Callery MP, et al., eds. *Mastery of Surgery*. 5th ed. Philadelphia, PA: Lippincott Williams & Wilkins; 2006.)

Rectocele

- An anterior invagination of the rectovaginal septum that is accentuated with straining to pass stool and may be associated with obstructed defecation (outlet constipation)
- Key diagnostic studies include:
  - Defecating proctogram
  - Anorectal manometry
  - Rectal volume studies (rectal physiology)
- Impaired rectal physiology may be amenable to biofeedback therapy
- Only rectoceles associated with obstructed defecation warrant surgical correction
- The surgical approach for rectocele repair may be transanal or transvaginal with imbrication of the rectovaginal septum for added support to the septum

24 | Abdominal Hernias

J.R. Salameh

A 35-year-old woman presents with a groin hernia. What type of hernia is it most likely to be?

An indirect inguinal hernia is the most common groin hernia in both men and women.

Groin Hernia

- Groin hernias are five times more common in males than in females
- Indirect inguinal hernias result from a persistently patent processus vaginalis
- Direct inguinal hernias are extremely rare in women
- Femoral hernias are more common in females but still rare overall
- Direct and indirect inguinal hernias are often indistinguishable on physical exam

Anatomy of the Abdominal Wall

- Layers of the abdominal wall (from superficial to deep)
  - Skin
  - Subcutaneous fat
  - Camper fascia (superficial and fatty)
  - Scarpa fascia (deeper and fibrous)
  - External oblique muscle
  - Internal oblique muscle
  - Transversus abdominis muscle
  - Transversalis fascia
  - Peritoneum
- Anatomy of the inguinal canal
  - Deep (internal) ring—entrance to the inguinal canal arising from the transversalis fascia
  - Superficial (external) ring—exit of the inguinal canal arising from the external oblique aponeurosis
  - Inguinal (Poupart) ligament—arises from external oblique and connects ASIS to pubic tubercle
  - Lacunar (Gimbernat) ligament—where the inguinal ligament splays out to insert on the pubic tubercle
  - Cooper (pectineal) ligament—an extension of the lacunar ligament that runs on the pectineal line of the pubic bone

Inguinal Hernias (Internal view)

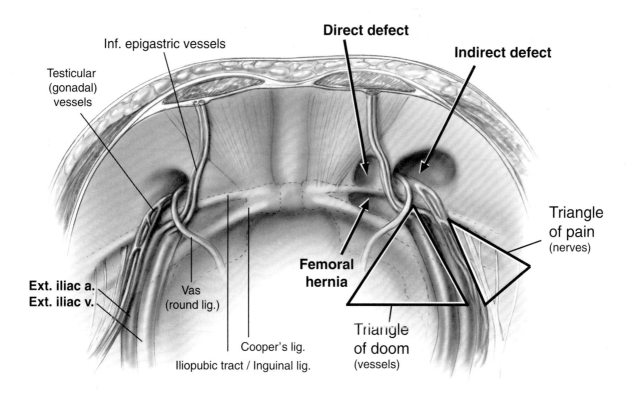

Inf. epigastric vessels

Testicular (gonadal) vessels

Direct defect

Indirect defect

Triangle of pain (nerves)

Femoral hernia

Ext. iliac a.
Ext. iliac v.

Vas (round lig.)

Cooper's lig.

Iliopubic tract / Inguinal lig.

Triangle of doom (vessels)

Repair through Preperitoneal Approach

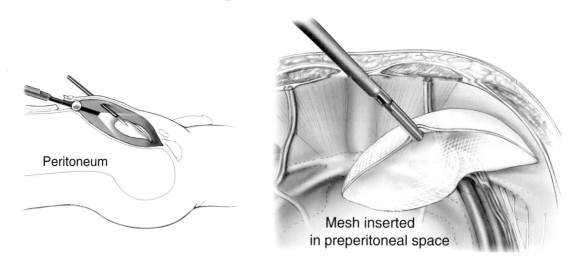

Peritoneum

Mesh inserted in preperitoneal space

A 50-year-old man presenting with an asymptomatic inguinal hernia asks you about the risk of incarceration. What it the likelihood that his hernia will incarcerate?

10% of inguinal hernias and 20% of femoral hernias present incarcerated. Direct inguinal hernias generally have a wide-necked sac (unless they pass through the external ring), which lowers their risk of incarceration.

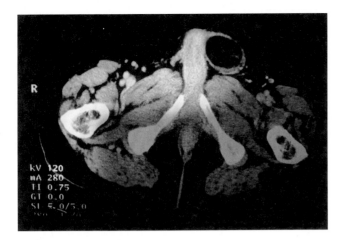

Left inguinal hernia. (With permission from Mulholland MW, Lillemoe KD, Doherty GM, Maier RV, Upchurch GR, eds. *Greenfield's Surgery*. 4th ed. Philadelphia, PA: Lippincott Williams & Wilkins; 2005.)

Management of an Incarcerated Hernia

- If the hernia is incarcerated without signs of strangulation (fever, leukocytosis, worsening tenderness, or skin erythema), reduction at the bedside can be attempted
- If the hernia has signs of strangulation, emergent herniorrhaphy (hernia repair) is required
  - Surgical mortality for a strangulated hernia with Child's C cirrhosis can be up to 50%
- Vigorous attempts at reducing an incarcerated hernia with a small neck may lead to "en masse" reduction resulting in ongoing compromise of the entrapped bowel

When operating on incarcerated or strangulated hernias, open the hernia sac to inspect the viability of its contents.

A frail, 75-year-old man with multiple significant comorbidities has a minimally symptomatic right inguinal hernia. He is deemed to have a prohibitive surgical risk. What is your recommendation?

Non-operative management with a truss for symptomatic relief.

Hernia Truss

- Can provide symptomatic relief
- Correct measurement and fitting are important to prevent incarceration within the truss
- Hernia control in approximately 30% of patients
- Complications include testicular atrophy, ilioinguinal or femoral neuritis, and incarceration

A Truss should NOT be used for femoral hernias due to the high incidence of strangulation.

A 54-year-old female presents with an acute, painful, non-reducible bulge on the right anteromedial thigh, below the inguinal ligament. What is the most likely diagnosis?

An incarcerated, or non-reducible, femoral hernia should be considered.

Femoral Hernia

- 5% of hernias overall
- Much more common in women

- Boundaries of the femoral canal:
    - Inguinal ligament (anterior)
    - Lacunar ligament (medial)
    - Cooper ligament (posterior)
    - Femoral vein (lateral)
- Surgical approach:
    - Anterior infrainguinal (mesh-plug repair)
    - Anterior inguinal (McVay repair)
    - Posterior preperitoneal (laparoscopic repair)
- If a hernia is not reducible at exploration, the inguinal ligament can be divided

---

A 14-month-old boy presents to emergency room with an incarcerated right inguinal hernia. What is the next step in management?

Hernia reduction, hospital admission, and a semi-elective repair in the future.

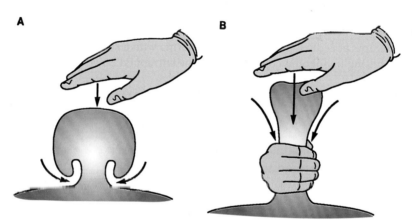

Hernia reduction (A) applying pressure directly to neck occludes neck (B) elongating neck while applying pressure allows reduction. (With permission from Mulholland MW, Lillemoe KD, Doherty GM, Maier RV, Upchurch GR, eds. *Greenfield's Surgery.* 4th ed. Philadelphia, PA: Lippincott Williams & Wilkins; 2005.)

Inguinal Hernia in Children
- High ligation and division of the hernia sac is indicated upon diagnosis
- Elective repair of reduced incarcerated hernias should be performed ASAP to avoid re-incarceration (16%)
- The incidence of developing a future contralateral inguinal hernia is 10% to 30%

A 2-month-old girl is noted to have a solid mass within an inguinal hernia. What is the most likely cause?

A normal ovary may present in an inguinal hernia sac in young girls. Beware of testicular feminization if the ovary appears abnormal or resembles a testicle (perform a biopsy and pelvic examination).

During an open repair of a right inguinal hernia, a bladder injury occurs. What was the most likely cause of the injury?

Failure to recognize the visceral component of a sliding hernia sac.

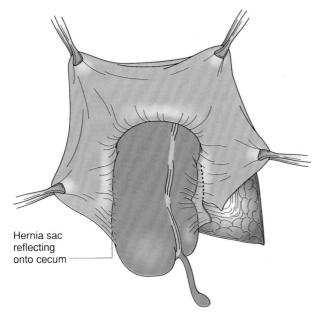

Sliding inguinal hernia being repaired through an open approach. (With permission from Mulholland MW, Lillemoe KD, Doherty GM, Maier RV, Upchurch GR, eds. *Greenfield's Surgery.* 4th ed. Philadelphia, PA: Lippincott Williams & Wilkins; 2005.)

Hernia sac reflecting onto cecum

Sliding Inguinal Hernia
- Visceral peritoneum of various organs comprises part of the wall of the hernia sac
- Common organs involved include the cecum, sigmoid colon, bladder, ovary, and fallopian tube
- Most sliding hernias are indirect hernias

A 43-year-old man presents with a persistently swollen and tender right testicle. Six weeks ago, he underwent a plug and patch repair of a large right indirect inguinoscrotal hernia. What is the most likely diagnosis?

Ischemic orchitis.

Testicular Atrophy after Hernia Repair
- Injury to the pampiniform venous plexus can cause venous thrombosis
- The resultant ischemic orchitis can cause testicular atrophy
- This complication is associated with the dissection of the indirect hernia sac distal to the pubic tubercle
- Orchiectomy is rarely necessary

A 51-year-old man presents with pain and numbness in the left upper lateral thigh after laparoscopic repair of a direct left inguinal hernia. What is the most likely diagnosis?

A tack injury to the lateral femoral cutaneous nerve.

Nerve Anatomy of the Groin

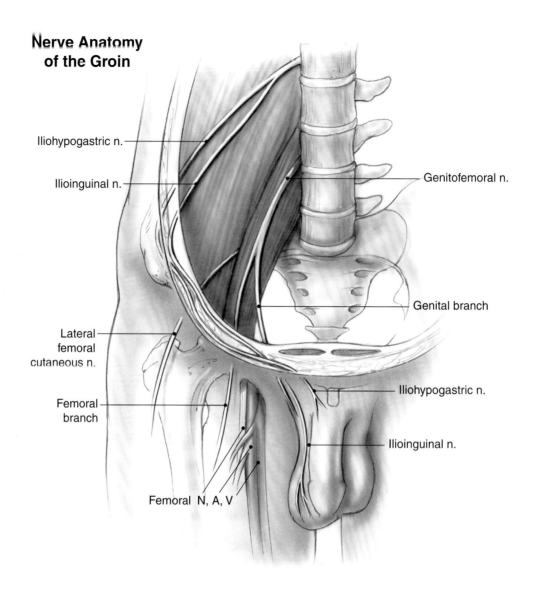

Iliohypogastric n.

Ilioinguinal n.

Genitofemoral n.

Genital branch

Lateral femoral cutaneous n.

Femoral branch

Iliohypogastric n.

Ilioinguinal n.

Femoral N, A, V

Nerve Injury Following Hernia Repair

- Common entrapment injuries during open repair include:
  - *Iliohypogastric nerve* (T12, L1)
    - Results in loss of sensation to the inguinal region and lower abdomen
  - *Ilioinguinal nerve* (most common) (L1)
    - Results in pain/numbness on ipsilateral side of penis, scrotum and inner thigh
    - Loss of cremasteric reflex
    - Need to watch for this nerve on top of the cord
  - Genital branch of *genitofemoral nerve* (L1, L2)
- *Lateral femoral cutaneous nerve* injury (L2, L3)
  - More likely with laparoscopic hernia repair
- Treatment is rest, analgesia, and infiltration/nerve block
- After one year of conservative measures, a nerve release, neurectomy, or laparoscopic removal of tacks may be indicated

Preperitoneal Space Danger Zones

- "Triangle of pain"
  - Delineated by the testicular vessels and iliopubic tract
  - Contains the femoral branch of the genitofemoral nerve, the femoral nerve, and the lateral femoral cutaneous nerve
- "Triangle of doom"
  - Delineated by the testicular vessels and vas deferens (apex at internal ring)
  - Contains the iliac artery, vein, and genitofemoral nerve

Osteitis of the Pubic Bone

- Point tenderness medial to incision and pain radiating to the base of the penis
- Caused by suturing/anchoring mesh into public tubercle
- Treated with NSAIDS, local injections, and observation

A 49-year-old man presents with a recurrent left inguinal hernia 1 year after a Liechtenstein hernia repair. The recurrent hernia is most likely to be what type of hernia?

Most recurrent inguinal hernias that develop after open anterior repair are direct hernias. A posterior preperitoneal approach (such as laparoscopic repair) is preferred to repair such hernias.

Recurrence of an Inguinal Hernia

- The incidence of recurrent hernia following a tension-free repair varies from 0.5% to 2%
- Recurrence of an indirect hernia in females is extremely unusual
- Repair of recurrent hernias is best achieved using a different approach from the initial repair to avoid areas of previous scarring and potential nerve injury
- In children, the recurrence rate for a standard sac ligation repair is 0.1%

A 92-year-old, thin, female nursing home resident presents with small bowel obstruction. What type of hernia should be suspected?

An obturator hernia is more common among elderly thin women.

Obturator Hernia

- Almost always on the right side
- Frequently presents with complete or partial small bowel obstruction (50% of cases)
- *Howship-Romberg sign* (50%) is obturator neuralgia upon extension, adduction, and medial rotation of the thigh
- A preoperative diagnosis is rare
- Explore and repair through a midline or supra-inguinal transverse incision

A 1-year-old female infant is referred for a 1.5 cm umbilical hernia. What is the next step in management?

Expectant management should be pursued for umbilical hernias less than 2 cm in diameter in young children.

Umbilical Hernia in Infants

- Occurs in 10% to 30% of live births
- More common in African-American than Caucasian infants
- Incarceration is rare
- If less than 2 cm in size, frequently close spontaneously; closure and repair should be delayed until approximately 4 years of age
- If larger than 2 cm, repair should be performed at the time of diagnosis

---

A 64-year-old woman with no history of prior abdominal surgery presents with a small reducible bulge in the right lower quadrant. A hernia defect cannot be clearly appreciated on physical exam. What is the most likely diagnosis?

Spigelian hernias occur at the lateral border of the rectus muscle.

Spigelian Hernia

- An abdominal wall hernia through transverse abdominis aponeurosis between the semilunar line (line of Douglas) and the lateral edge of the rectus muscle
- Nearly all occur below the arcuate (semicircular) line (the lower edge of the posterior rectus sheath, 3 to 6 cm below the level of the umbilicus)
- Ultrasound (and CT scan) can be used to verify the diagnosis
- Laparoscopy can occasionally be used in suspicious cases to diagnose and treat these hernias

Posterior View of Anterior Abdominal Wall

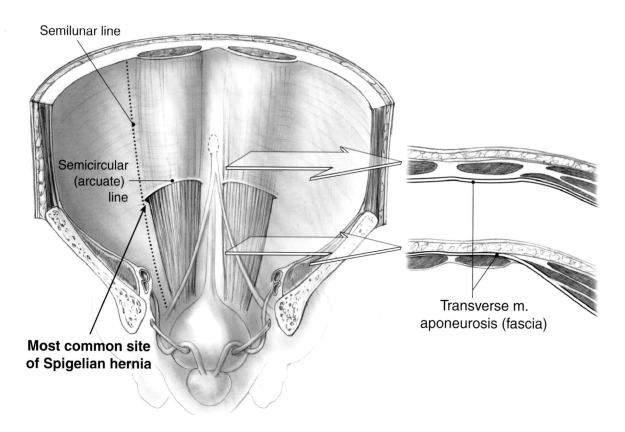

Semilunar line

Semicircular (arcuate) line

Most common site of Spigelian hernia

Transverse m. aponeurosis (fascia)

Spigelian hernias are usually small and interparietal; a fascial defect is often difficult to detect on exam because it is covered by the intact external oblique aponeurosis.

A 25-year-old woman presents with a bulge in her back below the 12th rib. What is the next step in management?

A lumbar hernia can occur through the superior lumbar triangle delineated by the 12th rib, internal oblique, and sacrospinalis muscle. Operative repair is indicated.

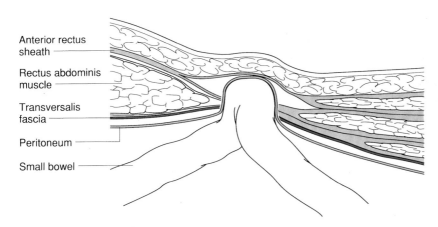

Anterior rectus sheath

Rectus abdominis muscle

Transversalis fascia

Peritoneum

Small bowel

Richter hernia. (With permission from Mulholland MW, Lillemoe KD, Doherty GM, Maier RV, Upchurch GR, eds. *Greenfield's Surgery.* 4th ed. Philadelphia, PA: Lippincott Williams & Wilkins; 2005.)

Named Hernias

Name	Description
Richter	Non-circumferential incarceration of bowel wall—can cause perforation without obstruction
Littre	Incarcerated hernia containing Meckel diverticulum
Grynfeltt	Through the superior lumbar triangle: 12th rib, internal oblique, and sacrospinalis
Petit	Through inferior lumbar triangle: Latissimus dorsi, external oblique, iliac crest
Petersen	Behind a Roux-limb; space between Roux-limb mesentery, transverse mesocolon, and retroperitoneum
Amyand	Acute appendicitis in an incarcerated inguinal hernia

A 54-year-old woman is admitted with an erythematous, non-reducible bulge at the site of a prior hysterectomy scar. She also has a fever, emesis, and abdominal distension. What is the most likely diagnosis?

Strangulated incisional hernia. Skin findings of infection (erythema, ulceration, and tenderness) are ominous signs of strangulation (ischemia).

Incisional Hernia

- Occurs after 10% to 15% of open abdominal operations
- The most common risk factor is the presence of a wound infection

> A 59-year-old multiparous woman presents with protrusion of a large mass through the perineum that is worsened by sitting or standing. What is the most likely diagnosis?

A perineal hernia is a very uncommon hernia that occurs when a hernia sac protrudes through the pelvic diaphragm.

Perineal Hernia

- Caused by congenital or acquired defects after abdominoperineal resection or perineal prostatectomy
- A bulge can be detected on bimanual rectal-vaginal examination
- Generally repaired through a transabdominal approach or a combined transabdominal and perineal approach

Sciatic Hernia

- Usual symptom is enlarging tender mass in the gluteal area ± bowel sounds
- Sciatic neuropathy and intestinal or ureteral obstruction may occur
- Can occur through the greater sciatic foramen, either above or below the piriformis, or through the lesser sciatic foramen

> A 65-year-old man undergoes an emergent sigmoidectomy with an end-colostomy. One year later, the patient presents with a large reducible bulge in the area of the colostomy. What is the most likely cause of this complication and what could have been done to prevent it?

Ostomies should be brought through the rectus muscle to prevent the development of a parastomal hernia.

Ostomy Brought Out Through Rectus Muscle

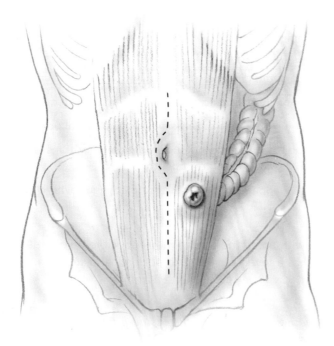

Reduces risk of parastomal hernia

25 | Surgical Oncology

Eric K. Nakakura

A 60-year-old woman has a 4 cm low-grade lower extremity soft tissue sarcoma with regional lymph node metastasis. What is the stage of her disease?

Stage III.

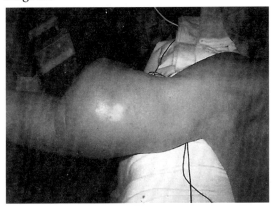

Large high-grade malignant histiocytoma. (With permission from Mulholland MW, Lillemoe KD, Doherty GM, Maier RV, Upchurch GR, eds. *Greenfield's Surgery*. 4th ed. Philadelphia, PA: Lippincott Williams & Wilkins; 2005.)

Soft Tissue Sarcoma

- Presents as a painless mass, which can be fast-growing
- Spreads hematogenously
- Lung is the most common site of metastatic spread
- Tumor grade is an important prognostic feature
- Staging System
    - Primary tumor
        - T1 ≤5 cm
        - T2 >5 cm (a: superficial, b: deep)
    - Regional lymph nodes (N0: none, N1: present)
    - Distant metastasis (M0: none, M1: present)
    - Histologic grade (G)
        - G1: Low-grade
        - G2: Intermediate grade
        - G3: High-grade
    - Stage grouping

Stage IA	T1a	N0	M0	G1,GX	
		T1b	N0	M0	G1,GX
Stage IB	T2a	N0	M0	G1,GX	
		T2b	N0	M0	G1,GX
Stage IIA	T1a	N0	M0	G2,G3	
		T1b	N0	M0	G2
Stage IIB	T2a	N0	M0	G2	
		T2b	N0	M0	G2
Stage III	T2a,b	N0	M0	G3	
		Any T	N1	M0	Any G
Stage IV	Any T	Any N	M1	Any G	

Characteristics of Benign and Malignant Soft Tissue Sarcomas

Feature	Benign	Malignant
Size	Small, well-circumscribed	Large, infiltrative
Location	Superficial, cutaneous	Deep, intramuscular
Cellularity	Slight to moderate	Moderate to marked
Cohesion	Cohesive	Discohesive, single cells
Nuclei	Uniform, vesicular chromatin	Pleomorphic, coarse chromatin
Necrosis	Absent	Present

Reprinted with permission from Kilpatrick SE, Geisinger KR. Soft tissue sarcomas: The usefulness and limitations of fine-needle aspiration biopsy. *Am J Clin Pathol.* 1998;110(1):50–68.

Grade is an important factor in predicting the outcome of soft tissue sarcomas and, unlike most other cancers, it is a part of the AJCC staging system. Less than 10% of adult soft tissue sarcoma patients exhibit lymph node metastasis.

A 50-year-old man has a 4 cm high-grade soft tissue sarcoma of the upper extremity that is completely excised with negative margins. Postoperatively, what adjuvant therapy is required?

There is no role for adjuvant therapy in this case.

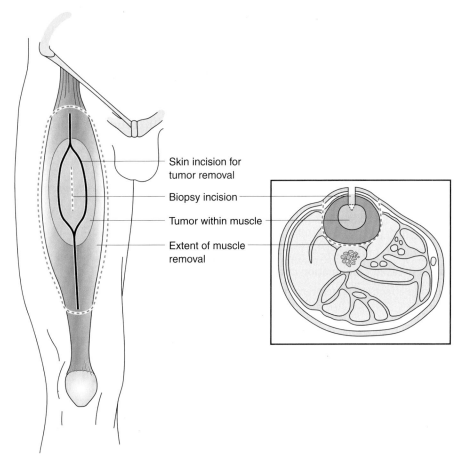

Skin incision for tumor removal

Biopsy incision

Tumor within muscle

Extent of muscle removal

Wide local excision for sarcoma. (With permission from Mulholland MW, Lillemoe KD, Doherty GM, Maier RV, Upchurch GR, eds. *Greenfield's Surgery*. 4th ed. Philadelphia, PA: Lippincott Williams & Wilkins; 2005.)

Treatment of Extremity or Trunk Soft Tissue Sarcoma

- Tumor <5 cm (low- or high-grade)
  - Complete excision with negative margins
- Tumor >5 cm (low-grade)
  - Complete excision and post-operative external beam radiotherapy (EBRT)
- Tumor >5 cm (high-grade)
  - Complete excision, brachytherapy (BRT), or post-operative EBRT
- Tumor >10 cm (high-grade)
  - Possible pre-operative chemotherapy, complete excision, and BRT or post-operative EBRT
- Chemotherapy is anthracycline (doxorubicin or epirubicin) and/or ifosfamide-based
- When possible resections should have a wide margin, preserving function
- Isolated metastases might be resected after multidisciplinary discussion

For primary extremity sarcomas, 5-year disease specific survival for low- and high-grade lesions is 95% and 66%, respectively.

A 55-year-old man with a metastatic gastrointestinal stromal tumor (GIST) is treated with Gleevec. What is the mechanism of action of Gleevec?

Gleevec is an oral tyrosine kinase inhibitor.

Gleevec (Imatinib mesylate, STI571)

- Inhibits c kit, platelet derived growth factor receptor, and Bcr-Abl receptor tyrosine kinases
- Approved for the treatment of GIST and chronic myelogenous leukemia

> A 65-year-old man with metastatic colon cancer receives treatment consisting of IV fluorouracil, leucovorin (folinic acid), and oxaliplatin (FOLFOX) together with avastin. What is the mechanism of action of avastin?

Avastin is a monoclonal antibody targeting vascular endothelial growth factor, which stimulates angiogenesis.

Avastin (Bevacizumab)

- Approved by the FDA for first-line treatment of metastatic colorectal cancer together with any fluorouracil-based combination chemotherapy regimen
- Serious side effects: GI perforation, wound dehiscence, arterial thromboembolism

> A 65-year-old woman with metastatic rectal cancer has evidence of disease progression during treatment with an irinotecan based regimen. What might be a reasonable next step in management?

Erbitux and irinotecan.

Erbitux (Cetuximab)

- A monoclonal antibody against epidermal growth factor receptor
- Approved by the FDA for metastatic colorectal cancer refractory to irinotecan-based chemotherapy

Irinotecan

- Inhibits topoisomerase I (an enzyme involved in DNA repair)

Fluorouracil

- Inhibits thymidylate synthase (a key enzyme of pyrimidine de novo synthesis/DNA synthesis)

Leucovorin

- Enhances inhibition of thymidylate synthase inhibition by fluorouracil

Oxaliplatin

- Forms adducts with DNA
- Frequently causes a sensory peripheral neuropathy

> A 40-year-old woman receives systemic adjuvant chemotherapy consisting of doxorubicin and cyclophosphamide (AC) for invasive breast cancer. What are the potential toxicities of this regimen?

Adriamycin (doxorubicin) is cardiotoxic and cyclophosphamide can cause hemorrhagic cystitis.

A 40-year-old woman with invasive breast cancer undergoes lumpectomy with breast irradiation. How is ionizing radiation believed to cause cells to lose their reproductive integrity?

Radiation is thought to act directly by targeting the DNA of dividing cells and indirectly with water to produce free radicals. Oxygen, the most important modifier of ionizing radiation, favors the formation of free radicals.

A 55-year-old man with colon cancer and a presumed isolated metastasis to the liver undergoes positron emission tomography (PET) to rule out additional sites of metastatic disease. What is the mechanism of PET scanning?

PET scanning is based on detecting glucose metabolism of neoplastic cells.

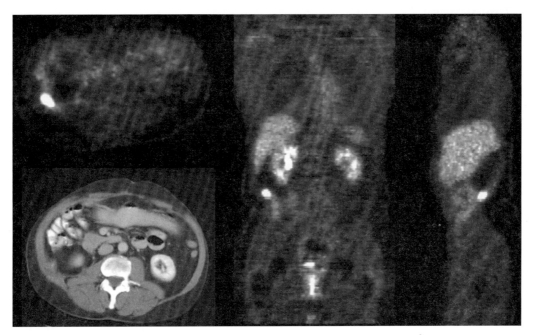

Positron emission tomography (PET) scan of a patient with recurrent colon cancer. (With permission from Mulholland MW, Lillemoe KD, Doherty GM, Maier RV, Upchurch GR, eds. *Greenfield's Surgery.* 4th ed. Philadelphia, PA: Lippincott Williams & Wilkins; 2005.)

Positron Emission Tomography

- A sensitive test for metastatic disease for some cancers
- Neoplastic cells exhibit accelerated glycolysis compared to normal cells
- Fluorodeoxyglucose (FDG) competes with glucose for uptake into cancer cells and remains trapped within them
- FDG-PET is a functional imaging technique

A 70-year-old man is diagnosed with adenocarcinoma of the pancreas. What is the most frequently mutated gene in pancreatic cancer?

Pancreatic cancer is most commonly associated with activating mutations of K-ras.

K-ras Mutation

- Mutated in more than 90% of conventional pancreatic cancers
- This is the highest prevalence of K-ras mutations in any tumor type
- Point mutations convert this proto-oncogene into an oncogene

p53 Mutation

- In response to DNA damage, p53 normally functions to arrest the cell before the G1/S transition, allowing DNA repair or apoptosis to occur
- In cells with inactivation of p53, G1 arrest does not occur and damaged DNA is replicated

Inactivation of p53 is the most common genetic event in human malignancy.

What are the common proto-oncogenes and what are their associated tumor types?

Proto-oncogenes

- K-ras
  - 12p
  - Soft tissue sarcomas, pancreatic and biliary cancer
- RET
  - 10q
  - MEN-2, medullary thyroid cancer
- c-myc
  - 8q
  - Breast, colon, cervical, and small cell carcinomas
- HER2/neu
  - 17q
  - Breast cancer, ovarian, gastric and oral cancers

What are the common tumor suppressor genes and what are their associated tumor types?

Tumor Suppressor Genes

- p53
  - 17p
  - Li-Fraumeni syndrome, sarcoma, breast cancer
- BRCA-1
  - 17q
  - Breast cancer, ovarian cancer
- BRCA-2
  - 13q
  - Breast cancer (male/female), pancreatic cancer, prostate cancer
- APC
  - 5q
  - FAP

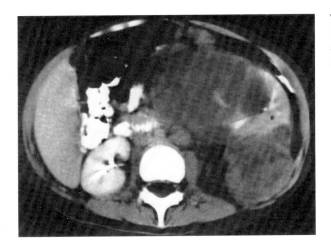

Wilms tumor. (With permission from Mulholland MW, Lillemoe KD, Doherty GM, Maier RV, Upchurch GR, eds. *Greenfield's Surgery*. 4th ed. Philadelphia, PA: Lippincott Williams & Wilkins; 2005.)

- WT1
  - 11p
  - Wilms tumor
- MENIN
  - 11q
  - MEN-1
- STK11
  - 19p
  - Peutz-Jeghers syndrome
- PTEN
  - 10q
  - Cowden syndrome
- VHL
  - 3p
  - von Hippel Lindau
- CDKN2
  - 9p
  - Familial atypical multiple mole melanoma syndrome, pancreatic cancer

What is the significance of the Deleted in Colorectal Cancer (DCC) gene in colorectal cancer patients?

Absence of DCC identifies a subgroup of patients who have stage II colorectal cancers with survival rates similar to stage III patients.

Deleted in Colorectal Cancer Gene

- Putative tumor suppressor gene on chromosome 18q
- May induce apoptosis in normal cells

A 30-year-old male presents for a screening colonoscopy. His father died of colorectal cancer when he was 40 and his brother recently had a colonoscopy with too many polyps to count. What is the genetic defect responsible for the family's mutation?

The patient has FAP and has a germline mutation in the APC gene.

APC Gene

- Tumor suppressor gene on chromosome 5q
- Inactivating mutations of the APC gene are present in over 80% of colorectal tumors

What selective COX-2 inhibitor is FDA-approved for management of patients with FAP in conjunction with endoscopic surveillance and surgery?

Celebrex (celecoxib).

COX-2 Gene

- Highly expressed in colorectal tumors
- COX-2 inhibition may work via restoration of apoptosis and inhibition of angiogenesis
- Celebrex reduces polyp number and polyp burden in patients with FAP

A 45-year-old female with a history of ER positive breast cancer status post mastectomy is placed on tamoxifen. Three months after starting the tamoxifen, she notes worsening right lower extremity swelling and pain. What are potentially serious complications of tamoxifen use?

DVT and PE are potential complications of tamoxifen use.

Complications of Tamoxifen

- Endometrial cancer
- Uterine sarcoma
- DVT/Pulmonary embolism
- Stroke
- Cataracts

A 65-year-old male with a history of colorectal cancer is status post right hemicolectomy. What tumor marker should be followed to monitor recurrence?

CEA.

Tumor Markers

Tumor	Cancer Marker
Pancreatic cancer	CA19-9
Colorectal cancer	CEA
HCC	α-fetoprotein
Prostate	PSA
Testicular cancer	hCG
Melanoma	Tyrosinase
HER2/neu	Breast cancer
Ovarian cancer	CA-125

26 | Melanoma

Sashank K. Reddy and Richard J. Redett

A 25-year-old female inquires about her risk factors for developing melanoma after her father was recently diagnosed with the disease. What are the risk factors for melanoma?

Multiple controllable and uncontrollable risk factors have been identified for melanoma, including personal and family history, skin color, presence of dysplastic nevi, and immune status.

Risk Factors for Melanoma

- Incidence of melanoma in Caucasians in the United States is approximately 25/100,000 annually in men and 17/100,000 in women
- Patients with light skin (Fitzpatrick type I), freckling, blue eyes, red hair are at higher risk for developing melanoma
- The risk of melanoma increases with the number of benign or atypical nevi
- The odds ratio of developing melanoma in patients with 100 or more nevi is 7.7 compared with patients with 0 to 4 nevi
- 10% of patients with melanoma have a family member with melanoma
- A history of five or more severe sunburns in childhood doubles melanoma risk
- A prior melanoma increases the risk of developing a second melanoma by 8.5 fold
- A prior non-melanoma skin cancer increases the risk of developing a melanoma skin cancer by approximately threefold
- Patients with compromised immune systems are at higher risk for developing melanoma
- Genetic causes predisposing to melanoma
  - Xeroderma pigmentosum
  - Tenfold increased risk of melanoma in patients with mutations in cell cycle regulatory genes CDKN2A or CDK4
  - Familial atypical multiple mole syndrome—almost 100% risk of melanoma
    - Also associated with increased risk of pancreatic cancer

Patients at higher risk for melanoma are those with a history of melanoma, two or more relatives with melanoma, lighter skin, dysplastic nevi, history of blistering sunburn as a child, and immune compromise.

A mother brings in her 4-year-old son with an 8-cm congenital nevus and inquires about any risk of malignancy. What is the appropriate response?

The child has a risk of developing malignancy. Based on size, congenital nevi may progress to invasive melanoma.

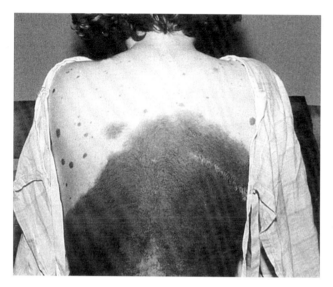

Large congenital nevus. (With permission from Mulholland MW, Lillemoe KD, Doherty GM, Maier RV, Upchurch GR, eds. *Greenfield's Surgery.* 4th ed. Philadelphia, PA: Lippincott Williams & Wilkins; 2005.)

Congenital Nevi

- 1% of children are born with congenital nevi
- Lifetime risk of progression from congenital nevus to melanoma is dependent on the lesion's size
- Classified as small <1.5 cm, medium-sized 1.5 to 20 cm, and large >20 cm
- Lesions <1.5 cm have a less than 1% chance of progressing to melanoma
- Lesions >20 cm have a 4.5% to 10% lifetime risk of progressing to melanoma
- Many of these will develop into melanoma in the first few years of life and therefore early excision is warranted

There is a spectrum of management strategies for congenital nevi based on size: large lesions (greater than 20 cm) should be excised early in life, while small lesions (less than 1.5 cm in size) have a minimal chance of progression and should be carefully observed.

A 45-year-old male has a 1.5-mm-thick melanoma on his right arm, without any axillary lymphadenopathy or abnormalities on chest X-ray. His liver function tests are normal. CT scans of the abdomen and pelvis are obtained and are negative for any distant metastases. What is this patient's TNM classification?

This patient's lesion has an American Joint Committee on Cancer (AJCC) TNM classification of T2, N0, M0.

Melanoma TNM Classification

- Based on the American Joint Committee on Cancer (AJCC) classification
- **Tumor (T)**

- T1 = Depth of 1 mm or less
  - For T1 lesions, T status is further designated "a" or "b" based on $<$ or $\geq$ 1 mitosis/mm^2
- T2 = 1 to 2 mm
- T3 = 2 to 4 mm
- T4 = >4 mm
- For all lesions, T status is further designated "a" or "b" based on ulcerated or non-ulcerated
- **Node (N)**
  - N0 = No affected nodes
  - N1 = One affected node
    - T status is further designated "a" or "b" based on micro- or macrometastases
  - N2 = Two or three nodes or in-transit lesion with negative LNs
    - T status is further designated "a," "b," or "c" based on micro- or macrometastases, or in-transit lesion with negative LNs
  - N3 = Four or more nodes; matted LNs or in-transit lesion with positive LNs
- **Metastasis (M)**
  - M0 = No metastases
  - M1a = Distant skin or distant lymph node metastases
  - M1b = Any lung metastases
  - M1c = All other visceral metastases or distant metastases, or any patient with any metastases with an elevated LDH
- Further subdivisions exist based on metastasis size

A 50-year-old male with a 2-mm-thick melanoma on his leg has two enlarged inguinal lymph nodes. A chest X-ray is normal. What is his clinical stage?

This patient's lesion has an American Joint Committee on Cancer (AJCC) TNM classification of T2, N2, M0, which is classified as clinical stage III.

Melanoma Staging

- Based on TNM classification of disease
- Staging should be used following complete excision of the primary melanoma and clinical and radiologic evaluation for metastases
  - Stage 0: in situ disease only
  - Stage I: T1 or T2; no nodal disease
  - Stage II: T2 with ulceration, or T3 or T4; no nodal disease
  - Stage III: Any nodal disease
  - Stage IV: Any metastatic disease
- All stage II tumors need sentinel lymph node biopsy
- All stage III tumors need full LN dissection
- Need to include superficial parotidectomy for anterior H&N melanomas

Nodal disease is stage III and any metastatic disease is stage IV.

Yes. The Breslow scale is based on tumor depth in millimeter and is simple and frequently used, especially for prognosis. The Clark system is based on histologic depth of invasion of the tumor, although its use is more historic.

Other Pathologic Classifications for Melanoma

- Breslow Thickness Scale
  - <0.75 mm
  - >0.75 to 1.5 mm
  - >1.5 to 4.0 mm
  - >4.0 mm
- The Breslow system uses melanoma depth as the sole criteria of melanoma. The second and third levels of thickness are grouped together for treatment purposes
- Clark classification
  - Level I: In situ (epidermis only)
  - Level II: Penetrates papillary dermis
  - Level III: Reaches papillary-reticular dermis border
  - Level IV: Penetrates reticular dermis
  - Level V: Into subcutaneous tissue

A 50-year-old man presents with a new diagnosis of melanoma. What does the workup of this patient entail, and what are the different types of melanoma?

The initial workup of a patient with melanoma should begin with a search for metastatic disease. Melanoma is generally divided into four main types: Superficial spreading, nodular, lentigo maligna, and acral lentiginous.

Evaluation and Categories of Melanoma

- Excisional biopsy of the lesion, with a narrow 1- to 2-mm margin of adjacent normal-appearing skin is recommended
- An incisional biopsy may be acceptable for larger lesions
- The initial workup includes a careful exam looking for other lesions
- The most common location is the trunk (in men) and legs (in women)
- Additional staging using a chest X-ray, liver function tests, and a CT scan of the abdomen and pelvis should be performed in patients with a positive sentinel node or with clinically evident nodal disease
- CT scans of the brain and chest should be obtained if distant disease is suspected
- In decreasing frequency, the most common sites of metastases are skin > lung > liver > brain > bone

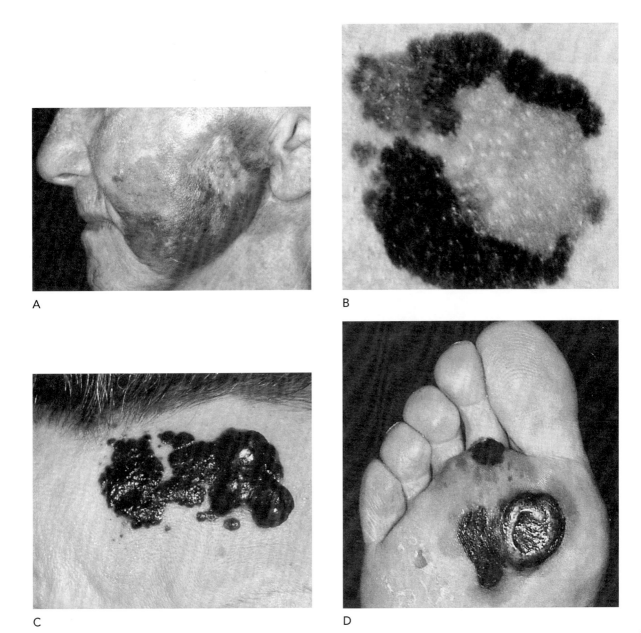

Types of melanoma: (A) lentigomaligna; (B) superficial spreading; (C) nodular; and (D) acral lentiginous. (With permission from Mulholland MW, Lillemoe KD, Doherty GM, Maier RV, Upchurch GR, eds. *Greenfield's Surgery*. 4th ed. Philadelphia, PA: Lippincott Williams & Wilkins; 2005.)

Types of Melanoma

- **Superficial spreading melanoma** (60%)
  - Initial radial growth followed by a vertical phase
  - Least aggressive
- **Nodular melanoma** (15%)
  - Aggressive due to a characteristic rapid vertical phase
  - Most likely to have metastases at the time of diagnosis
  - May present with a blue toned nodule

- **Lentigomaligna melanoma** (10%)
  - Found often in sun-exposed regions in elderly patients (can arise from Hutchinson freckle)
  - Decreased propensity for metastatic spread
- **Acral lentiginous melanoma** (rare)
  - Aggressive type with a poor prognosis
  - May appear as a pink or red nodule (amelanotic melanoma)
  - Often found on palms, soles, and nail beds (subungual)
  - More commonly affects dark-skinned populations

Nodular melanoma is the type most frequently associated with early metastases at the time of diagnosis.

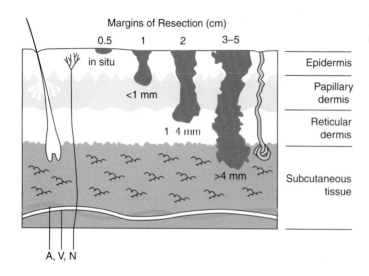

Melanoma invasion and recommended margins for resection.

Treatment of Melanoma

- Wide excision is the treatment of choice
  - 1 cm margins for lesions <1 mm
  - 1 to 2 cm margins for lesions 1 to 2 mm
  - 2 cm margins for lesions 2 to 4 mm
  - 2 to 3 cm margins for lesions >4 mm
- Sentinel node biopsy is the standard of care for all localized tumors >1 mm deep or > 0.75 mm with high-risk characters such as ulceration, mitotic rate $\geq 1/mm^2$, and Clark level IV/V (without clinically positive nodes)
- Nodal status is the most powerful predictor of survival
- Positive sentinel node requires completion lymph node dissection
- Clinically positive lymph nodes require a completion lymph node dissection
- There is no role for Mohs surgery in the management of melanoma
- Interferon has been shown to increase 5-year survival (from 36% to 47%) in node positive, stage III disease
- Toxicities of interferon are neurologic and hematologic
- High-dose interleukin 2 for metastatic melanoma and achieves durable responses (in 16% of patients)
- Ipilimumab (anti-CTLA-4 mAB) and Vemurafenib (BRAF inhibitor) for surgically refractory or metastatic melanoma

A 32-year-old golfer presents with melanoma of the nail bed. What is the treatment of choice for his disease?

Subungual melanoma has a poor prognosis and should be treated with amputation at the proximal interphalangeal (PIP) joint.

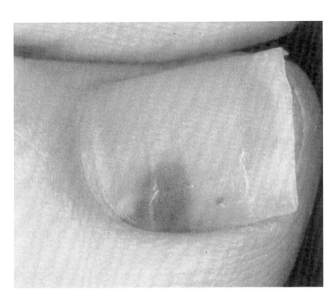

Subungual melanoma. (With permission from Mulholland MW, Lillemoe KD, Doherty GM, Maier RV, Upchurch GR, eds. *Greenfield's Surgery.* 4th ed. Philadelphia, PA: Lippincott Williams & Wilkins; 2005.)

Melanoma of the Fingers and Toes

- Carries a poor prognosis
- The first toe is the most common site
- No role for a sentinel node biopsy
- Often requires an amputation one phalanx proximal to the melanoma

A 53-year-old man has a T3, N0, M0 melanoma in the preauricular region. No cervical lymphadenopathy is found. What is the most appropriate management?

Management for this patient includes wide local excision with superficial parotidectomy, and sentinel lymph node biopsy.

Melanoma of the Head and Neck

- Melanomas are approximately 3.5 times more likely to occur in the face than in the non-head and neck skin
- The above patient has a stage II melanoma with no cervical lymphadenopathy
- Positive sentinel lymph nodes are found in between 10% and 21% of patients with head and neck melanoma
- Neck dissection is indicated in patients with stage II disease and positive nodal metastases detected on sentinel lymph node biopsy

Micrometastases to the lymph nodes will occur in 30% to 40% of patients with intermediate-thickness melanoma of the head and neck. Sentinel lymph node biopsy is indicated and, if positive, should be followed by a formal neck dissection.

A patient presents with a biopsy-proven 2.8-mm deep melanoma on his right arm and no palpable lymphadenopathy. What margin do you recommend to the patient for wide local excision?

The tumor should be excised with a 2-cm margin on all sides; this patient should also be offered sentinel lymph node biopsy.

27 | Non-melanoma Skin Cancer

Sashank K. Reddy and Richard J. Redett

A 42-year-old woman presents with a lesion on the helix of her right ear that is suspicious for squamous cell carcinoma (SCC). What are the risk factors for non-melanoma skin cancers?

Risk factors for non-melanoma skin cancers can be divided into host and environmental factors.

Risk Factors for Skin Cancer

- Host factors
  - A low melanin concentration in the skin (melanin protects against UV radiation)
  - Genetic disorders: Xeroderma pigmentosum, porokeratosis, nevoid basal cell syndrome, and albinism
  - Precursor lesions: Nevus sebaceous of Jadassohn, actinic keratoses, and cutaneous horns
- Environmental factors
  - UV-B is carcinogenic through direct photochemical damage to cutaneous DNA
  - UV-A potentiates the effects of UV-B
  - Ionizing radiation at high doses
  - Chemical carcinogens (polycyclic aromatic hydrocarbons, nitrogen mustard, chronic arsenic exposure, and psoralens)

A 58-year-old man presents with a 7-mm nodular basal cell carcinoma (BCC) on his forehead. What is the most appropriate management of this lesion?

The most appropriate treatment is surgical excision with a 5-mm margin.

Basal Cell Carcinoma

- BCC is the most common form of skin cancer
- Account for 80% of non-melanoma skin cancers
- Originates from epidermis—basal epithelial cells and hair follicles

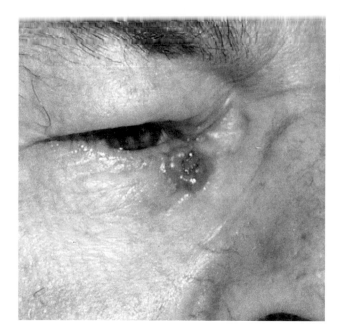

Basal cell carcinoma. (With permission from Mulholland MW, Lillemoe KD, Doherty GM, Maier RV, Upchurch GR, eds. *Greenfield's Surgery.* 4th ed. Philadelphia, PA: Lippincott Williams & Wilkins; 2005.)

- Risk factors
  - Blond or red hair, blue or green eyes, fair skin, ultraviolet light exposure, smoking, immunosuppression, and exposure to ionizing radiation, coal tar, and arsenic
- Genetic factors that predispose to BCC
  - Xeroderma pigmentosum
  - Nevoid BCC syndrome (Gorlin syndrome)
  - Bazex syndrome
  - Rombo syndrome
  - Albinism
- Hyperactivation of the sonic hedgehog (SHH) pathway is commonly found in BCC. Loss of function mutations in the SHH inhibitor patched homolog 1 (PTCH1) have been implicated in familial and sporadic BCC.
- p53 mutation in 50% of sporadic BCCs
- Can occur anywhere on the body but 80% occur on the head and neck, particularly on the nose
- BCCs grow slowly and less than 1% metastasize
- The classic lesion—nodular BCC—presents as a slow-growing, translucent, elevated nodule
- Other variants include sclerosing, superficial, and ulcerating

Treatment of Basal Cell Carcinoma

- Management options include surgical resection, Mohs surgery, electrodessication and curettage, cryotherapy, radiotherapy, laser phototherapy, and topical agents
  - Electrodessication, cryosurgery, and laser phototherapy are destructive and do not permit pathologic review
- Mohs micrographic surgery is the treatment of choice for high-risk lesions and for many facial BCCs
- Electrodissection and curettage are the treatment of choice for small (<2 mm) lesions with 5-year cure rates of 95%

- Surgical excision of superficial and nodular BCC can have 5-year cure rates of 99% for lesions on the trunk and 92% or greater for lesions on the face depending on size
- Radiotherapy can be used in poor surgical candidates or for tumors in areas that are difficult to excise
- Topical imiquimod is FDA approved for small (<2 cm) superficial BCCs that are not on the head
- Vismodegib, a hedgehog pathway inhibitor, has been FDA approved for metastatic BCC or BCC otherwise refractory to surgery or radiation

BCC is the most common cancer of the body, and is characterized by a pearly white lesion with a rolled border and underlying telangiectasia. These lesions rarely metastasize, but can be locally aggressive and have a predilection for local recurrence.

A 50-year-old man presents with a 2.5 × 1.5 cm SCC of the lip, with pain in the distribution of the right mental nerve. The patient has a 2.0-cm palpable node in his right neck. Radiographic workup is negative for metastatic disease. What is the next step in management?

This patient has pain in the distribution of the mental nerve, suggesting invasion of adjacent structures. A local excision should be performed with a regional lymphadenectomy.

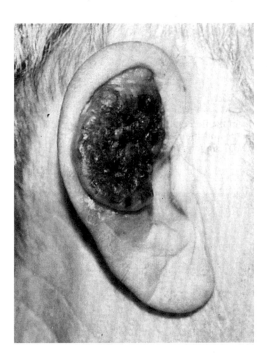

Squamous cell carcinoma. (With permission from Mulholland MW, Lillemoe KD, Doherty GM, Maier RV, Upchurch GR, eds. *Greenfield's Surgery.* 4th ed. Philadelphia, PA: Lippincott Williams & Wilkins; 2005.)

Squamous Cell Carcinoma

- Second most common non-melanoma skin cancer accounting for 15% to 20%
- Most commonly found on the head and neck
  - Head and neck (especially lower lip) lesions are common in men and lower leg lesions in women
- Presents as papules, plaques, or nodules with hyperkeratosis or ulceration
- Central ulceration is typical of poorly differentiated SCCs

- Grows faster than BCCs and can metastasize
- The risk of SCC seems to correlate with cumulative sun exposure as opposed to BCC and melanoma, which correlate more with episodic exposure to intense sunlight
- Risk factors
  - UVB exposure is the major risk factor; UVA also plays a role
  - Ionizing radiation exposure
  - Immunosuppression
  - Actinic keratosis
  - Human papillomavirus infection
  - Burns—SCC arising in a burn wound is known as Marjolin ulcer
  - Chronic, non-healing wounds
  - Genetic predisposition—Xeroderma pigmentosum, epidermolysis bullosa, albinism
- Mutations in p53 are common
- Bowen disease—SCC in situ
  - 10% turn into invasive SCC
  - Treatment: Excision with negative margins
- Erythroplasia of Queyrat—SCC of the penis
  - Red, velvety plaque
- Diagnosis
  - Biopsy—punch, shave, or excisional
  - Pathology: Atypical keratinocytes with keratin pearls

Treatment of Squamous Cell Carcinoma

- Options include surgical resection, Mohs surgery, electrodessication and curettage, cryotherapy, radiotherapy, laser phototherapy, and topical agents
- Cryotherapy, electrodissection, and radiation are reserved for Bowen disease and superficial SCC
- Surgical excision is recommended for larger lesions or those extending into subcutaneous tissues
- Surgical excision can achieve a 5-year cure rate of 92% in primary SCCs
- Margins of 4 mm are recommended for small lesions without high-risk features, with larger margins required for larger, more concerning lesions
- Mohs surgery is recommended for high-risk SCCs, particularly in cosmetically sensitive areas
- Lymph node biopsy is indicated for patients with palpable disease

---

A 45-year-old woman presents with a lesion on her right arm that has grown rapidly over the period of 2 months. The lesion is plaque-like with central ulceration. Biopsy demonstrates a keratoacanthoma. How should this be managed?

Keratoacanthomas are benign lesions that are often mistaken for SCCs.

Keratoacanthoma

- Benign lesions with rapid growth
- Have rolled edges and are filled with keratin

- Are not malignant, but are easily mistaken with SCC due to their appearance
- Treatment
    - Often involute spontaneously over months
    - If small, can excise
    - If large, biopsy and observe

A 54-year-old man with a long history of an ulcerated burn scar presents with a non-healing wound at the margin of the scar. What is the most appropriate management?

The lesion should be biopsied to rule out Marjolin ulcer.

Marjolin Ulcer

- An SCC arising from a chronic wound, particularly a pressure sore, fistula, or burn scar
- The tumor generally begins at the margin of the wound and grows slowly over years
- Any suspicious mass should be biopsied
- Marjolin ulcers have a higher tendency to metastasize than other SCCs
- Treatment is a complete excision of the lesion and regional lymph node dissection if lymphadenopathy is present

An SCC arising within a chronic wound, also known as a Marjolin ulcer, requires surgery.

A 70-year-old man presents with a 2 cm × 3 cm flat lesion on his lower cheek that has a "stuck-on" appearance. He has had this lesion for many years, although when it first appeared 30 years ago it was much smaller and has gradually grown. On examination, he has multiple similar lesions across his body; he reports his father had similar lesions. What is the appropriate management of this lesion?

The lesion can be observed without intervention.

Seborrheic Keratosis

- Most common benign epithelial tumor
- Increased occurrence with advancing age
- Often hereditary
- Grow slowly over time, with a "stuck-on" appearance
- Frequently multiple lesions across the body
- No malignant potential
- In contrast, actinic keratoses (or solar keratosis) are pre-malignant lesions found in sun-damaged skin (0.1% to 16% per lesion per year incidence of progression to SCC)

A 65-year-old man presents with a 1-cm firm, pink mass on his cheek and a palpable cervical lymph node. The lesion is biopsied and reveals a Merkel cell carcinoma. What is the most appropriate management?

Surgical excision with a 3-cm margin should be performed with a superficial parotidectomy and ipsilateral neck dissection.

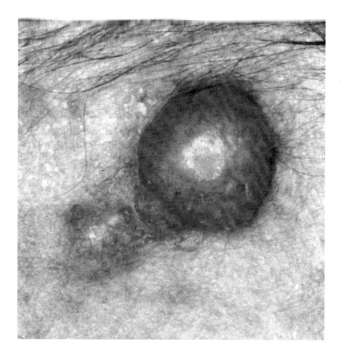

Merkel cell carcinoma. (With permission from Mulholland MW, Lillemoe KD, Doherty GM, Maier RV, Upchurch GR, eds. *Greenfield's Surgery*. 4th ed. Philadelphia, PA: Lippincott Williams & Wilkins; 2005.)

Merkel Cell Carcinoma

- Neuroendocrine lesion of the dermis
- Rare malignancy that arises in the dermis of elderly patients
- More commonly affects Caucasians and more common in men than women
- Associated with a virus Merkel cell polyoma virus in 75% of cases
- Locally aggressive and can extend into the subcutaneous tissue
- Diagnosis
  - Immunohistochemical staining for neuron-specific enolase and neurofilament protein
  - Histology reveals sheets of oval cells with indistinct borders that invade the deep dermis
- Wide local excisions are indicated
- Lymph node dissection is indicated for a palpable lymph node
- Five-year survival is 45% with localized disease, 25% with metastatic disease

Merkel cell carcinoma is a rare malignancy that requires aggressive resection.

A 25-year-old woman presents with a 1.5-cm firm, raised nodule on her left thigh that began as a plaque. A biopsy of the lesion is performed and confirms dermatofibrosarcoma protuberans. What is the next step in management?

Dermatofibrosarcoma should be treated like a true sarcoma. Apply general sarcoma principles to this disease and surgically excise with a wide 2- to 4-cm margin. Mohs can be applied to evaluate the margin at the time of surgery.

Dermatofibrosarcoma Protuberans

- A rare dermatologic form of fibrohistiocytic sarcoma
- Occurs mostly in young adults (20 to 40 years old)
- Local extension may be present (characteristic of sarcomas) and the lesion may extend beneath normal-appearing skin

- Excise with WIDE (2 to 4 cm) margins and consider Mohs to evaluate margins
- Recurrence common

Dermatofibrosarcoma protuberans is found in young adults and, like most sarcomas, it requires a wide excision and often recurs.

> A 30-year-old female presents with edema and swelling in her axilla. The area is also weeping serous fluid. What is the appropriate management?

Hidradenitis should be initially treated with antibiotics and improved hygiene.

Hidradenitis Suppurativa
- Caused by occlusion and abnormal epithelial cycling in follicular units
- Infections of the apocrine sweat glands may also be involved
- Usually occurs in the axilla or groin
- Cultures often fail to yield organisms; when lesions are superinfected, most common organisms are *Streptococcus* and *Staphylococcus*
- Treatment
  - Antibiotics and improved hygiene
  - Surgery may be necessary if disease is refractory to antibiotics
  - Infliximab has been shown to be effective for moderate to severe hidradenitis in clinical trials; data for other anti-tumor necrosis factor agents are less clear
  - Oral retinoids have also shown benefits

> A 42-year-old male presents with a painful, subungual blue nodule. The nodule is 7 mm and her symptoms are exacerbated by cold weather and washing her hands in cold water. What is the appropriate management?

The lesion is a Glomus tumor and should be excised either via nail bed or via a lateral approach if it is at the nail margin.

Glomus Tumor
- Presents as a painful, subungual blue nodule <1 cm
- Symptoms are exacerbated by cold
- Most often affects women between 30 and 50 years
- Treatment: Excision

> A 15-year-old male presents with a large red lesion on his neck and worsening fatigue and swelling in his lower extremities. How should this be managed?

Large hemangiomas that do not involute can lead to congestive heart failure (CHF) due to shunting of blood and should be embolized or surgically excised.

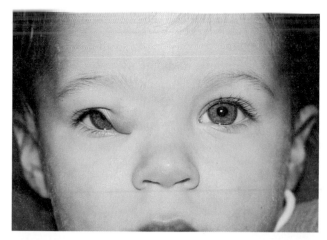

Hemangioma. (A) Hemangioma medial upper eyelid. The lesion impairs the visual access and should be treated to prevent long term vision problems. (B) Partially treated upper eyelid hemangioma. (With permission from Mulholland MW, Lillemoe KD, Doherty GM, Maier RV, Upchurch GR, eds. *Greenfield's Surgery*. 4th ed. Philadelphia, PA: Lippincott Williams & Wilkins; 2005.)

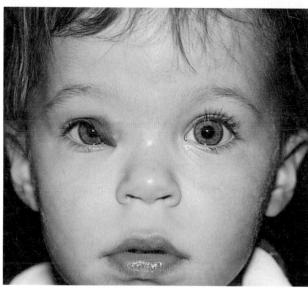

Hemangioma

- The most common tumor of infancy
- Are present at birth and usually spontaneously involute during first 2 years of age are usually not present at birth but may appear within a couple of weeks
- Types of hemangioma
  - Capillary—usually involute
  - Cavernous—less likely to involute
- Symptoms
  - Usually asymptomatic
  - Association with PHACE syndrome (posterior fossa brain anomalies, hemangioma, arterial lesions, cardiac anomalies, eye anomalies)
  - Kasabach-Merritt syndrome—consumptive coagulopathy → thrombocytopenia
    - Not associated with true hemangioma of infancy
    - More common with kaposiform hemangioendothelioma
  - CHF
  - Airway impairment (if large and in neck) and visual impairment if around orbit or in eyelid
  - Bleeding or ulcerations

- Treatment
  - Non-surgical: Intralesional steroid injections, systemic steroids
  - Interferon-alpha is a second-line treatment
  - Embolization
  - Laser or cryotherapy
  - Surgical excision or beta blockers

> A 53-year-old male with a history of ulcerative colitis (UC) presents with a necrotic ulcer on his leg with purple, edematous borders. What is the diagnosis and treatment?

Pyoderma gangrenosum, a skin condition associated with UC, is initially treated with systemic steroids and cyclosporine.

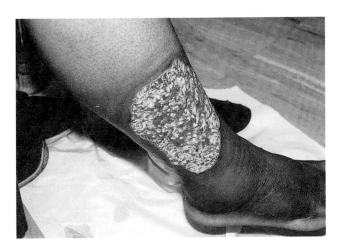

Pyoderma gangrenosum. (With permission from Mulholland MW, Lillemoe KD, Doherty GM, Maier RV, Upchurch GR, eds. *Greenfield's Surgery.* 4th ed. Philadelphia, PA: Lippincott Williams & Wilkins; 2005.)

Pyoderma Gangrenosum

- Presents with a rapidly enlarging necrotic ulcer with purple, edematous borders
- Usually in the lower extremities
- Associated with UC, ileitis, arthritis, leukemia, and lymphoma
- Treatment
  - Treat underlying disease if possible
    - If associated with UC, some patients respond to colectomy
  - Most can be treated medically with systemic steroids and cyclosporine
  - If large, may need surgical excision and skin graft although care should be taken as surgical trauma can worsen wound

28 | Breast Disease

Lisa Jacobs

During a simple mastectomy, what anatomic boundaries of the breast define the resection?

- Superior: Clavicle
- Inferior: Inframammary crease
- Medial: Sternum
- Lateral: Latissimus dorsi muscle
- Posterior: Fascia of the pectoralis major muscle

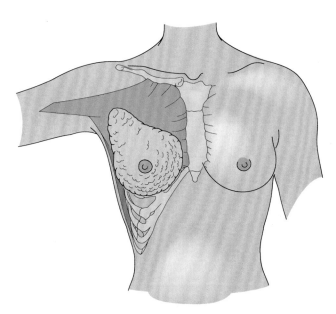

Boundaries of resection for a mastectomy. (With permission from Mulholland MW, Lillemoe KD, Doherty GM, Maier RV, Upchurch GR, eds. *Greenfield's Surgery.* 4th ed. Philadelphia, PA: Lippincott Williams & Wilkins; 2005.)

Internal Structure of the Breast

- There are 15 to 20 lobes of glandular tissue
- The lobes are interdigitated throughout the breast and drain into the lactiferous ducts and sinuses in the retroareolar area

459

- There is a retromammary bursa posterior to the breast tissue and anterior to the pectoralis major muscle fascia
- The subcutaneous fascia extends through the breast tissue to the skin overlying the breast and provides support to the breast (Cooper ligaments)

Polythelia and Polymastia

- The milk line extends from the axilla to the groin
- Polythelia is accessory nipples along the milk line
- Polymastia is accessory breast tissue along the milk line
- Amastia is the absence of one or both breasts
  - It is differentiated from Poland syndrome by the presence of the chest wall musculature in amastia (absent in Poland syndrome)

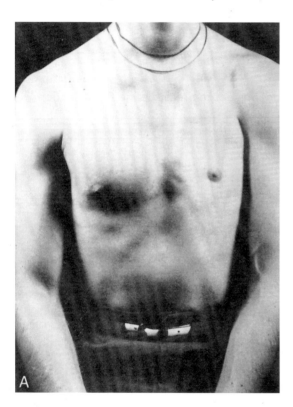
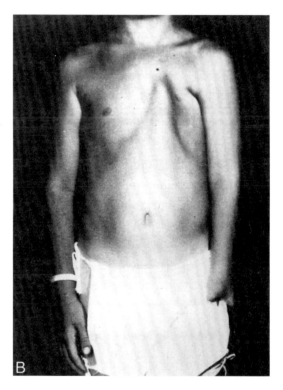
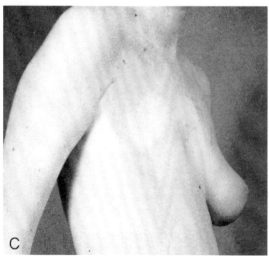

Poland syndrome. (With permission from Mulholland MW, Lillemoe KD, Doherty GM, Maier RV, Upchurch GR, eds. *Greenfield's Surgery*. 4th ed. Philadelphia, PA: Lippincott Williams & Wilkins; 2005.)

Poland Syndrome

- Absence of the musculature of the shoulder girdle (pectoralis major and pectoralis minor) and malformation of the ipsilateral upper limb
- Other findings may include partial absence of the external oblique and serratus anterior, hypoplasia or complete absence of the breast or nipple, costal cartilage and rib defects, hypoplasia of subcutaneous tissues of the chest wall, and brachysyndactyly
- Usually unilateral
- Higher incidence in females than males
- The most common component is breast hypoplasia

Breast Changes in Pregnancy

- Early in pregnancy, the breast increases in volume, which is associated with breast tenderness
- The terminal ductal lobular unit undergoes extensive hyperplasia and formation of new ductules
  - Occurs mostly in the first half of pregnancy
- The secretory activity of the breast is increased in the later months of pregnancy
- In the postpartum lactating female, the breast tissue is stimulated by prolactin and produces colostrum initially, followed by breast milk

---

A 25-year-old woman presents with a red painful area in her breast. She is 6 weeks postpartum and is breastfeeding. What is the most likely diagnosis?

Mastitis is the most likely diagnosis given the recent history of breastfeeding and the sign of a local infection (pain); however, it is important to consider a diagnosis of inflammatory breast cancer in any patient with breast redness (especially in the absence of signs or symptoms of infection).

Mastitis

- Most commonly occurs in the lactating female and results from an area of unexpressed milk that becomes secondarily infected
- Mastitis is treated with oral antibiotics and continuation of breastfeeding
- Warm compresses and breast massage can also be used to try to express the trapped milk
- Mastitis can proceed to become a breast abscess, which must be treated by drainage, either through repeated aspirations or incision and drainage
- The most common organisms of mastitis and breast abscess are *Staphylococcus aureus* (most common) and *Streptococcus* species
- If there are any systemic signs of infection, the patient should be started on antibiotics and a workup for inflammatory breast cancer should be initiated

If the diagnosis of breast abscess or mastitis is made, a full evaluation of the breast should be completed once the symptoms resolve.

A 40-year-old woman presents with severe pain in the lateral half of the breast. Physical examination reveals a painful cord. What are the most likely diagnosis and treatment?

Mondor disease is a superficial thrombophlebitis of the veins of the anterior thoracoabdominal wall (the lateral thoracic vein, the thoracoepigastric vein, or the superficial epigastric vein).

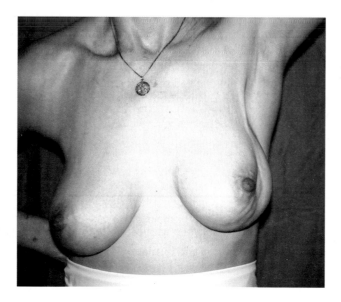

Mondor disease. (With permission from Mulholland MW, Lillemoe KD, Doherty GM, Maior RV, Upchurch GR, eds. *Greenfield's Surgery.* 4th ed. Philadelphia, PA: Lippincott Williams & Wilkins; 2005.)

Mondor Disease

- Most common at the lower outer quadrant of the breast
- May be associated with local inflammatory states, previous surgery, trauma, or strenuous exercise
- It is NOT associated with neoplasm
- If any suspicious mass is identified on physical examination, it should be biopsied
- Treat with nonsteroidal anti-inflammatory drugs (NSAIDs)

Therapy for Mondor disease is supportive with analgesics and warm compresses. The pain and cord usually resolve within 2 to 8 weeks.

A 25-year-old female presents to the office complaining of bilateral breast pain. The pain is cyclic and is associated with her menstrual cycle. What should she do?

Cyclic mastodynia is treated with cessation of caffeine intake and smoking as well as the use of NSAIDs.

Mastodynia

- Cyclic mastodynia
  - Most often benign
  - Pain is associated with the menstrual cycle and most often fibrocystic disease
  - Treatment is with a supportive bra, NSAIDs, decreased caffeine intake, and smoking cessation
- Continuous mastodynia
  - Often represents an acute or subacute infection
  - If new onset, do a bilateral mammogram if the patient is over 30 or bilateral whole breast ultrasound if the patient is under 30 to rule out cancer

What is the significance of unilateral bloody nipple discharge in a young pregnant woman in the late second trimester?

Bloody nipple discharge in a pregnant patient may be physiologic but requires an evaluation to rule out malignancy.

Nipple Discharge

- Most nipple discharge is benign
- All patients with new nipple discharge should have a bilateral mammogram and ultrasound of the retroareolar area
- Bloody nipple discharge
  - Most is benign and is secondary to an intraductal papilloma or papillomatosis
  - 10% of patients with a bloody nipple discharge have breast cancer
  - Treatment: Galactogram and excision of ductal area
- Green discharge
  - Usually secondary to fibrocystic disease
  - If cyclic and non-spontaneous, do not need to do excision—just reassure patient
- Serous discharge
  - Concerning for cancer, especially if coming from only one duct or spontaneous
  - Treatment: Excisional biopsy of ductal area
- Spontaneous discharge
  - No matter what color or consistency, spontaneous discharge is worrisome for cancer
  - All patients need a biopsy

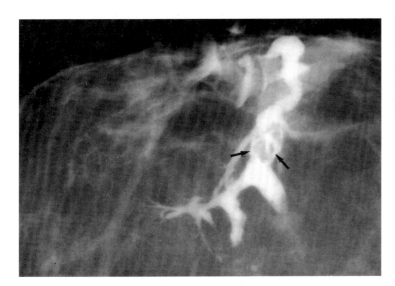

Ductogram demonstrating an intraductal papilloma. (With permission from Mulholland MW, Lillemoe KD, Doherty GM, Maier RV, Upchurch GR, eds. *Greenfield's Surgery.* 4th ed. Philadelphia, PA: Lippincott Williams & Wilkins; 2005.)

If the workup of bloody discharge is negative and the discharge persists, the ductal system should be excised to rule out malignancy.

A 36-year-old woman presents with a complaint of a new breast mass. What should the initial workup include?

Imaging studies include ultrasound and mammogram (with shielding if pregnant) and a physical examination. If the abnormality is suspicious by imaging or physical examination, a core needle biopsy should be performed.

A New Breast Mass

- A history, physical exam, and ultrasound are appropriate first steps
- A mammogram can be performed in a young woman if the breasts are not markedly dense
- If a simple cyst is suspected, a cyst aspiration can be performed in the office
  - If the mass resolves completely after the aspiration and the fluid is not bloody, the area can safely be followed with serial physical exams
- If an ultrasound documents a simple cyst, it can safely be followed clinically
- Solid lesions can be followed with imaging and physical examination if they are small and have classic characteristics of benign lesions
- All complex cysts or solid lesions that are not classically benign should undergo a core needle biopsy if possible
  - If a core needle biopsy is not possible, an excisional biopsy should be performed

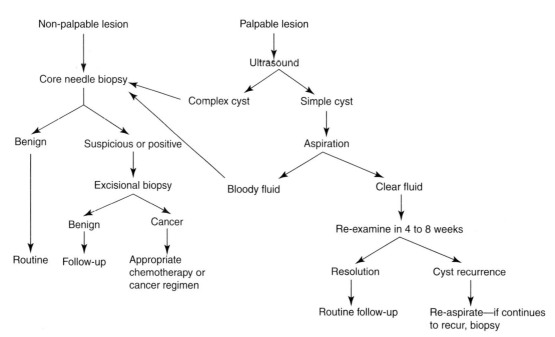

(With permission from Mulholland MW, Lillemoe KD, Doherty GM, Maier RV, Upchurch GR, eds. *Greenfield's Surgery.* 4th ed. Philadelphia, PA: Lippincott Williams & Wilkins; 2005.)

An ultrasound should be performed for evaluation of all palpable breast lesions.

A 24-year-old female presents with a firm, mobile mass in her left breast. What is the most likely diagnosis?

A benign fibroadenoma.

Fibroadenoma

- Benign mass made of stromal and glandular elements
- Most common breast lesion in women <30 years

- Are firm, mobile masses
- May have single or multiple and can be bilateral (10%)
- Often have pain in these lesions with the menstrual cycle
- Can enlarge during pregnancy
- Should have workup above

Fibrocystic Disease

- Benign disease associated with proliferation of fibrous tissue → cysts and nodularity of breasts
- Most common breast lesion overall
- Most commonly found in women aged 30 to 50 years
- Have firm, mobile breast masses that become tender during the menstrual cycle
- Treatment
  - Control pain by minimizing caffeine intake
  - Symptoms improve post-menopause

> A 48-year-old woman presents with a new palpable breast mass. Her mammogram and ultrasound are normal. What is the most appropriate next step?

If the mass is clinically suspicious, a core needle biopsy should be performed. Mammogram and ultrasound can miss up to 20% of all breast cancers.

Mammography

- Mammograms have a 50% false-positive rate over 10 years
  - Only about 20% of biopsies performed because of an abnormal mammogram have significant pathology
- Magnification views can be used to help define microcalcifications
- If a density is seen on mammography, compression views can be used to help differentiate the nature of the abnormality

If the density effaces on compression then it is probably benign.

Ultrasound Findings Suspicious for Malignancy

- Irregular shape
- Rough uneven border
- Heterogeneous internal echoes
- Posterior shadowing indicating that the lesion is solid and not cystic
- No lateral shadows or hyperechoic border
- Masses that are taller than they are wide
- Disrupted fascial planes

Mammographic Findings Suspicious for Malignancy

- Asymmetric density
- Any new mass
- Microcalcifications
  - Clustered
  - Stellate pattern
  - Pleomorphic

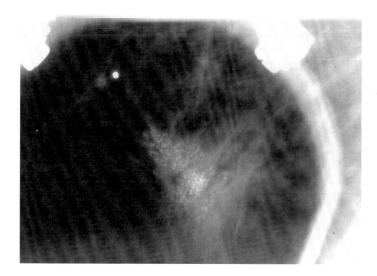

Mammogram with clustered microcalcifications. (With permission from Mulholland MW, Lillemoe KD, Doherty GM, Maier RV, Upchurch GR, eds. *Greenfield's Surgery.* 4th ed. Philadelphia, PA: Lippincott Williams & Wilkins; 2005.)

All new breast masses in postmenopausal women should have a histologic (tissue) diagnosis.

A 63-year-old woman is noted to have a mammographic abnormality upon routine screening. What is the next step in management?

- *Compare the mammogram to previous mammograms.*
- *Perform magnification and spot compression views.*
- *Perform an ultrasound evaluation of the area if there is a density present on mammogram.*

Follow-Up of an Abnormal Mammogram

- All mammograms are interpreted using the Breast Imaging Reporting and Data System
  - BIRADS 0: Needs additional imaging
  - BIRADS 1: Completely normal mammogram
  - BIRADS 2: Abnormality that is benign (e.g., simple cyst, duct ectasia, and benign calcifications)
  - BIRADS 3: Abnormality that is probably benign (e.g., unchanged calcifications and density that resolves with compression)
  - BIRADS 4: Abnormality that is possibly malignant (e.g., new calcifications and new density that persists with compression)
  - BIRADS 5: Abnormality that is probably malignant (e.g., new highly suspicious calcifications and new highly suspicious density)
  - BIRADS 6: Known malignancy present

BIRADS 1 and 2 mammographic lesions are followed with yearly screening.

BIRADS 3 mammographic lesions should have repeat imaging in 6 months.

BIRADS 4 and 5 mammographic lesions should be biopsied.

A 53-year-old woman presents for evaluation following a mammogram, which was significant for a small cluster of microcalcifications in her left breast. She does not have any masses on physical exam. What is the next step in management?

When available, a stereotactic core needle biopsy is minimally invasive and can sometimes provide a diagnosis; it is often preferable to a needle-guided excisional biopsy as an initial step in management.

Biopsy Approaches for Evaluating Breast Abnormalities

- Stereotactic core needle biopsy is most utilized for microcalcifications
  - This technique uses mammographic guidance to perform a core needle biopsy
- Ultrasound-guided core needle biopsy is used when the lesion is visible on ultrasound
- Palpation-directed core needle biopsy can be performed for palpable lesions
- A fine needle aspiration (FNA) is adequate for simple cyst aspiration and biopsy of a suspicious axillary node, but not much else
- For suspicious lesions, a core needle biopsy can provide enough tissue to differentiate between an in situ vs. invasive tumor and for tumor markers such as estrogen and progesterone receptors and Her-2-neu
  - When possible, core needle biopsy is preferable to excisional biopsy to reach a diagnosis
  - This results in a reduced positive margin rate and allows for axillary staging, which reduces the total number of surgeries required for management
- When a core needle biopsy is not possible, an excisional biopsy can be performed, either with wire localization, image guidance, or palpation directed
- An incisional biopsy has very limited indications in the management of breast tumors

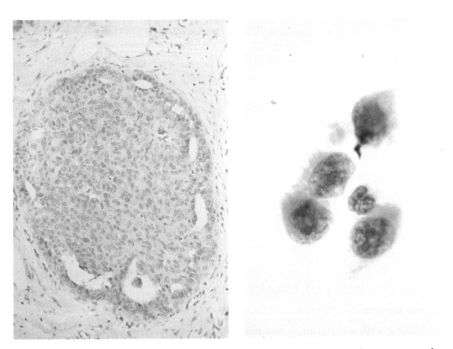

Comparison of (A) core needle and (B) FNA biopsy specimens. (With permission from Mulholland MW, Lillemoe KD, Doherty GM, Maier RV, Upchurch GR, eds. *Greenfield's Surgery.* 4th ed. Philadelphia, PA: Lippincott Williams & Wilkins; 2005.)

If inflammatory breast cancer or Paget disease is suspected, a punch biopsy of the suspicious skin should be performed.

> A 38-year-old woman with a breast mass has a core needle biopsy of a mammographic abnormality demonstrating a radial scar. What is the next step in management?

A radial scar is one of the histologic findings that should be followed with an excisional biopsy.

Histologic Findings on Core Needle Biopsy That Require Excisional Biopsy

- Radial scar
- Atypical hyperplasia
- Lobular carcinoma in situ (LCIS)
- Discordant biopsy (i.e., the pathologic findings are not consistent with the imaging studies or physical examination findings)
- Papillary lesion

An excisional biopsy is a term sometimes used interchangeably with lumpectomy, partial mastectomy, and breast preservation. In the context of nearly all breast cancers, these procedures should have adequate clear margins (usually 1 to 2 cm), a sentinel node biopsy (unless nodes are palpable), and be coupled with postoperative radiation.

Histologic Findings on Core Needle Biopsy That Do Not Require Excisional Biopsy

- No increased risk of breast cancer
  - Duct ectasia
  - Fibrocystic breast disease
  - Apocrine metaplasia
  - Cysts
  - Fibroadenoma
  - Fibrosis
  - Usual duct hyperplasia
  - Mastitis
  - Periductal mastitis
  - Squamous metaplasia
- Slightly increased risk (1.5 to 2.0 times normal)
  - Florid epithelial hyperplasia
  - Sclerosing adenosis

Histologic Characteristics of Breast Cancer

- Monomorphic pattern
- Nuclear crowding with a variation in nuclear size
- Chromatin clumping
- Prominent nucleoli

Indian filing (malignant cells forming a line) is the classic histologic finding of lobular carcinoma.

> A 35-year-old woman in the second trimester of pregnancy has a new diagnosis of Stage I breast cancer. What is the appropriate recommendation?

- Surgery and chemotherapy are safe in the second and third trimesters
- Radiation therapy should be deferred until the pregnancy is complete
- The surgery can*not* include sentinel lymph node biopsy using isosulfan blue dye

Breast Cancer and Pregnancy

- Breast cancer in pregnancy is associated with a poor prognosis
- Although pregnancy and lactation are not directly responsible, pregnant woman are commonly diagnosed at a later stage than non-pregnant women, and the worse prognosis is most likely due to the delay in diagnosis and treatment
- Termination of the pregnancy does not change the prognosis of the breast cancer

> How long should pregnancy be delayed after the diagnosis of a successfully treated breast cancer?

Pregnancy following breast cancer is generally deferred until at least 2 years after diagnosis. However, if the patient is on adjuvant hormonal therapy, pregnancy is not recommended until that treatment course is complete, usually 5 years. A subsequent pregnancy does not affect recurrence even with node-positive disease.

Chemotherapy and Pregnancy

- Chemotherapy does not increase the rate of birth defects in subsequent pregnancies
- Ovarian failure and infertility from chemotherapy is drug-, dose-, and age-dependent

Alkylating agents such as adriamycin are most likely to result in infertility.

> A 55-year-old woman has a history of right breast cancer 2 years prior. She was treated with a modified radical mastectomy. She now presents with a mammographic abnormality in the contralateral breast. How should she be evaluated at this time and what is the likely diagnosis?

The workup of a contralateral breast cancer should include what is routine for all abnormal mammograms. The likely diagnosis is a benign process; however, all women with breast cancer have an increased risk in the contralateral breast.

Contralateral Breast Cancer

- Risk factors include a history of breast cancer (especially LCIS)
- The risk of bilateral breast cancer increases as the age at first diagnosis decreases
    - Women diagnosed under the age of 50 have a 13.3% risk of bilateral breast cancer
    - Women diagnosed over the age of 50 have a 3.5% risk of bilateral breast cancer
- The question important to staging is whether a contralateral breast cancer represents a second primary or metastasis from the original breast cancer
    - The new tumor should be considered a second primary cancer if:
        - There is an in situ component in the tumor
        - The new tumor has a different histology from the original tumor

- The new tumor should be considered metastasis if:
  - There is widespread metastatic disease
  - There is direct extension across the midline
- If there is no compelling evidence that the cancer is a metastasis, it is assumed to be a second primary and therefore has a better prognosis
- If felt to be a metastasis from the contralateral breast, a staging workup should be completed to rule out widespread metastatic disease

A general estimate of risk of a second primary breast cancer is 0.5% per year.

Ten years following a left-sided mastectomy, a woman develops angiosarcoma of her left arm. What is the most likely cause?

Angiosarcoma of the skin and soft tissue of the arm can develop in the presence of chronic lymphedema (Stewart-Treves syndrome). It was originally described in patients treated with a radical mastectomy but can occur in any patient with lymphedema.

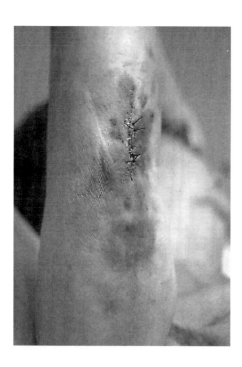

Stewart-Treves syndrome. (With permission from Mulholland MW, Lillemoe KD, Doherty GM, Maier RV, Upchurch GR, eds. *Greenfield's Surgery.* 4th ed. Philadelphia, PA: Lippincott Williams & Wilkins; 2005.)

Stewart-Treves Syndrome
- The initial presentation is the appearance of a painless bruise or purple nodule on the arm
- The time interval between axillary dissection and development of angiosarcoma averages 10.5 years
- 60% have received post-mastectomy radiation therapy
- 75% of cases involve the upper arm, but it can also occur on the forearm, elbow, chest wall, and shoulder
- The tumor always involves the dermis and subcutis
- Median survival = 19 months
- Treatment often requires amputation due to the size of the lesion and the poor functional quality of the arm, but wide local excision can be attempted for small lesions

Angiosarcoma should be suspected with any painless bruise or purple nodule on an arm with chronic lymphedema.

> What histologic diagnosis is associated with the greatest risk of local recurrence of breast cancer?

Ductal carcinoma in situ (DCIS) is associated with a significant risk of local recurrence.

Ductal Carcinoma In Situ

- The presence of DCIS carries an increased future risk of invasive breast cancer of approximately 1% per year
- Standard treatment choices include lumpectomy plus radiation therapy OR simple mastectomy
  - Some advocate eliminating radiation therapy in low-grade lesions that have been resected with greater than 2-mm margins
- There is a 2% incidence of axillary node involvement
- Prognostic features include tumor grade and comedo type
  - Comedo type (has central necrosis): often has a higher mitotic rate
  - Noncomedo type (lacks central necrosis): has a lower mitotic rate; is often estrogen receptor-positive
- Tamoxifen is used for chemotherapy
  - Side effects include an increased risk of endometrial cancer and deep vein thrombosis in postmenopausal women

Tamoxifen decreases the recurrence of DCIS by 40% and invasive cancer by 30%.

> What is the most common cause of clustered microcalcifications on routine mammogram in a young woman?

Ductal carcinoma in situ.

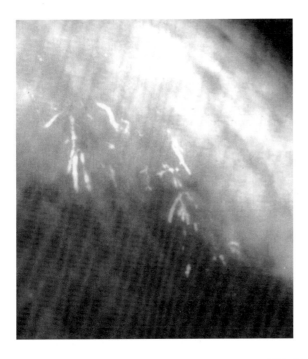

Mammogram typical for DCIS. (With permission from Mulholland MW, Lillemoe KD, Doherty GM, Maier RV, Upchurch GR, eds. *Greenfield's Surgery.* 4th ed. Philadelphia, PA: Lippincott Williams & Wilkins; 2005.)

Lobular carcinoma in situ.

Lobular Carcinoma In Situ

- Considered to be a marker of increased risk and not a premalignant lesion
  - 10-fold increased risk of development of breast cancer in either breast
  - 21% risk of invasive breast cancer over 35 years with a higher rate of bilateral breast cancer
  - The most common subsequent malignancy is infiltrating ductal CA, although infiltrating lobular CA also occurs more commonly in patients with LCIS than in the general population
- If diagnosed on core needle biopsy, an excisional biopsy should be performed to identify any potential adjacent invasive malignancy
- If diagnosed on excisional biopsy, no further treatment is warranted
  - A positive margin does NOT affect recurrence rate
- Usually, there are no abnormalities on physical exam or mammogram with LCIS—it is an incidental finding
- A prophylactic simple mastectomy is an option
  - It has no proven survival benefit
  - If a prophylactic simple mastectomy is performed, it should be bilateral
- Tamoxifen reduces the risk of invasive breast cancer by 50%

LCIS does not need to be resected with negative margins.

Mastectomy Resection Margins

- Simple mastectomy: Removal of all breast tissue
  - Performed for LCIS or DCIS if mastectomy is desired
  - Performed for people with genetic disposition to breast cancer (e.g., BRCA 1 and BRCA 2) with no evidence of malignant disease who desire prophylactic mastectomy
  - Used in conjunction with sentinel lymph node biopsy for patients with invasive disease
- Modified radical mastectomy
  - The most common type of mastectomy performed for malignant disease with known positive lymph nodes
  - Removal of all breast tissue, pectoralis fascia, and level I and II lymph nodes
- Radical mastectomy
  - Now rarely performed
  - Removal of all breast tissue and pectoralis major and minor with axillary lymph node dissection

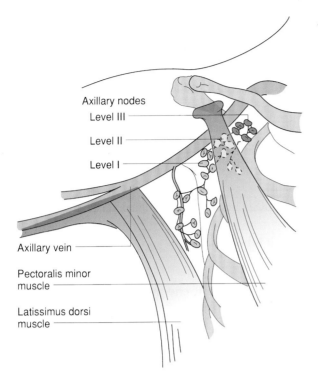

Axillary lymph node levels. (With permission from Mulholland MW, Lillemoe KD, Doherty GM, Maier RV, Upchurch GR, eds. *Greenfield's Surgery*. 4th ed. Philadelphia, PA: Lippincott Williams & Wilkins; 2005.)

Axillary Lymph Node Levels in Breast Cancer

- Level I: Lateral to pectoralis major
- Level II: Deep to pectoralis major
- Level III: Medial to pectoralis minor
- Rotter nodes: Nodes between the pectoralis major and minor
- 97% of lymph drainage is to the axillary nodes with the other 3% going to internal mammary nodes
- Cancer in supraclavicular nodes represent N3 disease

A 45-year-old woman presents with a painless area of breast enlargement and redness. She has a normal mammogram. What is the best next step?

Perform a skin biopsy to rule out inflammatory breast cancer, a very serious condition often underappreciated by clinicians.

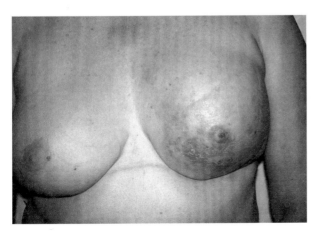

Inflammatory breast cancer. (With permission from Mulholland MW, Lillemoe KD, Doherty GM, Maier RV, Upchurch GR, eds. *Greenfield's Surgery*. 4th ed. Philadelphia, PA: Lippincott Williams & Wilkins; 2005.)

Inflammatory Breast Cancer

- The clinical triad for diagnosis is painless breast enlargement with redness and skin thickening
  - A "peau d'orange" appearance of the skin overlying the breast is caused by edema
- The diagnosis is clinical and can be confirmed with skin biopsy of the inflamed skin
  - Beware: A negative skin biopsy does NOT eliminate the diagnosis
- Systemic signs and symptoms of an infection may indicate mastitis or a breast abscess
  - An ultrasound can rule out a fluid-filled abscess cavity
- Imaging studies should be done to identify the underlying breast malignancy
- Pathology demonstrates dermal lymphatic invasion
- Treatment includes neoadjuvant chemotherapy followed by a modified radical mastectomy, even if there is a complete clinical response
- Do NOT perform a sentinel lymph node biopsy as it is not reliable
- Five-year survival is now 40% with neoadjuvant therapy

The treatment of inflammatory breast cancer is neoadjuvant chemotherapy, modified radical mastectomy, and post-mastectomy radiation therapy.

A 45-year-old woman presents with a well-circumscribed 5-cm rubbery mobile mass. What diagnosis must be ruled out?

Cystosarcoma phyllodes tumors are typically rapidly enlarging, sharply demarcated, and freely mobile tumors in women.

Cystosarcoma Phyllodes Tumor

- Presentation is usually a mobile nontender nodular breast mass
- Is a cousin of fibroadenoma
  - Clinically, phyllodes tumors are larger (median size 4 to 5 cm), present in older patients (median age 45), and grow faster than fibroadenomas
  - Cytology is unreliable in distinguishing between the two
- A 3-cm margin is recommended for resection, which often results in a mastectomy due to the large size of the tumor at presentation
- Axillary node dissection is only done for clinically positive nodes
- 1% of these tumors are metastatic
- There is no survival benefit to undergoing radiation therapy or chemotherapy

Like most sarcomas, phyllodes tumors have a high rate of local recurrence (15% to 60%) usually due to inadequate initial excision. The treatment for local recurrence is re-excision.

A 50-year-old woman presents with a 3-month history of rash on her right nipple. She has identified no other abnormalities in her breast. On breast imaging there is an area of microcalcification in the retroareolar area. How should this patient be managed?

The history is suspicious for Paget disease of the breast with an underlying malignancy. The patient should have a punch biopsy of the abnormal area of the areola and a core needle biopsy of the microcalcifications. If the areola is not involved but the nipple shows changes, excision of a segment of nipple can be accomplished with a small eclipse-shaped excision.

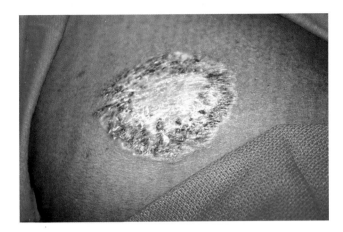

Paget disease of the nipple. (With permission from Mulholland MW, Lillemoe KD, Doherty GM, Maier RV, Upchurch GR, eds. *Greenfield's Surgery.* 4th ed. Philadelphia, PA: Lippincott Williams & Wilkins; 2005.)

Paget Disease

- Presents as nipple erythema, scaling, and erosions of the areola and surrounding skin
- Paget cells do NOT invade the dermal basement membrane and are therefore a form of carcinoma in situ
- Paget disease is often associated with an underlying invasive cancer, even though a mass may only be present in 50% of cases
- Treatment is based on the underlying malignancy, which is usually an infiltrating ductal carcinoma or DCIS
- A simple mastectomy is often performed, and a nodal evaluation is based on suspicion for invasion
- Breast conservation therapy is sometimes possible, but *the entire nipple-areolar complex must be removed*

What is the proper management of infiltrating lobular carcinoma?

Treated with the same local treatment options as ductal carcinoma: either breast preservation with radiation therapy OR a total mastectomy. Axillary staging is completed with a sentinel lymph node biopsy and completion node dissection in most cases with positive lymph nodes.

Lobular Carcinoma

- Indian filing on histology
- More commonly multifocal and multicentric
- High risk of bilaterality (6% to 28%)
- The presence of signet ring cells indicates a worse prognosis

A 56-year-old woman undergoes a right mastectomy and postoperatively notes weak internal rotation and abduction of her right arm as well as difficulty doing pull-ups. What is her diagnosis?

Thoracodorsal nerve injury.

Nerve	Innervation	Consequence of Damage to Nerve
Thoracodorsal	Latissimus dorsi	Weak internal rotation and abduction of the arm and weakness with pull-ups
Long thoracic	Serratus anterior	Winged scapula
Pectoral nerves (medial and lateral)	Pectoralis major—both nerves Pectoralis minor—medial nerve only	Muscle atrophy
Intercostobrachial nerve	Sensory	Numbness of upper, inner aspect of arm including axilla

A 45-year-old woman presents with an enlarged axillary node. A biopsy of the node reveals adenocarcinoma. What are the next steps in the evaluation of this patient?

Mammogram of bilateral breasts and additional imaging as deemed necessary, including ultrasound and possible MRI of the breast.

Management of a Solitary Positive Axillary Node

- Imaging as above
- Evaluation of the node for estrogen receptors, progesterone receptors, and HER2/neu receptors
  - If the tumor is estrogen and progesterone receptor positive then the primary is probably breast cancer
- Discuss the histology with the pathologist to determine if it is consistent with a breast primary
  - Lymphoma is the most common cause of primary axillary adenopathy
- If it is truly an unknown primary breast cancer, a modified radical mastectomy is indicated
  - When the breast is resected, the primary is found on pathology 68% to 95% of the time
- A metastatic workup should be completed prior to initiation of therapy if there are more than four positive nodes (since Stage IV disease would be treated differently)
- An alternative option for management of the breast in the case of unknown primary is axillary dissection with whole breast radiation therapy
- If the primary lesion is identified, then it is managed by standard techniques
- The overall prognosis of the patient is unchanged whether or not the primary is identified in the breast prior to surgery

For a positive axillary node with an unknown primary in the breast, a modified radical mastectomy is indicated.

A 35-year-old woman presents with a new breast mass that she noticed 2 months ago on self-examination that has not gone away. Imaging and a core needle biopsy reveal an infiltrating ductal carcinoma that is 7 cm in size. What are the management options?

The patient should receive surgery, chemotherapy, and radiation therapy, but the management options for the breast should be discussed with the patient. The options include:

- Total mastectomy with sentinel lymph node biopsy with completion axillary dissection with positive nodes
- Total mastectomy with sentinel lymph node biopsy with completion axillary dissection with positive nodes with reconstruction
- A partial mastectomy (breast conservation) with sentinel lymph node biopsy and completion axillary node dissection for positive nodes if neoadjuvant chemotherapy is successful in decreasing the tumor size

Neoadjuvant Therapy

- There has been no proven survival benefit
- The only advantage to neoadjuvant chemotherapy is to increase the breast preservation rate
- The disadvantage to neoadjuvant chemotherapy is that staging is incomplete
  - The original nodal status and the original tumor stage may be unknown
  - This has implications on the recommendation of sentinel lymph node biopsy and postoperative radiation therapy
- Patients who have a complete response to neoadjuvant chemotherapy are in a favorable group: Overall survival is improved compared to those that do not have a complete response when matched by pretreatment stage

---

What is the difference between multicentric and multifocal disease?

Multicentric disease is two separate foci involving more than one quadrant of the breast. Standard treatment of multicentric disease is mastectomy.

Multifocal disease is two separate foci within the same quadrant of the breast. Treatment is mastectomy or breast preservation with radiation therapy.

Following trauma to the breast in a patient with a silicone implant, a rupture of the implant is suspected. What is the best test to obtain?

MRI is the best test for a silicone implant rupture.

A 52-year-old man presents with bilateral breast enlargement. What is the most likely cause?

The most common cause of gynecomastia in men is physiologic.

Male Gynecomastia

- Gynecomastia occurs at three time points in the male: the neonatal period, adolescence, and late adulthood
  - Gynecomastia in the neonatal period is due to maternal and placental hormones and regresses spontaneously
  - Gynecomastia in the adolescent period
    - Occurs in a 40% to 60% of pubertal boys
    - Prepubertal gynecomastia should be evaluated for possible endocrine pathology

- Gynecomastia in adult males
  - Increases in the age range of 50 to 69
  - Is thought to be due to alterations in the serum testosterone to estrogen ratio
  - The rate decreases over the age of 70, which is thought to be due to decreasing body fat
- Risk factors for gynecomastia in the adult male include
  - Obesity
  - Estrogen excess states (hermaphroditic, gonadal tumors, germ cell tumors, lung cancer, hepatocellular cancer, and adrenal cortical neoplasms)
  - Androgen deficiency states (aging, hypogonadism from genetic abnormalities, or secondary testicular failure)
  - Medications (spironolactone)
- Treatment is for symptomatic cases and includes subcutaneous mastectomy, treatment of the inciting event, or medications such as tamoxifen, clomiphene citrate, and danazol

Evaluation in the adult male should include a history and physical examination that includes a testicular exam, mammogram, and in some cases an endocrine profile.

A 45-year-old male presents with a discrete subareolar mass. What is the appropriate management?

Similar to female breast cancer: physical exam, imaging, and core needle biopsy.

Male Breast Cancer
- Male breast cancer comprises approximately 1% of all breast cancers
- Klinefelter syndrome is a risk factor (3% risk in these patients)
- Presents approximately 10 years later than female breast cancer (average age of 64)
- Bilateral male breast cancer occurs in about 2% of all cases
- Mammography can be useful
- Men present at more advanced stage, usually with a palpable subareolar mass
- Outcomes are the same as for females (stage for stage)
- The pathology is consistent with ductal carcinoma in nearly every case
  - Lobular carcinoma is very rare but can be seen with Klinefelter syndrome
- Bloody nipple discharge is rare
- BRCA2 mutations are common (20%)

Treatment for Male Breast Cancer
- The surgical management of male breast cancer usually requires a mastectomy
  - Breast conservation for small tumors may be possible
  - If breast conservation is chosen, as in women, it will always be accompanied by radiation therapy
- The majority are estrogen receptor or progesterone receptor positive (65% to 95%)
  - Therefore, tamoxifen is an effective treatment, although loss of libido and impotence may be dose-limiting side effects
  - Chemotherapy should be considered with positive nodes and no metastatic disease, or with a high risk primary tumor and negative nodes

- Hormonal manipulation, either with orchiectomy or tamoxifen, is important in the management of metastatic disease
- The need for adjuvant chemotherapy should be determined by the pathology of the primary tumor and the nodal status

What is the most common initial site of metastatic breast cancer?

Metastasis to bone is characteristic of breast cancer.

A 55-year-old woman presents for a second opinion regarding management of her newly diagnosed 6-cm breast cancer. Her first surgeon recommended a mastectomy. When is breast preservation contraindicated?

Contraindications for Breast Conservation Surgery
- Size >5 cm (unless neoadjuvant chemotherapy is used to reduce the size of the primary tumor)
- If there is a contraindication to radiation therapy
- Large tumor to breast size ratio
- Central lesions or Paget disease
  - Occasionally, breast preservation can be used, but the nipple areolar complex is usually sacrificed in what is called a central mastectomy
- Multicentric disease
  - In-breast recurrence risk of 25% to 40% vs. 11% for unicentric disease
- Inability to follow up with mammography either due to a difficult to follow mammogram (dense breasts or multiple microcalcifications) or poor compliance
- Total mastectomy does not lead to better survival compared to breast preservation (partial mastectomy/lumpectomy with radiation therapy)
- There is a lower local recurrence risk with total mastectomy (1% to 5%) when compared with partial mastectomy/lumpectomy with radiation therapy (approximately 15%)

The choice of operation for the breast does not alter the recommendation for chemotherapy.

A 43-year-old woman presents with a new breast cancer diagnosed on her initial screening mammogram. The tumor is 3 cm in size and she has a firm mobile palpable node. How should the patient's axilla be managed?

The patient should be offered breast preservation or mastectomy and a level I and II axillary node dissection. Another option would be to perform an FNA of the axillary node to definitively establish the presence of nodal involvement.

Axillary Node Dissection
- The standard axillary node dissection for breast cancer is a level I and II node dissection (defined as removal of the fat pad inferior to the axillary vein and posterior and lateral to the pectoralis minor muscle)

- It is currently only performed in those patients with a failed sentinel lymph node biopsy, a positive sentinel lymph node, or palpable axillary nodes with a positive fine needle aspirate
- 30% of breast cancer patients with clinically negative nodes will have positive nodes on histologic examination
- 20% of cancers <1 cm in size (T1b) will have positive nodes
- Level I and II axillary node dissection is effective for local control in the axilla
- An axillary node dissection requires drain placement
- Possible complications include seroma, wound infection, numbness of the posterior aspect of the upper arm, injury to the long thoracic nerve (serratus anterior/winged scapula) or thoracodorsal nerve (latissimus dorsi), decreased range of motion of the shoulder and lymphedema
  - The lymphedema rate is 15% to 25%
  - Hypesthesia of the upper inner arm is common and is due to injury to the intercostal brachial nerve
- The local recurrence risk after axillary node dissection is 3% to 4%

Pectoralis major muscle atrophy is uncommon, but when it occurs, is due to injury to the medial and lateral pectoral nerves.

Sentinel Lymph Node Biopsy

- Standard of care for the management of breast cancer with a clinically negative axilla
- Indicated for breast cancers >1 cm
- Not recommended in patients with previous axillary surgery
- Usually removes two to three lymph nodes
- Techniques include isosulfan blue dye only, radiosulfur colloid only, or a combination of both
  - The combination of both provides a higher success rate at identification of the sentinel lymph node with a lower false-negative rate
- Provides the same prognostic information with fewer complications as compared with a standard axillary dissection
- Complications, while less frequent than for axillary node dissection, include seroma, hematoma, wound infection, injury to nerves, and lymphedema. The lymphedema rate is 1% to 5%.
- The local recurrence risk and survival compared to standard axillary dissection is the same

A sentinel lymph node biopsy is only indicated in patients with clinically negative lymph nodes.

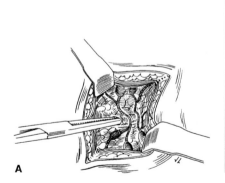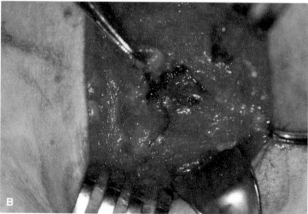

Sentinel lymph node biopsy. (With permission from Fischer JE, Bland KI, Callery MP, et al., eds. *Mastery of Surgery.* 5th ed. Philadelphia, PA: Lippincott Williams & Wilkins; 2006.)

A 30-year-old woman with scleroderma underwent a mastectomy for a 1.5-cm breast cancer. What was the most likely reason for the mastectomy?

A contraindication to perform radiation therapy can be a reason to proceed to mastectomy as the surgical treatment, since breast conservation for cancer requires postoperative radiation for comparable survival results.

Radiation Therapy Indications Following Breast Conservation Surgery

- All patients with breast cancer treated with breast conservation should receive radiation therapy to reduce the local recurrence risk in the breast
    - There are few exceptions such as low-grade DCIS with a greater than 2-mm margin
- Patients with only LCIS do not receive radiation therapy

Prior radiation therapy to the chest for any malignancy excludes the possibility of performing radiation, and thus, the ability to perform breast conservation surgery for cancer.

Radiation Therapy Indications Following Mastectomy

- Four or more positive lymph nodes
    - The management of patients with one to three positive nodes is controversial
- Matted axillary nodes
- All T4 breast cancers
    - T4: Any size with
        - Extension to the chest wall, not including the pectoralis major muscle
        - Edema or ulceration of the skin of the breast or satellite skin nodules confined to the ipsilateral breast
        - Inflammatory cancer
- Positive resection margins
- Reconstruction options are limited in these patients

A 55-year-old woman with a history of breast cancer who underwent a partial mastectomy 10 years ago recently underwent a mastectomy for a 1-cm breast cancer recurrence. What was the most likely reason for the mastectomy?

Inability to perform radiation therapy.

Contraindications to Radiation Therapy

- Scleroderma or other connective tissue disease (e.g., Raynaud phenomenon and Sjogren syndrome)
- Previous radiation therapy to the chest (e.g., for breast cancer and lymphoma)
- Pregnancy

If a patient is diagnosed with breast cancer late in pregnancy, radiation therapy can be deferred until the postpartum period.

Complications of Radiation Therapy

- Fatigue
- 0.1% to 0.2% risk of a radiation-induced malignancy
- A tender, red, firm, or swollen breast for weeks following treatment
- Desquamation of the skin
- The long-term result is a breast that is more firm and appears smaller than the contralateral breast

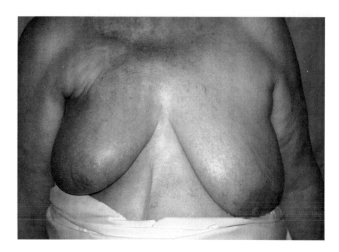

Skin changes following radiation therapy. (With permission from Mulholland MW, Lillemoe KD, Doherty GM, Maier RV, Upchurch GR, eds. *Greenfield's Surgery*. 4th ed. Philadelphia, PA: Lippincott Williams & Wilkins; 2005.)

A 40-year-old premenopausal woman presents with a 1.5-cm node-negative infiltrating ductal carcinoma. The management of the breast was a partial mastectomy. What adjuvant therapy is recommended?

Chemotherapy and radiation therapy.

Adjuvant Therapy for Breast Cancer

- Adriamycin based regimens are commonly used for 4 to 8 cycles but these have an increased rate of cardiac toxicity in the long term
  - Taxane-based regimens are an alternative to adriamycin-based regimens if cardiac toxicity is a concern
- Herceptin is used for patients with a positive HER2 receptor
- Whole breast radiation therapy follows chemotherapy

A 75-year-old patient undergoes a lumpectomy and sentinel node biopsy for a T1N0M0 infiltrating ductal breast cancer. The tumor size is 0.8 cm and estrogen receptors are positive and progesterone receptors are negative. The lymph nodes are negative for disease. What is the next step in management?

Women over the age of 70 can be treated with breast preservation without radiation therapy if the margins are clear and the patient will receive adjuvant hormonal therapy.

Selective Estrogen Receptor Modulators

- **Tamoxifen**
  - Competitively inhibits estradiol binding to the estrogen receptor
  - Proven to decrease recurrence and mortality in receptor-positive patients
  - Inhibits hepatic cytochrome P450 activity
    - May interact with warfarin, calcium channel blockers, erythromycin, and cyclosporin
  - The most common side effects are vasomotor (hot flushes) and signs of decreased estrogen such as vaginal dryness and loss of libido
  - Patients taking tamoxifen also have an increased risk of developing deep venous thrombosis, uterine cancer, and cataracts
- **Raloxifene**
  - Mechanism not completely understood
  - Possibly reduces risk of breast cancer in women at increased risk
  - Used only as a chemopreventive agent and not as a therapeutic agent for patients diagnosed with breast cancer
- **Aromatase Inhibitors**
  - Aromatase inhibitor that blocks conversion of aromatizable steroids to estrogen
  - Both steroidal and nonsteroidal types
  - More effective than tamoxifen in the treatment of breast cancer
  - Side effects include muscle and joint aches and menopausal symptoms

---

If one of your female patients had a sister with bilateral breast cancer at the age of 42, what is your patient's risk of development of breast cancer?

Approximately 50%.

Risk Factors for Breast Cancer

- Early menarche
- Late menopause
- Nulliparity or first birth >30 years of age
- Hormone use (most importantly hormone replacement therapy)
- Family history for breast cancer (especially premenopausal first degree relatives)

Strategies for Women at Increased Risk for Breast Cancer

- Close observation with early mammogram starting 10 years prior to the age of the youngest first degree relative at the time of diagnosis
- Monthly breast self-examination, and clinical breast examination every 6 months
- Prophylactic mastectomy (either subcutaneous or total) reduces the risk of developing breast cancer by 96%
- Tamoxifen 20 mg daily for 5 years has been shown to reduce the risk of breast cancer in a high-risk population by 49%
- Annual screening breast MRI

Candidates for Prophylactic Mastectomy

- Patients with a family history compatible with hereditary breast cancer
- A known carrier of a BRCA1 or BRCA2 mutation
- A young patient with a unilateral early stage breast cancer treated with mastectomy and one additional risk factor
- Biopsy-proven LCIS
- A woman at increased risk for development of breast cancer that is difficult to follow with physical examination or breast imaging

Remember that LCIS is simply a "marker" of cancer and not cancer itself.

A woman whose mother died of breast cancer is found to be BRCA positive. What is her risk of developing breast cancer?

Approximately 60% to 80% given a positive family history AND a positive BRCA test.

Breast Cancer Genes

- BRCA
  - Autosomal dominant inheritance
  - Accounts for 5% of breast cancer in the United States
  - Characterized by early age at onset and propensity for bilaterality
  - BRCA1 (chromosome 17q)
    - Associated with an 80% risk of breast cancer and 40% risk of ovarian cancer
    - Maternal or paternal inheritance
    - Males with the gene do not have a significantly increased risk of breast cancer (only act as carriers)
    - Prophylactic TAH/BSO may be indicated
  - BRCA2 (chromosome 13q)
    - No increased risk of ovarian cancer
    - Males with the gene have an increased risk of developing breast cancer
    - The risk of breast cancer in a woman with the gene is 60%
- Other diseases associated with breast cancer
  - Li-Fraumeni syndrome
  - Ataxia-telangiectasia
  - Cowden disease
  - Peutz-Jeghers syndrome
  - Muir-Torre syndrome (Lynch type II syndrome)

Most patients diagnosed with breast cancer do not have any genetic abnormalities.

29 Breast Reconstruction

P. Pravin Reddy and Joshua L. Levine

A 42-year-old female underwent mastectomy with sentinel node biopsy for ductal carcinoma in situ of the left breast. She insists on having an immediate reconstruction without a prostheses/implant. What are her options?

Currently less than 20% of women undergoing mastectomy pursue reconstruction. According to a federal law in place since 1998, patients may choose the manner in which to undergo breast reconstruction following oncologic procedures. If no radiation is planned following mastectomy, immediate breast reconstruction with a deep inferior epigastric perforator (DIEP) flap represents the best ideal method of reconstruction.

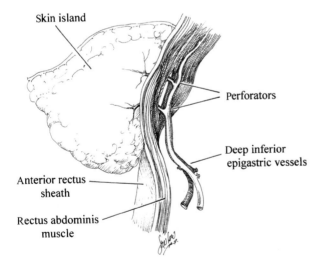

DIEP flap. (With permission from Fischer JE, Bland KI, Callery MP, et al., eds. *Mastery of Surgery.* 5th ed. Philadelphia, PA: Lippincott Williams & Wilkins; 2006.)

Deep Inferior Epigastric Perforator Flap

- The rectus abdominis muscle is preserved in its entirety including motor innervation
- The flap is based on the *deep inferior epigastric artery* perforator system and transferred using microsurgical techniques
- Flap survival in experienced hands is as high as 98%
- The recipient vessels are the *internal mammary/thoracic* vessels or the *thoracodorsal* vessels
- Previous abdominal surgery usually does not preclude the DIEP flap

485

- DIEP flaps are not indicated in patients having undergone liposuction of the abdomen or a previous transverse rectus abdominis myocutaneous (TRAM) flap
- Autologous tissue reconstruction yields superior results in restoring a breast with natural texture and symmetry to the contralateral breast
- Complications of surgery include immediate flap failure, complete or partial flap loss, fat necrosis, hematoma, infection, and seroma

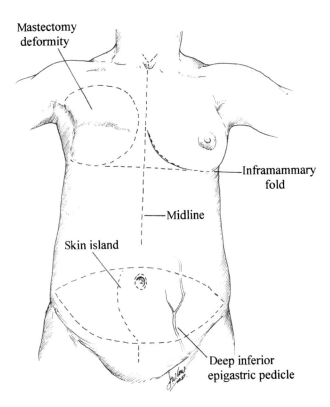

Surgical planning for DIEP flap. (With permission from Fischer JE, Bland KI, Callery MP, et al., eds. *Mastery of Surgery.* 5th ed. Philadelphia, PA: Lippincott Williams & Wilkins; 2006.)

A 37-year-old female underwent mastectomy with sentinel node biopsy for ductal adenocarcinoma of the right breast. Her tumor size was 6 cm and she agrees to have radiation therapy. She insists on having a reconstruction without a prostheses or implant. What are her options?

Radiation therapy, although well tolerated by the DIEP flap, may result in loss of flap volume, contracture of the skin envelope thus distorting the reconstructed breast, a severe skin reaction, and pigment changes. Delayed reconstruction with a DIEP flap represents the best treatment option as the rectus abdominis muscle is spared. Excision of radiated skin may also be required.

A 57-year-old female underwent mastectomy and the plastic surgeon you are working with plans to perform a TRAM flap to reconstruct the breast. What artery is used for this method of reconstruction?

The TRAM flap is a pedicled flap based on blood supply from the superior epigastric artery.

Transverse Rectus Abdominis Myocutaneous Flap

- The flap necessarily sacrifices the rectus abdominis muscle and results in functional loss
- Long-term complication may include ventral abdominal hernia, troubling abdominal bulges, and instability of the trunk
- Less tissue can be reliably transferred with the TRAM flap compared to the DIEP flap

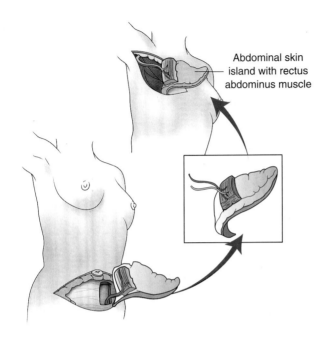

Abdominal skin island with rectus abdominus muscle

Free TRAM flap. (With permission from Mulholland MW, Lillemoe KD, Doherty GM, Maier RV, Upchurch GR, eds. *Greenfield's Surgery.* 4th ed. Philadelphia, PA: Lippincott Williams & Wilkins; 2005.)

A 39-year-old woman underwent a partial left mastectomy and seeks reconstruction. What method of reconstruction is best applied in this situation?

The extended latissimus dorsi (ELD) myocutaneous flap is best applied to reconstruction of partial mastectomy defects.

Extended Latissimus Dorsi Myocutaneous Flap

- May be used in conjunction with a prostheses, or implant, to fully reconstruct the breast mound
- Applied as a pedicled myocutaneous flap based on the *thoracodorsal* vessels
- Sacrifice of the latissimus dorsi (LD) muscle may compromise upper extremity function in the form of weakness and early fatigue with arm extension and weak internal/external rotation
- An alternative to the ELD flap is to reconstruct partial defects with perforator flaps thus preserving the LD (e.g., *thoracodorsal artery perforator flap* or *lateral thoracic skin flap* based on intercostal perforators)

A 46-year-old woman has tissue expanders placed following a mastectomy. How long will the tissue expanders remain in place?

Breast reconstruction with implants usually occurs in two stages. The first stage entails tissue expansion for several weeks followed by exchange of the expander to a permanent implant.

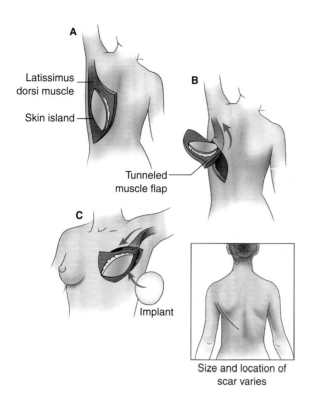

LD flap. (A) An appropriately sized skin island based on the latissimus dorsi muscle is designed. (B) The pedicled myocutaneous flap based on the thoracodorsal vessels is rotated anteriorly and inset into the mastectomy defect to recreate the breast mound. (C) It is common practice to place a tissue expander or implant beneath the latissimus flap in order to create an adequately projecting breast mound. The donor site scar may be adjusted in order to camouflage it within the bra line (*boxed diagram*). (With permission from Mulholland MW, Lillemoe KD, Doherty GM, Maier RV, Upchurch GR, eds. *Greenfield's Surgery*. 4th ed. Philadelphia, PA: Lippincott Williams & Wilkins; 2005.)

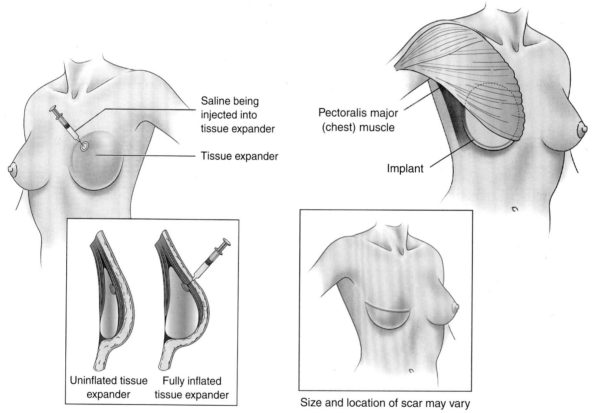

Breast reconstruction with implants. (A) Placement of tissue expander. (B) Placement of implant. (With permission from Mulholland MW, Lillemoe KD, Doherty GM, Maier RV, Upchurch GR, eds. *Greenfield's Surgery*. 4th ed. Philadelphia, PA: Lippincott Williams & Wilkins; 2005.)

Tissue Expanders and Implants

- Immediate or delayed reconstruction following mastectomy is performed by creating a submuscular pocket with elevation of the *pectoralis major* and *serratus anterior* muscles
- A tissue expander is inserted into the pocket followed by primary skin closure
- After allowing 4 weeks for tissues to stabilize, second stage reconstruction is performed by replacing the tissue expander with either saline or silicone permanent implants
- Recruitment of soft tissues then occurs over the subsequent 6 to 8 weeks until adequate breast volume is achieved
- Nipple areolar reconstruction is typically accomplished with local flaps and tattooing
- Reconstruction may be performed in a single stage in cases of small breast volumes
- Possible complications of reconstruction with prostheses include infection leading to loss of implant, capsular contracture, implant extrusion or exposure, and device failure
- Silicone-gel filled implants are subject to high failure rates after 10 to 15 years
- High-dose chemotherapy may result in increased complications following immediate breast reconstruction with prostheses
- Tissue expanders tolerate radiation therapy but may have to be deflated prior to initiating radiation therapy
- Radiation results in increased rates of capsular contracture

30 | Anesthesia

Jeremy D. Kukafka and Lee A. Fleisher

A 32-year-old male presents to the emergency department after sustaining multiple gunshot wounds to the abdomen. The patient's abdomen is distended and he is disoriented. His blood pressure is 100/64 and heart rate is 143. The patient is intubated in the trauma bay following the administration of propofol and succinylcholine. His blood pressure then falls precipitously and he suffers a cardiac arrest. What was the likely cause of his cardiac arrest?

Propofol is an intravenous anesthetic which causes a decrease in systemic vascular resistance (SVR). This patient was in severe hemorrhagic shock and his blood pressure was maintained by peripheral vasoconstriction and tachycardia. Propofol caused a decrease in sympathetic responsiveness and directly caused vasodilatation, resulting in severe hypotension and cardiac arrest. Propofol should be used with extreme caution in the hypovolemic patient.

Choosing an Intravenous Anesthetic

- Intravenous anesthetics are most commonly used to induce anesthesia
- Inhaled (volatile) anesthetics are most commonly used in the maintenance of anesthesia
- Inhaled (volatile) anesthetics can be used to induce anesthesia (inhalational induction), and intravenous anesthetics can be used in the maintenance of anesthesia (total intravenous anesthesia[TIVA])
- Intravenous anesthetics vary in their effects on the cardiac, pulmonary, and central nervous systems
- Choice of anesthetic should be individualized to the patient's needs, hemodynamic physiology, and the clinical scenario

Propofol

- Rapid onset and offset of action
- Antiemetic
- Decreases SVR
- Acts as a mild cardiac depressant

- Causes dose-dependent respiratory depression
- Decreases cerebral blood flow and intracranial pressure (ICP)
- Lacks analgesic (pain) effects
- Decreases postoperative nausea and vomiting

Propofol is a popular intravenous anesthetic due to its rapid onset and offset of action, as well as its antiemetic properties. However, it should be used with caution in clinical situations when peripheral vasodilatation is to be avoided, such as severe hypovolemia or aortic stenosis.

Thiopental

- Rapid onset of action
- Slower offset of action than propofol, especially after repeated doses
- Decreases SVR
- Decreases cerebral blood flow and ICP
- Causes dose-dependent respiratory depression

Etomidate

- Rapid onset of action
- Slower offset of action than propofol
- Does NOT affect SVR
- Ideal in patients with cardiovascular instability or when vasodilation would be detrimental
- Decreases cerebral blood flow and ICP
- Can cause adrenocortical suppression

Etomidate is an ideal intravenous agent for use in the setting of hypovolemic or hemorrhagic shock, but may still lead to hypotension secondary to reduction in sympathetic tone.

Ketamine

- Induces a dissociative anesthesia
- Can cause unpleasant hallucinations
- Usually given with a benzodiazepine to prevent hallucinations
- Acts as a sympathomimetic, increasing heart rate and blood pressure
- Maintains ventilatory drive
- Increases cerebral blood flow and ICP
- Has potent analgesic properties

Ketamine should be avoided in patients with increased ICP, a ruptured globe, or those at risk for coronary ischemia. It has been used in hemorrhagic shock to maintain sympathetic tone, although it can result in hypotension in situations where endogenous sympathetic reserve is depleted. Ketamine is also useful as an induction agent when maintenance of spontaneous negative inspiratory pressure is indicated, as in the physiology of an anterior mediastinal mass.

	Propofol	Etomidate	Thiopental	Ketamine
Respiratory depression	Yes	Yes	Yes	Supports respiratory drive
Systemic vascular resistance	Decreased	No change	Decreased	Increased (decreased if endogenous catecholamines are depleted)
Analgesic effect	No	No	No	Yes
Nausea and vomiting	Decreased	Increased	No change or increased	No change
Cerebral blood flow	Decreased	Decreased	Decreased	May increase
Intracranial pressure	Decreased	Decreased	Decreased	May increase
Adrenocortical suppression	No	Yes	No	No

A 6-year-old girl presents to the operating room for an open reduction and internal fixation of a fractured femur. The patient is extremely anxious and uncooperative. How would you induce anesthesia?

An inhalation induction uses a volatile anesthetic to induce anesthesia and can be accomplished without intravenous access.

Inhaled (volatile) Anesthetics

- Usually used to maintain anesthesia
- May also be used to induce anesthesia
- Dosage is expressed in percent concentration of inhaled gas
- All inhaled (volatile) anesthetics cause some degree of vasodilatation and myocardial depression
    - Nitrous oxide has the most hemodynamically stable pharmacodynamics
- Choice of volatile anesthetic
    - Titratability
        - Desflurane is the most titratable, followed by sevoflurane
    - Airway irritability
        - Sevoflurane causes the least airway irritation and is readily used for the induction of anesthesia
        - Desflurane is associated with the most airway irritability
    - Effect on closed air spaces
        - Nitrous oxide readily diffuses from the blood to closed air spaces, causing either expansion or an increase in pressure
- Nitrous oxide should be avoided in situations where an increase in volume or pressure of an enclosed air space should be avoided, such as middle ear surgery, bowel obstruction, a closed pneumothorax, or the presence of intravascular gas.

Minimum Alveolar Concentration

- Defined as the partial pressure of inhaled anesthetic that prevents movement in response to a surgical incision in 50% of the population
- Used to determine the appropriate dosage and to compare potencies of volatile anesthetics
- The concept of Minimum Alveolar Concentration (MAC) is additive. Certain factors reduce or increase the MAC of a given inhalational anesthetic agent. Examples include:
  - Potency of a volatile agent
  - Age
  - Patient temperature
  - Concurrent drug administration
  - Ethanol and illicit substance use
  - Pregnancy

A 33-year-old healthy woman is about to undergo an emergent abdominal laparoscopy for ovarian torsion. The patient last ate a full meal 3 hours prior to presentation in the operating room. What strategy should be used for induction and intubation?

Adults who have eaten within 6 to 8 hours of general anesthesia are at increased risk for aspiration. When an operation is urgent or emergent, a rapid-sequence induction with propofol and succinylcholine can be used. The anesthesiologist compares the potential risk of aspiration with the potential risk of delaying surgery.

Rapid Sequence Induction

- Used to decrease the risk of aspiration prior to intubation
- A mask with 100% oxygen is placed over the patient's mouth and nose
  - Replaces the gas in the patient's lungs with oxygen (denitrogenation)
- The patient is then given an intravenous induction agent (e.g., propofol, etomidate, thiopental, ketamine) along with succinylcholine, providing rapid onset of anesthesia and muscle paralysis
  - A rapidly acting non-depolarizing muscle relaxant (such as rocuronium) may be used if succinylcholine is contraindicated
- Cricoid pressure is applied prior to induction
  - The cricoid cartilage is a circumferential ring, and applying pressure compresses the esophagus posterior to it
  - Cricoid pressure reduces the likelihood of passive regurgitation/aspiration of gastric contents
  - Cricoid pressure can also improve visualization of vocal cords, although this is best achieved by applying pressure to the thyroid cartilage
- Once fasciculations from the succinylcholine are seen, the patient is intubated and the airway secured
- Positive pressure mask ventilation is avoided to prevent delivering air into the stomach, which would increase the risk for aspiration

---

A 29-year-old construction worker who presented after a fall from a ladder with paraplegia and multiple fractures is going to the OR for revision of his external fixation. It is 6 days after his fall. What paralytic should you avoid in this patient?

Succinylcholine. Due to his spinal trauma, there is upregulation of his acetylcholine receptors. Succinylcholine administration would likely result in hyperkalemia.

Succinylcholine

- Rapid onset and offset of action
- Binds, depolarizes, and non-competitively inhibits acetylcholine receptors at the neuromuscular junction (NMJ)
- Metabolized by plasma pseudocholinesterases
  - An extended clinical effect is seen in patients with atypical plasma pseudocholinesterases
- Fasciculations usually occur and can cause postoperative myalgias
- Causes an acute transient increase in plasma potassium level
  - Increase in plasma potassium level is related to the number of acetylcholine receptors at the NMJ
  - Patients with increased receptors at the NMJ are at increased risk for hyperkalemia
    - Spinal cord injury
    - Burns
    - Immobility
    - Neuromuscular disorder such as muscular dystrophy
    - However, succinylcholine may be given to patients in renal failure with normal potassium levels

Non-Depolarizing Neuromuscular Blockers

- Act by competitively antagonizing the acetylcholine receptor at the NMJ
- Each depolarizing neuromuscular blockers (NMB) has its own unique profile based on
  - Onset of action
    - Rocuronium has a fast onset
  - Duration of action
  - Hemodynamic effects
    - Pancuronium causes tachycardia by vagolysis
  - Metabolism
    - Most non-depolarizing NMBs are metabolized by the liver and/or kidney
    - Cisatracurium degrades spontaneously in plasma and is useful in patients with liver and kidney failure

Monitoring Effects of Non-Depolarizing Neuromuscular Blockers

- An electric current is placed over a peripheral nerve, and the corresponding muscle is observed
- The standard is to administer four pulses of current at a set frequency (train-of-four)
- The fewer the number of twitches, the greater the neuromuscular blockade

Reversal of Non-Depolarizing Neuromuscular Blockers

- Non-depolarizing NMBs act by competitive inhibition
- By increasing the concentration of acetylcholine in the NMJ, it is possible to clinically reverse the effects of the NMB
- The patient must have at least one visible twitch when testing the train-of-four
- An acetylcholinesterase inhibitor is used
  - Acetylcholinesterase inhibitors can increase the amount of acetylcholine at muscarinic receptors as well, resulting in bradycardia
  - An anticholinergic agent (i.e., atropine or glycopyrrolate) must be given with the acetylcholinesterase inhibitor (i.e., neostigmine or edrophonium) to prevent this bradycardia

A 28-year-old male presents to the operating room for elective shoulder surgery. The anesthesiologist recommends performing an interscalene block for postoperative pain control. 30 cc of 0.5% ropivacaine is injected around the brachial plexus via the interscalene groove in the patient's neck. Shortly after injection, the patient comments on a ringing sound in his ears and begins to seize. What should you do next?

The patient's seizure is due to local anesthetic toxicity. Treatment includes monitoring and maintaining the patient's airway, oxygenation, ventilation, and circulation. Administer a benzodiazepine, barbiturate, or propofol to stop the seizure.

Mechanism of Local Anesthetics

- Prevent propagation of nerve impulses by blocking sodium channels
- Act by entering neurons in the neutral uncharged form and then block sodium channels from within the cell

Local anesthetics do not work well when infiltrated into an acidic, infected area (such as an abscess) because the local anesthetic molecules become charged and cannot enter the nerve cell.

Type of Local Anesthetic

- Ester anesthetics
  - Metabolized by plasma pseudocholinesterases
  - Can cause allergic reaction in patients allergic to para-aminobenzoic acid
  - Examples include tetracaine, procaine, and chloroprocaine
- Amide anesthetics
  - Metabolized by the liver
  - Should be used cautiously in patients with liver failure
  - Examples include lidocaine, bupivacaine, and ropivacaine

Patients who present with an allergy to ester local anesthetics (e.g., patients who have a history of a reaction to procaine at the dentist) may be safely administered a preservative-free amide local anesthetic.

Local Anesthetic Toxicity

- Central nervous system
  - Perioral numbness (can be the first symptom in awake patients)
  - Tinnitus
  - Slurred speech
  - Vertigo
  - Seizures
    - Treatment is maintenance of the patient's airway, oxygenation, ventilation, circulatory support, and administration of a benzodiazepine, barbiturate, or propofol to stop the seizure

- Cardiovascular
  - Profound hypotension
  - Cardiac depression
  - Degree of cardiac toxicity
    - Bupivacaine > ropivacaine > lidocaine
    - Duration of local anesthetic cardiac toxicity parallels duration of action
      - Bupivacaine ~ ropivacaine > lidocaine
      - Bupivacaine-induced cardiac toxicity can be refractory to pharmacologic treatment and may require cardiopulmonary bypass
  - Local anesthetic cardiac toxicity can be refractory to catecholamines and cardiac defibrillation. Treatment may require intravenous lipid emulsion or cardiopulmonary bypass. Intravenous lipid emulsion is thought to preferentially remove the lipid-soluble local anesthetic out of the myocardium and into the lipid emulsion
- Toxic doses

	Plain solution (mg/kg)	Solution with epinephrine (mg/kg)
Lidocaine	4–5	7
Bupivacaine	2.5	3

The first sign of lidocaine toxicity is perioral numbness and tinnitus in the conscious patient.

A 27-year-old man presents to the operating room for removal of a testicular varicocele. The anesthesiologist and patient decide on spinal anesthesia. Bupivacaine is injected into the subarachnoid space at the L4–L5 interspace. A T4 level block is achieved and the operation is performed successfully. How did the bupivacaine reach the T4 level if it was injected at L4?

The injected bupivacaine was hyperbaric, meaning that its density is higher than the density of cerebrospinal fluid. The hyperbaric bupivacaine was injected into the subarachnoid space at the L4-5 level and the patient was placed in the supine position. The dense bupivacaine then drifted cephalad along the thoracic kyphosis to the T4 spinal level.

Strategies for Neuraxial (Spinal/Epidural) Anesthesia
- Determine the spinal nerve root which innervates the region to be anesthetized
  - T4: Cesarean section, testicular surgery
  - T6: Lower abdominal surgery (i.e., appendectomy)
  - T10: Hip surgery, vaginal delivery
  - S2–S5: Anal surgery
  - Determine required speed of onset
  - Determine desired duration of action and titratability of anesthesia

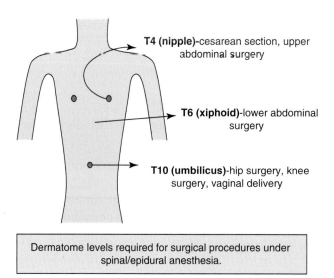

T4 (nipple)-cesarean section, upper abdominal surgery

T6 (xiphoid)-lower abdominal surgery

T10 (umbilicus)-hip surgery, knee surgery, vaginal delivery

Dermatome levels required for surgical procedures under spinal/epidural anesthesia.

Spinal Anesthesia

- Rapid onset of action
- Local anesthetic (possibly combined with an opioid) is injected into the subarachnoid space
- Duration of action determined by properties of local anesthetic
- The addition of epinephrine can extend duration of action
- Technique
  - Injected into the subarachnoid space below the conus medullaris (L1-2)
  - Injected solutions are isobaric, hypobaric (mixed with sterile water), or hyperbaric (mixed with dextrose)
  - The patient is then positioned so gravity and spine curvature cause the local anesthetic to reach the desired level
    - A patient undergoing hemorrhoidectomy can be injected with hypobaric tetracaine into the subarachnoid space at the L4–L5 level while in the prone-jackknife position. The local anesthetic will migrate caudally against gravity to anesthetize the sacral nerve roots
- A catheter can be placed into the subarachnoid space as a continuous infusion, but this is not common

Epidural Anesthesia

- Local anesthetic (possibly combined with an opioid) is injected via a catheter placed in the epidural space
- The epidural space is a potential space located deep to the ligamentum flavum and superficial to the dura
- The injected solution diffuses across the dura to reach the spinal cord and nerve roots
- By injecting a large volume into the epidural space, a large region may be blocked
- Since the catheter is left in place, epidural anesthesia is useful for long procedures and for the treatment of postoperative pain, including patient-controlled epidural analgesia

Side Effects of Spinal and Epidural Anesthesia

- Sympathectomy
  - T1–L2 give rise to the sympathetic nervous system
  - T1–T4 give rise to cardioaccelerator fibers
  - Blocking these levels can lead to hypotension and bradycardia

- Post-dural puncture headache
  - Postural in nature
    - Severity increases when sitting up
    - Severity decreases when supine
  - Treatment options
    - Hydration
    - Caffeine therapy
    - Epidural blood patch
- Total spinal anesthesia
  - Caused by a high level of spinal anesthesia
  - May cause a total sympathectomy and severe hypotension
  - May block phrenic nerve roots, resulting in respiratory arrest
  - Treatment
    - Secure airway, oxygenation, and ventilation
    - Support circulation with volume administration, vasopressors and inotropes
    - Administer an amnestic agent, such as midazolam, since the patient is still fully aware during a high spinal

---

A pulmonary artery (PA) catheter is placed in a 60-year-old man in the intensive care unit because of signs and symptoms of cardiogenic shock. The hemodynamic parameters show a low cardiac index and a high PA diastolic pressure and high PA occlusion pressure. What drug would you like to give to improve his left ventricular function but avoid tachycardia?

Milrinone.

Cardiovascular Drugs

Inotropes

- Milrinone
  - Inotrope and vasodilator
  - Decreases SVR and pulmonary vascular resistance (PVR), and an increases cardiac output (CO)
  - Phosphodiesterase inhibitor
- Epinephrine
  - Mixed beta and alpha agonist
  - Increases SVR and CO
  - May be arrhythmogenic
- Isoproterenol
  - A nonselective beta-1 and beta-2 adrenergic agonist
  - Increases CO and decreases SVR and PVR
  - Chronotrope and may be arrhythmogenic

- Dobutamine
  - Mainly acts on beta-1 adrenergic receptors, but also has minor agonist effects on beta-2 adrenergic and alpha-adrenergic receptors
  - Has more inotropic and chronotropic activity than isoproterenol
- Dopamine
  - Inotropic and chronotropic beta-1 adrenergic activity at lower doses (3 to 10 µg/kg/min)
  - Alpha-1 adrenergic activity predominates at higher doses (>10 µg/kg/min)
- Ephedrine
  - Indirectly acting sympathomimetic
  - Releases endogenous catecholamines
  - Increases CO and SVR

Vasopressors

- Phenylephrine
  - Alpha agonist
  - Increases SVR and may increase PVR
- Norepinephrine
  - Mixed alpha and beta agonist
  - Predominantly acts to increase SVR and may increase PVR
- Vasopressin
  - Acts on vasopressin receptors
  - Increases SVR

Vasodilators

- Nicardipine
  - Calcium channel blocker
  - More potent arterial vasodilator than venous vasodilator
- Nitroprusside
  - Venous and arterial vasodilator, decreasing SVR and PVR
  - Side effect is *cyanide toxicity* following several days of continuous use
- Nitroglycerin
  - More potent venous vasodilator

A 62-year-old woman presents to the preoperative clinic prior to an elective colectomy for colon cancer. She has a history of coronary artery disease with a prior myocardial infarction 4 years ago that was treated with angioplasty and a stent in the left circumflex artery. The patient currently is asymptomatic and walks two miles, three times per week. Does the patient need further coronary evaluation prior to her surgery?

The patient is scheduled for elective surgery and has had coronary revascularization within the past 5 years. Since then, she has not had any recurrence of symptoms and has a good exercise tolerance (>4 METs). Therefore according to the American College of Cardiology (ACC)/American Heart Association (AHA) guidelines, the patient may proceed to surgery without further coronary evaluation.

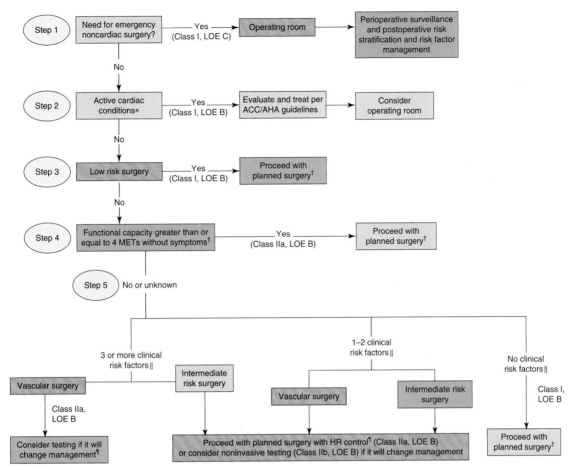

(Reprinted with permission from Fleisher LA, Beckman JA, Brown KA, et al. ACC/AHA 2007 guidelines on perioperative cardiovascular evaluation and care for noncardiac surgery. *Circulation.* 2007;116:e418-e500. Copyright © 2009 Wolters Kluwers Health, Inc.)

American College of Cardiology/American Heart Association Guidelines for Preoperative Cardiovascular Evaluation for Noncardiac Surgery

- Evidence suggests that preoperative coronary revascularization solely for the purpose of getting the patient through surgery is of no benefit. (CARP trial)
  - Risk of preoperative coronary revascularization is comparable to the risk of surgery itself
  - CABG should be reserved for those patients who require revascularization independent of surgery
- Patients currently on beta-blockers for an old myocardial infarction should have the medications continued throughout the perioperative period

An 8-year-old girl is having a tonsillectomy. Shortly after induction of anesthesia with propofol and succinylcholine, the patient becomes tachycardic and the end-tidal carbon dioxide level begins to increase. Her temperature is noted to be 102°F. How could this have been avoided?

This patient might have had a positive family history of malignant hyperthermia, which would have resulted in the avoidance of succinylcholine and volatile anesthetics. These agents are known to trigger malignant hyperthermia in susceptible patients.

Malignant Hyperthermia

- Autosomal dominant disorder with variable penetrance
- Defect of the ryanodine receptor, which controls calcium release in skeletal muscle
- Triggering agents
  - Succinylcholine
  - Potent volatile anesthetics
    - Not nitrous oxide
- Sequence of events
  - Uncontrolled calcium release
  - Uncontrolled skeletal contraction
  - Extreme hypermetabolic state
  - Severe acidosis
  - Rhabdomyolysis
  - Hyperkalemia
  - Possible renal failure
  - Possible cardiac dysrhythmia/cardiac arrest
  - Possible disseminated intravascular coagulation
- Management
  - Prevention with a detailed patient and family history
    - Neuromuscular disorders, such as muscular dystrophy, can be associated with malignant hyperthermia
  - Avoid triggering agents
    - May use TIVA or regional anesthesia
  - Treatment
    - Stop all potential triggering agents
    - Hyperventilate lungs with 100% oxygen
    - Dantrolene (2.5 mg/kg) IV every 10 minutes to a maximum dose of 10 mg/kg
    - Ice to cool patient
    - Treat metabolic/electrolyte abnormalities
    - Hydrate and diurese to avoid rhabdomyolysis-induced renal failure

---

A 33-year-old healthy woman is having an elective laparoscopic cholecystectomy. Minutes after insufflation of the peritoneum, there is an abrupt drop in blood pressure and end-tidal carbon dioxide. What is the most likely cause?

While insufflation alone can cause hypotension via decreasing venous return to the heart, a carbon dioxide embolism classically presents with the sudden onset of hypotension and decreased end-tidal carbon dioxide during abdominal insufflation.

Differential Diagnosis of a Sudden Drop in End-Tidal Carbon Dioxide

- Disconnection of the ventilator tubing or mucous plugging
- Pulmonary embolism, either gas or thrombus
- Profound vasovagal response
- Myocardial event

- Tension pneumothorax
- Any cause of an abdominal compartment syndrome (excessive intra-abdominal pressure leads to decreased venous return)
    - Abdominal hemorrhage
    - Significant edema
    - Ascites
    - Insufflation

There is a broad differential diagnosis for decreased end-tidal carbon dioxide. A sudden decrease in expired carbon dioxide can represent an acute decrease in CO with impending cardiac arrest. An increase in end-tidal carbon dioxide either represents alveolar hypoventilation, or increased carbon dioxide production or absorption.

Venous Gas Embolus

- Associated with procedures that could introduce gas into the venous system
    - Laparoscopy
    - Laser tumor resection
    - Craniotomy
    - Cardiac surgery
    - Vascular surgery
    - GI endoscopy
    - Hepatic resection
    - Venovenous bypass during liver transplantation
- Causes
    - Carbon dioxide embolism can occur with the creation of a pneumoperitoneum
        - Carbon dioxide enters the circulation through vascular tears or raw surfaces of vascular-rich tissue such as the liver
- Treatment
    - Release of pneumoperitoneum and flush field with saline
    - Position patient head down
    - Hyperventilate with 100% oxygen
    - Inotropic support to augment right ventricular contractility
    - Aspirate air through a central line in the right atrium

SUGGESTED READINGS

McFalls EO, Ward HB, Moritz TE, et al. Coronary-artery revascularization before elective major vascular surgery. *N Engl J Med.* 2004; 351:2795–2804.

Fleisher LA, Beckman JA, Brown KA, et al. ACCF/AHA focused update on perioperative beta blockade incorporated into the ACC/AHA 2007 guidelines on perioperative cardiovascular evaluation and care for noncardiac surgery. *Circulation.* 2009; 120:e169–e276.

31 Critical Care I: Principles of Management

Samir M. Fakhry and Joseph V. Sakran

A 60-year-old male with a history of hypertension and a colon mass underwent a 4-hour right colon resection under general anesthesia for adenocarcinoma of the colon. The estimated blood loss was 800 mL and intra-operative urine output was 150 mL. The anesthesiologist had placed a right internal jugular catheter and administered 3,000 mL of normal saline and 1 unit of packed red blood cells (pRBCs). Preoperative evaluation revealed that the patient had a hematocrit of 40% and a normal serum creatinine. Admission to the ICU was requested because the patient was slow to awaken from anesthesia and was hypothermic (35.4°C). He arrived in the ICU on mechanical ventilation. Vital signs in the first hour included BP 110/50, HR 120, urine output of 25 mL for the hour, and a temperature of 35.4°C. The patient is not moving. What are the next steps in management?

Re-warming and close hemodynamic monitoring are important principles. Multiple priorities must be addressed concurrently. Support for organ function, analgesia/sedation, and fluid and electrolyte management are priorities that must be addressed on an ongoing basis.

Initial Management of the Postoperative Intensive Care Unit Patient

- Chest X-ray is needed to evaluate the placement of the central venous catheter (CVC) and endotracheal tube (ETT)
- An arterial blood gas (ABG) to assess ventilation/oxygenation
- A complete blood count and chemistry panel are indicated to evaluate blood loss and check electrolytes
- A fluid challenge may be warranted. One liter of normal saline or lactated Ringer (NOT hypotonic fluid, which will cause hyponatremia) should be given as a bolus and urine output monitored. At least 30 to 50 mL (0.5 to 1 mL/kg) of urine per hour is generally desirable
- Restoring a normal temperature is important and can be accomplished by using external warming devices, warm IV fluids, humidified air delivered by the ventilator, and raising the temperature of the patient's room
- Residual neuromuscular blockade can be evaluated using a "Train-of-Four" nerve stimulator. Once the patient has regained motor function and sedation has begun to wear off, the ventilator may be adjusted to allow the patient to participate in ventilation

A 52-year-old female patient underwent a prolonged operative procedure for perforated diverticulitis. She was found to have significant contamination of her peritoneal cavity and required a sigmoid resection and colostomy. In the perioperative period, she demonstrated evidence of infection with fever, tachycardia, and two episodes of hypotension from which she was resuscitated with crystalloids. Postoperatively, she was placed in the ICU and continued to require full mechanical ventilation support. Attempts at weaning have resulted in a rapid respiratory rate with desaturation to 90% on pulse oximetry. Her chest X-ray reveals bilateral pulmonary infiltrates. Her white blood cell (WBC) count is 14,000 and her hematocrit is 24%. ABG determination shows a pH of 7.35, a PaO_2 of 65, and a $PaCO_2$ of 48 on intermittent mandatory ventilation with settings of: rate = 12/minute, tidal volume = 800 mL, FiO_2 = 0.65 and PEEP = 5 cm H_2O. The patient is awake and appears uncomfortable with poor synchronization with the ventilator. Her preoperative weight was 90 kg. What is the patient's diagnosis and what are the next steps in management?

The patient has evidence of acute respiratory distress syndrome (ARDS). She will benefit from a ventilator strategy consistent with the ARDS network (ARDSnet) guidelines using low tidal volumes and low ventilator pressures. This patient should be placed on a lower tidal volume of 550 mL and her ventilator rate increased in order to improve her ventilation and oxygenation.

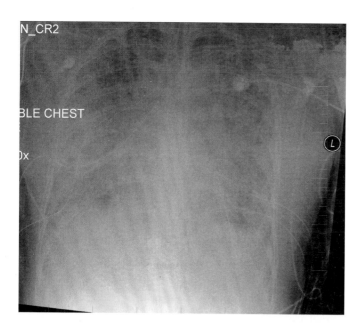

Chest X-ray of a patient with acute respiratory distress syndrome (ARDS). (With permission from Fischer JE, Bland KI, Callery MP, et al., eds. *Mastery of Surgery.* 5th ed. Philadelphia, PA: Lippincott Williams & Wilkins; 2006.)

The Acute Respiratory Distress Syndrome

- The diagnosis requires the following:
    - A predisposing condition (most frequently sepsis)
    - Bilateral patchy pulmonary opacities or infiltrates on chest X-ray
    - Acute onset of respiratory distress
    - A PaO_2/FiO_2 ratio <200
    - Low total static compliance
    - Normal pulmonary capillary wedge pressure
- Important to differentiate ARDS from pulmonary edema secondary to poor left ventricular function or congestive heart failure

- Most readily distinguished with a pulmonary artery catheter
- Chest X-ray imprecise to differentiate
- Trans-esophageal echocardiography can assess cardiac function by measuring ventricular filling
- The most effective strategy for the patient with ARDS is the implementation of the ARDSnet protocol for mechanical ventilation
  - Tidal volumes of approximately 6 mL/kg and plateau pressures of 30 mmHg or less
  - In a prospective randomized trial, this protocol resulted in improved outcomes
- Steroid use is contraindicated in ARDS patients
- Mortality remains high (30% to 40%) and is related to the underlying condition

ARDS manifests as bilateral diffuse patchy infiltrates on chest X-ray in the absence of pulmonary edema (absence of pulmonary edema is defined as a pulmonary capillary wedge pressure <18 mmHg).

In the above-mentioned patient, a hematocrit of 24 is noted in the postoperative period. After adjusting the patient's mechanical ventilator and providing her with adequate sedation and analgesia, her heart rate is 80 bpm with a blood pressure of 120/80 mmHg and a urine output of 55 mL per hour. She has no evidence of acidosis and has good tissue perfusion. Should the patient receive blood transfusion? How should analgesia and sedation be managed?

No transfusion is indicated in this patient as long as her hemoglobin (Hb) exceeds 7 mg/dL (i.e., a hematocrit above 21%) in the absence of hemodynamic instability, a suspicion of ongoing bleeding or active myocardial ischemia.

Assessing the Need for a Blood Transfusion

- Blood transfusion in the hemodynamically stable patient without active myocardial ischemia is not required for a hemoglobin >7 mg/dL (hematocrit >21%)
- In younger patients, blood transfusions above these levels worsen the outcome
- Patients who have expected or ongoing bleeding or active myocardial ischemia should receive a blood transfusion as indicated for their situation
- Adherence to the "transfuse to 10/30" rule is not justified

The above-mentioned patient continues to improve and is weaned down to minimal settings on the ventilator (PS 40/5/5)? What parameters can be used to assess her readiness to be extubated?

The Tobin index (rapid shallow breathing index RSBI), negative inspiratory force, tidal volume, and cuff leak.

Weaning to Extubation

- Mental Status
  - The ability of patients to follow commands indicates a higher probability they will be able to protect their airway
- A "spontaneous breathing trial" on a T-piece or C-PAP allows assessment of patient's readiness for extubation
  - "Tobin index" (rapid shallow breathing index): Respiratory Frequency to Tidal Volume ratio (F/V_T); F in breaths per minute, V_T in liters
  - An accurate measure of the likelihood of successful extubation (no other test or variable shown to be predictive)

- An index of less than 105 is generally associated with a high likelihood of successful extubation
- The index was intended to accurately select patients for *extubation*– Patients with a tracheostomy do not require calculation of their F/V_T ratio as they can simply undergo a trial off the ventilator and be reconnected if they fail
  - Negative inspiratory force
    - Useful adjunct but not a good predictor of successful extubation on its own
    - Gives an indication of the patient's strength and ability to take their own breath
    - < -25 is desirable for extubation
  - Cuff leak test
    - ETT cuff is deflated and either the patient breathes around the ETT or the ventilator delivers a breath part of which leaks around the ETT
    - A positive cuff leak suggests no swelling in the trachea
    - Not entirely reliable

A 32-year-old man is admitted to the ICU following an extensive abdominal procedure for resection of a large tumor. His blood loss was estimated at 1,500mL. He received large volumes of crystalloids as well as blood, fresh frozen plasma and platelets in the operating room. Upon arrival to the intensive care unit, he is ventilated and oxygenating well, his blood pressure is 90/50 mmHg, his heart rate 125 bpm and he has minimal urine output. His hematocrit is 37%. What is the optimal choice of fluid for volume resuscitation in this patient?

Crystalloids are the preferred fluid for resuscitation in this patient. There is no demonstrated advantage to the use of albumin or other colloids. In this patient, it would also be prudent to monitor the hematocrit as crystalloid resuscitation proceeds.

Electrolyte Content of Commonly Used Intravenous Crystalloid Solutions

Solution	Electrolyte (mEq/L)						
	Na+	K+	Ca2+	Mg2+	Cl⁻	HCO_3^-	
0.9% NaCl	154	–	–	–	154	–	
0.45% NaCl	77	–	–	–	77	–	
0.33% NaCl	56	–	–	–	56	–	
0.2% NaCl	34	–	–	–	34	–	
Lactated Ringer	130	4	4	–	109	28	
3.0% NaCl	513	–	–	–	513	–	
5.0% NaCl	855	–	–	–	855	–	

(With permission from Mulholland MW, Lillemoe KD, Doherty GM, Maier RV, Upchurch GR, eds. *Greenfield's Surgery*. 4th ed. Philadelphia, PA: Lippincott Williams & Wilkins; 2005.)

IV Fluids

- There has been no advantage of albumin over saline in resuscitation in critically ill patients found in a large prospective randomized data
- A Cochrane meta-analysis suggested that the use of albumin resulted in worse outcomes

- A liter of lactated Ringer provides 25 mL of bicarbonate through the conversion of lactate to bicarbonate in the liver
- Normal saline has a larger quantity of chloride but no bicarbonate
- Patients who receive large volumes of normal saline are likely to develop a hyperchloremic metabolic acidosis
  - Normal saline hyperchloremic compared to serum (154 mEq/L compared to 100 mEq/L)
  - As larger volumes of normal saline are administered, the serum chloride progressively rises
  - Metabolic acidosis likely due to a reduction in the strong anion gap by an excessive rise in plasma chloride as well as high renal bicarbonate elimination
- Patients receiving large volumes of lactated Ringer often become hyponatremic since lactated Ringer contains 130 mEq of sodium per liter
- The choice of crystalloid fluid is often related to the presence or absence of acidosis and the patient's chloride level
- Normal saline is the only fluid that is universally compatible with blood products. Using normal saline obviates the need for switching IV fluids and lines whenever blood is transfused.
- The initial hematocrit in patients who have had recent bleeding may not adequately reflect the true amount of blood loss and will frequently fall as resuscitation is completed
- End points of resuscitation in most patients should be the return of vital signs to normal, a urine output of at least 30 to 50 mL/hour, absence of metabolic acidosis from tissue hypoperfusion (which can be measured with serial lactates), and the return of normal capillary refill

The above patient remains hypotensive despite aggressive resuscitation. A pulmonary artery catheter is placed for closer monitoring. The following values are returned: CO = 10, SV = 40, PCWP = 9, CVP = 1, SVR = 1,800. What is the appropriate next step in management?

The patient remains hypovolemic and should be given more fluid resuscitation.

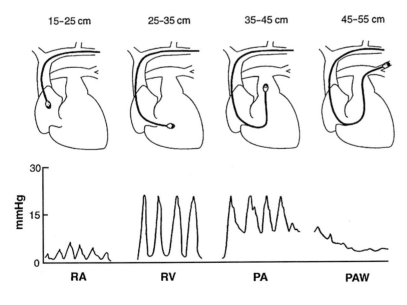

Pressure waveforms with pulmonary artery catheterization. (With permission from Fischer JE, Bland KI, Callery MP, et al., eds. *Mastery of Surgery.* 5th ed. Philadelphia, PA: Lippincott Williams & Wilkins; 2006.)

Pulmonary Artery (Swan-Ganz) Catheter

- Placing the catheter
  - Zone 3 of the lungs is the optimal positioning
  - There is dependent flow of blood in zone 3 and venous P > alveolar P → pressure is more accurately reflected for the left atrium (LA)
  - If the catheter tip is in zone 1 or 2, it reflects alveolar, not LA pressure
  - Relative contraindications: Previous pneumonectomy, left bundle branch block

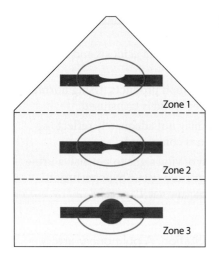

Zones of the lung.

- Pulmonary artery catheter normal values

Parameter	Normal values	Miscellaneous
Cardiac output	4–8 L/min	
Cardiac index	2–4 L/min/m²	Calculated by CO/body surface area
Stroke volume	40–50 mL/m²	
Pulmonary artery pressure	15–30/8–15 mmHg	
PCWP	6–12 mmHg	– Reflects filling pressure of LV – Can be distorted by pulmonary HTN, aortic regurgitation, mitral stenosis, mitral regurgitation, high PEEP and poor LV compliance
CVP	1–6 mmHg	– Reflects filling pressure of RV – Low levels useful for initial fluid resuscitation but otherwise unreliable – Aids in diagnosis of RV infarct and tamponade – Non-myocardial factors that increase CVP include kinking of catheter, vasoconstrictive drugs, positive-pressure ventilation, pneumothorax, flail chest, tamponade, and PE
SVR	900–1,200 dynes/cm²	

- Approximate distances to wedge
  - R SC: 45 cm
  - R IJ: 50 cm
  - L SC: 55 cm
  - L IJ: 60 cm
- Complications
  - Hemoptysis post-pulmonary artery catheter placement → concerning for pulmonary artery perforation
    - Pull catheter back slightly and inflate balloon
    - Increase PEEP
    - If bleeding does not resolve, may need lobectomy
  - Heart block
  - Thrombosis
  - Bacterial endocarditis

Should the above patient be placed on stress gastritis prophylaxis and if so what is the preferred modality or agent?

This patient should receive stress gastritis prophylaxis. There are a number of acceptable options including sucralfate, H2 blockers, and antacids titrated to an alkaline gastric pH.

Gastritis Prophylaxis

- The pathophysiology of stress gastritis relates to underperfusion of the stomach and gut; it is therefore a type of organ failure
- Stress gastritis is NOT due to excess acid production in the stomach
- More aggressive resuscitation of ICU patients has resulted in significantly fewer cases of stress gastritis
- The diagnosis is best established by upper GI endoscopy—diffuse erosions will be seen in the mucosa of the stomach
- Stress gastritis prophylaxis is indicated for patients with:
  - Mechanical ventilation
  - Steroid therapy
  - Burn
  - Shock
  - Coagulopathy
- Stress gastritis prophylaxis is not indicated in patients who are simply NPO after routine surgery

---

A 70-year-old woman is admitted to the ICU following upper abdominal surgery. She is on mechanical ventilation and the anesthesia team reports that she aspirated gastric contents at the time of intubation. She is hemodynamically stable at this time. What are appropriate interventions for the aspiration episode?

Decompression of the stomach with an NG tube, suctioning the pharynx and the airway, and providing supplemental oxygen and mechanical ventilation as needed are appropriate interventions after an episode of aspiration.

Aspiration

- Most episodes result in a transient chemical pneumonitis, which may manifest as arterial oxygen desaturation
- A minority of patients become supra-infected with bacteria
- "Prophylactic" antibiotics are not indicated for simple aspiration
- Steroids are contraindicated
- There is no utility in obtaining a sputum culture initially
- Treatment is supportive

Bronchoscopy should be reserved for severe cases of aspiration complicated by segmental occlusion of airways and lobar collapse that are unresponsive to standard suctioning and chest physiotherapy.

Several days later, the above patient is still on mechanical ventilation. She has poor IV access and a CVC needs to be placed. What organisms are most frequently isolated from the bloodstream of ICU patients and what are appropriate precautions and techniques to ensure the lowest possible central line associated bloodstream infection (CLABSI) rate?

The organisms most commonly isolated from the blood of ICU patients are coagulase negative Staphylococcus and Staphylococcus aureus. Adherence to CDC recommendations for hand washing, full sterile precautions (sterile gown, sterile gloves, cap, large sterile sheet), chlorhexidine skin preparation, antimicrobial impregnated CVCs, and the use of a pre-procedure checklist have been shown to decrease CLABSI rates.

Central Line Associated Blood Stream Infection

- Over half of coagulase negative *Staphylococcus* and *Staphylococcus aureus* isolates are now methicillin resistant
- Empiric antibiotic coverage for critically ill patients suspected of having bacteremia from CLABSI should include:
  - Vancomycin (or other drug effective against MRSA)
  - Broad-spectrum coverage to include gram negative organisms

CDC Guidelines for the Placement of Central Venous Catheters

- 2% chlorhexidine preparation for skin antisepsis
- Sterile barriers including a cap, mask, sterile gown, sterile gloves, and a large sterile sheet, for the insertion of CVCs or guidewire exchanges

Catheter Management

- CVCs coated with minocyclin and rifampin are superior to those coated with chlorhexidine/silver sulfadiazine and are associated with a dramatically lower rate of CLABSI
- Do not routinely replace CVCs when there are no signs of infection
  - A wire exchange of the CVC with semi-quantitative culture of the catheter tip can help establish the diagnosis of CLABSI without the risks associated with a new CVC placement
- The diagnosis of CLABSI is established with:
  - Fever, tachycardia, elevated white blood cell count, and other signs of infection with no alternative infectious source
  - A positive peripheral blood culture
  - A catheter tip segment growing over 15 colonies of the same organism on semi-quantitative culture on an agar plate

- Resolution of the infection with removal of the CVC and appropriate antibiotics
- If purulence is detected at the catheter insertion site and the patient has signs of infection, cultures need not be performed—the CVC should be removed

A 60-year-old man underwent an abdominal aortic aneurysm repair. He required re-intubation shortly after arriving in the ICU. Three days later, he continues to require ventilator support and now has a fever, an elevated white blood cell count, a new infiltrate on chest radiograph and purulent sputum. What is the patient's diagnosis and what is the effective therapy?

The most likely diagnosis is ventilator-associated pneumonia (VAP). Appropriate therapy is broad-spectrum antibiotic coverage initially which is then modified to a narrower spectrum based on culture results.

Ventilator-Associated Pneumonia

- The most common nosocomial infection in the surgical ICU
- Strategies for prevention ("The VAP bundle")
    - Elevate the head of the bed to 30 to 45 degrees
    - Subglottic suctioning
    - Do not change ventilator circuit more than every 48 hours
    - Comprehensive oral cleaning regimen, e.g., with chlorhexidine
- Caused by aspiration of oropharyngeal pathogens or leakage of secretions containing bacteria around the ETT cuff
- Early onset VAP (first 4 days of hospital stay) usually involves a community-type organism
- Late onset VAP (after the first 4 days) has a higher incidence of multi-drug-resistant organisms
    - Gram positive organisms (including MRSA)
    - Aerobic gram negative organism (*P. aeruginosa, K. pneumoniae, Acinetobacter* species)
- Anaerobes are uncommon in VAP
- Fungi and viruses are uncommon in immunocompetent patients
- Early, appropriate, broad-spectrum, antibiotic therapy should be prescribed with adequate doses to optimize antimicrobial efficacy
- "De-escalation" of antibiotics should be considered once culture data are available
- A shorter duration of antibiotic therapy (5 to 7 days) is adequate for most patients with uncomplicated VAP who initially received appropriate therapy and have had a good clinical response
- A delay in treatment of VAP or the use of inappropriate and/or inadequate antibiotic therapy is associated with increased mortality

The patient in the above case study continues to have a fever and an elevated white blood cell count. Two days later, he develops hypotension, tachycardia, and altered mental status. His temperature rises to 39°C and his WBC is now 24,000. His urine output falls to below 20 mL/hour. ABG determination reveals hypoxemia and a metabolic acidosis. What is the patient's diagnosis?

The patient has developed the systemic inflammatory response syndrome (SIRS) and has progressed to septic shock. He requires aggressive management of multiple simultaneous priorities and is at high risk of complications and death.

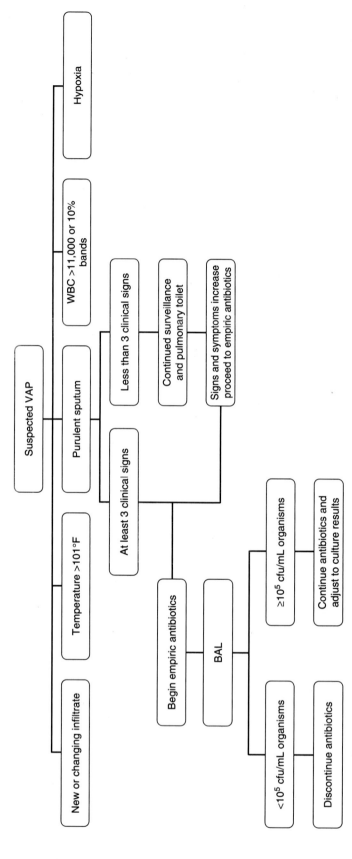

Diagnosis and treatment of ventilator-associated pneumonia (VAP). (With permission from Fischer JE, Bland KI, Callery MP, et al., eds. *Mastery of Surgery.* 5th ed. Philadelphia, PA: Lippincott Williams & Wilkins; 2006.)

Systemic Inflammatory Response Syndrome

- SIRS criteria
    - Body temperature <36°C or >39°C
    - Heart rate >90 bpm
    - Respiratory rate >20 or $PaCO_2$ <32
    - WBC count <4,000 or >12,000
    - If two or more of these criteria are met, the patient has SIRS
- A significant number of patients (especially after injury or in the postoperative period) develop SIRS with no infectious cause identified
    - Majority improve over time
- Sepsis is defined as SIRS with an infectious cause
- Patients who have hypotension in addition to the above findings are considered to be in "septic shock"

Treatment of Patients with Septic Shock

- Begin resuscitation immediately using crystalloid with goal CVP 8–12, MAP ≥65 and UOP >0.5 mL/kg/hour
- Obtain at least two sets of blood cultures
- Start broad-spectrum antibiotics within 1 hour of recognizing septic shock
    - Reassessment and de-escalation of antibiotics once culture results available
    - Duration of therapy is usually 1 week
    - Duration of therapy may be longer if patient is immunocompromised or has another potential source of infection identified
- Attempt to identify the infectious source as quickly as possible and within the first 6 hours
    - Evaluate for effective source control, including possible drain placement or surgical drainage
- The preferred vasopressor is norepinephrine. Vasopressin (0.03 to 0.04 units/minute) is an alternative to norepinephrine or may be added to it
    - If blood pressure is unresponsive to these agents, epinephrine may be added
    - Dobutamine may be useful for patients with myocardial dysfunction evidenced by low cardiac output and elevated filling pressures
    - Low-dose dopamine for "renal protection" is unsubstantiated and should be avoided
- Studies are divided on the use of steroids in patients with sepsis
- Recombinant activated protein C is no longer recommended for sepsis
- Transfusion is reserved for a hemoglobin of <7 to 8 mg/dL in the absence of acute hemorrhage
- Low tidal volume and limitation of plateau pressure for mechanical ventilation of ARDS
- Avoid neuromuscular blockade
- Maintain normal blood glucose levels (<150 mg/dL)
- Bicarbonate is not useful in patients with pH >7.15
- Deep vein thrombosis prophylaxis
- Stress ulcer prophylaxis

Critical Care II: Perfusion and Shock

Albert Chi

Assuming adequate cardiac function, what is the most effective way to improve oxygen delivery in a 60-kg septic patient with a hemoglobin of 8.0, oxygen saturation of 97%, an arterial blood gas of pH = 7.33, PaO_2 = 65, $PaCO_2$ = 42, and a stroke volume of 55?

Transfusion to a hemoglobin level of 10 mg/dL.

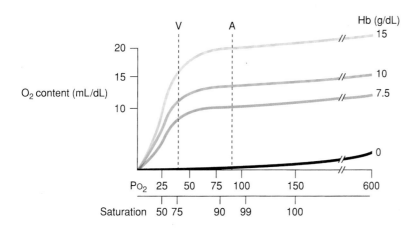

Oxygen content as a function of hemoglobin. (With permission from Mulholland MW, Lillemoe KD, Doherty GM, Maier RV, Upchurch GR, eds. *Greenfield's Surgery.* 4th ed. Philadelphia, PA: Lippincott Williams & Wilkins; 2005.)

Oxygen Delivery

- Options to improve oxygen delivery include increasing hemoglobin, PaO_2, SaO_2, and stroke volume
    - PaO_2 = amount of unbound oxygen in arterial blood—measured by arterial blood gas
    - SaO_2 = amount of oxygen bound to hemoglobin—measured by pulse oximetry
- Oxygen delivery = arterial oxygen content (CaO_2) × cardiac output (CO)
    - CO = heart rate (HR) × stroke volume (SV)
    - CaO_2 = [(Hgb × 1.39) × SaO_2] + [PaO_2 × 0.0031]
        - 1.39 = amount of oxygen in milliliter carried by each gram of fully oxygenated Hgb
        - 0.0031 = solubility of oxygen in plasma
    - Oxygen delivery= {[(Hgb × 1.39) × SaO_2] + [PaO_2 × 0.0031]} × HR × SV

Increasing the hemoglobin in an anemic patient is usually the best way to improve oxygen delivery.

Oxygen Extraction

- Calculated as the difference between the arterial and venous oxygen content divided by the arterial oxygen content
- The pulmonary arteriole is the site of the lowest oxygen saturation in the body

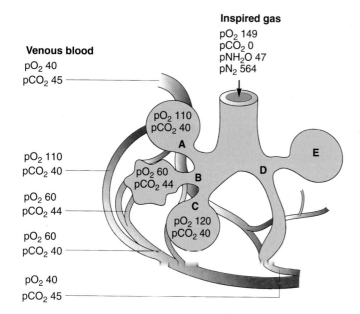

Inspired gas
pO_2 149
pCO_2 0
pNH_2O 47
pN_2 564

Venous blood
pO_2 40
pCO_2 45

pO_2 110
pCO_2 40

pO_2 60
pCO_2 44

pO_2 60
pCO_2 40

pO_2 40
pCO_2 45

pO_2 110
pCO_2 40

pO_2 60
pCO_2 44

pO_2 120
pCO_2 40

Variables affecting pulmonary gas exchange: (A) normal gas exchange, (B) hypoventilation, (C) decreased diffusion, (D) alveolar collapse, (E) shunting of blood flow away from normally ventilated alveolus. (With permission from Mulholland MW, Lillemoe KD, Doherty GM, Maier RV, Upchurch GR, eds. *Greenfield's Surgery.* 4th ed. Philadelphia, PA: Lippincott Williams & Wilkins; 2005.)

- Oxygen delivery:consumption ratio is 5:1
  - Oxygen consumption is usually supply independent
  - Oxygen consumption changes only when low levels of delivery are reached

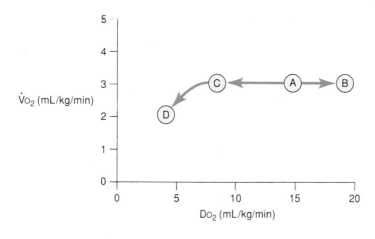

$\dot{V}O_2$ (mL/kg/min)

DO_2 (mL/kg/min)

Oxygen consumption is supply independent except for very low oxygen delivery states. (With permission from Mulholland MW, Lillemoe KD, Doherty GM, Maier RV, Upchurch GR, eds. *Greenfield's Surgery.* 4th ed. Philadelphia, PA: Lippincott Williams & Wilkins; 2005.)

- SvO_2—saturation of venous blood
  - Normally is 65% to 75%
  - Increased SvO_2
    - AV shunt
    - Decreased oxygen extraction—sepsis, cirrhosis, cyanide toxicity, hyperthermia, paralysis, coma, sedation
    - Hyperbaric O_2
  - Decreased SvO_2
    - Occurs with increased oxygen consumption or decreased delivery

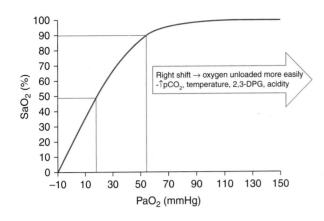

Oxygen dissociation curve. The oxygen dissociation curve is shifted to the right with increased pCO_2, acidity, 2,3-DPG (2,3-diphosphoglycerate), and temperature, thus favoring oxygen unloading to the tissues in times of physiologic stress. Bohr effect is a right shift with increased CO_2.

Right shift → oxygen unloaded more easily -↑pCO_2, temperature, 2,3-DPG, acidity

A 60-kg man presents with a closed fracture of his left femur. He is awake and somewhat anxious. His blood pressure is 110/80 and his heart rate is 100 bpm. What is his estimated blood loss?

His clinical picture is consistent with class II shock, corresponding to an estimated 15% to 30% blood volume loss (750 to 1500 mL). The initial alteration in hemorrhagic shock is increased diastolic pressure.

Hypovolemic Shock

	Class I	Class II	Class III	Class IV
% Blood loss	<15%	15–30%	30–40%	>40%
Volume loss	<750 cc	750–1,500 cc	1,500–2,000 cc	>2,000 cc
Blood pressure	Normal	Normal	↓	↓
Pulse pressure	Normal	↓	↓	↓
Pulse	Normal	Normal to ⇑	⇑	⇑ ⇑
Mental status	Alert	Mildly anxious	Confused	Lethargic
Resuscitation	Crystalloid	Crystalloid	Crystalloid and blood	Crystalloid and blood

A 50-year-old woman is 6 hours status post an exploratory laparotomy and closure of a perforated duodenal ulcer which was undiagnosed for 24 hours prior to operation. She remains intubated and has undergone a massive fluid resuscitation. The nurse informs you that the patient is now oliguric and has high peak airway pressures. What is the next step in management?

Immediate decompressive laparotomy is indicated for abdominal compartment syndrome.

Abdominal Compartment Syndrome

- An acute increase in intra-abdominal pressure
- Common causes include
  - Intra-abdominal or retroperitoneal bleeding
  - Post-resuscitation visceral edema

- Aggressive intra-abdominal packing
- Excessive tension of the wound at the time of closure (usually manifests immediately)
- Signs
    - Increasing peak airway pressure secondary to elevated diaphragm and decreased compliance
    - Oliguria (blood flow to and from kidney is decreased)
    - Increased abdominal girth and abdominal tension
    - Increased central venous pressure (CVP)
    - Hypotension secondary to decreased venous return
- This is a clinical diagnosis, but may be confirmed by checking bladder or gastric pressure (>20 mmHg), which suggests the presence of increased abdominal pressures
- Treatment is a prompt decompressive laparotomy

A 32-year-old man has progressive renal failure in the ICU. What are the indications for hemodialysis?

Classic indications for hemodialysis include hyperkalemia, fluid overload (resistant to diuretic therapy), acute intoxication/toxic ingestion (EtOH, toxic agents), and a uremic syndrome (especially when uremic pericarditis is present)

- **Mnemonic AEIOU**
    - Acid–base problems (severe acidosis or alkalosis)
    - Electrolyte problems (hyperkalemia)
    - Intoxications
    - Overload, fluid
    - Uremic symptoms

A 72-year-old man is noted to be hypotensive following an emergent laparotomy for perforated diverticulitis. His heart rate is 120 bpm, systolic blood pressure is 80 mmHg, temperature is 38.5°C, and he is oliguric. A pulmonary artery catheter is placed and his cardiac output is found to be 6.0 L with a systemic vascular resistance of 1,500 dyn·second/cm⁵. What is the most likely etiology of his shock?

Hypovolemia. In the postoperative period, this may be due to under-resuscitation or bleeding.

A 24-year-old man with a gunshot injury to the abdomen underwent an extensive bowel resection. Blood loss was approximately 1.5 L and he received 5 L of fluids during the operation. A pulmonary artery catheter revealed a cardiac output of 12 L and a systemic vascular resistance of 500 dyn·second/cm⁵. What is the most likely etiology of his hemodynamic instability?

These parameters indicate a hyperdynamic state consistent with septic shock or a profound systemic inflammatory response syndrome. Fluid resuscitation and vasopressor support of the peripheral vasculature are necessary.

A 74-year-old man who underwent a lower extremity bypass procedure is found to have a cardiac output of 3.7, a heart rate of 90 bpm, and a systemic vascular resistance of 2,000 dyn·second/cm^5. What is the most likely intervention required?

An increase in CVP, PCWP, and SVR with a decrease in cardiac output is classic for cardiogenic shock, most likely secondary to a myocardial event. Improving cardiac function with inotropic agents (dobutamine, dopamine, etc.) is critical once tension pneumothorax and tamponade are ruled out. These conditions should be ruled out in this case given the markedly elevated systemic vascular resistance.

Pulmonary Artery Catheters

- Allow measurement of right atrial, pulmonary artery, and pulmonary artery occlusion pressures as well as cardiac output and mixed venous O$_2$ saturations
- Pulmonary artery P are measured at the tip of a non-occluded PA catheter
- Pulmonary artery occlusion P
  - Can be measured once the balloon is positioned in a medium-sized pulmonary artery
  - Used to assess PVR, pulmonary edema, intravascular volume status, LV preload, and LV performance

Pulmonary Artery Catheter Parameters in Shock

- Hypovolemic: Low CVP/PCWP, low CI, high SVRI
- Vasogenic: Low CVP/PCWP, high CI, low SVRI
- Cardiogenic: High CVP/PCWP, low CI, high SVRI
  - Right heart failure: High CVP, CVP ≥ PCWP
    - High right atrial pressure, low CI, high PVRI
  - Left heart failure: High PCWP, PCWP > CVP

Acronyms

CVP: Central venous pressure	LAP: Left atrial pressure
CI: Cardiac index	LVEDP: Left ventricular end diastolic pressure
SVRI: Systemic vascular resistance index	PADP: Pulmonary artery diastolic pressure
PVRI: Pulmonary vascular resistance index	PCWP: Pulmonary capillary wedge pressure
RAP: Right atrial pressure	PA: Pulmonary artery

Type of shock	Blood pressure	Heart rate	Cardiac output	Systemic vascular resistance	Pulmonary capillary wedge pressure
Hypovolemic	↓	⇧	Normal or ↓	⇧	⇧
Septic	↓	⇧	⇧⇧	↓↓	↓ or ⇧
Cardiogenic	↓	Normal or ↓	↓↓	⇧	⇧
Neurogenic	↓	↓	Normal or ↓	↓	↓

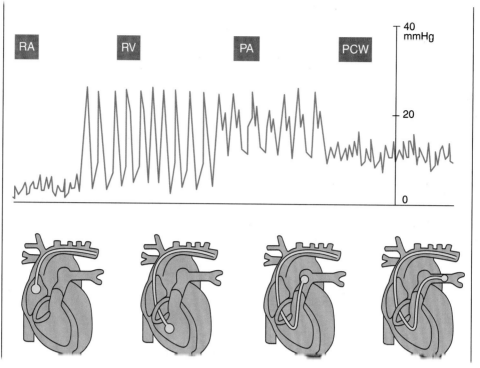

PA catheter pressure waveform characteristics during passage through the heart. (Reprinted with permission from Anaesthesia UK, © 2005.)

- **Normal Hemodynamic Parameters**
  - MAP—70 to 110 mmHg
  - SVR—900 to 1200 dynes/cm^2
  - PVR—80 to 120 dynes/cm^2
  - CO—4 to 7 L/min
  - DO$_2$—700 to 1,400 mL/O$_2$/m^2
  - VO$_2$—180 to 280 mL/O$_2$/m^2
  - O$_2$ extraction—20% to 30%
  - CaO$_2$—16% to 22%
- Vasogenic shock includes septic, anaphylactic, and neurogenic shock
- Other conditions
  - Cardiac tamponade
    - Equalization of diastolic pressure: CVP = PADP = PCWP
  - Mitral stenosis
    - Large "a" wave, PCWP = LAP > LVEDP
  - Mitral regurgitation
    - Large "v" wave, PCWP = LAP > LVEDP
  - Aortic regurgitation
    - LVEDP > LAP = PCWP

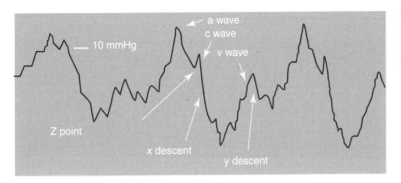

Waveforms of central venous pressure monitoring. (Reprinted with permission from WebMD, Copyright © 2013 by WebMD LLC.)

Electrical event (EKG)	Mechanical event	Right atrial pressure wave (normal RAP is 2 to 6 mmHg)
80–100 ms after P wave	RA systole	a wave
	RA diastole	x descent
After QRS	Tricuspid valve closure	c wave
After peak of T wave	RA filling/tricuspid valve closed	v wave
	RA emptying at opening of tricuspid valve/onset of right ventricle diastole	y descent

33 | Trauma I: Principles of Trauma Care

Samir M. Fakhry, Adesola Akinkuotu, and Joseph V. Sakran

A 20-year-old man presents to the trauma center following a high-speed motor vehicle crash. He was reportedly the unbelted driver of a high-speed vehicle when he went off the road and struck a tree. He was found by rescuers outside the vehicle unconscious and unresponsive. He had a deformity of his right thigh. Upon arrival in the trauma bay, the patient had a blood pressure of 100/50, a heart rate of 120 bpm, and oxygen saturation of 89% on 50% FiO_2. His Glasgow Coma Scale (GCS) is 5. What are the initial steps in the management of this patient?

The Advanced Trauma Life Support (ATLS) protocol consists of evaluating the patient for airway, breathing, and circulation (ABCs). Non-intubated patients with respiratory distress or airway compromise or abnormal mental status (GCS ≤8) should be intubated.

Airway

- Evaluation of the airway is the highest priority for a trauma patient
  - Can the patient talk?
  - Chest auscultation
  - CO_2 detector
  - Pulse oximetry
- Endotracheal intubation should be accomplished while maintaining in-line stabilization of the cervical spine
- Verify correct endotracheal tube position for patients intubated in the field
- Patients with severe facial trauma or a difficult airway should undergo cricothyroidotomy

Breathing

- If breath sounds are absent on one hemithorax, a pneumothorax should be suspected
- If the patient is hemodynamically unstable with absent breath sounds on one side of the chest, they should undergo
  - Emergency needle decompression followed by chest tube placement or
  - Emergent chest tube placement
  - If patient has worse oxygenation after chest tube placement, they may have a tracheobronchial injury, in which case, the chest tube should be clamped and they should be main stem intubated on the unaffected side

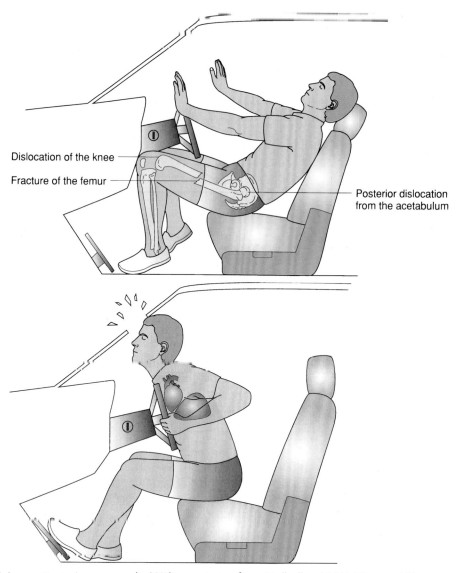

Dislocation of the knee

Fracture of the femur

Posterior dislocation
from the acetabulum

Injury patterns in a car crash. (With permission from Mulholland MW, Lillemoe KD, Doherty GM, Maier RV, Upchurch GR, eds. *Greenfield's Surgery.* 4th ed. Philadelphia, PA: Lippincott Williams & Wilkins; 2005.)

- If there is >1,500 mL of initial output or >200 mL/hour of output for the first 4 hours or >2,500 mL over the first 24 hours, the patient should have a thoracotomy
- In a hemodynamically stable patient, a chest X-ray should be obtained
- Physical examination by auscultation can be misleading in 20% to 30% of patients

Circulation

- All multi-trauma patients should have two large-bore IVs placed in the peripheral veins of the upper extremities
- Central venous lines are generally beneficial in unstable patients
- In patients with penetrating thoraco-abdominal injury, central venous access above and below the injury is preferred
- Alternatives include a saphenous vein cut-down at the ankle or groin
- An intraosseous infusion device can also be used for access, especially for small children and infants
- Patients who are hypotensive or in hemorrhagic shock should be resuscitated using 2 to 3 L of isotonic crystalloid solution as the initial volume challenge

- Patients who continue to be hemodynamically unstable following this challenge should be given uncrossmatched blood
- Two units of O⁺ blood are appropriate for males and women who are not of childbearing age, while O⁻ should be used for women of childbearing age
- An appropriate response to fluid resuscitation is return of blood pressure and heart rate to normal
- Patients who continue to be in shock should undergo appropriate diagnostic evaluation emergently or be taken to the operating room for further resuscitation and control of bleeding
- If patient has distended neck veins, muffled heart sounds, and hypotension, i.e., Beck triad, they may have cardiac tamponade and need emergent pericardiocentesis or thoracotomy to evacuate the blood
  - An echo will initially show impaired diastolic filling of the right atrium
  - Note: Pericardiocentesis blood typically does not clot
- Patients who have sustained a spinal cord injury (especially above the first thoracic vertebrae) may present with a low blood pressure
  - They are in *"spinal shock"*
  - Systolic blood pressure is typically 80 to 90 mmHg with a normal heat rate or bradycardia
  - Urine output is usually high
  - Extremities are warm and well perfused (in hemorrhagic shock they are vasoconstricted with cool, mottled extremities)
  - Vasopressors are sometimes used for peripheral vasoconstriction—should generally be reserved for cases where tissue perfusion is impaired. This is generally accomplished with the use of alpha agonists, such as phenylephrine.
  - Other causes of shock (especially hemorrhage) may be present along with hypotension from spinal cord injury

Disability

- Neurologic examination
- Pupillary response
- Glasgow Coma Score

Exposure

- Multi-trauma patients should have all clothing removed for complete exposure
- Protect the entire spine until there is enough evidence to show that the spine is not injured
- The patient should be in a cervical collar and log-rolled to evaluate their back

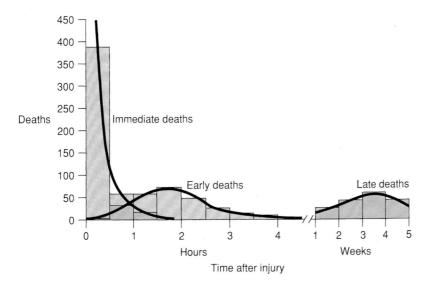

Three periods of peak mortality after injury. (With permission from Mulholland MW, Lillemoe KD, Doherty GM, Maier RV, Upchurch GR, eds. *Greenfield's Surgery.* 4th ed. Philadelphia, PA: Lippincott Williams & Wilkins; 2005.)

An unidentified male is dropped off at the ER door by a vehicle that then speeds away. He has sustained a gunshot wound to the right thigh just above the knee. His BP is 90 systolic and his HR is 130. He is conscious and complaining of pain. While he is being prepared for surgery, resuscitation for his hemorrhagic shock is initiated. Describe the early steps in fluid resuscitation.

Direct pressure applied to the external wound may be helpful. A tourniquet can be used in cases of overwhelming bleeding for short periods of time. Place two large bore IV catheters in the upper extremities. Rapidly infuse 2 to 3 L of isotonic crystalloid solution. If vital signs do not respond, start type O blood (O negative for females of child bearing age).

Blood Volume Resuscitation

- Control of bleeding via application of direct pressure to wounds, stabilization of fractures (splints, traction including the pelvis), etc.
- Pelvic stabilization can be achieved via external fixation devices including a binder or sheet passed around the pelvis and tied over the pubic symphysis to minimize pelvic expansion
- Tourniquets to control bleeding secondary to penetrating injury to the extremities are useful for the short term as a temporizing measure
- Blood loss should be replaced using the 3 to 1 rule: Replace blood loss with equal volumes of packed red blood cells and give three times the blood loss volume in crystalloid solution
  - Example: A blood loss of 1,000 mL would require 1,000 mL of packed red blood cells (approximately 3 units) and 3,000 mL of lactated Ringer's or normal saline solution
- While lactated Ringer's solution is often the initial fluid of choice in trauma, saline is universally compatible with blood products and is preferred with concomitant transfusions
- Large volumes of normal saline solution will result in a hyperchloremic metabolic acidosis, which may confuse the end point of the resuscitation
  - An elevated serum chloride will distinguish this condition from metabolic acidosis resulting from underperfusion of the tissues

Transfusion Guidelines for Fresh Frozen Plasma

- The major indication for fresh frozen plasma (FFP) is abnormal coagulation parameters
- FFP and platelet transfusion should be reserved for specific indications and should NOT be administered "prophylactically"
- Consider giving FFP with a congenital deficiency of AT-III, prothrombin, factors V, VII, IX, X, and XI, protein C, protein S, plasminogen, or antiplasmin
- FFP is indicated for bleeding due to an acquired deficiency from warfarin, vitamin K deficiency, liver disease, massive transfusion, or disseminated intravascular coagulation

The most common cause of diffuse "oozing" is hypothermia, underscoring the importance of keeping the patient warm.

Transfusion Guidelines for Platelets

- Transfuse for platelet count ≤10,000 platelets/mm³ (for prophylaxis)
- Transfuse for platelet count ≤50,000 platelets/mm³ for microvascular bleeding ("oozing") or before a planned procedure
- Transfuse for demonstrated microvascular bleeding and a precipitous fall in platelets
- Transfuse patients in the operating room who have had complicated procedures or have required more than 10 units of blood AND have microvascular bleeding
- Transfuse patients with documented platelet dysfunction (e.g., prolonged bleeding time greater than 15 minutes, abnormal platelet function tests), petechiae, purpura, microvascular bleeding ("oozing"), or before an elective procedure

Massive Transfusion Protocol

- Drawing on recent military experience, many centers are employing massive transfusion protocols for patients with acute, large volume blood loss
- Resuscitation with pRBCs and FFP in a ratio of 1:1 or 1:2 is frequently recommended
- Platelets are usually added in a ratio of 1:1 with ongoing severe bleeding

A 40-year-old man falls 35 m. Evaluation at the trauma center reveals three broken ribs on his left and a grade 3 splenic injury with fluid in the left upper quadrant of his abdomen. Nonoperative management is chosen and he is admitted to the surgical service. What should he be told regarding his prognosis?

Nonoperative management will be successful in most patients with blunt splenic injury, thus avoiding splenectomy.

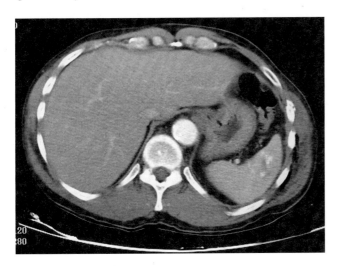

CT scan of the abdomen showing splenic injury with contrast extravasation ("blush") within the spleen. (With permission from Mulholland MW, Lillemoe KD, Doherty GM, Maier RV, Upchurch GR, eds. *Greenfield's Surgery.* 4th ed. Philadelphia, PA: Lippincott Williams & Wilkins; 2005.)

Management of Blunt Splenic Trauma

- The grade of the injury is directly related to the chance of failure of nonoperative management
  - Nonoperative management consists of bed rest, serial exams, and serial hemoglobins
  - Nonoperative management has generally failed if the patient becomes unstable, has a persistently falling hemoglobin despite ongoing blood transfusion, or develops worsening findings on abdominal exam—such patients should have emergent splenectomy
- In hemodynamically stable patients with contrast extravasation in the spleen (a vascular "blush"), angiography with embolization is the treatment of choice
- Hemodynamically unstable patients are generally not candidates for non-operative management
- Splenic salvage maneuvers (cautery, argon beam coagulator, topical hemostatic agents, suture repair, mesh wrap, hemisplenectomy) are rarely utilized

Management of Blunt Hepatic Trauma

- Majority of cases managed non-operatively
  - Conservative management the same as for blunt splenic trauma
- In hemodynamically stable patients with contrast extravasation, angiography with embolization is a treatment option
- Surgical management
  - Manual compression of the liver parenchyma (critical in major liver injury to allow anesthesia to catch up with resuscitation)—perform with packing of right upper quadrant (RUQ)

- Occlusion of the portal triad thereby compressing the portal vein and hepatic artery (the Pringle maneuver) is indicated for massive bleeding
- Continued bleeding despite a Pringle maneuver suggests retrohepatic source (hepatic vein or inferior vena cava)
- Direct suturing with a large blunt needle using absorbable suture material is often effective
- Perform finger fracture hepatotomy to expose lacerated vessels and ducts and selectively ligate them
- Omental packing can be placed in potential space of liver laceration to prevent bleeding
- Common bile duct injury
    - If <50% diameter → use stent
    - If >50% diameter →choledochojejunostomy
- Hepatic resection is associated with a high mortality and is typically not recommended unless the dissection has already been performed by the injury
- Consider the use of atriocaval shunt to achieve control for retrohepatic venous injuries

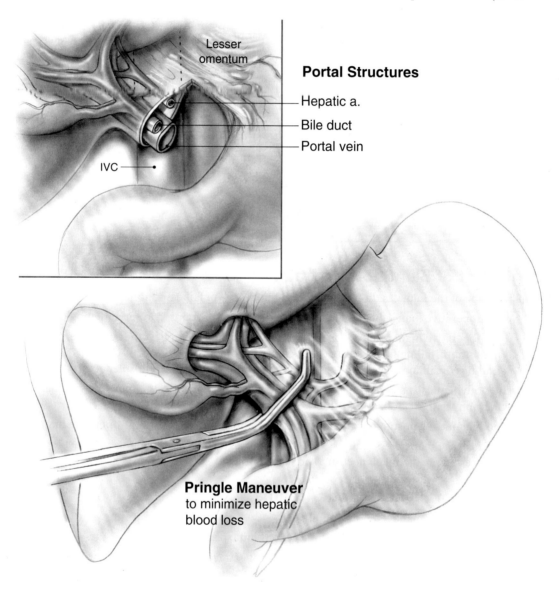

The portal triad consists of the hepatic artery, the portal vein and the common bile duct known as the Pringle Maneuver, cross-clamping of the portal triad can provide control of liver hemorrhage not originating from the hepatic veins and the retro-hepatic vena cava.

- If bleeding persists and is only controlled with direct pressure and the patient is coagulopathic, acidotic and/or hypothermic, perihepatic packing, compressing the liver wound between chest wall, diaphragm, and retroperitoneum should be employed ("damage control")—the patient is then taken to the ICU for resuscitation and re-warming with return to the OR after 24 to 48 hours for removal of packs and control of residual bleeding

Management of Blunt Pancreatic Trauma

- May be asymptomatic at presentation
- Serum amylase or lipase is not useful in excluding pancreatic injury at presentation
- CT may detect blunt pancreatic injury but a normal appearing CT does not exclude injury
- Management is frequently dictated by whether or not there is injury to the pancreatic duct
  - No ductal injury
    - If patient stable, expectant management may be best option
    - If patient becomes symptomatic, repeat CT scan and drain fluid collection if present
  - Ductal disruption
    - More likely to require surgery
    - Occasionally, can use ERCP to place a stent over injury
    - Location of injury will dictate operation
      - Ductal injury at or distal to the neck will require a distal pancreatectomy
      - Concern for ductal injury proximal to the neck that cannot be determined intraoperatively should be treated with wide drainage and postoperative ERCP with possible stenting
    - Whipple should NOT be performed emergently
- Overall, less aggressive surgical intervention results in better outcomes with drainage being associated with better results than resection

---

A 58-year-old woman presents with left hemiplegia after a high-speed motor vehicle crash. She is alert and responsive. Her head CT scan is negative. What is the next step in her management?

Spiral CT angiography of the neck vessels should be performed. A negative CT angiogram of the neck has an extremely high true negative predictive value and no further work-up is required if the CT angiogram is negative. Intimal dissection with luminal compromise is frequently documented as the abnormality in symptomatic patients but asymptomatic patients may also have highly significant lesions. Transection with pseudoaneurysm formation as well as arteriovenous fistulas can also occur. Treatment with anti-thrombotics is the treatment of choice when surgical repair cannot be accomplished. Accumulating data have demonstrated that neck vessel injury in blunt trauma is more common than previously thought. Patients at risk for neck vessel injury can be identified using screening criteria.

Screening Criteria for Blunt Cervical Vessel Injury

- Lateralizing neurologic deficit (not explained by head CT)
- Infarct on head CT scan
- Cervical hematoma (nonexpanding)
- Massive epistaxis
- Anisocoria/Horner's syndrome
- Glasgow Coma Score ≤8 without significant CT findings
- Cervical spine fracture
- Basilar skull fracture
- Severe facial fracture (Le Forte II or III only)

- "Seatbelt sign" above clavicle
- Cervical bruit or thrill
- In some reports, severe upper thoracic trauma is associated with blunt cervical vessel injury

Penetrating Neck Trauma

- Symptoms
  - Carotid injury: Expanding or pulsatile hematoma; neurologic symptoms
  - Esophagus/pharynx: Crepitus, oropharyngeal bleeding
  - Trachea/larynx: Subcutaneous emphysema, stridor, dyspnea
- Diagnosis
  - Penetrating injuries that don't penetrate the platysma require no further diagnostic or therapeutic intervention
  - Location of the penetrating injury is classified by zone and guides diagnostic workup in hemodynamically stable patients

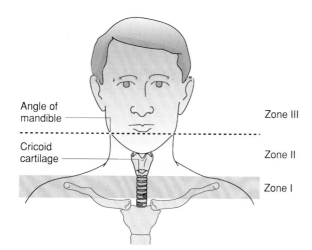

Angle of mandible

Cricoid cartilage

Zone III

Zone II

Zone I

Zones of the neck. (With permission from Mulholland MW, Lillemoe KD, Doherty GM, Maier RV, Upchurch GR, eds. *Greenfield's Surgery*. 4th ed. Philadelphia, PA: Lippincott Williams & Wilkins; 2005.)

Recent studies suggest that CT angiography of the neck and chest is a useful alternative to the above diagnostic tests

- Treatment
  - Patients who are hemodynamically unstable should be taken emergently to OR
  - Carotid injury: If there is an expanding hematoma, explore immediately
  - Never probe a neck wound or hematoma without proximal and distal control
  - Esophageal/pharyngeal injury
    - If pharyngeal injury contained, can be observed

Zones of the neck	Location	Tests
1	Clavicle → cricoid	Angiography, bronchoscopy, rigid esophagoscopy, and contrast esophagogram
2	Cricoid → angle of mandible	Angiography, tracheo-bronchoscopy, rigid esophagoscopy, and contrast esophagogram
3	Angle of mandible → base of skull	Angiography and laryngoscopy/pharyngoscopy

- If esophageal injury <24 hours, can close primarily and place drains
- If esophageal injury >24 hours, create a "spit" fistula (to divert stream), drain the area of the leak widely (include chest tube), and place a gastrostomy tube

---

Three patients are brought to the ED after a "shoot-out" with police. *Patient #1* sustained a trans-temporal gunshot wound (GSW) to the head. His GCS in the field was 4 and he was intubated. He presents to the ED with a GCS of 3T. *Patient #2* sustained a GSW to the left chest, just lateral to his left nipple. He is complaining of shortness of breath. Vital signs are: BP 110/70, HR 114, RR 28, and oxygen saturation of 93% on room air. *Patient #3* sustained a GSW to the abdomen at the level of the umbilicus. He is complaining of abdominal pain. His vital signs are: BP 95/40, HR 120, RR 30 oxygen saturation 96% on room air. You (the surgeon) and an ED physician are available to care for them along with two nurses and a respiratory therapist. In what order should these three patients be prioritized?

Patient #3 requires immediate operative intervention and should be taken to the OR by the surgeon as an emergency. Patient #2 requires immediate left thoracostomy tube placement, which can be accomplished by the ED physician. Patient #2 should be put on a 100% FiO$_2$ facemask, given IV fluid resuscitation, and a single dose of antibiotics (first generation cephalosporin). Patient #1 has a highly lethal lesion. He requires supportive care (mechanical ventilation, IV fluids, antibiotics) while he undergoes head CT scan to determine the extent of injury.

Management of Gunshot Injuries

- Patients with abdominal gunshot wounds have >90% chance of having a surgically correctable lesion and should go to the OR
- A small subgroup of these patients (such as those who are stable with tangential injuries) may benefit from an abdominal CT scan to determine the need for operative intervention
  - Such selective management should be done by experienced surgeons at trauma centers capable of performing serial abdominal exams
- Patients with gunshots to the chest who survive to arrive in the ED are likely a select group, since injury to the heart and great vessels is associated with a high mortality
- Decompression of hemothorax and/or pneumothorax is a high priority and should be accomplished for all patients expeditiously
- Unstable patients require immediate operative intervention

A 27-year-old man presents to the ED following a bar fight. He has an odor of alcohol. His vital signs are normal but he is drowsy and makes incomprehensible sounds when awakened or stimulated. Following completion of a primary and secondary survey the only finding in addition to his altered mental status is a 3-cm laceration just to the left of the umbilicus. What is the appropriate diagnostic and therapeutic approach?

There are a number of options available for the evaluation of the patient. Since his mental status (and thus, the reliability of his abdominal exam findings) is poor, observation cannot be utilized in this case. The remaining options would include local wound exploration, diagnostic peritoneal lavage, or exploratory laparoscopy.

Management of Abdominal Stab Wounds

- For stab wounds below the nipple line, consider both thoracic and abdominal injury
- An abdominal CT scan is not sensitive for small bowel injury and a "negative" abdominal-pelvic CT scan does not rule out intra-peritoneal injury

- Exploratory laparotomy/laparoscopy is indicated for any ONE of the following three criteria:
  - Hemodynamic instability
  - Significant abdominal distention
  - Peritonitis
- Evisceration of abdominal contents (most commonly omentum or bowel) through a stab wound is a relative indication for surgical exploration
  - Although not all of these patients will have an injury, most trauma surgeons will explore patients with evisceration
- Non-operative management of stab injuries to the abdomen can be considered when ALL of the following three criteria are met
  - Hemodynamic stability
  - A soft, non-tender, and non-distended abdomen
  - The patient has a normal mental status and is cooperative
- Only 30% to 50% of these patients have an intra-abdominal injury that requires surgical correction
- Local wound exploration is an effective option
  - The wound is explored locally by instilling local anesthesia, followed by enlarging the wound to allow careful dissection through the tissue planes, following the stab wound but not interfering with its path and ultimately determining whether the stab wound has penetrated the fascial layers and/or peritoneum
  - If there has been fascial and/or peritoneal penetration, the patient is then taken to the operating room for exploration
- Patients with stab wounds to the back who are hemodynamically stable without significant abdominal distention or peritonitis can be managed with triple contrast abdominal-pelvic CT scan, which will frequently delineate the path of the injuring object as well as organ injury

---

A 55-year-old woman was involved in a high-speed motor vehicle crash. She was the restrained front seat passenger and the vehicle was struck on her side by a large truck. There was significant intrusion into the vehicle, resulting in prolonged extrication. The patient has not been conscious since the crash. Initial vital signs at the scene were a blood pressure of 40 mm Hg systolic with an agonal heart rate. The patient was intubated at the scene. Cardiopulmonary resuscitation (CPR) was begun when the patient lost her vital signs as she was being loaded in the ambulance. CPR was continued for 30 minutes during transport. Upon her arrival to the trauma center, she had ongoing CPR without vital signs, fixed and dilated pupils, and no electrical activity on ECG. What is the next step in this patient's management?

The patient should be declared dead.

Cardiopulmonary Resuscitation
- Patients who have sustained cardiopulmonary arrest in the field after blunt trauma and require pre-hospital CPR for longer than 5 minutes have a negligible chance of survival
- Patients who have sustained penetrating trauma and who have undergone more than 15 minutes of pre-hospital CPR also have no reasonable chance of survival
- Emergency department thoracotomy should be reserved for patients who have sustained penetrating trauma and have had less than 15 minutes of pre-hospital CPR
- Exceptions include patients suspected of having pericardial tamponade despite the absence of vital signs on arrival in the trauma bay
- Emergency department thoracotomy for the blunt trauma patient who has already undergone CPR for longer than 5 minutes is futile

- Exceptions to the above recommendation include the pediatric patient, patients with complicating factors such as hypothermia or patients suspected of having a medical cause such as a myocardial infarction as the inciting event

> A 25-year-old male is involved in a roll-over car crash. He never lost consciousness, but upon presentation, his upper front teeth and maxilla are freely mobile. What type of fracture does he have?

A Le Fort I fracture. Treatment is reduction, stabilization, and intra-maxillary fixation.

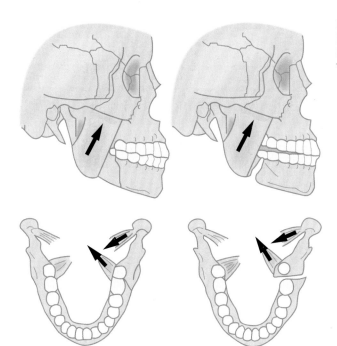

Le Fort fractures. (With permission from Fischer JE, Bland KI, Callery MP, et al., eds. *Mastery of Surgery.* 5th ed. Philadelphia, PA: Lippincott Williams & Wilkins; 2006.)

Le Fort Fractures

- Le Fort I fracture
  - Maxillary fracture that separates the upper jaw and maxilla from the face
  - Treatment is reduction, stabilization, and intra-maxillary fixation
- Le Fort II fracture
  - Nasomaxillary fracture that separates the nasomaxillary complex from the upper face
  - Often results on a downward force on the upper nose
  - Treatment is the same as for a Le Fort I fracture
- Le Fort III fracture
  - Separates the face from the base of the skull
  - Treatment: Suspension wiring to frontal bone; may also need external fixation

34 | Trauma II: Traumatic Injuries

Lisa M. Kodadek and Diane A. Schwartz

A 35-year-old man with significant mandibular trauma presents in respiratory distress and is coughing up blood. An intubation attempt is unsuccessful secondary to distorted anatomy and copious bleeding in the oral cavity. What is the next step?

A surgical airway should be performed in any trauma patient where quick endotracheal intubation is not possible.

Cricothyroidotomy

- Indicated for upper airway obstruction, failed intubation, or maxillofacial trauma
  - Specific maxillofacial trauma of concern includes fracture of the larynx and any injury causing edema of the glottis
- Procedure
  - Identify the cricothyroid membrane just caudal to the thyroid cartilage (Adam's apple)
  - Make a 2- to 4-cm transverse incision over and through the cricothyroid membrane
  - Insert a finger into the incised membrane opening
  - Use manual pressure to control bleeding from anterior jugular veins if a laceration occurs
    - Sacrifice these vessels if necessary
    - Use suture ligation once airway is secure
  - Dilate the tracheal opening wide enough to admit a no. 6 tracheostomy tube
  - Insert the tracheostomy tube, remove the obturator, insert the inner cannula, and insufflate the cuff
  - Connect the Ambu bag and confirm placement by auscultation, oxygen saturation, and end-tidal CO_2

What is an absolute contraindication for performing a diagnostic peritoneal lavage (DPL)?

A planned emergent laparotomy for any reason.

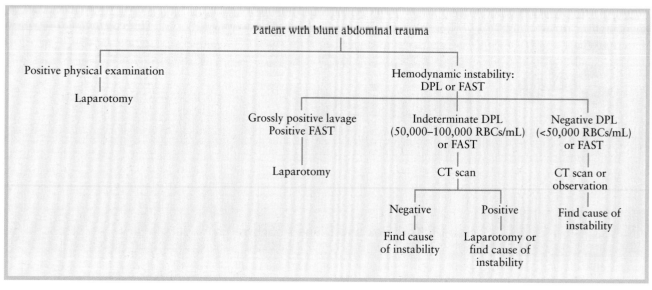

Management of blunt abdominal trauma (With permission from Mulholland MW, Lillemoe KD, Doherty GM, Maier RV, Upchurch GR, eds. *Greenfield's Surgery.* 4th ed. Philadelphia, PA: Lippincott Williams & Wilkins; 2005.)

Diagnostic Peritoneal Lavage

- Historically useful for a rapid assessment of abdominal injury requiring surgery
- Has been replaced by focused assessment with sonography for trauma (FAST), which is used in hemodynamically unstable patients to localize hemorrhage to a body cavity
- Sometimes used in developing countries where ready access to ultrasound technology or CT is not available
- Occasionally considered in hemodynamically unstable obese patients where FAST is technically challenging
- Procedure
    - Make a small vertical midline incision down to the linea alba below the umbilicus
        - In patients with pelvic fractures or hematoma, or women who are pregnant, make the incision above the umbilicus
    - Insert a sterile Foley catheter aimed toward the pelvis and aspirate directly
        - The presence of gross blood or any enteric contents at this point is an indication to abort the procedure and prepare the patient for a laparotomy
    - Inject 10 cc/kg (up to 1 L) of warm crystalloid, wait for 5 to 10 minutes, and drain
        - Drainage of at least 30% of the initial liter of fluid is necessary before sending the specimen for cell count
        - Patient may need to be log-rolled or positioned in reverse Trendelenburg to allow adequate drainage
    - Send fluid for cell count and amylase
- Any ONE of the following indicates a "positive DPL" mandating surgery:
    - Gross blood on initial aspiration
    - Enteric contents on initial aspiration
    - 100,000 red blood cells per cubic mm
    - 500 white blood cells per cubic mm
    - Amylase >175
    - Any bile or urine

A positive DPL is associated with no significant injury in up to 30% of patients; thus, it is not frequently used and is becoming replaced by other diagnostic modalities (FAST, CT in conjunction with physical exam).

A 28-year-old man presents to the emergency room following a bicycle crash. He is coherent but complains of abdominal pain. On presentation his blood pressure was 84/40 mmHg, which remained low at 95/50 mmHg following rapid infusion of 2 L of lactated Ringers through two large-bore IVs. What is the next step in management?

A chest X-ray (CXR) should be obtained to ensure appropriate triage of body cavities. Emergent laparotomy is indicated for any unstable patient with signs or symptoms of an abdominal source. At the time of operation, based on suspicion of the mechanism of injury, several maneuvers can be used to achieve exposure of critical organs. A CT scan should not be performed since the patient is unstable (given his episode of hypotension that did not resolve with IV fluid administration).

Exploring an Abdomen Full of Blood

- Pack all four quadrants
- Expose the diaphragmatic hiatus for supraceliac aortic clamping if necessary
- If there is a hematoma at the diaphragmatic hiatus making exposure of the aorta difficult, then access the aorta through a left thoracotomy
- Systematically remove the packs and define bleeding
- Use the Mattox maneuver to expose the supramesocolic aorta
- Use the Cattell maneuver to expose the inferior vena cava
- If the injury is localized to the infrarenal aorta, the supraceliac clamp can be moved down to the infrarenal position

Supraceliac Aortic Control

- Enter the lesser sac through the gastrohepatic ligament (beware of a replaced or accessory left hepatic artery)
- Retract the esophagus and stomach to the left, exposing the right crus
- Expose the supraceliac aorta by separating the two limbs of the right crus
- Clear medial and lateral walls bluntly (not circumferentially) and place the clamp on the aorta

Mattox Maneuver

- Provides access to the left retroperitoneum (aorta, left kidney, and ureter)
- Take down the left white line of Toldt and extend it up from the sigmoid colon to the splenic flexure
- Mobilize the spleen
- Reflect the viscera medially (to the right)
- This technique is also known as a lateral to medial visceral sweep

Cattell Maneuver

- Provides access to the right retroperitoneum (inferior vena cava, right kidney, and ureter)
- Incise the peritoneal reflection from the ileocecum to the hepatic flexure

Never perform a CT scan on an unstable patient.

A 17 year old unrestrained driver of a motor vehicle crash arrives to the emergency department. He has a GCS of 5, pulse of 110, blood pressure at 120/94 mmHg, a large open fracture of the left lower extremity, and bruising over his chest and abdominal wall. What is the next step in management?

First, endotracheal intubation is indicated for airway protection. Next, perform a CXR and FAST to rule out hemorrhage in other compartments that can exacerbate hypotension and make intracranial pressure (ICP) worse. Then, correct his hypotension and hypoxemia before addressing the closed head injury, which will require an ICP monitor to titrate cerebral perfusion. It is critical to correct hypovolemia with adequate fluid replacement before giving mannitol or hypertonic saline (either can be used for elevated ICP).

Glasgow Coma Scale

- Used on all patients who present as traumas as an objective way of recording their level of consciousness
- Maximum score: 15
- Minimum score: 3
- (Scoring system table in Chapter 1)

Head Trauma

- Epidural hematoma
  - Due to rupture of the middle meningeal artery
  - Initial presentation: Initial brief loss of consciousness followed by a lucid interval
  - Have a lens-shaped hematoma
  - Treatment: Emergent craniotomy, evacuation of hematoma

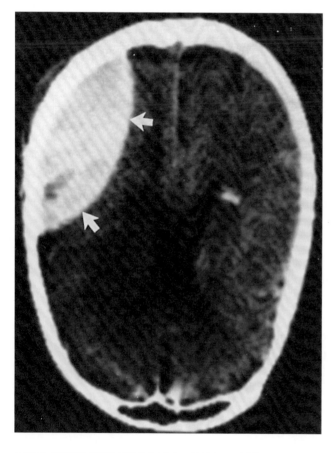

CT of epidural hematoma. (With permission from Mulholland MW, Lillemoe KD, Doherty GM, Maier RV, Upchurch GR, eds. *Greenfield's Surgery.* 4th ed. Philadelphia, PA: Lippincott Williams & Wilkins; 2005.)

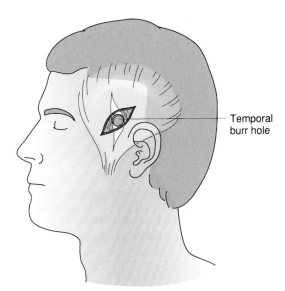

Location for the creation of a burr hole. (With permission from Mulholland MW, Lillemoe KD, Doherty GM, Maier RV, Upchurch GR, eds. *Greenfield's Surgery*. 4th ed. Philadelphia, PA: Lippincott Williams & Wilkins; 2005.)

Temporal
burr hole

- Subdural hematoma
  - Due to rupture of bridging veins between the dura and arachnoid
  - Initial presentation: Either asymptomatic, or progressive lethargy, CN VI palsy depending on the size
  - Have a crescent-shaped hematoma
  - If patient does not have symptoms, they can be observed with serial neurologic exams and/or CT scans
  - If patient is symptomatic, will need emergent craniotomy and decompression

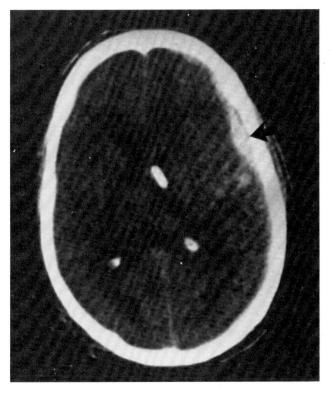

Subdural hematoma. (With permission from Mulholland MW, Lillemoe KD, Doherty GM, Maier RV, Upchurch GR, eds. *Greenfield's Surgery*. 4th ed. Philadelphia, PA: Lippincott Williams & Wilkins; 2005.)

- Subarachnoid hemorrhage (SAH)
  - Trauma is the most common cause of an SAH
  - Have blood in subarachnoid space (base of brain along cerebral gyri)
  - Treatment: Keep ICP low and prevent secondary injury
- Intraparenchymal hematoma
  - Due to tearing of intraparenchymal capillaries
  - Have parenchymal hematoma and may have mass effect
  - Treatment: Observation or craniotomy if deteriorates

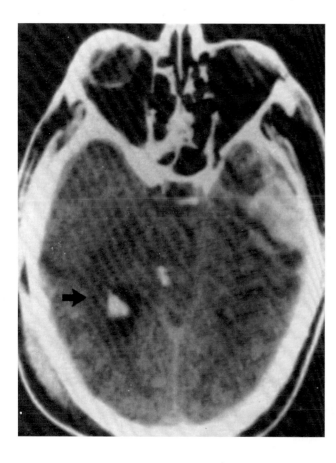

Contusion and associated intracerebral hematoma. (With permission from Mulholland MW, Lillemoe KD, Doherty GM, Maier RV, Upchurch GR, eds. *Greenfield's Surgery.* 4th ed. Philadelphia, PA: Lippincott Williams & Wilkins; 2005.)

- Traumatic brain injury is the leading cause of morbidity and mortality in trauma patients
  - Give seizure prophylaxis for 1 week in this patients—typically 1 g Keppra BID
- Elevated ICP
  - Goal ICP <20 mmHg
  - Need to avoid hypotension to keep cerebral perfusion pressure >60
    - Cerebral perfusion pressure = MAP – ICP
    - Have breakdown of autoregulation of cerebral perfusion pressure at <50 mmHg and >150 mmHg
    - Peak ICP occurs at 48 to 72 hours post-injury
  - Management
    - Increased venous drainage
      - Straighten neck to improve venous drainage
      - Keep head of bed >30°

- Decrease cerebral blood flow
  - Neuromuscular paralysis
  - Hyperventilation (to $PaCO_2$ of 30) causes arterial vasoconstriction
- Decrease cerebral edema
  - Mannitol
  - Hypertonic saline
- With acute herniation, 30 mL of 23% NS can be used
  - Administer through a central line
  - Decreases ICP by 50%
  - Effect sustained for 8 hours
  - Arrange for emergent neurosurgical intervention

A 24-year-old man presents after falling from the third story of a building. He has neck pain but is otherwise coherent and has a normal neurological exam. What is the next step in management?

Pain versus no pain is the first decision point in the management of potential neck injuries in conscious patients. In this patient, he should be immediately immobilized and a neck CT should be performed.

Cervical Spine Management

- The C-spine can be cleared if ALL of the following NEXUS study criteria are met:
  - No intoxication (the patient is alert and awake with no mental status changes)
  - No neurologic deficits
  - No neck pain
  - No "distracting" injuries (injuries that would distract the patient from pain in their neck)
  - Neck exam is normal (no tenderness on midline palpation with a full range of motion, not limited by pain)
- If there are any neurologic deficits attributable to a possible C-spine etiology or the CT is abnormal, an MRI and neurosurgical consult are indicated

Cervical Spine Fractures

- C1 fracture (Jefferson fracture)
  - Usually causes instability of the cervical spine, but the patient does not have any neurologic deficits
  - Fracture of anterior and posterior arches with lateral displacement
  - Treatment: Halo brace
- C2 fracture (Hangman fracture)
  - Often seen in motor vehicle collisions
  - Bilateral pedicle fracture
  - Due to hyperextension of the neck
  - Treatment: Halo brace

- C2 odontoid fracture
  - Type I. Fracture of the tip of the dens—is a stable fracture that just requires C collar
  - Type II (base of dens) and type III (body of C2)
    - Unstable fractures
    - Treatment: Open reduction, internal fixation (ORIF) or fusion
- Fractures at or above C3 are associated with respiratory failure

Thoracolumbar Spine Fractures
- Compression (wedge) fracture
  - Are stable fractures
  - Treatment: Thoracolumbosacral orthosis (TLSO) brace
- Chance fracture
  - Often seen when people are wearing a lap seatbelt due to hyperflexion injury
  - Fracture through the vertebral body, pedicles, and lamina
  - Up to 40% associated with occult pancreatic or bowel injury due to mechanism of injury
  - Treatment: ORIF
- Burst fracture
  - Due to axial loading
  - Unstable fracture involving the vertebral body
  - Treatment: ORIF
- Lesions at or above T5 are associated with neurogenic shock secondary to loss of sympathetic output

Management of any life-threatening problem is a higher priority than the C-spine.

A 51-year-old man presents to the emergency room after a fall. He has a GCS of 15 and complains of back pain. He is hemodynamically stable and has two large-bore IVs in place. A CT scan demonstrates a retroperitoneal hematoma in the pelvis. What is the next step in management?

Conservative management with close monitoring is the treatment of choice for stable pelvic and lateral abdominal retroperitoneal hematomas secondary to blunt trauma.

Associated Injuries in Zones of the Peritoneum

Zone	Location	Associated Injuries
1	Central retroperitoneum	Pancreaticoduodenal injuries or major abdominal vascular injury
2	Flank or perinephric area	Injuries to the genitourinary tract or to the colon (i.e., with penetrating trauma)
3	Pelvis	Pelvic fractures
(With permission from Mulholland MW, Lillemoe KD, Doherty GM, Maier RV, Upchurch GR, eds. *Greenfield's Surgery.* 4th ed. Philadelphia, PA: Lippincott Williams & Wilkins; 2005.)		

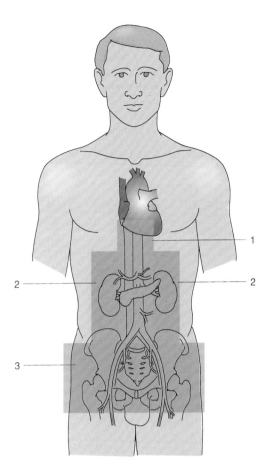

Zones of the retroperitoneum. (With permission from Mulholland MW, Lillemoe KD, Doherty GM, Maier RV, Upchurch GR, eds. *Greenfield's Surgery.* 4th ed. Philadelphia, PA: Lippincott Williams & Wilkins; 2005.)

Retroperitoneal Hematomas in Blunt Trauma

- All of the following criteria must be met in order to manage retroperitoneal hematomas non-operatively:
    - The hematoma was caused by blunt trauma
    - The patient is hemodynamically stable
    - The hematoma is located lateral to the psoas muscle or in the pelvis
- For zone 2 (lateral) hematomas, obtain a CTA
    - If there is no hilar injury, the patient can be observed
    - Urine leaks can be controlled with drains
- Stable pelvic and some retrohepatic hematomas can be observed
- Central and portal hematomas (zone I) should be explored
- Pericolic hematomas should be explored (cannot exclude colonic wall injury)

Retroperitoneal hematomas caused by penetrating injury in any zone, with limited exception for zone 2 injury in hemodynamically stable patients, should be explored in the operating room.

A 28-year-old male arrives with pulse of 120, blood pressure of 80/40, and pelvic instability following a fall from a height of 14 feet. A pelvic X-ray confirms an open book fracture. There do not appear to be any other injuries. What is the next step in management?

Temporize with a pelvic binder while you ensure airway, breathing, and circulation are stabilized. Also, look for other injuries requiring operative management and call for blood and FFP (fresh frozen plasma) as needed. Then, perform emergent angioembolization followed by external pelvic fixation.

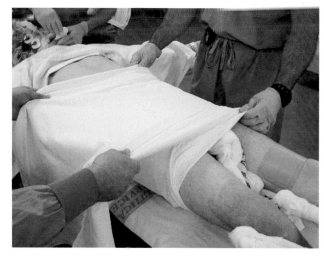

External pelvic stabilization. (A) Demonstrates use of a sheet as an external pelvic binder for temporary stabilization of a pelvic fracture. (B) Demonstrates the pelvic binder in place and secured with clamps. (With permission from Mulholland MW, Lillemoe KD, Doherty GM, Maier RV, Upchurch GR, eds. *Greenfield's Surgery*. 4th ed. Philadelphia, PA: Lippincott Williams & Wilkins; 2005.)

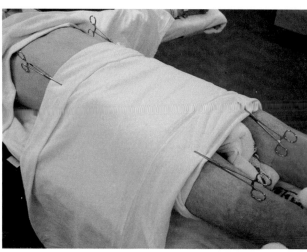

Pelvic Fractures

- If the patient is hemodynamically unstable, exclude thoracic and intra-abdominal causes
- An unstable patient with a negative diagnostic peritoneal lavage (DPL)/FAST can be managed with external fixation in ED and angioembolization
- An unstable patient with a positive DPL/FAST should undergo operative management
  - Repair intra-abdominal injuries
  - Perform pre-peritoneal packing since intra-abdominal packing does not help pelvic bleeding
  - Angioembolization if necessary
  - Rectosigmoidoscopy if stable to rule out rectal injury
  - External or internal fixation
- All patients with pelvic fractures should be evaluated for rectal injury

A 14-year-old female arrives hemodynamically stable after sustaining a single direct kick by a horse to her epigastrum. A CT scan performed on initial assessment at an outside hospital demonstrates a periduodenal hematoma. What is the next best diagnostic test?

An upper GI study can delineate a duodenal perforation.

Periduodenal Hematomas Identified on Computed Tomography

- If the patient is unstable, explore the hematoma surgically
- If stable, evaluate for a leak using gastrograffin followed by a barium swallow study
- If no leak is seen, observe the patient for approximately 2 weeks
- If symptoms of gastric outlet obstruction occur during observation, exploration may be required

Periduodenal Hematomas Identified at Exploration

- Always explore to evaluate for a laceration/perforation
- If laceration/perforation is identified with an associated pancreatic head hematoma, then cannulate the ampulla of Vater through the laceration and perform a retrograde cholangiopancreatography to evaluate for pancreatic injury

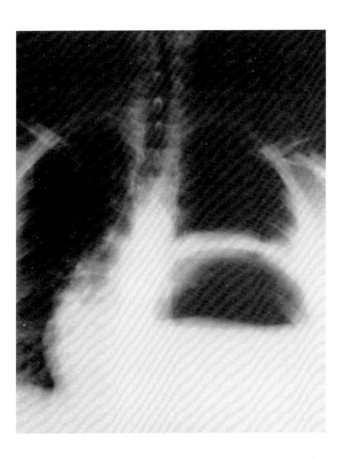

Rupture of the left hemidiaphragm. (With permission from Mulholland MW, Lillemoe KD, Doherty GM, Maier RV, Upchurch GR, eds. *Greenfield's Surgery.* 4th ed. Philadelphia, PA: Lippincott Williams & Wilkins; 2005.)

Diaphragmatic Injuries

- Up to 25% of left thoracoabdominal penetrating injuries will have a diaphragmatic injury
- Diaphragmatic injury cannot be appropriately evaluated by imaging—suspicion should be high for these types of injuries
- Some centers advocate laparoscopy for left-sided penetrating injuries between the nipple and costal margin
- Left-sided diaphragmatic injuries need to be repaired secondary to future risk of herniation through the injury

Gastric Trauma

- Assess grade
  - Grade 1: Contusion, hematoma, or partial-thickness laceration
  - Grade 2: Laceration of the:
    - GE junction or pylorus (size <2 cm)
    - Proximal 1/3 of the stomach (size <5 cm)
    - Distal 2/3 of the stomach (size <10 cm)
  - Grade 3: Laceration of the:
    - GE junction or pylorus (size ≥2 cm)
    - Proximal 1/3 of the stomach (size ≥5 cm)
    - Distal 2/3 of the stomach (size ≥10 cm)
  - Grade 4: Tissue loss or devascularization of <2/3 of the stomach
  - Grade 5: Tissue loss or devascularization of >2/3 of the stomach

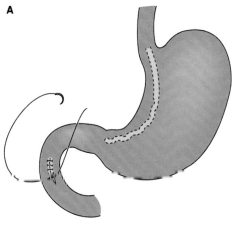

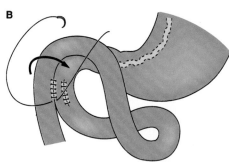

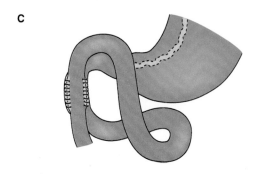

Jejunoileal patch for reinforcement of primary repair of duodenum. Panel (A) shows primary repair of duodenum. Panel (B) shows retrocolic loop of jejunum brought up to the area of concern. Panel (C) shows serosal patch repair. (With permission from Mulholland MW, Lillemoe KD, Doherty GM, Maier RV, Upchurch GR, eds. *Greenfield's Surgery.* 4th ed. Philadelphia, PA: Lippincott Williams & Wilkins; 2005.)

- Operative management
  - Grade 1 to 3: Primary closure
  - Grade 4 to 5: Resection of the distal stomach and devitalized proximal stomach with Billroth I or II or a Roux-en-Y reconstruction

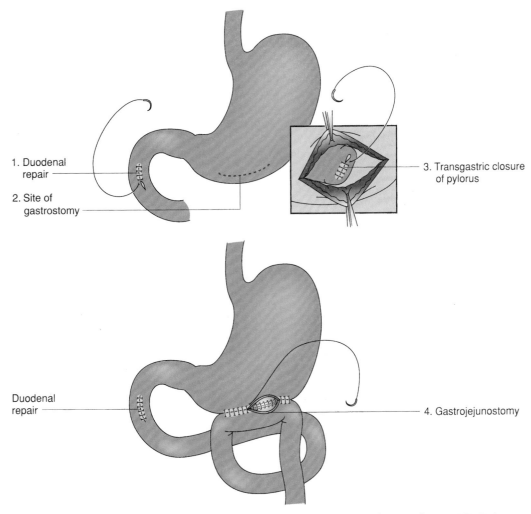

Pyloric exclusion for duodenal injury. (With permission from Mulholland MW, Lillemoe KD, Doherty GM, Maier RV, Upchurch GR, eds. *Greenfield's Surgery*. 4th ed. Philadelphia, PA: Lippincott Williams & Wilkins; 2005.)

Duodenal Trauma
- A simple laceration should be debrided and repaired with drains
- For complex lacerations with significant areas of devitalized tissue, consider:
  - Roux-en-Y duodenojejunostomy
  - Pyloric exclusion (duodenal diversion)
    - Oversew the pylorus closed through a gastrostomy then perform a gastrojejunostomy

Pancreas Trauma
- Surgical goals include achieving surgical hemostasis and placing drains for a pancreatic leak
- An intraoperative cholangiopancreatography or postoperative endoscopic retrograde cholangiopancreatography can be performed

- For a stable patient with a pancreatic duct injury in the body or tail, perform a distal pancreatectomy
- A Whipple procedure for trauma is rarely indicated and should not be performed in an unstable patient
- Consider placing a feeding jejunostomy or nasojejunal tube in any trauma patient with an anticipated prolonged ICU course

> A 19-year-old male presents to the emergency department 4 hours after suffering two gunshot wounds to the right thigh. One hour later, pulses are noted to be absent from the right foot. What is the next step in management?

An emergent operative exploration should be performed because of potential limb loss. An intraoperative angiogram can be performed if needed.

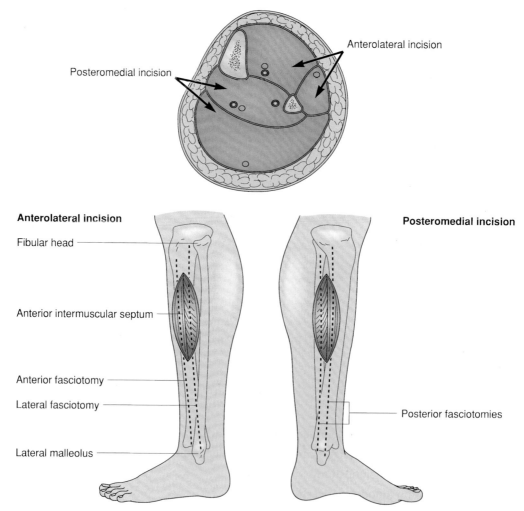

Surgical approach for fasciotomies. (With permission from Mulholland MW, Lillemoe KD, Doherty GM, Maier RV, Upchurch GR, eds. *Greenfield's Surgery*. 4th ed. Philadelphia, PA: Lippincott Williams & Wilkins; 2005.)

Extremity Trauma

- "Hard signs" requiring operative exploration
  - Active bleeding
  - Absent distal pulses
  - Expanding or pulsatile hematoma
  - Bruit/thrill
  - Distal ischemia
- An abnormal ankle-brachial index (ABI < 0.8) or neurological exam requires further evaluation (angiography or ultrasonography)
- When repairing the femoral artery, use the saphenous vein from the uninjured leg in case the femoral vein near the injured artery becomes compromised during the dissection
- Maintain a strong clinical suspicion for compartment syndrome in the early hours following surgery
  - Patients will usually complain of pain out of proportion to injury
  - Pain with passive stretch is one of the first clinical signs
  - Another early sign is numbness between the first and second toes with lower extremity injury
  - Loss of pulses is a late sign
- Prophylactic fasciotomy is recommended for:
  - 6 hours of ischemic time (due to concern for reperfusion injury)
  - Combined arterial and venous injury
  - Significant crush injury
  - Prolonged hypotension

For extremity trauma with a normal neurovascular exam and a normal ABI, no further workup is necessary.

A 25-year-old female presents to the emergency room after being the restrained driver in a head-on collision at 45 mph. Her heart rate is 125, BP is 90/60 and she is noted to have an unstable pelvis. An external fixation device is placed and she is taken to angiography for emergent embolization. After embolization, a Foley is placed and she is noted to have hematuria. What is the next step in management?

Since the patient is now stable, a CT cystogram can be performed to evaluate for a bladder injury.

Bladder Injury

- Can happen after blunt or penetrating trauma
- Often see these injuries with pelvic fractures
- Signs/symptoms: Hematuria, meatal blood
- Extraperitoneal bladder injury
  - Treat with urinary catheter drainage for 2 to 3 weeks
- Intraperitoneal injuries
  - Need immediate exploratory laparotomy and primary repair
  - After primary repair, continue Foley for 2 to 3 weeks

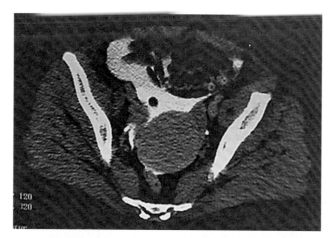

Intraperitoneal bladder injury. (With permission from Mulholland MW, Lillemoe KD, Doherty GM, Maier RV, Upchurch GR, eds. *Greenfield's Surgery.* 4th ed. Philadelphia, PA: Lippincott Williams & Wilkins; 2005.)

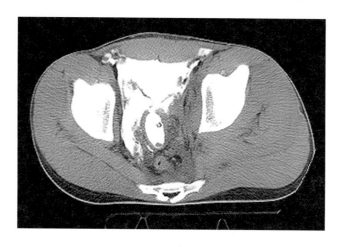

Extraperitoneal bladder injury. (With permission from Mulholland MW, Lillemoe KD, Doherty GM, Maier RV, Upchurch GR, eds. *Greenfield's Surgery.* 4th ed. Philadelphia, PA: Lippincott Williams & Wilkins; 2005.)

Renal Injury

- Most commonly associated with blunt trauma
- Symptoms: Hematuria, costovertebral angle tenderness
- Diagnosis: CT
    - EAST guidelines: IVP only used to check for second functioning kidney prior to nephrectomy, but does not change algorithm for nephrectomy if needed in the face of trauma
- Treatment
    - Non-operative for grade I–IV lesions
    - Grade V lesion: Partial or total nephrectomy

Ureteral Injury

- Symptoms: Similar to renal injury symptoms
- Treatment
    - Do primary repair immediately
    - Lower 1/3: Re-implant the ureter on the bladder
    - Upper 2/3: Re-anastamose over a stent
        - If >2 cm is missing, cannot perform a primary repair
            - Tie off both ends of the ureter and perform a ureteroureterostomy at a later time

Urethral Injury

- Symptoms: Blood at the urethral meatus, high-riding prostate on rectal exam, bruising of the perineum
- Do NOT attempt Foley placement!
- Diagnosis: Retrograde urethrogram
  - Performed with a small catheter placed in the tip of the urethra followed by dye injection
- Treatment
  - Suprapubic drainage or Foley placement if urology deems appropriate
  - Repair in 2 to 3 months
  - Early repair is associated with high rates of stricture and impotence

35 Thoracic Trauma

Edmund S. Kassis and Kathryn O'Keefe

A 24-year-old man is involved in a high-speed motor vehicle accident. He has an actively bleeding left arm wound, a deformed left humeral fracture, and ecchymoses over the anterior chest and abdomen. What is the next step in management?

Airway assessment is the first step in the management of all trauma patients.

Thoracic Trauma Management Begins with Airway Assessment

- Can the patient speak comfortably?
- Assess the endotracheal (ET) tube placed in field, including end tidal CO_2
- Maintain in-line traction
- If the airway is compromised, secure it with an ET tube or a surgical airway prior to advancing to the next step of the primary survey

Do not be distracted by the obvious injury and extremity bleeding. The ABCs are the priority for every trauma patient.

A 19-year-old man sustains a single stab wound to the left chest. On examination, his airway is patent, but he has decreased breath sounds on the left. He has a heart rate of 100 and a blood pressure of 130/80 mmHg. A chest tube is placed with immediate evacuation of 2 L of blood. What is the next step in management?

The patient should be taken to the operating room immediately for an exploratory left thoracotomy for bleeding.

Management of Traumatic Pneumothorax/Hemothorax

- Simple pneumothorax
  - Signs/symptoms
    - Decreased breath sounds on ipsilateral side
    - Tachycardia and tachypnea
    - Pleuritic chest pain

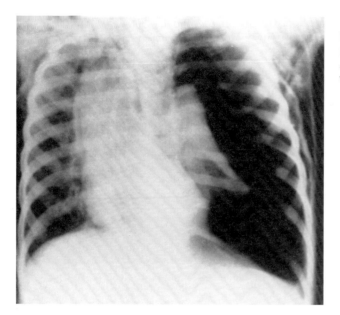

Tension pneumothorax. (With permission from Mulholland MW, Lillemoe KD, Doherty GM, Maier RV, Upchurch GR, eds. *Greenfield's Surgery.* 4th ed. Philadelphia, PA: Lippincott Williams & Wilkins; 2005.)

- Chest X-ray (CXR): No mediastinal shift
- Small pneumothoraces can be observed
- Large or expanding pneumothoraces mandate a chest tube
- Tension pneumothorax
  - Signs/symptoms
    - Jugular venous distention (JVD)
    - Tracheal shift
    - Hypotension
    - Narrowed pulse pressure
  - The diagnosis is made clinically—treatment should NOT be delayed to obtain a CXR
  - Treat with needle decompression followed by immediate chest tube placement
- Hemothorax
  - Blood in the chest cavity
  - Treat with a chest tube (use small tubes for air and large tubes for blood)
  - Blood will organize and clot in 3 to 10 days and may no longer drain; surgical evacuation via thoracoscopy (VATS) may be required to remove the blood at that point

Indications for Thoracotomy Following Chest Tube Placement

- Immediate drainage of 1500 mL of blood after chest tube placement
- Continued drainage of 250 mL/hour over 4 hours
- Drainage of 2500 mL in 24 hours
- Bright red arterial blood (much less likely to cease spontaneously)
- Significant air leak resulting in hypoxemia
- Persistent hemothorax despite adequate drainage with two chest tubes

If hemothorax is suspected, place a large chest tube (32 to 36 French) to prevent clotting.

A 30-year-old male is brought to the emergency department (ED) by paramedics after sustaining several gunshot wounds to the chest. In the field, he has a heart rate of 120 and a systolic blood pressure of 80. He is intubated. Upon entry to the trauma bay, he becomes asystolic. What is the next step in management?

An immediate ED thoracotomy is indicated for a sudden loss of vital signs with penetrating trauma to the chest.

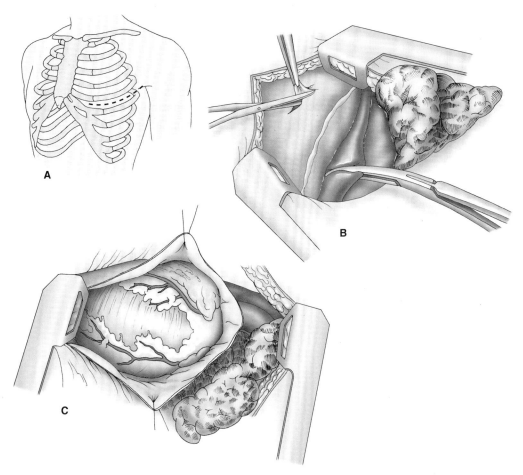

ED thoracotomy. (With permission from Fischer JE, Bland KI, Callery MP, et al., eds. *Mastery of Surgery.* 5th ed. Philadelphia, PA: Lippincott Williams & Wilkins; 2006.)

Indications for Emergency Department Thoracotomy

- Penetrating torso trauma with witnessed loss of vital signs in transit or in ED
- Blunt torso trauma with loss of vital signs in the ED
- Thoracotomy procedure
  - Identify the left fifth or sixth rib (just below the nipple line in men, just below the inframammary crease in women) and make an incision down to bone from the sternum to the posterior axillary line
  - Carry incision through subcutaneous tissue and muscle to enter the pleural space
  - Sweep the left lung away

- Bluntly dissect the mid descending thoracic aorta circumferentially and place an aortic cross-clamp
- Make a large longitudinal pericardiotomy medial to the phrenic nerve and examine heart for injuries
- Temporize any cardiac wounds with a stitch, a Foley balloon, or your finger
- For an arrested heart, begin cardiac massage and go to the operating room
- Occupational sharp injuries to clinicians are common during this procedure
- ED thoracotomy patients have a very poor prognosis

Indications for ED thoracotomy are limited. Avoid unnecessary invasive procedures that are of no benefit to the patient and place the healthcare team at risk.

A 55-year-old woman is involved in a high-speed motor vehicle accident. At the scene, she has a systolic blood pressure of 100, a heart rate of 110, and her GCS is 8. On arrival to the ED, she is intubated and intravenous access is secured. On examination she has bilateral breath sounds and JVD. What is the most appropriate next step in management?

An immediate pericardiocentesis is indicated to address a possible cardiac tamponade.

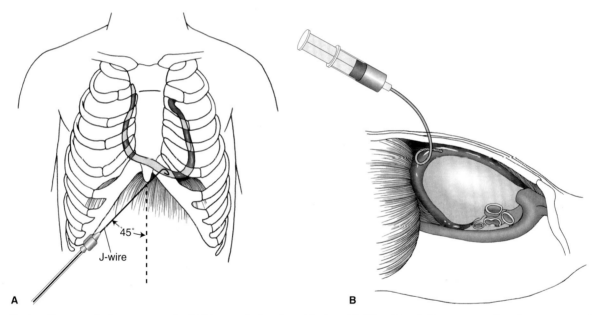

Pericardiocentesis for tamponade. (With permission from Fischer JE, Bland KI, Callery MP, et al., eds. *Mastery of Surgery.* 5th ed. Philadelphia, PA: Lippincott Williams & Wilkins; 2006.)

Cardiac Tamponade
- Seen in penetrating and blunt chest trauma
- The pericardium has poor compliance (stretch)
- Pericardial fluid decreases cardiac compliance resulting in decreased venous return and decreased cardiac output
- Signs/symptoms include:
  - Hypotension/tachycardia
  - JVD
  - Muffled heart tones

- Bilateral breath sounds (usually)
- Treatment
  - Pericardiocentesis or creation of a surgical pericardial window
  - Volume resuscitation

A 39-year-old woman presents to the trauma bay following a motor vehicle crash complaining of mild chest pain and abdominal pain. Her blood pressure is 92/50, heart rate is 116, and she has a seat belt mark on her chest. Her abdomen is diffusely tender and distended. A chest X-ray demonstrates a widened mediastinum. What is the next step in management?

An exploratory laparotomy should be performed immediately, before a CT scan or aortography. Workup of a possible aortic injury should be postponed until the life-threatening abdominal trauma is stabilized. It is rare for a blunt aortic injury to manifest as an acute decompensation during the initial trauma presentation, as the vast majority of patients die at the scene. The workup of a blunt cardiac injury should always be secondary to the initiation of prompt surgical treatment for any correctable life-threatening injuries.

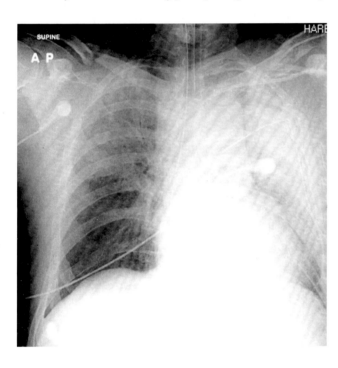

Traumatic aortic rupture. (With permission from Mulholland MW, Lillemoe KD, Doherty GM, Maier RV, Upchurch GR, eds. *Greenfield's Surgery*. 4th ed. Philadelphia, PA: Lippincott Williams & Wilkins; 2005.)

Blunt Thoracic Trauma

- **Pulmonary contusion**
  - Results from pulmonary hemorrhage and edema from a compression–decompression injury
  - Microvascular injury occurs with extravasation of blood/serum into the interstitial/alveolar space
  - Often seen with adjacent rib fractures and pulmonary lacerations
  - A common cause of morbidity
  - Diagnosis
    - CXR/CT
    - Signs/symptoms: Hypoxia, hypercarbia, respiratory acidosis
  - Treatment is supportive: Aggressive pain control, pulmonary toilet, and mechanical ventilation (if needed)

- Blunt cardiac injury
    - May result in ventricular, septal, and/or valvular injuries
    - The most common sign is sinus tachycardia
    - A normal ECG rules out blunt cardiac injury
    - An abnormal ECG merits 24 to 48 hours of observation and telemetry
    - Hemodynamically unstable patients with blunt cardiac injury should undergo echocardiography
    - Troponin and creatine phosphokinase tests are non-specific and not helpful
    - Sternal fracture is not predictive of blunt cardiac injury
- **Aortic Injury**
    - Injury most commonly occurs distal to the subclavian artery
    - Often result from deceleration forces at fixed/non-fixed aortic segments
    - 90% of patients die at the scene
    - The force of injury can cause a rare fracture of the first rib
    - Can present with hoarseness without laryngeal injury
    - CXR findings
        - Widened mediastinum
        - Blurring of outline of descending aorta
        - Opacification of the AP window
        - Widened left paraspinal stripe
        - Depression of the left mainstem bronchus
        - Tracheal deviation to the right
        - Esophageal deviation to the right (NG tube)
        - Right or left pleural cap
        - Left hemothorax without rib fracture
        - Right paratracheal stripe thickening
    - If any of the above CXR findings are identified, the patient should undergo immediate CT scan or angiography

Treat life-threatening problems (such as hypotension and acute abdomen) appropriately before working up an aortic injury, because aortic injuries are rare and often cause instant death. If a patient lives long enough to make it to the hospital with an aortic injury, then they can live long enough to have other immediate life-threatening injuries addressed first.

A 45-year-old man falls off a ladder and lands on his left side. On admission to the ED his airway is intact, he has diminished air entry on the left, and he has a grossly deformed, paradoxically moving left chest wall. What is the diagnosis?

A flail chest results in paradoxical movement of the flail segment with decreased air entry.

Flail Chest
- Three consecutive ribs that are fractured in two places
- Caused by large-force blunt chest trauma
- Treatment is supportive
    - Adequate analgesia (consider using epidural analgesia)
    - Aggressive pulmonary toilet
    - Ventilatory support may be necessary

An 18-year-old man presents after being stabbed in the left chest. He is alert and hemodynamically stable. On examination, he has an open wound through which air is being sucked in during inspiration. What is the treatment?

An open pneumothorax is treated with a sterile gauze secured on three sides and placement of a chest tube.

Open Pneumothorax

- An open wound into the chest through which air is sucked in during inspiration
- Needs to be at least 2/3 the size of the trachea to be physiologically significant
- Treatment
    - Initially, place sterile gauze secured on three sides
        - Prevents formation of a tension pneumothorax and allows lung to expand with inspiration
    - Chest tube

36 Burns

Vijay A. Singh

A 54-year-old man sustains a 4% flame burn to his right forearm during a cookout at his house. Upon examination, the wound is painful to touch with multiple blisters. Palpation of the wound shows good capillary refill. How would this type of wound be classified?

The burn should be classified as a superficial second-degree burn. These burns are typically hypersensate with good capillary refill and blisters. Treatment of these wounds is nonsurgical, and healing takes place within 3 weeks.

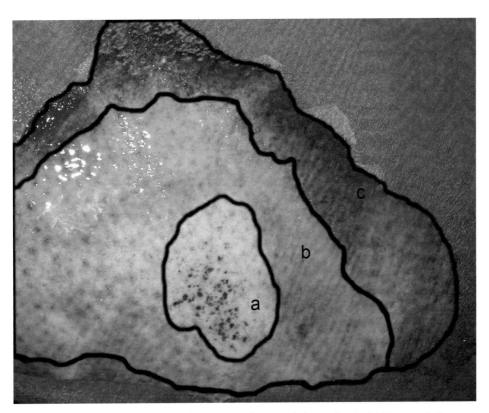

Burns of varying severity—zone of injury correlates with burn depth. (With permission from Mulholland MW, Lillemoe KD, Doherty GM, Maier RV, Upchurch GR, eds. *Greenfield's Surgery.* 4th ed. Philadelphia, PA: Lippincott Williams & Wilkins; 2005.)

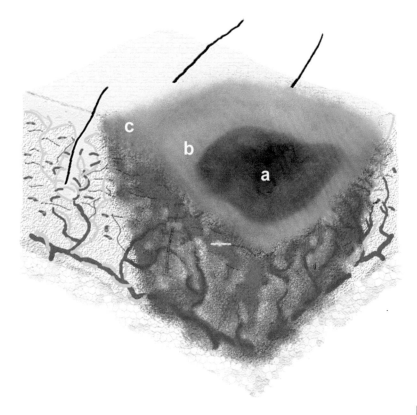

b

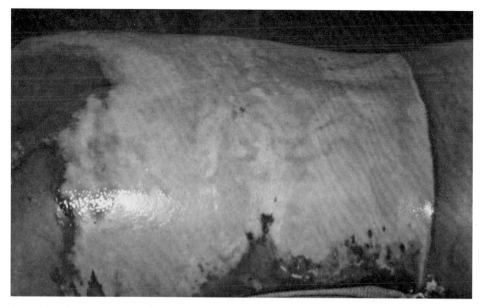

(Continued)

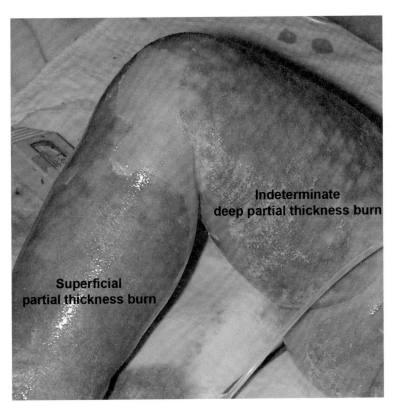

(Continued)

Burn Classification

- *First-degree burns* are limited to the epidermis
  - A long day in the sun
  - Have blanching erythema and pain
- *Second-degree burns* involve the epidermis and variable amounts of dermis
  - Superficial second-degree burns
    - Involve the epidermis and superficial dermis
    - Blisters are present
    - Burns are pink, moist, and tender
    - Healing takes place within 2 to 3 weeks, often with minimal scarring
  - Deep second-degree burns
    - Extend into deeper dermis
    - Skin is usually cherry red, mottled, or white
    - Long healing time and increased risk of infection
    - Greater potential for hypertrophic scar formation
    - Skin grafting is usually required
- *Third-degree burns*
  - Full-thickness damage to epidermis and dermis with extension into subcutaneous tissue
  - White or leather appearance

- Does not blanch
- Often painless due to nerve injury
- Debridement is necessary to remove necrotic tissue, which is prone to infection
- Subsequent skin grafting is always required (unless wound is very small)
  - *Fourth-degree burns*
    - Deep muscle, bone, or tendon are destroyed
    - Managed similar to third-degree burns

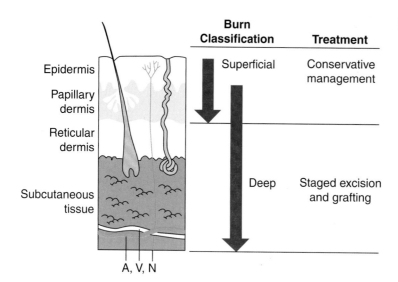

Burn classification and treatment.

Superficial versus Deep Classification

	Depth	Characteristics	Significance
Superficial	• First degree • Superficial second degree	• Wet, pink, or blistered • Painful • Blanches with pressure	• Intact dermal appendages (e.g., hair follicles and glands) allow regrowth of epidermis and healing in 2–3 wk
Deep	• Deep second degree • Third degree	• Appearance ranges from cherry red, mottled, white, non-blanching, to leathery, charred, or brown • May be insensate • Does not blanch with pressure	• Insufficient epithelial appendages; if healing occurs, it will be slow with resultant unstable skin, hypertrophic scarring, and contracture • Best treated with excision and grafting

Superficial burns may be treated conservatively, as opposed to deep burns, which require operative debridement.

A 68-year-old man injured in a house fire sustains facial burns. The examination reveals deep facial burns with evidence of carbonaceous sputum. What is the next step in management?

This patient should be intubated, stabilized, and transferred to a designated burn center. Carbonaceous sputum is a sign of inhalation injury and should be taken seriously because of the possibility of an impending airway emergency.

Inhalation Injury

- Caused by inhaling products of combustion (cyanide gas, carbon monoxide, burnt silk, paper, etc.)
- Three components of injury
  - Tissue hypoxia→ decreased oxygen carrying capacity of blood
  - Thermal injury→ upper airway edema in 18 to 24 hours
  - Lung injury→ obstructive atelectasis and bronchoconstriction
- Signs and symptoms—when to suspect inhalational injury
  - Loss of consciousness
  - Noxious chemicals involved
  - Carbonaceous sputum
  - Facial burns/singed nasal hairs/eyebrows
  - Hoarse voice
  - Erythema/swelling of oropharynx
- Diagnosis is made from any of the above findings with one of the following:
  - Carboxyhemoglobin >10%
  - Oxygen saturation <90%
  - Positive findings on laryngoscopy
  - Positive findings on bronchoscopy
  - High-probability V/Q scan
- Treatment: High-flow oxygen mask (intubate early as appropriate)
  - Oxygen will compete with carbon monoxide for hemoglobin binding
  - Carbon monoxide has a have life of hours (320 minutes on room air, 90 minutes on 100% oxygen, and 23 minutes on hyperbaric therapy)

Patients with facial and/or neck burns or other signs of inhalational injury should be intubated.

A 43-year-old woman presents with cutaneous eruptions on her face, chest, bilateral upper extremities, and abdomen (approximately 40% of total body surface area [TBSA]). These eruptions initially developed 3 days ago. In that time, the patient's wounds have rapidly evolved from a papular exanthem to confluent blisters with epidermal detachment. Also, there are multiple lesions noted in her oropharynx. The patient's history is significant for the recent restarting of Dilantin for epilepsy. What is her diagnosis?

This is a classic presentation of toxic epidermal necrolysis syndrome (TENS), which can mimic thermal injuries.

Toxic Epidermal Necrolysis Syndrome

- Rapidly evolving mucocutaneous reaction
- Characterized by widespread erythema, necrosis, and bullous detachment of the epidermis resembling scalding

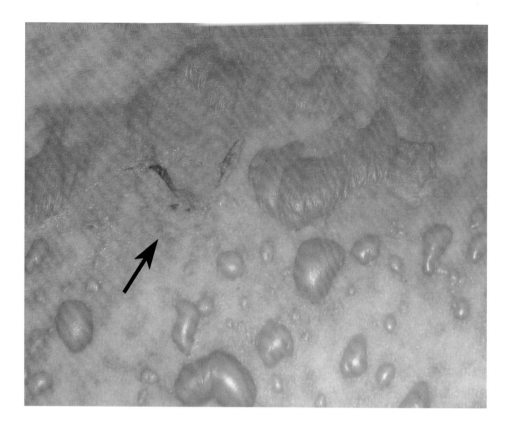

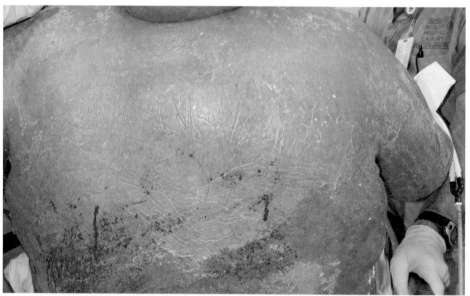

Toxic epidermal necrolysis. (With permission from Mulholland MW, Lillemoe KD, Doherty GM, Maier RV, Upchurch GR, eds. *Greenfield's Surgery*. 4th ed. Philadelphia, PA: Lippincott Williams & Wilkins; 2005.)

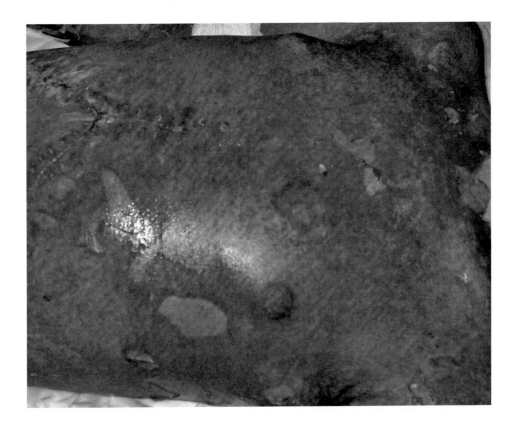

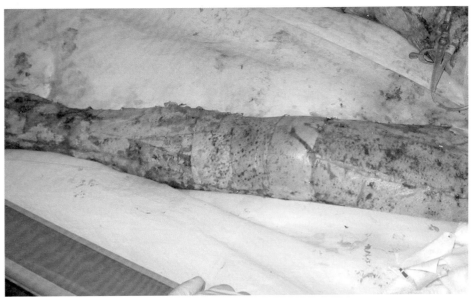

(Continued)

- Mainly attributed to build up of drug metabolites
- Associated with:
  - Sulfonamide antibiotics
  - Anticonvulsants (phenobarbital, phenytoin, carbamazepine, valproic acid)
  - Also reported with NSAIDs, allopurinol, vancomycin, corticosteroids, antiretrovirals
  - Some infections

- Classification is largely based on extent of epidermal detachment and morphology of skin lesion
  - Stevens-Johnson syndrome: Epidermal detachment less than 30% of body surface area involved with widespread erythematous or purpuric macules or flat atypical targets
  - TENS: Epidermal detachment greater than 30% of the body surface area in large epidermal sheets and without purpuric macules
- Mucosal lesions (oral, vaginal, conjunctival) are also evident
- Diagnosis
  - Nikolsky sign: Skin separation with horizontal traction
    - Due to dermal–epidermal separation
  - Definitive diagnosis is made on biopsy
    - Have keratinocyte necrosis at the dermal–epidermal junction
- Treatment is supportive—stop any possible offending drug
  - Do NOT give steroids
  - Prevent wound desiccation with topical antimicrobials and xenografts

TENS is a dermatologic abnormality that mimics burn injury and is mainly attributed to sulfonamides or phenytoin.

A 17-year-old student sustains a 50% TBSA gasoline burn. Upon examination, you find that the patient's bilateral upper extremity burn is circumferential. The area is white and tense. After acute resuscitation, what is the next step in therapy?

Urgent and proper placement of an escharotomy is required to prevent vascular or respiratory compromise in patients with restrictive burns.

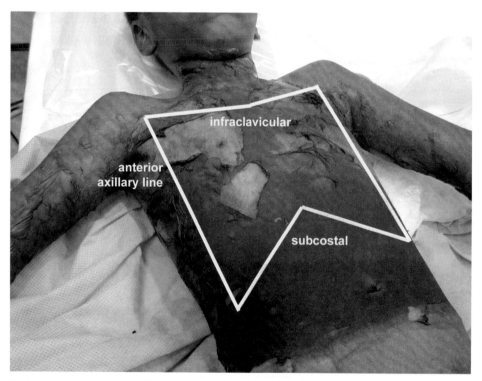

Escharotomy incisions. (With permission from Mulholland MW, Lillemoe KD, Doherty GM, Maier RV, Upchurch GR, eds. *Greenfield's Surgery.* 4th ed. Philadelphia, PA: Lippincott Williams & Wilkins; 2005.)

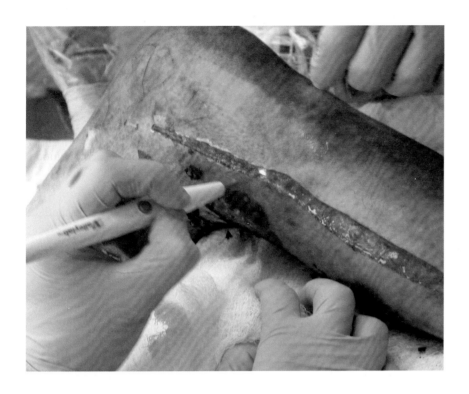

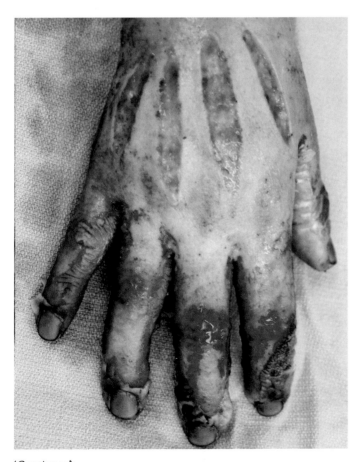

(Continued)

Escharotomy

- A longitudinal incision aimed at releasing tissue pressure to restore perfusion
- Common indications
  - Circumferential deep partial thickness or full thickness burns
  - Difficulty in ventilating patients with significant chest/torso burns
- Full-thickness incision
  - Must go through the entire depth of the burn to allow tissue expansion and a return of blood flow
- Particularly relevant to the neck, thorax, and extremities
- Extremity escharotomy: Place incisions on mid-medial and mid-lateral aspect of extremity and extend all the way distally
- Chest wall escharotomy: Place incisions at anterior axillary lines bilaterally which is connected by a subcostal incision (makes an "H" across chest)

When performing an escharotomy, general or topical anesthesia is not required.

A 25-year-old man spills ammonia on his hand and sustains a full-thickness burn to the dorsum of his right hand. On physical examination, the patient's hand is warm, tender, swollen, and has a mottled appearance with delayed capillary refill time. How do you treat this patient?

Copious irrigation of the affected region is the cornerstone treatment for most chemical injuries.

Chemical Burns

- Most chemical burns are more severe than the initial examination would suggest
- Unlike thermal burns, tissue loss can occur many hours after injury
- Alkalotic chemical burns produce deeper burns than acidotic burns due to liquefaction necrosis
- Acid burns produce coagulation necrosis
- For powder burns, wipe away powder before irrigation
- For tar burns, wipe away the tar with a lipophilic solvent
- For hydrofluoric acid burns, spread calcium on the wound
- Patients with chemical burns should be admitted if:
  - Injuries are deep and require excision
  - There is systemic manifestation of chemical toxicity
  - Chemical requires a specific antidote

Chemical burns should be irrigated with copious lukewarm water for at least 30 minutes after all saturated clothing is removed.

A 54-year-old man sustains an electrical burn to his right upper extremity after coming into contact with a power line, while picking cherries. Upon examination, the patient's right arm from the shoulder distally is white, hyposensate, and absent of capillary refill. Furthermore, no movement can be elicited from the involved area. Name two internal organs most susceptible to injury from an electrical burn?

Heart and kidneys—cardiac arrhythmias and rhabdomyolysis leading to acute renal failure are common problems after an electrical injury.

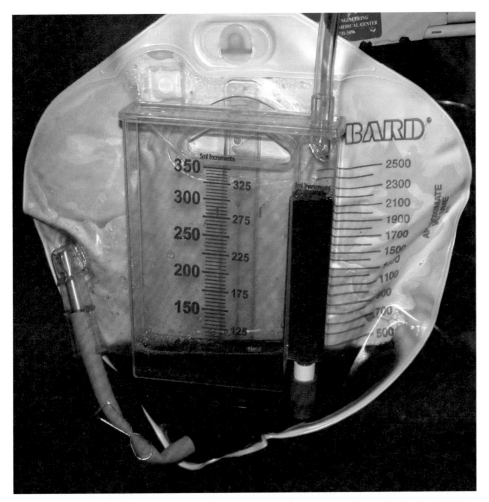

Myoglobinuria in a patient with rhabdomyolysis. (With permission from Mulholland MW, Lillemoe KD, Doherty GM, Maier RV, Upchurch GR, eds. *Greenfield's Surgery*. 4th ed. Philadelphia, PA: Lippincott Williams & Wilkins; 2005.)

Electrical Burns

- Can cause rhabdomyolysis and compartment syndrome
- Rhabdomyolysis can lead to acute renal failure
  - Standard therapy = aggressive fluid resuscitation and mannitol ± bicarbonate
  - In the acute phase, administer resuscitative IV fluids at a rate sufficient to maintain a urine output of at least 1 cc/kg/hour
  - Avoid lactated Ringer's because it has potassium (4 mEq/L)
- As with all burns, monitor closely for compartment syndromes
  - Burn patients who are at risk given massive fluid resuscitation and burn edema
  - Extremity compartment syndrome diagnosed by clinical suspicion or compartment pressures
    - Standard therapy = fasciotomies
  - Abdominal compartment syndrome diagnosed by clinical suspicion or bladder pressures
    - Manifests as increased airway pressures, hypotension, oliguria, and a tense abdomen
    - Standard therapy is surgical laparotomy, leaving abdomen open
- Cardiac monitoring is essential (cardiac enzymes × 3 + 12-lead ECG)

High transmission injuries often lead to irrevocable injury to the superficial and deep muscle layers of one or more compartments that may necessitate a fasciotomy.

A 33-year-old man has just undergone excision and autografting to his left forearm after suffering a deep-partial thickness grease burn while cooking. The grafted area is covered with a layer of fine mesh gauze. An eight-ply burn dressing is placed on top of the gauze and moistened with sulfamylon. What adverse affect may be anticipated?

Metabolic acidosis is the most common adverse effect seen with sulfamylon administration. Cessation of medication is required.

Sulfamylon (Mafenide Acetate)
- A carbonic anhydrase inhibitor
- Painful application
- Good eschar penetration
- Broad spectrum coverage, except fungal
- Comes in the form of a cream or solution
  - Sulfamylon cream
    - Topical agent indicated for adjunctive therapy for patients with second- and third-degree burns
    - Delivers antibacterial activity
    - Has deep tissue penetration
  - Sulfamylon solution
    - Adjunctive topical antimicrobial agent to control bacterial infection when used in moist dressing over meshed autografts on excised burns

A 45-year-old man of Middle Eastern descent had a second- and third-degree burns to 45% of his TBSA, which has been complicated by multiple wound infections. He recently underwent topical application of a new broad-spectrum antibiotic, which stained his skin black. Shortly after its application, he developed shortness of breath and cyanosis. How should his dressing change plan be modified based on these clinical findings?

The antibiotic is silver nitrate and the complication is methemoglobinemia. People with G6PD deficiency are at much higher risk for methemoglobinemia and silver nitrate should not be used in this patient population.

Silver Nitrate
- Broad spectrum
- Limited eschar penetration
- Painless application
- Stains skin black
- Can cause methemoglobinemia
  - Is contraindicated in patients with G6PD deficiency
- Can cause electrolyte imbalances including hyponatremia, hypochloremia, hypocalcemia, and hypokalemia

Silver Sulfadiazine (Silvadine)
- A topical antibiotic that gives prophylaxis against secondary infection (mainly *Staphylococcus aureus* and *Pseudomonas* species)
  - Broad spectrum—effective for *Candida*
  - Does not cover some forms of *Pseudomonas*

- Limited eschar penetration
- Painless application
- Can cause neutropenia and thrombocytopenia
- Do NOT use in patients with sulfa allergies

Bacitracin

- Bacitracin ointment provides good coverage against gram-positives
- Usually apply immediately after burns

There is no role for prophylactic oral antibiotics in any thermal injury. Burn wounds are diagnosed by biopsy with $>10^5$ organisms/g.

A 55-year-old male with chronic obstructive pulmonary disease sustains second- and third-degree burns to his face, chest, and bilateral upper extremities after smoking while on home oxygen. Approximately what percentage of his TBSA is burned?

For adult patients, the extent of TBSA burned can be initially estimated using the "rule of nines." In this case, 45% of his TBSA is burned.

Total Body Surface Area Burn Determination

- The "rule of 9s" is used to quickly approximate burn area
- Divides the body into units of surface areas divisible by nine, with the exception of the perineum
- The "rule of 9s" is used to guide initial resuscitation therapy

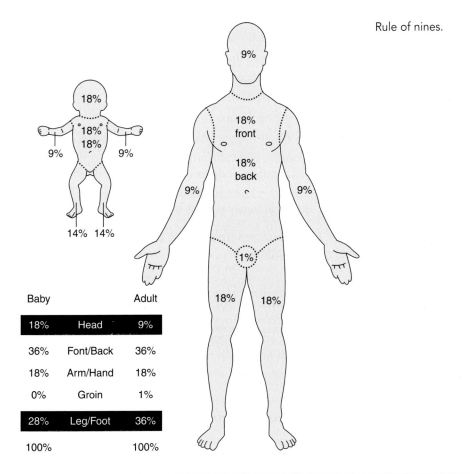

Rule of nines.

Baby		Adult
18%	Head	9%
36%	Font/Back	36%
18%	Arm/Hand	18%
0%	Groin	1%
28%	Leg/Foot	36%
100%		100%

Children have a disproportionately larger head in relation to their body when compared with adults—their head is 18% of the TBSA as opposed to 9%.

A 50-year-old man (90 kg) presents to the emergency department 2 hours after sustaining second- and third-degree burns to his chest and abdomen. How should this patient be resuscitated over the next 24 hours?

The TBSA for an adult's chest and abdomen is 18%. Total fluid needed over the first 24 hours is estimated with the Parkland formula, which is 4 times weight in kilogram times surface area burned = 6480 cc in this case. Half should be given in the initial 8 hours, and the second half over the subsequent 16 hours.

- *Fluids to be given in first 8 hours after injury: Half of 6480 cc = 3240 cc*
- *Fluids to be given over next 16 hours: Half of 6480 cc = 3240 cc*
- *This patient would receive 405 cc/h of IV fluids over the first 8 hours (3240/8) followed by 202 cc/h for the next 16 hours (3240/16).*

Burn Resuscitation

- Burn patients need aggressive resuscitation due to massive fluid loss
- The Parkland formula calculates an approximate fluid requirement for the initial 24-hour period

The Parkland Formula

4 × Weight (kg) × % TBSA burned

- The Parkland formula is a guide used for fluid resuscitation in thermal injuries
  - One half of the 24-hour volume requirement total should be given over the first 8 hours post injury
  - The second half should be given over the next 16 hours of the resuscitative period
  - Lactated Ringer's is the resuscitative fluid of choice in the first 24 hours
    - Colloid in the first 24 hours increases pulmonary complications
  - The 24-hour period begins at the time of the burn, not the time of presentation
  - TBSA burned includes only second- or third-degree burns
  - Titrate resuscitation based on urine output, central venous pressure, blood pressure, etc.
  - Although the Parkland formula is tested on exams, clinically, a urine output of 1 cc/kg/hour (or 2 to 4 mg/kg/hour in children) is the most accurate endpoint for burn resuscitation
    - The Parkland formula can grossly underestimate the amount of fluid required for resuscitation with inhalational injury, electrical injury or post-escharotomy

When calculating the amount of fluid to be given, remember that all calculations begin at the time of injury, not at the time of presentation.

A 3-year-old girl is brought in by her mother for an apparent scald burn from boiling water spilling onto her while playing near the stove. The burn is second-degree partial thickness on the anterior chest. The burn is estimated to be 8% of TBSA. Upon further examination, you note the wound has sharply demarcated margins with no splash markings. What is the next step in management?

Admit based on suspected child abuse given the sharply demarcated margins of the wound noted on physical exam.

Child Abuse

- Delayed presentation for medical care
- Conflicting stories
- Previous injury
- Sharply demarcated margins of burn
- Uniform depth
- Absence of splash marks
- Stocking or glove patterns

Child abuse accounts for 15% of burn injuries in children.

A 25-year-old woman presents to a local community hospital with superficial–partial thickness burns to 25% of her body from a house fire in which she was exposed to smoke for approximately 10 minutes. The patient denies shortness of breath, odynophagia, or any change in voice. What is the next step in management?

This patient should be stabilized and transferred to a designated burn center for treatment.

Criteria for Referral to a Burn Center

- Second- and third-degree burns >10% TBSA in patients aged <10 or >50 years
- Second- and third-degree burns >20% TBSA in all other patients
- Second- and third-degree burns to significant portions of hands, face, feet, genitalia, perineum, or skin overlying major joints
- Electrical and chemical burns
- Concomitant inhalation injury, mechanical traumas, preexisting medical conditions
- Any suspected child abuse or neglect

All patients must be hemodynamically stable before they are transferred from any facility.

A 35-year-old man who sustained third-degree burns to 75% of his body is about to undergo the first of multiple proposed operative procedures. The patient's current core body temperature is 35°C. What postoperative complications can you expect to occur?

Metabolic acidosis, coagulopathy, and increased rates of postoperative infection are known complications in the hypothermic patient. Metabolic acidosis is attributed to the decreased oxygen delivery that occurs due to the compromised overall perfusion and vasoconstriction that results from the hypothermic state. Coagulopathy is due to the accelerated microvascular thrombosis that is evident in sustained hypothermia.

Hypothermia

- Defined as a core temperature of less than 36°C for greater than 4 hours
- Burn patients are particularly susceptible due to a loss of the epidermal heat retention layer of the skin
- Treat with aggressive warming of fluids and inhaled air, and increased room temperature

Hypothermia is common in burn patients and is associated with an increased rate of postoperative infection.

A 62-year-old man is doing well in the hospital 1 week following a 30% burn during a house fire. Since the injury, the patient has had two operative debridement procedures with grafting and now is found to have an increasing WBC count to 20, temperature elevations to 103 degrees, oliguria, and hypotension. What is the most common source of sepsis in this patient?

Wound infection is common in burn patients and is the leading cause of morbidity and mortality.

Wound Infection

- Burn patients are immunocompromised leading to quick overpowering of host defenses and eventual sepsis
- Granulocyte chemotaxis and cell-mediated immunity are impaired in burn patients
- The burn wound is always a potential source of systemic infection until complete healing is accomplished
- Frequent clinical inspection of the wound itself and correlation with the clinical picture and quantitative tissue biopsy of suspicious lesions are often necessary
- Signs of burn wound infection
  - Peripheral edema
  - Conversion from second-degree → third-degree burns
  - Rapid eschar separation
- More than 100,000 (10^5) bacteria per gram of burned tissue signifies invasive infection

Pseudomonas is the most common organism in burn wound infection, followed by Staphylococcus, Escherichia coli, and Enterobacter. Pneumonia is the most common infection in burn patients and is the most common cause of death after inhalational injury.

A 48-year-old man has sustained full-thickness burns to his right lower extremity during a house fire. His burns are estimated at 12% of his body surface area. This patient will need excision and debridement. What is the best type of skin coverage for this patient?

Split-thickness skin grafts are ideal in burns because donor sites can be re-harvested many times.

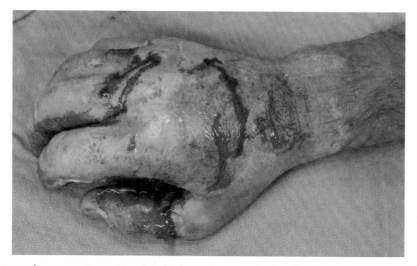

Full-thickness skin graft on a patient with a full-thickness burn to the hand. (With permission from Mulholland MW, Lillemoe KD, Doherty GM, Maier RV, Upchurch GR, eds. *Greenfield's Surgery.* 4th ed. Philadelphia, PA: Lippincott Williams & Wilkins; 2005.)

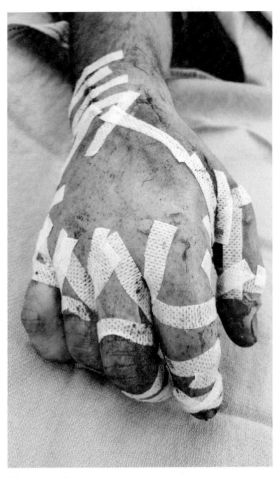

(Continued)

Principles of Burn Management

- Adequate nutrition
  - Caloric requirement = 25 kcal/kg/day + 30 kcal × (%TBSA burn)
  - Protein requirement = 1 g/kg/day + 3 g × (%TBSA burn)
  - Glucose is the best source of non-protein calories in burn patients
    - Burns use glucose in an obligatory fashion
- Complications after burns
  - Seizures—usually secondary to iatrogenic hypernatremia
  - Peripheral neuropathy—secondary to small vessel injury and demyelination
  - Curling ulcer—gastric ulcer that occurs with burns
  - Hypertrophic scar—wait 1 to 2 years for scar modification
  - Marjolin ulcer
    - Due to non-healing wound
    - Can have squamous cell cancer in these ulcers
  - Corneal abrasion—treat with topical antibiotics
- Wounds need serial excision and debridement
  - Try to excise deep second- and third-degree burns by 72 hours, except for wounds to face, palms, soles, and perineum, which should be delayed for 1 week
  - Local wound care between serial operations

- Three weeks until all dead tissue is excised
- Skin graft once wound is clean
  - Prior to skin graft, can use hemografts and xenografts to aid in healing
    - These decrease dessication, infection, protein loss, pain, water loss, and heat loss
    - They increase granulation tissue and can aid in quicker transition to skin grafting
  - Homografts (cadaveric tissue)
    - Last 2 to 4 weeks
    - These vascularize and are eventually rejected
  - Xenografts (porcine)
    - Last 2 weeks
    - Do not vascularize
  - Dermal substitutes—are not as good as homografts or xenografts
  - Most common reasons for skin graft loss is seroma or hematoma formation under the graft

Types of Skin Grafts

- Autograft
  - Skin grafts obtain nutrition through imbibition
  - Split-thickness skin graft
    - Comprised of epidermis only
    - Less likely to be rejected by the host
    - Are more likely to survive because graft is thinner and it is easier for imbibition and revascularization to occur
    - Higher rate of contraction
  - Full-thickness skin graft
    - Includes epidermis and dermis
    - More likely to be rejected by the host
    - Has a lower rate of contraction
    - Used for joints, face

Skin grafts are contraindicated if positive wound culture (>100,000 bacteria/g).

37 Gastrointestinal Hormones

Jordan E. Fishman and Adrian Barbul

A 48-year-old man presents to the emergency department with complaints of feculent discharge from his midline abdominal wound for 4 days. The patient had been discharged from the hospital approximately 1 week ago after undergoing a right hemicolectomy for cancer. After performing a full workup including a fistulogram, you diagnose the patient as having an enterocutaneous fistula. What medical therapy can be offered that will shorten the time needed for spontaneous closure of this fistula by lowering the rate of gastric and small bowel secretions?

Somatostatin is a polypeptide hormone produced throughout the gastrointestinal tract, as well as the central nervous system, that inhibits the secretion of many gastrointestinal hormones. This hormone plays a key role in limiting gastric emptying and small bowel digestive secretions.

Somatostatin

- Is secreted by the D cells of the pancreas, small bowel, colon, and stomach
- It is also secreted throughout the hypothalamus
- Binds to somatostatin receptors
- Is stimulated by the presence of gastric acid, fat, and protein in the duodenum (post-prandial state)
- Reduces smooth muscle contractions and blood flow within the intestine
- Suppresses the release of most gastrointestinal hormones, including: gastrin, cholecystokinin (CCK), secretin, motilin, vasoactive intestinal peptide (VIP), gastric inhibitory polypeptide, and enteroglucagon
- Opposes the effect of growth hormone-releasing hormone
- Reduces gastric secretions, gastric emptying, small bowel motility, small bowel digestive secretions, and colonic motility
- Non-gastrointestinal effects include inhibition of growth hormone and thyroid-stimulating hormone secretion
- Pharmacologic uses include treatment of enterocutaneous fistulas, pancreatic fistulas, carcinoid syndrome, and bleeding esophageal varices
- Octreotide is a long-acting somatostatin agonist

The migrating motor complex (MMC) is a cyclic pattern of intrinsic motor activity that travels from the stomach to the ileocecal junction. This helps to trigger peristaltic waves that facilitate the movement of indigestible substances, such as fiber, through the entire gastrointestinal tract. What important gastrointestinal hormone is critically involved in the MMC?

Motilin is a polypeptide hormone primarily secreted by the duodenum and jejunum.

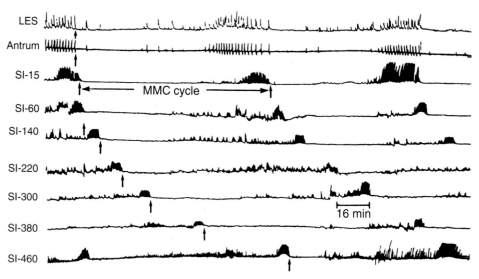

MMC. (With permission from O'Leary JP, Tabuenca A, eds. *Physiologic Basis of Surgery.* 4th ed. Philadelphia, PA: Wolters Kluwer Health/Lippincott Williams & Wilkins; 2007.)

Motilin

- Plays a large role in the initiation and coordination of the MMC
- Likely coordinates lower esophageal sphincter, stomach, and small intestine motility
- Erythromycin and related antibiotics act as non-peptide motilin agonists by binding at the M1 receptor and can be used as promotility agents
- Motilin is secreted into the circulation during the interdigestive state at intervals of roughly approximately 1.5 hours

Where in the gastrointestinal tract is secretin produced?

Secretin is produced in the crypts of Lieberkuhn of S cells located in the duodenum and proximal jejunum. Secretin regulates the pH of the duodenal contents by controlling gastric acid secretion and pancreatic bicarbonate production and secretion.

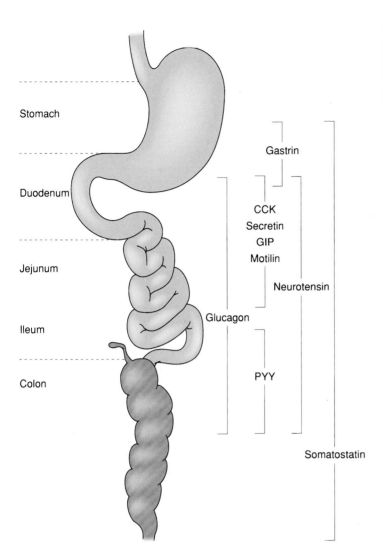

Locations of GI hormone secretions. (With permission from Mulholland MW, Lillemoe KD, Doherty GM, Maier RV, Upchurch GR, eds. *Greenfield's Surgery.* 4th ed. Philadelphia, PA: Lippincott Williams & Wilkins; 2005.)

Secretin

- Duodenal acidification stimulates release
- Activates bicarbonate-rich secretions from the pancreas, liver and duodenal Brunner glands, to neutralize gastric acid
- Inhibits antral G-cell–mediated gastrin release, thereby reducing gastric acid output

Paradoxically, in patients with gastrinoma, secretin stimulates gastrin release. This has led to the clinical application of secretin administration as a diagnostic maneuver for gastrinoma (Zollinger-Ellison syndrome). In patients who do not have a gastrinoma, secretin infusion will tend to decrease gastric acid secretion, whereas in patients with gastrinoma, secretin infusion increases gastric acid production.

Hormone	Location	Stimuli for release	Major activity
Gastrin	G cells in antrum of stomach	Antral distention, vagal stimulation, peptides, amino acids	Gastric acid and pepsinogen secretion
Somatostatin	D cells in antrum of stomach, pancreatic islets	Duodenal acidification	Inhibits gastrin and HCl release Inhibits pancreatic and gastric secretions Decreases gastrointestinal transit
Gastric inhibitory peptide	K cells in duodenum	Amino acids, glucose, acid in duodenum, and long-chain fatty acids	Decreases gastric acid secretion Increases insulin release
Cholecystokinin	I cells in duodenum and proximal jejunum	Amino acids, fatty acids, proteins	Gallbladder contraction and sphincter of Oddi relaxation Pancreatic enzyme secretion
Secretin	S cells in duodenum and proximal jejunum	Acid, fat, or bile in the duodenum	Pancreatic secretion of water and bicarbonate Alkalization of bile
Vasoactive intestinal peptide	Neuroendocrine cells throughout gastrointestinal tract	Acetylcholine (vagal mediated) and fat	Increases intestinal secretion of water and electrolytes Increases motility Inhibits gastrin release
Motilin	Duodenum and jejunum	Acid environment, vagal stimulation, gastrin-releasing peptide	Increases motility by activating the migrating motor complex
Ghrelin	Stomach	Fasting state	Triggers growth hormone release Believed to mediate hunger
Gastrin-Releasing Peptide (Bombesin)	Stomach and small bowel	Post-prandial state	Stimulates release of most GI hormones Believed to mediate satiety

A 32-year-old woman presents to clinic with a complaint of new onset abdominal discomfort ongoing for the past 2 weeks. The pain is described as a gnawing, burning pain felt in her epigastrium 2 hours after eating, and is relieved with oral intake. A urea breath test is positive and a subsequent endoscopy is performed which reveals a gastric ulcer. What gastrointestinal hormone is found to be significantly altered in this condition?

This patient's diagnosis is peptic ulcer disease secondary to Helicobacter pylori infection. Peptic ulcer disease is associated with abnormal gastrin secretion, causing either decreased or increased gastrin (and thus gastric acid) secretion.

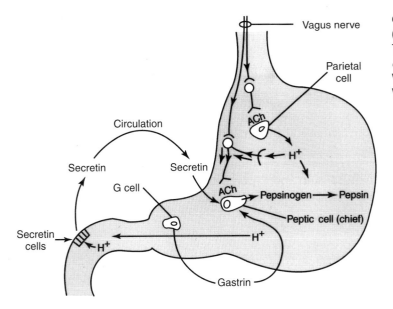

Gastric hormone secretion. (With permission from O'Leary JP, Tabuenca A, eds. *Physiologic Basis of Surgery.* 4th ed. Philadelphia, PA: Wolters Kluwer Health/Lippincott Williams & Wilkins; 2007.)

Gastrin

- Secreted from G cells in the antrum of the stomach and duodenum
- Released in response to partially digested proteins in the stomach (peptides and amino acids) and gastric distention
- Also released in response to the sight, smell, thought, or taste of food in the cephalic phase of digestion mediated by the vagus nerve
- Stimulates parietal cells of the stomach to secrete gastric acid via three pathways
  - Activation of the parietal cell CCK-B receptor, triggering direct acid secretion
  - Potentiation of histamine-mediated gastric acid secretion (H_2 receptor)
  - Increased secretion of histamine itself, further driving histamine-mediated gastric acid secretion
- Stimulates chief cells to secrete pepsinogen
- Promotes gastric and small bowel motility, inhibits pyloric contraction
- Trophic effect on gastric mucosa
- Inhibited by the release of somatostatin following duodenal acidification

> What are the actions of CCK?

- *CCK has five physiologic actions*
  - *Pancreatic enzyme secretion*
  - *Pancreatic fluid and bicarbonate secretion (through potentiation of secretin)*
  - *Contraction of the gallbladder*
  - *Relaxation of sphincter odd*
  - *Inhibition of gastric emptying (competitive inhibitor of gastrin)*

Cholecystokinin

- CCK is very similar in structure to gastrin (allows for competitive inhibition)
- Two roles

- Digestion
  - Stimulates pancreatic enzyme and bile expulsion from the gallbladder into the duodenum to facilitate fat emulsification and absorption
- Satiety
  - Mild hunger suppression from binding to CCK receptors distributed widely throughout the central nervous system (CNS)
  - CCK administration can cause nausea and anxiety, thus decreasing the desire to eat

---

A 65-year-old male with a history of hypertension and hyperlipidemia presents complaining of watery diarrhea. On further workup, he is found to have hypokalemia and achlorhydria. A tumor of what GI hormone can cause these symptoms?

A VIPoma causes WDHA syndrome (watery diarrhea, hypokalemia, and achlorhydria), also known as Verner-Morrison syndrome.

Vasoactive Intestinal Peptide

- Found throughout the entire gastrointestinal tract as well as the central nervous system
- Stimulates enteric (water and electrolyte), pancreatic (bicarbonate), and biliary secretions
- Dilates intestinal smooth muscle
- Inhibits gastrin-mediated gastric acid secretion
- Overproduction (as seen with the pancreatic endocrine tumor VIPoma) leads to prolonged watery diarrhea leading to dehydration and profound electrolyte abnormalities
- Symptoms can be treated with somatostatin

VIP acts mainly in a neuroendocrine fashion.

A 35 year old male presents to the clinic following extensive small bowel resections for multiple Crohn's disease-related small bowel obstructions. His recent clinical course is suggestive of short gut syndrome. What gastrointestinal hormone when exogenously administered may help promote mucosal growth and nutrient absorption?

Glucagon-like-peptide-2 (GLP-2) may help increase intestinal absorption in patients with short gut syndrome.

Glucagon-Like-Peptide-2

- Produced by L-type endocrine cells in the gastrointestinal tract
- Effects occur on both small intestinal and colonic cells
- Exogenously administered GLP-2 promotes small intestine and colon cell growth
- A recombinant analog (teduglutide) has shown promise in reducing TPN requirements for many patients with short gut syndrome

GLP-2 is FDA approved for the treatment of small bowel syndrome.

38 | Nutrition

Estefania de la Paz Nicolau, Kimberley Eden Steele, and Christopher L. Wolfgang

A 36-year-old morbidly obese female is involved in a car accident, sustaining a grade 2 liver laceration and bilateral femur fractures. A nutritionist is evaluating her to determine her daily caloric needs. She is 5' 3" tall and weighs 263 lbs. What weight should be used to calculate the patient's daily caloric needs?

When calculating the caloric needs of an obese patient (obesity is defined as 120% over the calculated ideal body weight [IBW]), the adjusted body weight should be used instead of the IBW. Using the adjusted body weight helps prevent overfeeding, because fat is not as metabolically active as muscle.

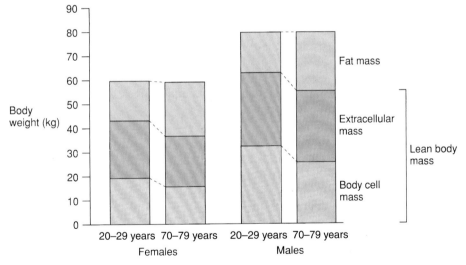

Body weight and lean mass in males and females. (With permission from Mulholland MW, Lillemoe KD, Doherty GM, Maier RV, Upchurch GR, eds. *Greenfield's Surgery*. 4th ed. Philadelphia, PA: Lippincott Williams & Wilkins; 2005.)

Ideal and Adjusted Body Weight

- IBW is calculated using the following formula:
  - Women: 100 lbs for 5'0" of height, plus 5 lbs for each inch over 5'0"
  - Men: 106 lbs for 5'0" of height, plus 6 lbs for each inch over 5'0"
  - For individuals shorter than 5'0" subtract 2 lbs for every inch under 5'0"

- Adjusted body weight = ((actual weight – IBW) × 0.25) + IBW
  - In the patient above, ((263 – 115) × 0.25) + 115 = 152 lbs

> A 27-year-old female develops an anastomotic leak 5 days after undergoing Roux-en-Y gastric bypass surgery. Conservative treatment with TPN is planned. Her weight on admission is 300 lbs, and her height is 5'. How should her caloric requirements be calculated?

There are three different methods for calculating caloric requirement: rough estimate, Harris-Benedict equation, and indirect calorimetry and Weir equation, each of which is described in further detail below.

1. Rough estimate
   - *25 kcal/kg/day* (35 kcal/kg/day for a critically ill or stressed patient)
2. Calculation of basal energy expenditure (BEE) using the *Harris-Benedict equation*:
   - Female BEE (kcal/day) = 655 + (9.6 × wt in kg) + (1.8 × ht in cm) – (4.7 × age)
   - Male BEE (kcal/day) = 66 + (13.7 × wt in kg) + (5 × ht in cm) – (6.8 × age)
   - NOTE: It is NOT necessary to memorize these formulas
   - Use actual body weight for non-obese or underweight patients
   - Use adjusted body weight for obese patients (>120% of IBW)
3. Calculation of BEE using indirect calorimetry and the Weir Equation
   - This method measures oxygen consumed in L/minute (VO_2) and carbon dioxide produced in L/minute (VCO_2) to estimate the 24-hour resting energy expenditure
   - BEE = [(3.9 × VO_2) + (1.1 × VCO_2)] × 1.44 – (2.8 × UUN)
   - UUN = 24-hour urinary urea nitrogen
   - Indications for use of indirect calorimetry
     - Multiple trauma victim
     - Severe sepsis
     - Failure to wean from ventilator
     - Morbid obesity
     - Poorly healing wounds
     - Burn patient
   - To account for the increased caloric requirements under stress, the BEE may be multiplied by a stress factor based on the patient's condition.
     - Low stress: 1.2
     - Moderate stress: 1.3
     - Severe stress: 1.5
     - Burns and sepsis: 2.0 to 2.5

> A 70-year-old female with a history of COPD on TPN has persistent difficulty weaning from the ventilator due to CO_2 retention. What nutritional modifications can be made to optimize her chances of extubation?

Indirect calorimetry may be used to determine the respiratory quotient (RQ) of this patient. The RQ can be used to adjust the nutritional composition of the TPN. For this case, it may be possible to reduce CO_2 production by decreasing the carbohydrate load in the TPN.

Respiratory Quotient

- RQ is a measure of energy expenditure
- RQ = Carbon dioxide produced (VCO_2)/oxygen consumed (VO_2)

RQ	Interpretation
<0.7	Starvation or underfeeding; ketosis
0.7	Metabolized substrate is mainly fat
0.8	Balanced mixture of fat and carbohydrates
1.0	Metabolized substrate is mainly carbohydrate
>1.0	Overfeeding; lipogenic state

It is important to keep the RQ between 0.7 and 1.0 to prevent fat accumulation in the liver and to alleviate potential respiratory distress secondary to excess glucose.

Which of the following two patients should the surgeon be more concerned about with regard to nutritional status: A well-appearing 35-year-old female with rheumatoid arthritis and a serum albumin level of 2.8, or a 64-year-old male with esophageal cancer preparing for transhiatal esophagectomy with an albumin of 2.8 and a BMI of 17.8?

The 35-year-old female with rheumatoid arthritis is most likely not malnourished. Visceral proteins (albumin, prealbumin, and transferrin), which are commonly used to estimate nutritional status, are influenced by many non-nutritional factors. This patient's low serum albumin (normal >3.5 g/dL) is likely due to chronic inflammation from her rheumatoid arthritis. The 64-year-old male with esophageal cancer, on the other hand, has an albumin <3.5 and is most likely malnourished from the disease process and his inability to eat. This is reflected in his low BMI of 17.8.

Assessment of Nutritional Status

- BMI and serum albumin are the most commonly used objective markers of nutritional status
- A preoperative BMI <18.5 kg/m² or albumin <3.5 g/dL is associated with increased morbidity
- *Serum albumin* is best used as an initial marker of the patient's overall nutritional status
  - It is not a good measure of acute changes in nutritional status because of its long half-life (21 days)
  - May be useful for assessment at the time of admission or in the outpatient clinic
- *Prealbumin* may be more useful for acute changes in nutritional status due to its short half-life (2 days)
- Albumin and prealbumin levels may be altered by factors not directly related to nutritional status.
  - Conditions that decrease serum albumin or pre-albumin include ascites, aggressive fluid resuscitation, inflammation, infection, stress, burns, hepatic failure, cancer, and hemorrhage
  - Conditions that increase serum albumin include transfusions, dehydration, and IV albumin administration
  - Conditions that increase serum pre-albumin include renal failure and steroid use
- *Transferrin* is another protein that can be used as a marker of a patient's nutritional status
  - Half-life of 8 to 10 days
  - Conditions that increase transferrin levels include chronic blood loss, iron deficiency, hepatic failure, dehydration, and chronic renal failure
  - Conditions that decrease transferrin levels include aggressive fluid resuscitation, chronic inflammation, pernicious anemia, and acute catabolic state (muscle breakdown)

What is the best estimate of protein metabolism in a critically ill patient?

Nitrogen balance, which can be calculated from nitrogen intake and output.

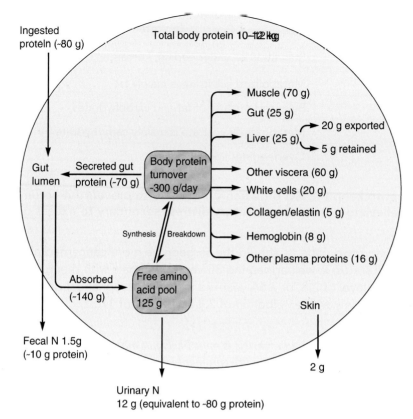

Whole body protein metabolism in a normal 70 kg man. (With permission from Mulholland MW, Lillemoe KD, Doherty GM, Maier RV, Upchurch GR, eds. *Greenfield's Surgery*. 4th ed. Philadelphia, PA: Lippincott Williams & Wilkins; 2005.)

Nitrogen Balance

- $N_{in} - N_{out}$ = (Total 24-hour protein intake/6.25) − (24-hour UUN + 4 g)
- Nitrogen intake is calculated from the enteral or parenteral intake given over 24 hours
- Nitrogen output is determined by measuring the amount of urea nitrogen in a 24-hour urine specimen (UUN)
- The addition of 4 g to the UUN is a "fudge factor" that takes into account 24-hour nitrogen loss from sources other than urine
- 6.25 g of protein contains 1 g of nitrogen
- In the critically ill patient, the goal is to achieve equilibrium
- A negative nitrogen balance indicates catabolism and means that more protein is being excreted than ingested
- A positive nitrogen balance indicates anabolism and means that more protein is being ingested than excreted, which usually occurs during the recovery phase of injury

---

A 24-year-old man with Crohn's disease complicated by an enterocutaneous fistula on chronic parenteral nutrition presents to your clinic with a new skin rash. What trace element deficiency might be responsible for the rash?

Zinc deficiency should be suspected in any patient on chronic TPN who develops a new skin rash.

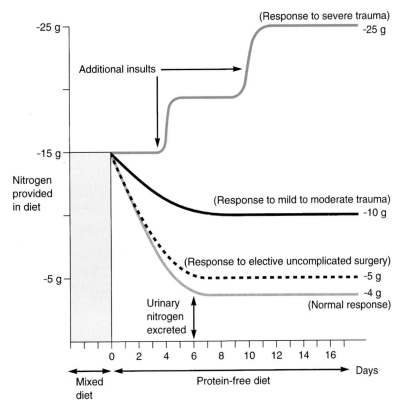

Response to starvation in normal, postoperative, and septic patients. (With permission from Mulholland MW, Lillemoe KD, Doherty GM, Maier RV, Upchurch GR, eds. *Greenfield's Surgery*. 4th ed. Philadelphia, PA: Lippincott Williams & Wilkins; 2005.)

Clinical Manifestations of Nutrient Deficiencies

Nutrient	Cellular role	Deficiency syndrome
Vitamin A	Photoreceptors, glycoprotein synthesis	Xerophthalmia, keratomalacia
Vitamin B1 (thiamine)	Carbohydrate metabolism	Beriberi, Wernicke-Korsadoff syndrome
Vitamin B2 (riboflavin)	Oxidation–reduction reactions	Cheilosis, angular stomatitis
Vitamin B3 (niacin)	Glycogen synthesis	Pellagra, dermatosis
Vitamin B6 (pyroxidine)	Protein metabolism	Convulsions in infancy
Vitamin B12 (cyanocobalamin)	Maturation of RBCs, neural function, DNA synthesis	Pernicious anemia, megaloblastic anemia, neuropathy
Vitamin C	Collagen synthesis	Scurvy
Vitamin D	Calcium and phosphorus absorption, mineralization	Rickets, osteomalacia
Vitamin K	Formation of prothrombin and other coagulation factors, bone proteins	Bleeding tendency, elevated PT
Biotin	Fatty acid synthesis	Dry skin, dermatosis, alopecia

(*Continued*)

Nutrient	Cellular role	Deficiency syndrome
Folate	Homocysteine, purine and pyrimidine metabolism, maturation of RBCs	Anemia, hyperpigmentation, hypercholesterolemia
Chromium	Promotion of glucose tolerance	Impaired glucose tolerance
Selenium	Component of glutathione peroxidase and thyroid hormone iodinase	Keshan disease (cardiomyopathy)
Copper	Enzyme component, hematopoiesis, bone formation	Hypochromic anemia, unresponsive to iron therapy
Zinc	Component of enzymes, skin integrity, wound healing	Dermatosis, glossitis
Omega-6 fatty acids	Prostaglandin synthesis, integrity of skin and cell membrane	Poor wound healing, dermatosis, increased risk of infection

What is the main fuel source of the small intestine?

Glutamine.

Glutamine

- The most abundant circulating amino acid
- Necessary for intra-organ nitrogen transport, maintenance of gut epithelial surfaces, and inhibition of bacterial translocation along the gut epithelium
- Involved in lymphocyte and macrophage production

Protein Digestion and Absorption

- Protein digestion begins in the stomach with pepsin
- Pepsin is formed by the action of acid on pepsinogen, which is secreted by gastric chief cells
- Pancreatic proteases are activated by enterokinase, which is located on the duodenal mucosa
- Most protein digestion takes place in the duodenum by pancreatic proteases and is complete by mid-jejunum
- The absorption of protein, in the form of amino acids, parallels that of digestion and is also complete by mid-jejunum

What is the main fuel source of the colon?

Short-chain fatty acids.

Fat Digestion and Absorption

- Ingested fat within the duodenum stimulates the release of cholecystokinin (CCK) from the proximal small bowel
- CCK stimulates the pancreas to release pancreatic lipases (lipase, cholesterol, esterase, and phospholipase)
- CCK also stimulates gallbladder contraction and the release of bile

- Bile emulsifies fats and facilitates the action of lipases
- Lipase hydrolyzes triglycerides to form free fatty acids and monoglycerides, which are absorbed by intestinal epithelium
- Long-chain fatty acids and cholesterol are incorporated into chylomicrons
- Short- and medium-chain fatty acids are bound to proteins (e.g., albumin) and transported to the liver via the portal system

A 45-year-old male with a history of ulcerative colitis is now status post total abdominal colectomy and end ileostomy. He is now having rectal pain and mucous secretions. What is the diagnosis and what should be done?

He has proctitis. Treatment is with a short-chain fatty acid enema. Because he has an end ileostomy, the colonocytes in the rectal stump are not receiving their main nutrient source.

What is the main fuel source of the brain?

Glucose.

Carbohydrate Digestion and Absorption
- Carbohydrate digestion begins in mouth by salivary amylase, and continues in duodenum with the addition of pancreatic amylase
- Amylases convert carbohydrate to oligosaccharides within the intestinal lumen
- Brush border associated oligosaccharidases convert oligosaccharides to mono- and disaccharides which are absorbed by intestinal epithelium

A 38-year-old male with a gunshot wound to the abdomen undergoes exploratory laparotomy. Postoperatively, he is placed on D5 half-normal saline at 125 mL/hour. How many kcal of energy will he receive in 24 hours?

There are 50 g of dextrose in each liter of this intravenous fluid. The patient will receive 3 L of fluid in 24 hours, for a total of 150 g of dextrose. One gram of dextrose yields 3.4 kcal. Therefore he will receive 150 × 3.4 = 510 kcal/day. The brain and red blood cells require a minimum of 100 g/day of glucose.

Energy Yields of Nutrients
- Fat: 9 kcal/g
- Protein: 4 kcal/g
- Carbohydrate: 3.4 kcal/g
- Alcohol: 7 kcal/g

A 58-year-old female is hospitalized for 6 days with a small bowel obstruction. Surgical therapy via an open laparotomy is now scheduled for the following day. Is this patient likely to benefit from perioperative TPN?

The patient will most likely not tolerate significant oral intake for another few days postoperatively, which will total greater than 10 days without nutrition. Therefore, the patient will benefit from the perioperative TPN, and it should be initiated.

A 28-year-old male involved in a high-speed auto collision sustained a devastating head injury and is now in the ICU with a poor mental state. What is the best route for nutrition?

If there are no contraindications, enteric feeding (gastric or post-pyloric) should be the first choice as a method of providing nutritional supplementation. This patient is at high risk for aspiration given his poor mental state; therefore, the best method of feeding would be a post-pyloric feeding tube with elevation of the head of the bed to 30° at all times.

Contraindications to Enteral Feeding

- Bowel obstruction
- Prolonged ileus
- Unable to obtain enteral access
- Severe pancreatitis
- High-output enterocutaneous fistula
- Short gut syndrome

Indications for Parenteral Nutrition

- A previously well-nourished patient without nutrition for 7 to 10 days
- Duration of illness anticipated to last longer than 7 to 10 days
- Malnutrition evidenced by >10% loss of body weight over 3 months
- Any malnourished patient with severe peritonitis, pancreatitis, thermal injury (>20% BSA), trauma, or other major illness

A 28-year-old female with perforated appendicitis undergoes pelvic drainage. Due to prolonged ileus, TPN is started via a peripherally inserted central catheter. You are called to her bedside because her arm is painful, red, and swollen, and there is exudate at the insertion site. What is the next step in management?

Phlebitis is inflammation of the vein secondary to mechanical, chemical, or infectious irritants. Mechanical phlebitis usually presents 24 to 72 hours after catheter insertion and can be managed with application of moist heat and arm elevation. If infection is suspected, in addition to heat and elevation, the treatment should also include removal of the catheter after obtaining blood cultures from it; the tip of the catheter should be sent for culture and sensitivities. If the arm is swollen, a duplex ultrasound should be performed to rule out venous thrombosis. If fungal infection or Pseudomonas is suspected, the catheter should be removed immediately.

A severely malnourished patient is suddenly found to be apneic 2 days following the initiation of TPN. What metabolic derangement is most likely to have caused this condition?

Hypophosphatemia is associated with refeeding syndrome.

Refeeding Syndrome

- Refeeding syndrome refers to the massive intracellular flux of phosphorous and potassium upon the introduction of nutrients into the system of a previously starved patient
- It begins approximately 1 to 2 days after initiating TPN, or 5 to 7 days after initiating enteral feeding

- Low serum phosphorous and potassium levels result, which can cause cardiomyopathy, decreased leukocyte chemotaxis, diaphragm dysfunction, seizures, thrombocytopenia, and hemolysis
- Inorganic phosphate is necessary for the processing of nutrients (especially glucose) in the production of ATP and nucleotides

Refeeding syndrome is prevented with aggressive phosphorus supplementation and gradual introduction of feeding (starting with 10 to 15 kcal/kg/day).

39 Wound Healing

Vijay A. Singh

A 39-year-old female sustained a large laceration to her right hand after punching a glass window 2 weeks ago. The initial wound measured 4 × 6 cm, but now is only 1 × 3 cm. What type of healing has occurred?

The healing in this patient occurred via secondary intention.

Types of Wound Healing

- Primary wound healing: The wound is closed within hours of injury
- Delayed primary wound healing: A contaminated wound is initially left open to prevent wound infection, and then closed 3 to 4 days later after host defense systems have debrided the wound
- Secondary wound healing: The wound left open and allowed to close by itself
  - Contaminated wounds, or wounds that are older than 24 hours, are frequently allowed to heal by secondary intention to help prevent wound infection

A 45-year-old male presents with a hypertrophic scar on his right hand after sustaining a burn 5 months ago. How do you differentiate between a hypertrophic scar and a keloid?

Hypertrophic scars remain confined to the traumatized area, whereas keloids extend pass the areas of trauma, projecting above the level of the surrounding skin.

Hypertrophic Scarring

- Occurs in areas of tension with poor approximation or where infection has occurred
- Typically occurs within the first month of injury
- Changes to brownish red or pale as it grows older
- Can be improved with topical or injectable glucocorticoid use
- Have better response to surgical resection than keloids
- No genetic disposition

597

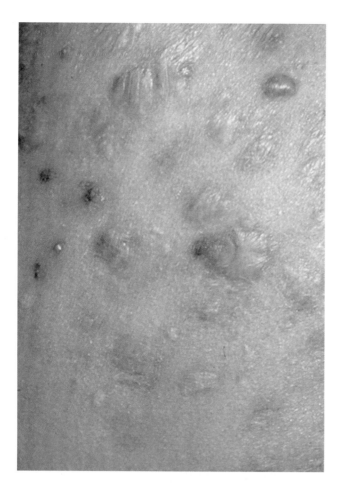

Hypertrophic scars. (With permission from Mulholland MW, Lillemoe KD, Doherty GM, Maier RV, Upchurch GR, eds. *Greenfield's Surgery*. 4th ed. Philadelphia, PA: Lippincott Williams & Wilkins; 2005.)

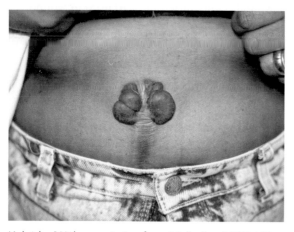 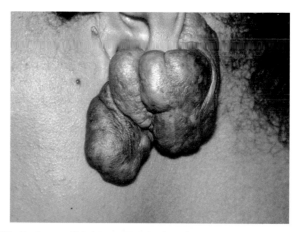

Keloids. (With permission from Mulholland MW, Lillemoe KD, Doherty GM, Maier RV, Upchurch GR, eds. *Greenfield's Surgery*. 4th ed. Philadelphia, PA: Lippincott Williams & Wilkins; 2005.)

Keloid

- Can occur anywhere
- Scar extends beyond the borders of the original scar tissue due to collagen deposition in adjacent tissue
  - Fibroblast collagen synthesis is 20 times normal
- Can be improved with topical or injectable glucocorticoid use
- Typically recur following surgical excision

- Can use radiation therapy in refractory cases
- Has a genetic disposition

Excessive scar tissue that forms hypertrophic scars or keloids usually develops within 6 to 8 weeks after the original injury.

A 45-year-old female presents with a hypertrophic scar on her left hand after sustaining a thermal injury approximately 1 year ago. What is the predominant collagen in scar tissue?

Type I is the predominant collagen type in a wound scar by day 3 or 4. The initial collagen in wounds is type III.

Collagen

- A protein polymer that acts as scaffolding for our bodies
- Has proline as every third amino acid
- Also has an abundant amount of lysine

Collagen type I	Major collagen found in skin, tendon, bone, dentin; primary collagen present in wound healing
Collagen type II	Specific for cartilage and vitreous humor
Collagen type III	In skin, muscles, and blood vessels
Collagen type IV	Basement membrane
Collagen type V	Widespread, particularly found in the cornea

- Type III collagen is the initial collagen in wound healing and is then replaced by type I collagen
- α-Ketoglutarate, vitamin C, oxygen, and iron are needed for hydroxylation of proline and subsequent cross-linking of proline residues
  - Scurvy is vitamin C deficiency
  - D-Penicillamine prevents collagen cross linking
- Maximum collagen accumulation at 2 to 3 weeks
- Afterwards, the amount of collagen remains the same but continued cross-linking improves collagen strength

Mutations in type I collagen produce osteogenesis imperfecta, which is characterized by deformed bones, short stature, and abnormalities of teeth.

A 64-year-old male had a ventral hernia repair performed 2 days ago. When will the wound achieve the greatest tensile strength?

Eight weeks. Wounds gradually increase their tensile strength as collagen deposition continues and scar remodeling takes place.

Tensile Strength

- After 3 weeks, tensile strength is only 15% to 30% of original strength
- After 6 weeks, tensile strength is 80% of original strength
- After 8 weeks, tensile strength is 90% of original strength

Tensile strength of any wound is never equal to pre-wound strength

After a motor vehicle accident, a patient is brought to the emergency room with multiple abrasions. Upon examination, the wounds are noted to be superficial. The wounds are irrigated, cleaned, and dressed with antibiotic ointment and dry gauze. Through what stages will these wounds proceed as they heal?

The four stages of wound healing are coagulation, inflammation, proliferation, and remodeling.

Stages of Wound Healing

- Coagulation (immediate)
    - Formation of clot and provisional wound matrix
    - Platelets aggregate and release inflammatory mediators and growth factors, particularly platelet-derived growth factor (PDGF) and transforming growth factor (TGF)
    - PDGF initiates chemotaxis of neutrophils, macrophages, and fibroblasts
- Inflammation (1 hour to 4 days)
    - Neutrophils and macrophages enter the wound for removal of necrotic debris and bacteria
    - Neutrophils phagocytose, debride, and produce proteinases, collagenases, and bactericidal proteins (but not growth factors)
    - Macrophages are the primary mediators of wound healing and the main source of growth factors; they modulate collagen deposition and organization
- Proliferation (3rd to 14th day)
    - Dominated by fibroblasts, collagen production, and angiogenesis
- Remodeling (3 weeks to 6 months)
    - Dynamic process of collagen deposition and resorption
    - Collagen becomes organized along lines of tension
    - Wound strength significantly increases during this stage

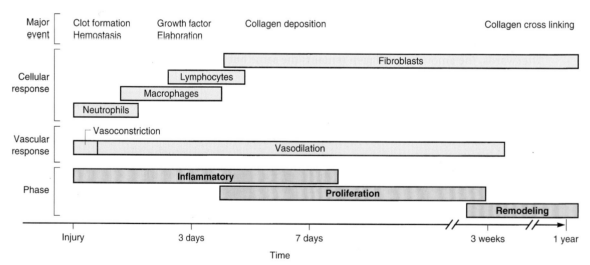

Wound healing phases and cell types. (With permission from Mulholland MW, Lillemoe KD, Doherty GM, Maier RV, Upchurch GR, eds. *Greenfield's Surgery.* 4th ed. Philadelphia, PA: Lippincott Williams & Wilkins; 2005.)

Cytokines in Wound Healing

- Interferon-γ
  - Source: Macrophages and T cells
  - Activates macrophages, polymorphonuclear neutrophils (PMNs), and fibroblasts
- Insulin-like growth factor-1
  - Source: Macrophages and fibroblasts
  - Activates fibroblasts and keratinocytes and increases collagen production
- Interleukin-2
  - Source: T cells
  - Triggers mitosis in fibroblasts
- PDGF
  - Source: Macrophages, platelets, and endothelial cells
  - Recruits PMNs, macrophages, and fibroblasts and stimulates angiogenesis
- Tumor necrosis factor-α
  - Source: PMNs
  - Overall activator of immune cells

Order of cell arrival in a wound (first to last): Platelets, PMNs, macrophages, fibroblasts, and lymphocytes.

A 40-year-old liver transplant recipient on chronic steroids has to undergo an open appendectomy. What can be given to improve wound healing?

Vitamin A (25,000 units per day) can improve wound healing in steroid-dependent patients.

Wound Healing in Patients

- Impediments to wound healing
  - Infection: Bacteria count >100,000 bacteria/g
    - Infection causes increase in cytotoxic oxidases and proteinases
  - Devitalized tissue: Retards granulation tissue formation
  - Radiation: Inhibits angiogenesis and causes fibrosis
  - Diabetes: Impedes early-phase response
  - Steroid therapy
    - Inhibits macrophages, PMNs, and collagen synthesis
    - Promotes a catabolic state
  - Albumin <3.0: Increases the risk of poor wound healing
  - Venous insufficiency
    - Have congested wound with heavy drainage
    - Poor immune cell penetration
  - Foreign bodies
    - Lead to a chronic inflammatory states
    - Cause adjacent fibrosis and predispose to infection

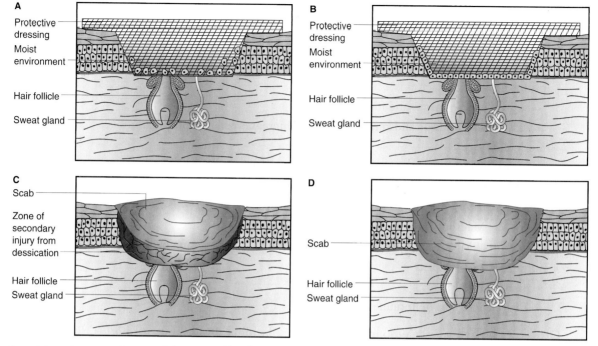

A moist environment is essential to wound healing. (With permission from Mulholland MW, Lillemoe KD, Doherty GM, Maier RV, Upchurch GR, eds. *Greenfield's Surgery*. 4th ed. Philadelphia, PA: Lippincott Williams & Wilkins; 2005.)

- Essentials to wound healing
  - Moist environment
  - Adequate oxygenation
  - Avoidance of edema
  - Removal of necrotic tissue

Smoking can have a detrimental effect on wound healing.

Platelets are known as the first response cell in wound healing. What are the products of platelet degranulation?

TGF-β and PDGF.

Contents of Platelet Granules
- PDGF: Chemoattractant
- TGF-β: Key component of tissue repair
- Beta-thrombomodulin: Binds thrombin
- Platelet aggregation factors: TXA2, thrombin, platelet factor 4
- Dense granules: Adenosine, serotonin, and calcium

Platelet degranulation also activates the complement cascade, specifically C5a, which is a potent chemoattractant for neutrophils.

40 | Antibiotics

J.W. Awori Hayanga, Nicholas F. Montanaro, and Robert A. Meguid

A 67-year-old gentleman was admitted to the intensive care unit following a suprarenal abdominal aortic aneurysm repair. His postoperative course was complicated by a pseudomonal ventilator-associated pneumonia and he failed to wean from the ventilator. At the time of operation, he had a prolonged aortic clamp time, postoperative hypotension and his creatinine had increased from a 0.8 to 3.5. Which antibiotic targeted against gram-negative rods is least advisable in the presence of deteriorating renal function? And how does this antibiotic work?

Aminoglycosides are nephrotoxic and should be avoided in the presence of renal impairment. In addition, they are unsuitable as SINGLE agent therapy against pseudomonas. They should ideally be used in combination with an extended-spectrum penicillin. Aminoglycosides block protein synthesis by inhibiting the 30s ribosome.

Classes of Bacteria

- Gram-positive cocci
  - *Staphylococcus* species: *Staph aureus, Staph epidermidi*
  - *Streptococcus* species: *Strep pneumonia, Strep pyogenes* (Group A *Strep*), *Strep agalactiae* (Group B *Strep*)
  - *Enterococcus* species
- Gram-positive bacilli
  - *Bacillus* species: *B. anthracis, B. cereus*
  - *Clostridia* species: *C. botulinum, C. difficile, C. perfringens, C. tetani*
  - *Lactobacillus* species
  - *Listeria monocytogenes*
  - *Nocardia* species
  - *Corynebacterium diptheriae*
- Gram-negative cocci
  - *Neisseria* species: *N. meningitidis, N. Gonorrhoeae*
- Gram-negative bacilli
  - *Citrobacter*
  - *Escherichia coli*
  - *Enterobacter*
  - *Klebsiella*

603

- *Proteus*
- *Pseudomonas*
- *Salmonella*
- *Serratia marcescens*
- *Shigella*
- Gram-negative coccobacillus
  - *Haemophilus influenzae*
- Anaerobes
  - *Clostridia* species, *Peptostreptococcus, Bacteroides, Actinomyces*
- Encapsulated bacteria
  - *Strep pneumonia, H.influenzae, Klebsiella pneumonia, N. Meningitidis*

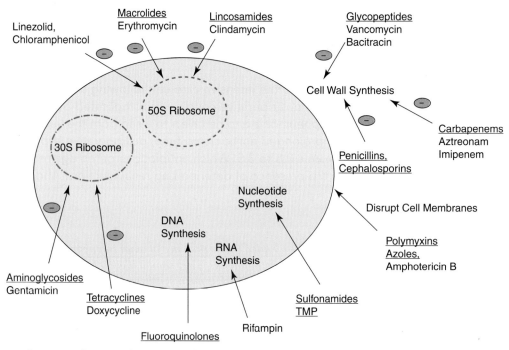

Mechanisms of action of various antibiotics. (With permission from O'Leary JP, Tabuenca A, eds. *Physiologic Basis of Surgery.* 4th ed. Philadelphia, PA: Wolters Kluwer Health/Lippincott Williams & Wilkins; 2007.)

Mechanism of Antibiotics

- Block bacterial cell wall synthesis by binding penicillin binding protein
  - Penicillins, cephalosporins, aztreonam, imipenem
- Block peptidoglycan synthesis
  - Vancomycin, bacitracin
- Block protein synthesis at the 50S ribosomal subunit
  - Macrolides, chloramphenicol, lincosamides
- Block protein synthesis at the 30S ribosomal subunit
  - Aminoglycosides, tetracyclines
- Block nucleotide synthesis
  - Sulfonamides, trimethoprim
- Block DNA topoisomerases
  - Fluoroquinolones

- Block mRNA synthesis
  - Rifampin
- Disrupt cell membranes
  - Polymixins
- Disrupt fungal cell membranes
  - Amphotericin B, azoles

A 25-year-old male with no significant past medical history presents with a painless, ulcerated lesion on his penis. He has been sexually active with 10 partners in the past 2 months and denies using any protection. He otherwise feels well. What antibiotic should be used to treat his infection and what is its mechanism of action?

The patient has syphilis, which is susceptible to penicillin. It is imperative that his infection be treated or he could progress to secondary and tertiary syphilis, which are more resistant to treatment. Testing and treatment should also be offered to his partners.

- **Penicillins**
  - Contain β-lactam ring
  - Penicillin G, Penicillin V, ampicillin, amoxicillin, carbencillin, methicillin, nafcillin, oxacillin, ticarcillin
  - Activity against *Streptococci, pneumococci, gonococci, meningococci,* spirochetes
  - Mechanism of action: Bactericidal
    - Inhibition of cell wall synthesis
    - Bind drug-specific receptors in bacterial cytoplasmic membrane (penicillin-binding proteins)
    - Inhibition of transpeptidases
    - Activation of autocatalytic enzymes
  - Resistance is via β-lactamases and is wide spread
    - β-lactamase inhibitors in combination with β-lactam antibiotics are used to combat resistance: Clavulinic acid, sulbactam, tazobactam.
  - Pharmacokinetics:
    - Varying degrees of oral absorption
    - Not metabolized
    - Excreted renally, except ampicillin and nafcillin, which are excreted in bile
    - Short half-lives (30 min to 1 hour)
  - Toxicity:
    - Allergic reactions
    - Nausea and diarrhea

A 57-year-old female with a history of hypertension and hyperlipidemia presents for a routine laparoscopic cholecystectomy. What class of antibiotic should she receive 1 hour to 30 minutes before the incision is made?

This is considered to be a clean GI type of operation, thus a first-generation cephalosporin will suffice. The purpose of the antibiotic is to prevent a surgical site infection.

- **Cephalosporins**
  - Also contain β-lactam rings
  - 1st generation: Cefazolin
    - Treat gram-positive cocci, *Proteus, E. coli, Klebsiella*
  - 2nd generation: Cefotetan, cefoxitin, cefuroxime
    - Treat gram-positive cocci, *H. flu, Enterobacter, Neisseria, Proteus, E. coli, Klebsiella, Serratia*
  - 3rd generation: Cefotaxime, ceftazidime, ceftriaxone
    - Treat serious gram-negative infections, meningitis
      - Ceftazidime: *Pseudomonas*
      - Ceftriaxone: *N. gonorrhoeae*
  - 4th generation: Cefepime, cefquinome
    - Treat serious gram-negative and gram-positive infections
    - Can cross the blood brain barrier
      - Cefepime: Nosocomial *Pseudomonas*
  - Mechanism of action: Bactericidal
    - Inhibition of cell wall synthesis
    - Bind drug-specific receptors in bacterial cytoplasmic membrane (penicillin-binding proteins)
  - Resistance is via β-lactamases or mutation of penicillin-binding proteins
  - Pharmacokinetics
    - Variable oral absorption
    - Not metabolized
    - Excreted renally, except ceftriaxone, which is excreted in bile
    - Short half-lives (30 min to 1 hour)
  - Toxicity
    - Allergic reactions—10% cross-reactivity with penicillin-allergic patients
- **Other β-lactam Antibiotics**
  - Aztreonam
    - Monobactam
    - Resistant to β-lactamases
    - Activity against *Klebsiella, Pseudomonas, Serratia*
    - Inhibits cell wall synthesis
    - Excreted renally
    - Not cross-reactive with penicillins
  - Imipenem
    - Carbapenem
    - Largely resistant to β-lactamases
    - Activity against gram-positive cocci, gram-negative bacilli, anaerobes
    - Administered with cilastatin to inhibit rapid renal inactivation
    - Partially cross-reactive with penicillins

A 39-year-old nurse with no significant past medical history presents with a red, painful, swollen nodule on her arm. On further evaluation, the nodule is fluctuant. You perform an incision and drainage (I&D) of the area and infected fluid is evacuated, but the patient continues to be febrile and have significant cellulitis. A culture of the fluid demonstrates methicillin resistant staph aureus (MRSA). What antibiotic should be used for initial treatment in this patient?

Vancomycin should be used initially until the sensitivities on the antibiotic susceptibility are available and she is clinically improving. These patients can often be transitioned to Bactrim or another sensitivity-specific antibiotic.

- **Vancomycin**
  - Activity against β-lactamase-producing *Staph aureus* and *C. difficile*
  - Mechanism of action: Bactericidal
    - Inhibition of cell wall mucopeptides
  - Resistance is rare
  - Pharmacokinetics:
    - Not orally absorbed
      - Can be used to treat bacterial enterocolitis
    - Wide tissue penetration
    - Not metabolized
    - Excreted renally
    - Dosing must achieve drug concentration within the therapeutic window
  - Toxicity:
    - Ototoxicity
    - Nephrotoxicity
    - "Red man" syndrome results from rapid infusion
- **Bacitracin**
  - Activity against aerobic gram-positive bacteria
  - Mechanism of action: Bactericidal
    - Inhibition of cell wall synthesis
  - Pharmacokinetics:
    - Topical use only
  - Toxicity:
    - Nephrotoxic

A 57-year-old female who is POD 1 status post laparoscopic gastric bypass surgery has a persistent cough. She had no episodes of emesis and no witnessed aspiration events. A chest X-ray demonstrates diffuse patchy infiltrates. On further questioning, the patient does remember that she was starting to have a cough and feeling more tired for the 2 days prior to surgery. She is diagnosed with a community-acquired pneumonia. What antibiotic should be used?

The patient had no evidence of aspiration and was only intubated for a couple of hours for her procedure. Her chest X-ray and story are most compatible with a community-acquired pneumonia. She should be treated with a macrolide antibiotic.

- **Macrolides**
  - Azithromycin, clarithromycin, erythromycin
  - Activity against aerobic gram-positive cocci bacteria
    - *Mycoplasma pneumoniae, Corynebacterium, C. trachomatis, Legionella pneumophila, Bordetella pertussis*
    - Azithromycin also active against *H. flu, M. catarrhalis, Neisseria*
    - Clarithromycin also active against *M. avium-intracellulare, H. pylori*
  - Mechanism of action: Bactericidal or bacteriostatic
    - Inhibition of protein synthesis
    - Erythromycin binds the 23S rRNA component of the 50S ribosomal subunit, resulting in blocking of the initiation complex and ribosomal translocation
  - Resistance is via multiple plasmid-mediated enzymes
  - Pharmacokinetics:
    - Azithromycin is cleared unmetabolized in urine
    - Clarithromycin is metabolized in the liver
    - Erythromycin is excreted in bile
  - Toxicity:
    - Hypersensitivity-based acute cholestatic hepatitis (rare)
    - Inhibition of cytochrome P450 by erythromycin, resulting in increased plasma levels of other drugs (e.g., warfarin, digoxin)
- **Chloramphenicol**
  - Broad-spectrum activity:
    - *Salmonella, H. meningitidis, H. flu* (some strains only)
  - Mechanism of action: Bacteriostatic
    - Inhibition of peptidyl transferase
    - Binds the 50S ribosomal subunit
  - Resistance is via formation of inactivating acetyl transferases
  - Pharmacokinetics:
    - Metabolized in liver
  - Toxicity:
    - Irreversible aplastic anemia (~1:30,000 patients)
    - Reversible bone marrow suppression
    - Gray baby syndrome when used in neonates
    - Inhibition of metabolism of phenytoin and warfarin

A 69-year-old otherwise healthy male undergoes an open right hemicolectomy for colon cancer. On post-operative day 4, he is noted to have increasing erythema around the incision site. He has no fluctuance and no purulent material can be expressed. He is otherwise afebrile and feeling well. He is allergic to penicillin. What antibiotic regimen should be started?

The patient may have a wound infection. As the patient is allergic to penicillin, thus clindamycin should be used if there is suspicion of cellulitis.

- **Lincosamides**
  - Clindamycin, lincomycin
  - Activity against aerobic gram-positive cocci, anaerobes
  - Mechanism of action: Bacteriostatic
    - Inhibition of protein synthesis
    - Erythromycin binds the 23S rRNA component of the 50S ribosomal subunit, resulting in blocking of the initiation complex and ribosomal translocation
  - Pharmacokinetics:
    - Orally absorbed
    - Wide tissue penetration
    - Metabolized in liver
    - Excreted renally and in bile
  - Risk of superinfection by *C. difficile* pseudomembranous colitis

A 37-year-old female with a history of Crohn's disease who is status post a small bowel resection complicated by multiple intra-abdominal abscesses and sepsis is started on a new antibiotic. One week after starting the antibiotic, the patient complains of increasing difficulty hearing and her creatinine also started to rise. What group of antibiotics has these side effects?

Aminoglycosides, which cover gram negative bacteria and are used for severe intra-abdominal sepsis, have side effects of irreversible ototoxicity and ATN.

- **Aminoglycosides**
  - Amikacin, Gentamicin, Neomycin, Streptomycin, Tobramycin
  - Activity against aerobic gram-negative bacteria
    - *E. coli, Enterobacter, Klebsiella, Proteus, Pseudomonas, Serratia*
  - Mechanism of action: Bactericidal
    - Inhibition of protein synthesis
    - Streptomycin binds the 30S ribosomal subunit, resulting in blocking of the initiation complex, misreading of mRNA, and disruption of polysomes
  - Resistance is via plasmid-mediated formation of various group transferases
  - Pharmacokinetics:
    - Not orally absorbed
    - Limited tissue penetration
    - Not metabolized
    - Excreted renally
    - Dosing must achieve drug concentration within the therapeutic window
  - Toxicity:
    - Irreversible ototoxicity
    - Acute tubular necrosis
    - Neuromuscular blockade resulting in respiratory paralysis at high doses
- **Tetracyclines**
  - Tetracycline, doxycycline
  - Activity against *Mycoplasma pneumoniae, chlamydiae, rickettsiae*

- Mechanism of action: Bacteriostatic
  - Inhibition of protein synthesis
  - Binds the 30S ribosomal subunit, resulting in blocking translation of Mrna
- Resistance is via decreased cellular uptake of the drug
- Pharmacokinetics:
  - Variable oral absorption
  - Metabolized in liver
  - Wide tissue distribution
  - Crosses placenta
- Toxicity:
  - Bone and teeth discoloration and irregularities in exposed fetus
  - Hepatic necrosis in patients with hepatic impairment
  - Photosensitivity in ultraviolet light

A 38-year-old male who suffered 3rd degree burns to 30% of his TBSA has been undergoing serial debridements of his wounds. He is noted to have a wound infection and topical antibiotics are started. 7 days later, he is noted to have pancytopenia. Which topical antibiotic used in burn wounds is associated with this side effect?

Sulfa antibiotics, including silver sulfadiazine, which is used in burn wound infections, have a risk of bone marrow suppression and pancytopenia.

- **Sulfonamides**
  - Sulfamethoxazole, sulfasalazine, silver sulfadiazine
  - Activity against gram-positive and gram-negative bacteria
    - Simple urinary tract infections, occular infections, burn infections (silver sulfadiazine), ulcerative colitis (sulfasalazine)
  - Mechanism of action: Bacteriostatic
    - Inhibition of folic acid synthesis
  - Resistance is plasmid-mediated
  - Pharmacokinetics:
    - Some tissue penetration
    - Metabolized in the liver
    - Excreted renally
  - Toxicity:
    - Granulocytopenia
    - Aplastic anemia
    - Thrombocytopenia
- **Trimethoprim**
  - Used in combination with sulfamethoxazole as TMP-SMX for treatment of complicated urinary tract infections, *H. flu* and *M. catarrhalis* sinusitis, *Aeromonas hydrophila* and *Pneumocystis carinii* pneumonia, *Shigella, Salmonella, Serratia*
  - Mechanism of action: Bacteriostatic
    - Inhibition of folic acid synthesis
    - In combination with sulfamethoxazole, the resulting sequential blockade of folate synthesis is bactericidal

- Resistance is via production of dihydrofolate reductase with reduced affinity for trimethoprim
- Pharmacokinetics:
    - Increased concentration in vaginal and prostatic fluids
    - Excreted renally
- Toxicity:
    - Granulocytopenia
    - Megaloblastic anemia
    - Leukopenia
    - Administration of folinic acid (leucovorin) may limit or reverse toxicity

---

A 14-year-old girl undergoes an uneventful laparoscopic appendectomy. However, on POD 2, she is complaining of burning with urination and is diagnosed with a UTI. She is given an antibiotic and feels significantly better. However, after resuming her normal activities, she has an acute rupture of her Achilles tendon. What antibiotic was she given that put her at risk for this orthopedic complication?

Fluoroquinolones, which are routinely used in management of uncomplicated UTIs, have a risk of tendon rupture and should not be used in children.

- **Fluoroquinolones**
    - Ciprofloxacin, norfloxacin, ofloxacin
    - Activity against gram-negative bacteria
        - *E. coli, N. gonorrhoeae, Klebsiella pneumoniae, Enterobacter, Salmonella, Shigella*
    - Mechanism of action: Bactericidal
        - Inhibition of bacterial topoisomerase II
    - Resistance is via altered drug sensitivity of DNA gyrase
    - Pharmacokinetics:
        - Orally absorbed
        - Wide tissue penetration except CNS
        - Metabolized
        - Secreted renally
    - Toxicity:
        - Mild symptoms
- **Rifampin**
    - Activity against *Mycobacterium*
        - Used with isoniazid (INH) against tuberculosis
        - Used with dapsone against leprosy
    - Mechanism of action: Bactericidal
        - Inhibition of mRNA synthesis
    - Resistance is via plasmid-mediated formation of various group transferases
    - Pharmacokinetics:
        - Orally absorbed
        - Wide tissue penetration including CNS
        - Metabolized by liver
        - Excreted fecally

- Toxicity:
  - Proteinuria
  - Induction of cytochrome P450, resulting in increased metabolism of other drugs
- **Polymixins**
  - Fatty acid-containing polypeptides
  - Activity against gram-negative bacteria
    - *Enterobacter, Pseudomonas*
  - Mechanism of action: Bactericidal
    - Interfere with lipopolysaccharides in cell membrane
  - Pharmacokinetics:
    - Topical use only
  - Toxicity:
    - Nephrotoxic (ATN)
    - Neurotoxic

A 35-year old female has short gut after multiple bowel resections for fistulizing Crohn's disease, and she is on long-term TPN. She presents to the hospital with hypothermia of 35 degrees and hypotension to 90s/50s. Broad-spectrum antibiotics are started, but her status continues to worsen. What should be added to the regimen?

Antifungals should be added due to likely fungemia. Azoles should be tried initially, but therapy should be broadened to Amphotericin B if her infection worsens.

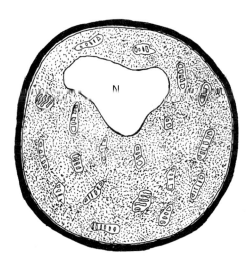

Fungal cell—different from bacteria in that it has a nucleus. (With permission from O'Leary JP, Tabuenca A, eds. *Physiologic Basis of Surgery.* 4th ed. Philadelphia, PA: Wolters Kluwer Health/ Lippincott Williams & Wilkins; 2007.)

- **Antifungals**
  - Amphotericin B
    - Used against systemic fungal infections
    - Can be used in conjunction with rifampin or tetracycline for synergistic effects
    - Mechanism of action:
      - Increases permeability of fungal cell membranes
    - Toxicity:
      - Hypokalemia
      - Nephrotoxicity
      - Hypotension
      - The liposomal preparation is associated with fewer side effects

- Azoles
  - Fluconazole, itraconazole, ketoconazole
  - Used against systemic fungal infections and for prophylaxis in patients with prolonged mechanical ventilation
  - Mechanism of action:
    - Inhibit synthesis of ergosterol, thus increasing permeability of fungal cell membranes
  - Pharmacokinetics:
    - Orally absorbed
    - Wide tissue penetration
    - Metabolized by liver (itraconazole, ketoconazole)
    - Excreted renally (fluconazole)
  - Toxicity:
    - Hepatotoxicity
    - Inhibition of cytochrome P450

What are drugs that have zero-order elimination?

Zero-order elimination is when a drug is eliminated at a constant rate. An example of a drug that undergoes zero-order elimination is phenytoin.

Pharmacokinetics

- Volume of distribution is the relationship of the drug dose to the plasma concentration.
  - V_d = Amount of drug in body/plasma drug concentration
- Clearance is the relationship of the rate of drug elimination to the plasma concentration.
  - CL = Rate of drug elimination/plasma drug concentration
- Half-life is the time required for the body to eliminate half of the drug dose from the body
  - $t_{1/2} = 0.7 \times V_d/CL$
  - 50% of the desired concentration is achieved after one half-life.
  - 94% of the desired concentration is achieved after four half-lives.

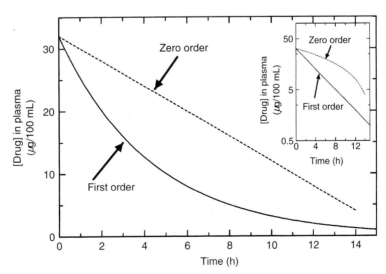

Zero and first order drug kinetics. (With permission from O'Leary JP, Tabuenca A, eds. *Physiologic Basis of Surgery.* 4th ed. Philadelphia, PA: Wolters Kluwer Health/Lippincott Williams & Wilkins; 2007.)

- Loading dose is a function of the desired plasma concentration (C_p), the volume of distribution and the bioavailability (F), and is NOT reduced for patients with impaired renal and hepatic function
  - Loading dose = $C_p \times V_d/F$
- Maintenance dose is a function of the desired plasma concentration (C_p), the clearance and the bioavailability (F), and IS reduced for patients with impaired renal and hepatic function
  - Loading dose = $C_p \times CL/F$
- Drug elimination can be either "zero-order" or "first-order"
  - Zero-order elimination follows a constant rate
    - Examples: Ethanol and phenytoin
  - First-order elimination is proportional to drug concentration and decreases exponentially
- Drug metabolism is either via phase I or phase II mechanisms in the liver
  - Phase I is reduction, oxidation, and hydrolysis, resulting in active metabolites (e.g., via cytochrome P450)
  - Phase II is acetylation, glucuronidation, and sulfation, resulting in inactive metabolites (conjugation reactions)

Forty minutes into a routine laparoscopic cholecystectomy for symptomatic cholelithiasis, you encounter bleeding and difficulty visualizing the important structures. You convert to an open procedure after 4 hours and take an additional 3 hours to complete the procedure. The patient had received a first generation cephalosporin antibiotic. When should he receive the next dose of antibiotics?

The next dose should be administered by the anesthesia team DURING the procedure of 4–6 hours following the initial dose.

Prophylactic Antibiotics in Surgical Practice

- Indicated for dirty, contaminated, clean-contaminated, or long/major cases
- Optional in small/clean cases where prosthetics are used (inguinal hernia repair)
- Not indicated for other clean small cases, except in some circumstances
- Administered within 1 hour prior to incision
- Consider redosing 4 to 6 hours after initial dose or for massive blood loss (given altered pharmacokinetics)
- There is no benefit in continuing prophylaxis beyond 24 hours following the operation
- Second generation cephalosporins are more effective in vitro against some strains of methicillin-sensitive *S. aureus*
- Clindamycin is often used for cephalosporin allergic patients
- Vancomycin may be considered in hospitals with a high prevalence of methicillin-resistant *S. aureus* (MRSA)
- In colorectal and obstetrics–gynecology cases, the pathogens are predominantly gram-negative anaerobes such as *Bacteroides* and *Enterococcus*
  - For these cases, there has been a demonstrated superiority for cefotetan over cefazolin and amoxicillin/clavulanate over metronidazole alone
- For colorectal surgery, new consensus guidelines recommend both a mechanical and oral antibiotic bowel prep before elective surgery
- Wound infections in clean elective operations are commonly caused by skin flora from the patient's skin
- Evidence to support the prevention of surgical site infections supports the following practices:
  - Using an electric razor to shave skin hair just prior to the operation
  - Patient washing the evening prior to the operation

- Avoiding hypothermia
- Tight glucose control

Strong evidence supports the practice that prophylactic antibiotics should be administered within 1 hour prior to the surgical incision.

A 46-year-old recidivist alcoholic returns to the emergency room with a bout of mild uncomplicated pancreatitis following a drinking binge. You are asked which antibiotic is best for acute pancreatitis.

Antibiotics are not indicated for uncomplicated pancreatitis. The administration of antibiotics in this and other settings where they have not been shown to be of benefit (e.g., extended prophylaxis) can be harmful to public health given the forecast epidemic of antimicrobial resistance which is predicted to significantly complicate surgery in future years.

A 76-year-old woman admitted for resection of a large retroperitoneal sarcoma had an ICU hospitalization complicated by prolonged intubation requiring tracheostomy as well as renal failure and critical illness polyneuropathy. She developed a new temperature of 39.0 °C overnight and was cultured. How should the appropriate antibiotic be selected?

Empiric therapy in the ICU setting should be broad, covering the gram-negative non-fermenters (Pseudomonas, Acinetobacter, and Stenotrophomonas) as well as MRSA. Therapy should be largely based on local antibiotic resistance patterns.

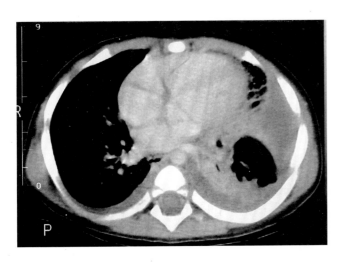

Pneumonia that developed into an empyema. (With permission from Mulholland MW, Lillemoe KD, Doherty GM, Maier RV, Upchurch GR, eds. *Greenfield's Surgery.* 4th ed. Philadelphia, PA: Lippincott Williams & Wilkins; 2005.)

Ventilator-Associated Pneumonia (VAP)

- Greater than 10,000 organisms on a qualitative culture obtained via BAL
- Is seen after patients have been on the ventilator for >48 hours
- Once BAL is performed, prophylactic antibiotics should be commenced empirically based on local antibiotic resistance patterns
- One common choice is the combination of vancomycin (to cover potential MRSA and other gram-positive bacteria) and piperacillin-tazobactam (to cover gram-negative bacteria)
- Combination coverage ("double covering") may be useful for ill patients in the first few days of treatment
- Antibiotics should be tailored appropriately based on sensitivities

- To prevent VAP, make sure ventilated patients are being managed with bundle of interventions (The VAP bundle)
  - Head of bed at ≥30 degrees
  - Mouth hygiene
  - Subglottic endotracheal suctioning
  - Sedation breaks

Community-Acquired Pneumonia
- Most commonly caused by *Strep pneumoniae*
- Other common pathogens include *M. pneumoniae*, *Legionella*, *Chlamydophila* (formerly *Chlamydia*) *pneumoniae*, and *H. flu*
- Empiric therapy may consist of either a macrolide, doxycycline, or an anti-pneumococcal fluoroquinolone
- Other antibiotic regimens in clinical practice include amoxicillin or amoxicillin/clavulanate

> A 75-year-old male who is 2 weeks status post gastrectomy complicated by a wound infection for which he was treated with clindamycin presents with 5 days of diarrhea and malaise. What treatment should be initiated?

Clostridium difficile colitis is a common infection following antibiotic use, especially with clindamycin. Initial treatment is with oral vancomycin or vancomycin enemas. IV metronidazole can be added for refractory infections. If colitis progresses, patient may need fecal allotransplant (via enema) or a total colectomy.

C. difficile Colitis
- Spread as a spore
- Most commonly follows recent antibiotic use as the antibiotics kill the normal, healthy colonic bacteria
- Symptoms: Diarrhea, abdominal pain
- Diagnosis: *C. difficile* toxin, pseudomembranous colitis on colonoscopy
- Treatment
  - Initial: Oral vancomycin
  - Severe: Oral vancomycin, vancomycin enemas, IV flagyl
  - Severe, recurrent: Fecal injection (allotransplant) via enema
  - Toxic megacolon, sepsis, perforation: Emergent surgical exploration

> A 85-year-old lucent male underwent an open left hemicolectomy for a perforated diverticulitis. That evening, you are called to the bedside for altered mental status and fever of 41 °C. When you examine the patient, you note that he has thin, gray drainage coming from his wound. What is the next step in management?

The patient should be taken emergently to the OR for debridement of his necrotizing wound infection. The very high temperature immediately following surgery is a rare and ominous finding, especially if the patient did not have a fever preoperatively.

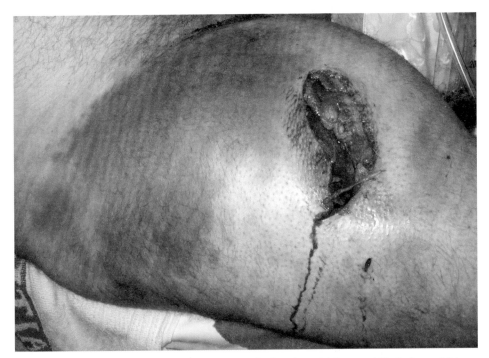

Necrotizing fasciitis. (With permission from Mulholland MW, Lillemoe KD, Doherty GM, Maier RV, Upchurch GR, eds. *Greenfield's Surgery*. 4th ed. Philadelphia, PA: Lippincott Williams & Wilkins; 2005.)

Necrotizing Fasciitis

- Spreads to all layers of the tissues including skin and muscle, sometimes within hours
- Can be seen in the immediate post-operative period
- Symptoms: Crepitance, pain, "dishwater drainage"
- An unusually strong malodor can be the presenting sign
- Pathogens: Most often polymicrobial; if it involves a single pathogen, is often Strep Pyogenes
- Treatment
  - Excision of all infected dead tissue, i.e. tissue that does not bleed when cut
  - Broad spectrum antibiotic therapy—commonly used agents include penicillin, gentamicin, clindamycin, or metronidazole

41 Cell Biology

Debashish Bose, Justin B. Maxhimer, and Catherine Pesce

An 8-year-old boy develops bacterial meningitis and is treated with penicillin. What is the mechanism of action of this medication?

All β-lactam antibiotics inhibit bacterial cell wall synthesis by interfering with a transpeptidase reaction that covalently links amino acid residues in the cell wall. Bacterial cell walls are made of peptidoglycans that are chains of polysaccharides and polypeptides. Blockage of cell wall synthesis results in cell death; thus, β-lactam antibiotics are bactericidal.

Plasma Membrane Composition

- The basic structure of all cell membranes is the *phospholipid bilayer*
- It consists of two leaflets of phospholipid molecules whose fatty acyl tails form the *hydrophobic* interior of the bilayer while their polar, *hydrophilic* head groups line both surfaces
- The outer surface of the cell generally has a negative charge created by terminal residues on oligosaccharide chains, such as sialic acid
- 40% of the plasma membrane consists of *lipid*
  - The most common lipids are phospholipids (specifically phosphatidylcholine and phosphatidylethanolamine), glycolipids, and cholesterol
  - The more cholesterol in the membrane, the greater the membrane fluidity
- 60% percent of the plasma membrane consists of *protein*
  - Integral membrane proteins can be attached to one side of the membrane or span the entire membrane (transmembrane protein)

Cell Membrane

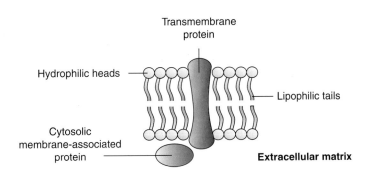

Plasma Membrane Proteins

- **Transmembrane** proteins
  - Have one or more portions that span the phospholipid bilayer
  - This group includes *receptor* molecules linked to intracellular enzymes, *transport* molecules, and *ion channels*
  - Most are linked to the bilayer through covalent bonds
  - While the majority of transmembrane proteins are in an α-helical configuration, *porins* are transmembrane proteins composed of antiparallel β-strands arranged in a barrel shape
  - Specific transmembrane proteins provide hydrophilic paths for ions involved in electrical signaling, primarily Na^+, K^+, Ca^{2+}, and Cl^-
  - The amino acid sequence in specific regions of these proteins determines the selectivity for specific ions
- **Peripheral** proteins
  - Do not interact with the hydrophobic core of the bilayer; instead, they are usually bound to the membrane indirectly by interactions with other transmembrane proteins or directly with lipid polar head groups
  - Examples include proteins that link the cytoskeleton to membrane junctions (e.g., *actin*, *protein kinase* **C**)
  - Interactions take place through non-covalent bonds

Cell Transport and Electrolyte Concentrations

- There are two basic types of cell transport: diffusion and active transport
- *Diffusion* is driven by concentration gradients (does not require energy in the form of ATP)
  - Simple diffusion: Usually hydrophobic substances such as oxygen, carbon dioxide, and urea
  - Facilitated diffusion: Carrier-mediated, thus limited by the number of carrier proteins
- *Active transport* requires ATP
- There are three major types of transport proteins
  - *ATP-powered pump* are ATPases that use the energy of ATP hydrolysis to move ions across a membrane against their electrochemical gradient
    - The Na^+/K^+-ATPase pumps 3 Na^+ ions out and 2 K^+ ions into the cell per ATP hydrolyzed
    - The Ca^{2+}-ATPase pumps 2 Ca^{2+} ions out of the cell (or into the sarcoplasmic reticulum in muscle cells) per ATP hydrolyzed
    - These pumps create an intracellular ion milieu of high K^+, low Na^+, and low Ca^{2+} that is very different from the extracellular fluid milieu of low K^+, high Na^+, and high Ca^{2+}
  - Ion channels: Catalyze movement of specific ions down their electrochemical gradient
    - An example is the *potassium channel* which allows K^+ to move across the membrane down its concentration gradient
    - While the Na^+/K^+-ATPase pumps K^+ ions into the cytosol from the extracellular medium and thus generates the K^+ concentration gradient, it is the movement of K^+ ions down their concentration gradient from the cytosol outward through the "resting K^+ channels" that generates the negative membrane potential of about -70 Mv
  - Transporters: Facilitate movement of specific small molecules or ions, such as glucose, amino acids, Na^+, and H^+
    - *Uniporters* transport a single type of molecule *down* a concentration gradient
    - *Symporters* transport one molecule *against* a concentration gradient, driven by movement of one or more ions down an electrochemical gradient *in the same direction*
    - *Antiporters* transport one molecule *against* a concentration gradient, driven by movement of one or more ions down an electrochemical gradient *in the opposite direction*

Electrolyte Concentrations

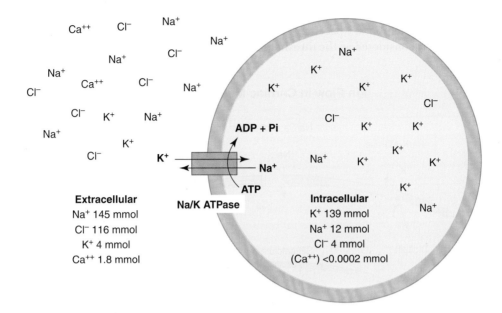

Extracellular
Na⁺ 145 mmol
Cl⁻ 116 mmol
K⁺ 4 mmol
Ca⁺⁺ 1.8 mmol

Na/K ATPase

Intracellular
K⁺ 139 mmol
Na⁺ 12 mmol
Cl⁻ 4 mmol
(Ca⁺⁺) <0.0002 mmol

An 80-year-old man is rushed to the emergency room as a trauma patient after falling down a flight of stairs. On arrival, his EKG demonstrates cardiac bigeminy with normal sinus complexes followed by wide complexes. He also has nausea, vomiting, and is disoriented. The paramedics in the field report that he has a history of diabetes, hypertension, and congestive heart failure. On arrival, the nurse asks you which lab tests to order.

In addition to head trauma, one must consider digitalis toxicity in this patient. Thus, in addition to obtaining a full electrolyte panel, it may be helpful to send a digoxin level.

Digoxin Toxicity

- The cardiac glycosides digoxin and digitoxin inhibit the Na/K ATPase, known as the "sodium pump"
    - Inhibition of the pump leads to positive inotropy by (1) increased intracellular sodium and (2) reduced calcium expulsion through a calcium-sodium exchanger
    - The increase in free calcium leads to greater contractility in the cardiac sarcomere
- Digoxin is toxic at levels greater than 2 ng/mL, and toxicity is usually manageable by withholding further drug administration
    - Signs and symptoms of digitalis toxicity include visual and GI disturbances, and cardiac arrhythmias such as premature ventricular contractions (PVCs) and bigeminy
    - For these patients, electrolytes, especially potassium, calcium, and magnesium, must be closely monitored along with withdrawal of glycoside therapy
    - For treatment of more serious arrhythmias, lidocaine is preferred
- Severe digitalis intoxication is usually accompanied by hyperkalemia and depressed automaticity
    - The administration of antiarrhythmics such as quinidine and procainamide are contraindicated in digoxin toxicity, but short-acting beta-adrenergic blockers such as esmolol can be considered for supraventricular tachyarrhythmias
    - Calcium channel blockers are contraindicated as they inhibit renal excretion of digoxin
    - Likewise, cardioversion should be reserved for ventricular fibrillation because glycoside-induced arrhythmias can be made worse

- Administration of digitalis-specific antibodies (DSFab; commercially: Digibind or DigiFab) is first line therapy for cardiac manifestations of digoxin toxicity
- Lidocaine and phenytoin are preferred for ventricular tachycardia and/or fibrillation
- Insertion of a temporary pacemaker catheter is viable for severe digitalis toxicity, but should be carefully considered as the threshold for ventricular arrhythmias may be lowered

Ion Flow in Cardiac Muscle

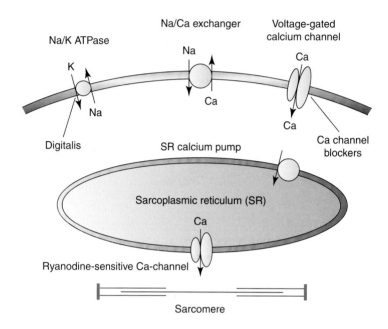

You see a 56-year-old woman in clinic after a right hemicolectomy in which 2 of 17 lymph nodes are positive for colonic adenocarcinoma. You tell her that she needs chemotherapy and that 5-fluorouracil will likely be one of the agents used to treat her. What is the mechanism of action of 5-fluorouracil?

A metabolite of 5-fluorouracil (5-FU) called 5-fluoro-2′-deoxyuridine-5′-phosphate (FdUMP) complexes with thymidylate synthase, an enzyme required for the synthesis of thymine nucleotides. This results in inhibition of DNA synthesis. 5-FU also interferes with RNA processing and function. Thus, cytotoxicity of 5-FU is based on both DNA and RNA effects. Its main side effects are myelosuppression and mucositis. It is a cell cycle-dependent anticancer drug.

Which is the most variable phase of the cell cycle?

G1 is a part of the cell cycle in interphase, and it is the most variable phase.

The Cell Cycle

- The cell cycle is composed of a long *interphase* (G_1, S, G_2) and a short *mitosis (M)* phase
- Interphase:
  - G_1 phase prepares cell for entry into S phase, or the cell enters G_0 if cellular conditions are not right
    - G_0 may be irreversible (terminal differentiation) or reversible
    - The restriction point, R, is a point in G_1 after which the cell is committed to DNA synthesis

- S phase: DNA synthesis occurs and two sister chromosomes are generated
- G$_2$ phase: a quiescent phase in which the cell prepares for entry into mitosis
- RNA and protein synthesis occur during both the G$_1$ and G$_2$ phases

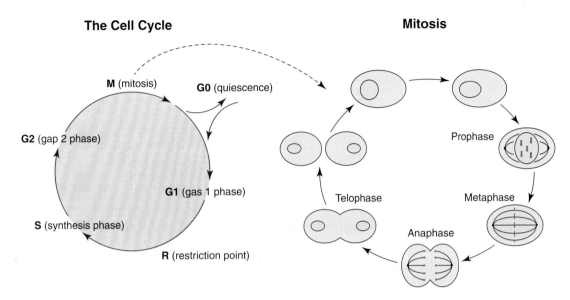

Cell cycle and mitosis.

- Mitosis: Cell division
  - **Prophase**
    - The chromosomes shorten, the nucleolus disappears, the nuclear envelope disappears, and the spindle apparatus forms
    - The centrioles replicate and move toward opposite ends of cell
    - The shortened chromosomes, known as identical chromatids, are held together by the centromere
  - **Metaphase**
    - The chromosomes move toward the center of the cell and the centromeres align at the equatorial plate
    - The centromeres attach to spindle fibers from the spindle apparatus
    - The centromeres of each chromatid duplicate
  - **Anaphase**
    - The chromatids migrate to opposite poles
    - The chromatids are now referred to as chromosomes
  - **Telophase**
    - The chromosomes decondense
    - Each cell forms a nucleolus and nuclear envelope

The M phase of the cell cycle is most susceptible to radiation therapy.

A 46-year-old woman has blood streaked bowel movements. Her mother and two siblings have had colon cancer, all before 50 years of age. A colonoscopy 7 years prior was negative for tumor or polyps. Which hereditary trait does this patient most likely have?

Lynch I syndrome is one of the two main types of hereditary nonpolyposis colorectal carcinoma (HNPCC). HNPCC families carry mutations in the genes responsible for a mismatch repair. This leads to the accumulation of mutations and microsatellite instability, both of which contribute to the rapid progression of tumors in HNPCC.

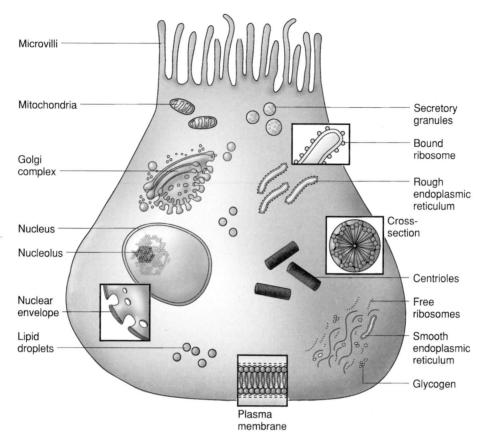

Microvilli

Mitochondria

Golgi
complex

Nucleus

Nucleolus

Nuclear
envelope

Lipid
droplets

Secretory
granules

Bound
ribosome

Rough
endoplasmic
reticulum

Cross-
section

Centrioles

Free
ribosomes

Smooth
endoplasmic
reticulum

Glycogen

Plasma
membrane

Typical epithelial cell. (With permission from Mulholland MW, Lillemoe KD, Doherty GM, Maier RV, Upchurch GR, eds. *Greenfield's Surgery.* 4th ed. Philadelphia, PA: Lippincott Williams & Wilkins; 2005.)

Components of the Nucleus

- **Nuclear envelope**
  - Composed of a double-membrane
  - The outer membrane of the nuclear envelope sometimes has *ribosomes* attached that may be continuous with the *endoplasmic reticulum*
  - Traffic in and out of the nucleus is regulated by pore complexes composed of a cylindrical structure called the annulus, which forms the rim, and an inner central granule
- **Nucleolus**
  - Primary function of the nucleolus is the generation of ribosomes, composed of proteins and ribosomal RNA
  - The *fibrillar* zone is where ribosomal RNA is transcribed
  - The *granular* zone has sites where the ribosomal RNA is condensed with ribosomes and proteins in order to form pre-ribosomal subunits
  - The subunits are transported to the cytoplasm, where they are assembled into free ribosomes or membrane-bound ribosomes, which become attached to the rough endoplasmic reticulum involved in the protein synthesis
  - Ribosomes are composed of 50S and 30S subunits
- **Chromatin:** DNA and protein complex
- **Matrix:** Involved in replication, transcription, and posttranscriptional processing and transport
- DNA replication and transcription take place in the nucleus
- Translation and posttranslational processing occur in the rough endoplasmic reticulum, Golgi complex, or free ribosomes in the cytoplasm

> A 15-year-old woman develops a urinary tract infection and is given a course of ciprofloxacin. Where does this medication have its action?

Ciprofloxacin inhibits DNA gyrase, which is involved in DNA replication.

DNA Replication

- DNA replication begins at the *origin of replication*
- *DNA gyrase*, a topoisomerase, relieves supercoiling in DNA by creating a transient break in the double helix
- The *leading strand* provides the backbone for continuous DNA synthesis
- The *lagging strand* provides for discontinuous, *Okazaki fragment* production
- *DNA polymerase* synthesizes DNA in the $5' \rightarrow 3'$ direction of both strands
- DNA ligase seals the Okazaki fragments
- Transcription of messenger RNA from DNA occurs by assembly of complementary base pairs on the DNA template one nucleotide at a time, which is catalyzed by RNA polymerase
- Still in the nucleus, the initial transcript then undergoes posttranscriptional processing
  - This consists of capping of the 5' end and polyadenylation of the 3' end
- The product is a stretch of RNA with both introns (noncoding segments) and exons (which contain the coding for proteins)
- *Introns* are removed from the RNA transcript by splicing
- The resulting messenger RNA is moved to the cytoplasm where it binds to ribosomes to begin translation

DNA Replication

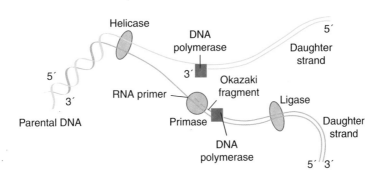

> Which amino acids are essential for a postoperative, critically ill patient who has not eaten for 1 week?

The essential amino acids are so named because humans cannot synthesize them and they must be provided in the diet. They are arginine, histidine, isoleucine, leucine, lysine, methionine, phenylalanine, threonine, tryptophan, and valine.

Translation

- Messenger RNA (mRNA) is transcribed from DNA and is exported to the ribosomes, either in cytosol or in the endoplasmic reticulum (ER)
- The ribosomes begin the process of translation, in which the mRNA acts as a template for the production of proteins from amino acids

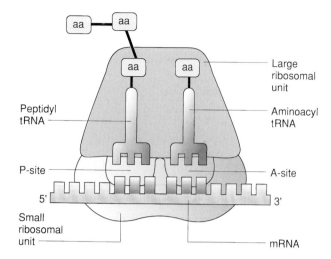

(With permission from Mulholland MW, Lillemoe KD, Doherty GM, Maier RV, Upchurch GR, eds. *Greenfield's Surgery.* 4th ed. Philadelphia, PA: Lippincott Williams & Wilkins; 2005.)

The Genetic Code

- Amino acids are synthesized and attached to transfer RNAs (tRNA) which pair specific amino acids with specific mRNA sequences
- Sequences occur in triplets called codons
- Any given string of ribonucleotides, therefore, gives rise to three reading frames which specify how the codons are "read"
- The codon AUG is an initiation codon, and it encodes the amino acid methionine.
- Codons UAA, UAG, and UGA are stop codons
- An mRNA sequence with 50 or more codons without a stop codon is known as an open reading frame
- The three ribonucleotide sequence on the tRNA that recognizes and binds to the codon on the mRNA is known as the anticodon
- This binding occurs by the formation of hydrogen bonds between complementary nucleotides
- The process of coupling amino acids with appropriate tRNAs occurs by a process known as activation of amino acids
- Aminoacyl-tRNA synthetases couple tRNAs with amino acids in an ATP-dependent enzymatic process that is catalyzed by magnesium

On postoperative day 7 after undergoing a low anterior colon resection, a 63-year-old male tests positive for vancomycin-resistant enterococcus (VRE) upon surveillance culture of his stool. He is started on oral linezolid. What is the mechanism of action of this medication?

Linezolid inhibits the 50S ribosomal subunit involved in protein synthesis.

The Ribosome

- In the next stage of translation, initiation occurs when a ribosomal subunit binds to the mRNA
- Ribosomes are generally composed of 60S and 40S subunits
- The first subunit bound to mRNA is the smaller 40S subunit
- This is followed by binding of the tRNA corresponding to the initiation codon AUG, which encodes the amino acid methionine
- The 60S subunit then binds the mRNA to begin the process of polypeptide synthesis
- These steps require energy, in the form of GTP, and the assistance of proteins known as initiation factors

- Of note, the corresponding prokaryotic ribosomal components are 50S and 30S, which are the targets of some antibiotics
- The initial methionine amino acid begins the polypeptide
- Polypeptide synthesis progresses in the **N** to C-terminal direction when referring to amino acid orientation
- The subsequent *elongation* phase consists of the sequential recruitment of activated amino acids to the ribosome-mRNA complex and the formation or peptide bonds, a process that is catalyzed by ribosomal RNA, or a ribozyme
- This process also requires GTP and protein elongation factors
- Translation is terminated when the complex encounters one of the three stop codons
- Protein release factors assist in the cleavage of the final amino acid-tRNA bond, the dissociation of the ribosomal complex, and the release of the generated polypeptide
- The process of translation often takes place with clusters of ribosomes known as polysomes simultaneously translating the same mRNA strand

> A nurse comes to your office concerned that a colleague has been having hypoglycemic spells. She suspects that her colleague is injecting herself with insulin. What study can you use to elucidate this situation?

Insulin is initially synthesized as a single polypeptide chain (preproinsulin) that has an N-terminal signal sequence that directs its processing once secreted. This signal sequence is cleaved off and the resulting proinsulin is stored in secretory granules. Disulfide bonds form between the A and B peptide portions of the precursor molecule. When insulin secretion is triggered by elevated blood glucose, the molecule is cleaved such that the C peptide is removed and the active insulin molecule, consisting of A and B peptides linked by disulfide bonds, is released. The proinsulin concentration is less than 20% of total immunoreactive insulin, while in patients who have an insulinoma, this rises to 30% to 60%. Exogenous insulin administration is diagnosed when a patient presents with the triad of hypoglycemia, a low plasma C-peptide level, and high insulin levels.

Post-Translational Modification

- Polypeptide chains synthesized by ribosomes assume a natural, energy-conserving three-dimensional shape by folding to maximize hydrogen bonds, ionic and van der Waals interactions, and hydrophobic interactions
- However, many will be further processed by cleavage, modification of targeting sequences, modification of amino- and carboxy terminals, and addition of side chains that ultimately change the shape of the protein
- These modifications have effects on targeting, protein activation and function, protein–protein interactions, and protein degradation

Protein Targeting

- In the endoplasmic reticulum (ER) of human cells, proteins destined for membranes or secretion are designated by a signal sequence, usually consisting of 15 to 30 amino acids at the amino-terminal end recognized by the signal recognition particle
- This results in the temporary halting of translation as the peptide emerges from the ribosomal complex, and brings the nascent peptide to receptors in the ER membrane and the peptide translocation complex
- This complex guides the peptide into the lumen of the ER in an ATP-dependent process
- Here, glycosylation, removal of signal sequences, and other modifications occur
- Two classic biochemical ways of adding carbohydrate side chains are via N-linked (to asparagine) and O-linked (to serine or threonine) glycosylation

- N-linked carbohydrates are added in the ER
- O-linked carbohydrates are added in the Golgi complex
- Cysteine residues in polypeptide chains are often linked covalently to other cysteine residues located elsewhere in the peptide sequence via disulfide bonds in such a way that they stabilize the tertiary structure of a protein molecule
- Proteins in eukaryotic cells are targeted for destruction by the covalent attachment of ubiquitin to the protein in an ATP-dependent manner
- A determinant of protein half-life is the specific amino-terminal amino acid on the protein (after the amino-terminal end has been processed)

The Cytoskeleton

- Cell shape and activity are supported by a dynamic network of protein filaments constituting the cytoskeleton
- The cytoskeleton is an important component of cell–cell interaction
- The three main types of filaments are actin, intermediate filaments, and microtubules

Actin

- Globular subunits make up filaments that have polarity
- Free monomeric and filamentous actin are in a dynamic equilibrium, constantly adding to one end and being degraded off of the other end of the actin chain
- Single chains of actin form an actin filament by pairing in a helical structure

Skeletal Muscle

- In a unit known as a *sarcomere*, actin forms thin filaments which are attached on one end to a structure known as a Z-disk
- Between these thin actin filaments, myosin forms thick filaments with globular myosin heads

Skeletal Muscle

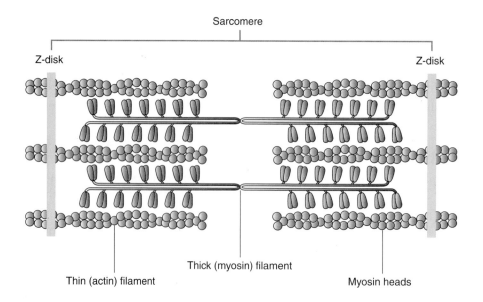

Sarcomere

Z-disk · Z-disk

Thick (myosin) filament

Thin (actin) filament · Myosin heads

- Muscle contraction is produced by shortening of the sarcomere, resulting from an ATP and Ca^{2+}-dependent ratcheting of the myosin heads along the actin filaments
- This brings the thick and thin filaments into a more closely overlapped configuration, shortening the sarcomere

The serial organization of sarcomeres in the muscle allows the entire muscle to contract
- The organization of the muscle, sarcomeres, and thick and thin filaments is the basis of the stretch-dependent generation of force by muscles
- If the muscle is too stretched out, there are few contacts between myosin heads and actin filaments, so the generation of contraction is weak
- If there is too much overlap, the amount of contraction the muscle can generate is limited
- In heart muscle, this trade-off is described by the Frank-Starling curve
- Actin also plays an important role in cell shape, including forming the core of structures such as microvilli in intestinal epithelium

Intermediate Filaments

- A group of proteins that form filaments on the order of 10 nm thick
- There are four types: Type I (Keratins), Type II (vimentin, desmin, glial fibrillary protein), Type III (neurofilaments), and Type IV (nuclear lamins)
- Intermediate filaments are involved in stabilizing the structure of the nucleus as well as the cytosol

Microtubules

- Microtubules are hollow fibers formed by 13 parallel protofilaments made up of "A" and "B" tubulin subunits
- Microtubules form the mitotic spindle as well as the structural core of cilia, flagella and neuronal axons

A patient with a small bowel obstruction is being managed conservatively with nasogastric decompression. He becomes febrile and has rigors. What is the most likely mechanism of his symptoms?

Bacterial translocation through ischemic bowel walls results from compromised blood supply to the affected area of bowel. Intraluminal pressure from the obstruction becomes greater than the perfusion pressure of the arteries and capillaries supplying the intestinal mucosa, leading to compromised mucosal viability and breakdown of the tight junctions between cells. Local inflammation also makes the endothelial cells of the local microvasculature leaky. All of this facilitates the free migration of bacteria through the bowel mucosa and into the bloodstream and lymphatic system. Symptoms of sepsis ensue.

Cell–Cell Interactions

- Aside from cell membrane receptor activities, cells interact with each other through *junctions* and interactions with the *extracellular matrix*
- This is especially well-studied in epithelial tissue where cells are organized in sheets and have apical and basal polarity
- Underlying the cell layer is a connective tissue layer known as the basement membrane
- The epithelial cells communicate with each other and are supported through junctions and interactions with the basement membrane

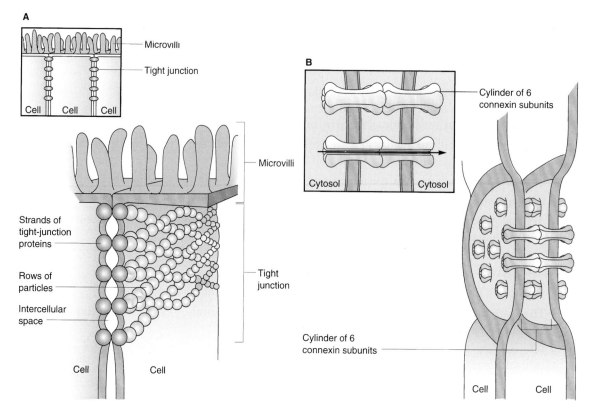

Tight junction. (With permission from Mulholland MW, Lillemoe KD, Doherty GM, Maier RV, Upchurch GR, eds. *Greenfield's Surgery.* 4th ed. Philadelphia, PA: Lippincott Williams & Wilkins; 2005.)

Tight Junctions

- Exclusive to epithelial tissue, these are interlocking ridges on the cell surfaces that occlude the intercellular space
- In forming a belt known as the *zonula occludens* near the apical border of the cells, tight junctions keep epithelia selectively permeable to macromolecules, ions, and water-soluble molecules
- A variety of integral membrane proteins form these anastomosing ridges

Adhering Junctions

- In epithelia, just deep to the zonula occludens is a zonula adherens, or adhesion belt
- In the zonula adherens, cells are connected by contact between cell membrane glycoproteins, transmembrane proteins and proteins on the inner surface of the cell membrane that constitute a major anchorage site of cytoskeletal microfilaments
- Included in this group are desmosomes and hemidesmosomes which form adhesion plaques connecting cells to each other or to the extracellular matrix

Gap Junctions

- While these connections also form protein complexes that bridge the intercellular gap, the significance of the gap junction is the presence of connexons, proteins that form tubes or pores that traverse the intercellular gap
- These channels allow the passage of macromolecules, ions, etc.
- Gap junctions are critical to the passage of waves of excitation through cardiac and smooth muscle cells

Integrins

- A family of transmembrane proteins that link the cytoskeleton to the extracellular matrix
- Composed of "A" and "B" subunits that combine to form specific receptors for certain components of the extracellular matrix, such as fibronectin, laminin, and vitronectin
- They connect with intracellular intermediate filaments and other components of the cytoskeleton
- An interesting aspect of integrins lies in their ability to mediate "inside-out" signaling, whereby the affinity of the integrin receptor for an extracellular ligand is modified by changes in the intracellular portion of the cell
- This occurs, for example, in monocytes and neutrophils, which increase their affinity for endothelial cell adhesion molecules by modifying integrin molecules
- Other cellular adhesion molecules (CAM) include the cadherins, selectins, NCAM, and ICAM, which play roles in the interaction of leukocytes with endothelial cells during inflammation

---

An elderly, hypotensive woman with severe acute pancreatitis is anxious and disoriented and breathing rapidly. What is a possible acid–base disorder responsible for her symptoms?

Metabolic acidosis results in a compensatory drive leading to hyperventilation. This patient's hypotension is resulting in a metabolic acidosis because of tissue hypoperfusion. This results in a shift from aerobic to anaerobic metabolism in hypoxic tissues, and the production of lactic acid.

Cell Metabolism

- Proteins, lipids, and polysaccharides are broken down into smaller molecules before they are utilized by the cell as either a source of energy or as building blocks for other molecules

Catabolism of Proteins, Fats, and Carbohydrates

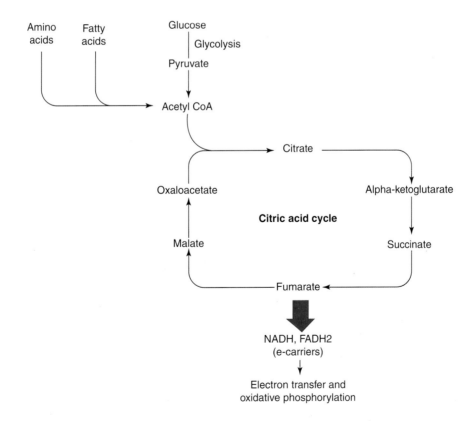

Glycolysis

- Oxidation of glucose is known as glycolysis
    - Glucose is oxidized to either lactate or pyruvate
    - Under aerobic conditions, the dominant product in most tissues is pyruvate and the pathway is known as aerobic glycolysis
    - When oxygen is depleted, for instance during prolonged vigorous exercise, the dominant glycolytic product in many tissues is lactate and the process is known as anaerobic glycolysis
- Glycolysis converts glucose into two molecules of pyruvate
    - During this formation, two forms of activated carrier molecules, ATP and NADH, are produced without the use of molecular oxygen
    - Glycolysis involves a sequence of 10 reactions, each catalyzed by an enzyme, allowing the energy from oxidation to be stored in activated carrier molecules in the form of 6 ATPs and 2 NADHs
    - The NADH generated during glycolysis is used to fuel mitochondrial ATP synthesis via oxidative phosphorylation, producing either two or three equivalents of ATP depending upon whether the glycerol phosphate shuttle or the malate-aspartate shuttle is used to transport the electrons from cytoplasmic NADH into the mitochondria
    - The net yield from the oxidation of 1 mole of glucose to 2 moles of pyruvate is, therefore, either 6 or 8 moles of ATP
    - Complete oxidation of the 2 moles of pyruvate, through the TCA cycle and electron transport chain, yields an additional 30 moles of ATP
    - The total yield from the complete oxidation of 1 mole of glucose to CO_2 and H_2O is either 36 or 38 moles of ATP
- In aerobic metabolism, the pyruvate produced by glycolysis is rapidly decarboxylated by a complex of enzymes located in the mitochondria called pyruvate dehydrogenase
    - One molecule of CO_2, one molecule of NADH, and one molecule of acetyl CoA are produced in this process
    - Under aerobic conditions, pyruvate in most cells is further metabolized via the TCA cycle.
    - Normally, during aerobic glycolysis, the electrons of cytoplasmic NADH are transferred to mitochondrial carriers of the oxidative phosphorylation pathway generating a continuous pool of cytoplasmic NAD^+
- Under anaerobic conditions, and in erythrocytes under aerobic conditions, pyruvate is converted to lactate by the enzyme lactate dehydrogenase (LDH), and the lactate is transported out of the cell into the circulation
    - The conversion of pyruvate to lactate provides the cell with a mechanism for the oxidation of NADH (produced during the G3PDH reaction) to NAD^+, which occurs during the LDH catalyzed reaction
    - This reduction is required since NAD^+ is a necessary substrate for G3PDH, without which glycolysis ceases

TCA Cycle

- The bulk of ATP used by many cells to maintain homeostasis is produced by the oxidation of pyruvate in the TCA cycle
- During this oxidation process, reduced NADH and reduced $FADH_2$ are generated
- NADH and $FADH_2$ are principally used to drive the process of oxidative phosphorylation, which is responsible for converting the reducing potential of NADH and $FADH_2$ to high energy phosphate in ATP
- The fate of pyruvate depends on the cell energy charge
- In cells or tissues with a high energy charge pyruvate is directed toward gluconeogenesis, but when the energy charge is low pyruvate is preferentially oxidized to CO_2 and H_2O in the TCA cycle, with generation of 15 equivalents of ATP per pyruvate

The Citric Acid Cycle

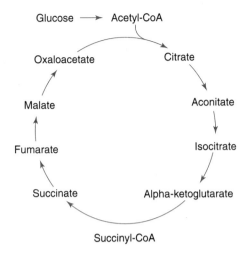

A 56-year-old chemistry professor is found to be hypotensive with multiple PVCs, abdominal pain, and diarrhea. He was found in his laboratory with an open bottle of an unknown chemical in his hand. He recently lost his grant. What is the next step in management?

Among the toxic agents possible in this patient, one must consider arsenic. Urine should be sent for arsenic levels, and dimercaprol (British anti-Lewisite) should be administered. Arsenic is toxic secondary to enzyme inhibition due to sulfhydryl groups as well as its chelation activity, which poisons mitochondrial oxidative phosphorylation. Lethal doses are in the range of 100 to 300 mg. Arsenic toxicity may also be relevant in the cancer patient population, e.g. in acute promyelocytic leukemia, and in patients taking certain non-Western/traditional medicines.

Electron Transport Chain

- The last step in the degradation of a glucose molecule during which the major portion of energy is released
- The electron transport chain (ETC) is embedded in the inner membrane of the mitochondria
- The electron carriers NADH and $FADH_2$ transfer electrons that they have gained from oxidizing other molecules to the electron transport chain
- As electrons pass along this chain of electron acceptor and donor molecules, they decrease to successively lower energy states, and liberated energy is used to pump H^+ ions across the inner mitochondrial membrane creating a gradient
- This gradient serves as a source of trapped energy, ultimately utilized to phosphorylate ADP to ATP

A 45-year-old female underwent a Roux-en-Y gastric bypass without complications. One year later she develops bilateral paresthesia of her toes, calf muscle tenderness, and foot-drop. She is diagnosed with dry beriberi, a manifestation of thiamin deficiency. How is thiamin absorbed?

Thiamin (Vitamin B$_1$) is absorbed from the lumen of the small intestine by active transport. Alcoholism, intestinal bypass, and other causes of chronic protein–calorie malnutrition are risk factors for the development of thiamin deficiency. An advanced deficiency primarily affecting the cardiovascular system is known as "wet beriberi," while a deficiency primarily affecting the nervous system is referred to as "dry beriberi."

Protein Synthesis and Metabolism

- The *liver* is the major site of *nitrogen metabolism* in the body
- All tissues have some capability for synthesis of the non-essential amino acids, amino acid remodeling, and conversion of non-amino acid carbon skeletons into amino acids and other derivatives that contain nitrogen
- In times of dietary surplus, the potentially toxic nitrogen in amino acids is eliminated via transamination, deamination, and urea formation, while the carbon skeletons are generally conserved as carbohydrate via gluconeogenesis or as fatty acid via fatty acid synthesis pathways
- Amino acids fall into three categories: glucogenic, ketogenic, or glucogenic and ketogenic
- Glucogenic amino acids are those that give rise to a net production of pyruvate or TCA cycle intermediates, such as α-ketoglutarate or oxaloacetate, all of which are precursors to glucose via gluconeogenesis
  - All amino acids except lysine and leucine are at least partly glucogenic
  - Lysine and leucine are the only amino acids that are solely ketogenic, giving rise only to acetyl-CoA or acetoacetyl-CoA, neither of which result in net glucose production
  - A small group of amino acids (isoleucine, phenylalanine, threonine, tryptophan, and tyrosine) give rise to both glucose and fatty acid precursors and are characterized as being glucogenic and ketogenic
- Finally, it should be recognized that amino acids have a third possible ketogenic fate; during times of starvation, the reduced carbon skeleton is used for energy production (oxidized to CO_2 and H_2O)

Amino Acid Degradation

- An important function of enzymes is amino acid degradation by removal of α-amino groups so that the nitrogen can be incorporated into other compounds or excreted
- The reactions occur through transamination, oxidative deamination, and amino acid oxidase
- **Transamination**
  - The first step in the catabolism of most amino acids
  - The transfer of the α-amino group from an amino acid to α-ketoglutarate results in the production of an α-ketoacid (derived from the original amino acid) and glutamate
    - α-ketoglutarate plays a unique role in amino acid metabolism by accepting the amino groups from other amino acids, thus becoming glutamate
  - Transaminases (also known as aminotransferases) catalyze this reaction, and each aminotransferase is specific for one or a few amino group donors
  - All aminotransferases require pyridoxal phosphate, which is covalently linked to the lysine of the enzyme
  - Pyridoxal phosphate becomes pyridoxamine phosphate upon receipt of the amino group of an amino acid
  - The pyridoxamine form of the coenzyme then reacts with an α-keto acid to form an amino acid and regenerate pyridoxal phosphate
- **Oxidative deamination**
  - Results in liberation of the amino group as free ammonia
  - These reactions occur in the kidney and liver, resulting in the formation of α-keto acids and ammonia
  - α-keto acids can enter the TCA cycle, while ammonia can enter the urea cycle
  - These reactions are catalyzed by glutamate dehydrogenase, which is found in both the mitochondria and the cytosol

- Glutamate is the only amino acid that undergoes rapid oxidative deamination, using NAD or NADP as a coenzyme
- **Amino acid oxidase**
  - The L- and D-forms of amino acid oxidase remove amino groups from L- and D-amino acids, respectively
    - L-amino acid oxidase is primarily involved in deamination of lysine
    - Both enzymes also produce an α-keto acid
  - Amino acids are categorized by the final products of the pathways of their degradation
  - Ketogenic amino acids are degraded to either acetyl CoA (e.g., isoleucine, leucine, tryptophan) or acetoacetyl-CoA CoA (leucine, lysine, aromatic amino acids), which can give rise to ketone bodies
  - Glucogenic amino acids are degraded to pyruvate (e.g., alanine, glycine, serine) or TCA cycle intermediates (valine, leucine, glutamate, etc.), which can give rise to glucose

---

A cirrhotic patient is obtunded and has a significantly elevated ammonia level. What amino acid is essential if the patient is to clear the ammonia?

Glutamate, by virtue of being the main amino acid available for oxidative deamination in humans, serves as a "sink" for amino terminal nitrogens in protein metabolism and funnels ammonia into the urea cycle for excretion. The enzymes for urea synthesis are only found in the periportal hepatocytes, hence the impairment of nitrogen excretion in liver failure.

The Urea Cycle

- Urea is the major disposal form of amino groups derived from amino acids
- It accounts for about 90% of the nitrogen-containing compounds of urine
- The urea cycle occurs exclusively in the liver—urea is produced by the liver and excreted through the kidneys
- There are two nitrogens in the urea molecule: one is supplied by NH_3 (through the oxidative deamination of glutamate) and the other is supplied by aspartate (through transamination)
- Urea is produced by the liver and excreted through the kidneys
- The first two reactions leading to the synthesis of urea occur in mitochondria and the rest in the cytosol
- Formation of carbamoyl phosphate by carbamoyl phosphate synthase I is driven by cleavage of two moles of ATP. Ammonia is incorporated into carbamoyl phosphate with CO_2. The formation of carbamoyl phosphate is markedly increased by the presence of amino acids, particularly arginine
- Ornithine and citrulline are basic amino acids
  - Ornithine is regenerated in each urea cycle just like oxaloacetate is regenerated during the TCA cycle
  - Ornithine plus carbamoyl phosphate gives citrulline which is transported into the cytosol
- The α-amino group of aspartate donates the second nitrogen and citrulline condenses with aspartate to form arginosuccinate
- Arginosuccinate is cleaved to yield arginine and fumarate.
  - Arginine forms a precursor to urea and fumarate goes into the TCA cycle
  - Fumarate provides the link between the urea cycle and the TCA cycle
- Arginine is cleaved into ornithine and urea
  - Urea is a highly soluble, nontoxic compound that enters the blood and is excreted in the urine
  - Ornithine may then enter mitochondria

- The levels of the urea cycle enzymes fluctuate with changes in feeding patterns.
  - With a protein-free diet, urea excretion accounts for only 60% of total urinary nitrogen (compared to 80% in the normal diet), and the levels of all urea cycle enzymes decline
  - With a high-protein diet or during starvation (gluconeogenesis from amino acids is high), the levels of urea cycle enzymes increase several-fold

The Urea Cycle

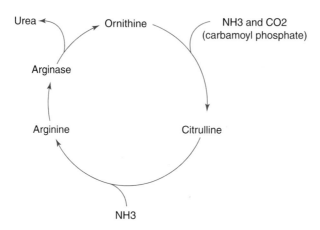

Nucleic Acid Metabolism
- Nucleic acids are important intracellular signaling molecules and coenzymes as well as the single most important means of coupling endergonic to exergonic reactions
- Nucleic acids also store genetic information in the form of DNA and RNA
- RNA is composed of nucleotides containing a phosphoribosyl component and either one of the aromatic bases adenine (A), guanine (G), cytosine (C), with uracil (U) substituted in RNA instead of thymine (T) in DNA
- These aromatic bases come in two forms: pyrimidines (T, C, U) and purines (A, G), which can be distinguished by their nitrogen-containing aromatic ring structures
- Nucleotides are derived from biosynthetic precursors of carbohydrate and amino acid metabolism, and from ammonia and CO_2
- The *liver* is the major organ of de novo synthesis of all four nucleotides
- De novo synthesis of pyrimidines and purines follows two different pathways
  - Pyrimidines are synthesized first from aspartate and carbamoyl-phosphate in the cytoplasm to the common precursor ring structure *orotic acid*, onto which a phosphorylated ribosyl unit is covalently linked
  - Purines are first synthesized from the sugar template onto which the ring synthesis occurs
- Degradation is only complete for pyrimidines, whereas purines are excreted from the body in the form of uric acid

---

Which vitamins are fat soluble?

Vitamins A, D, E, and K.

Fatty Acid Metabolism
- The blood is the carrier of triacylglycerols in the form of VLDLs and chylomicrons, fatty acids bound to albumin, amino acids, lactate, ketone bodies, and glucose

---

- Most lipids in the plasma are found in the form of lipoproteins, 90% in association with *very low density lipoproteins* (VLDLs)
- A small but significant portion of triglycerides are available in plasma as *free fatty acids* (FFAs)
- Stored triglycerides in adipose tissue are made available by lipases, releasing glycerol which can be used in the liver to make glucose
- Fat released into the blood stream comes in the form of chylomicrons
- Newly absorbed fat from the bowel is absorbed through specialized lymphatics known as lacteals
- Triglycerides are subsequently incorporated into intermediate, low and high density lipoproteins, or IDLs, LDLs, and HDLs
- LDLs carry most of the plasma cholesterol
- At the cellular level,
    - LDL is taken up by cells by an LDL receptor and the formation of coated pits
    - After lysosomal hydrolysis, free cholesterol is released
    - Cholesterol becomes part of the cell membrane, is stored in ester forms, and suppresses endogenous cholesterol synthesis by inhibiting HMG CoA-reductase

> Two years after primary resection of an abdominal mass that turned out to be a gastrointestinal stromal tumor (GIST), a recurrence is found at the hilum of the liver. The patient asks you about options for chemotherapy for GIST tumors.

ST1571, also known as Gleevec or imatinib mesylate, is a tyrosine kinase inhibitor that demonstrates activity against specific kinases (ABL, BCR-ABL, KIT) and the platelet derived growth factor receptor (PDGFR). Its basis for activity against GIST tumors is the inhibition of KIT, which is mutated to be constitutively active in 75% to 90% of GIST tumors. The overall response rate to ST1571 in metastatic GIST is 60%.

How Signal Transduction Works

- Signal transduction at the cellular level refers to the movement of signals from outside the cell to inside
- The movement of signals can be simple, like that associated with receptor molecules of the acetylcholine class
    - Receptors constitute channels which, upon ligand interaction, allow signals to be passed in the form of small ion movement, either into or out of the cell
    - These ion movements result in changes in the electrical potential of the cells that, in turn, propagate the signal along the cell
- More complex signal transduction involves the coupling of ligand–receptor interactions to many intracellular events
    - These events include phosphorylation by tyrosine kinases and/or serine/threonine kinases
    - Protein phosphorylation changes enzyme activities and protein conformations
- The eventual outcome is an alteration in cellular activity and changes in the program of genes expressed within the responding cells

Receptors

- There are three general classes of signal transducing receptors: receptors with intrinsic enzymatic activity, G-protein coupled receptors, and steroid and growth factor receptors
- Receptors with intrinsic enzymatic activities
    - Include tyrosine kinases (e.g., PDGF, insulin, EGF and FGF receptors), tyrosine phosphatases (e.g., CD45, protein of T cells and macrophages), guanylate cyclases (e.g., natriuretic peptide receptors) and serine/threonine kinases (e.g., activin and TGF-b receptors)

A Ligand-triggered ion channel (acetylcholine receptor at nerve–muscle junction)

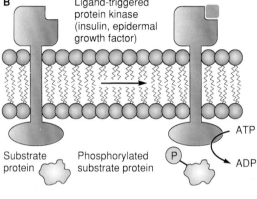

Ligand binding site

Ligand

Ion

Exterior

Cytosol   Receptor protein

B Ligand-triggered protein kinase (insulin, epidermal growth factor)

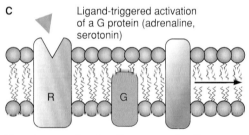

ATP

ADP

Substrate protein

Phosphorylated substrate protein

P

C Ligand-triggered activation of a G protein (adrenaline, serotonin)

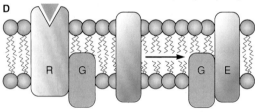

R   G

Receptor protein

Inactive G signal-transducing protein

Inactive response enzyme (adenylate cyclase, phospholipase)

D

R   G   G   E

Activated form of G protein

Activated G activates enzyme that generates "second messengers," such as cAMP or inositol 1,4,5-triphosphate

Types of cell surface receptors. (With permission from Mulholland MW, Lillemoe KD, Doherty GM, Maier RV, Upchurch GR, eds. *Greenfield's Surgery.* 4th ed. Philadelphia, PA: Lippincott Williams & Wilkins; 2005.)

- Receptors with intrinsic tyrosine kinase activity are capable of autophosphorylation as well as phosphorylation of other substrates
- **G-Protein Coupled Receptors (GPCRs)**
    - Receptors that are coupled, inside the cell, to GTP-binding and hydrolyzing proteins (termed G-proteins)
    - Receptors that interact with G-proteins all have a structure that is characterized by 7 transmembrane spanning domains and are termed serpentine receptors
    - Examples of this class are the adrenergic receptors, odorant receptors, and certain hormone receptors (e.g., glucagon, angiotensin, vasopressin, and bradykinin)
- **Steroid** and **Growth Factor Receptors**
    - Receptors that are found intracellularly and, upon ligand binding, migrate to the nucleus where the ligand–receptor complex directly affects gene transcription

Types of Receptors and Signaling

- **Receptor Tyrosine Kinase**: Many receptors that have intrinsic tyrosine kinase activity as well as the tyrosine kinases that are associated with cell surface receptors, contain tyrosine residues that, upon phosphorylation, interact with other proteins of the signaling cascade
- **Non-Receptor Protein Tyrosine Kinase**: There are numerous intracellular protein tyrosine kinases (PTK) that are responsible for phosphorylating a variety of intracellular proteins on tyrosine residues following activation of cellular growth and proliferation signals. There are two distinct families of non-receptor PTKs
    - The archetypal PTK family is related to the Src protein, which was first identified as the transforming protein in Rous sarcoma virus
    - Subsequently, a cellular homolog was identified as c-Src
    - The second family is related to the Janus kinase (Jak)
    - Most of the proteins of both families of non-receptor PTKs couple to cellular receptors that lack enzymatic activity themselves
        - This class of receptors includes all of the cytokine receptors [e.g., the interleukin-2 (IL-2) receptor] as well as the CD4 and CD8 cell surface glycoproteins of T-cells and the T-cell antigen receptor (**TCR**)
- Receptor Serine/Threonine Kinases: The receptors for the TGF-β superfamily of ligands have intrinsic serine/threonine kinase activity
    - There are more than 30 multifunctional proteins of the TGF-β superfamily that also includes the activins, inhibins, and the bone morphogenetic proteins (BMPs)
    - This superfamily of proteins can induce and/or inhibit cellular proliferation or differentiation and regulate migration and adhesion of various cell types
    - The signaling pathways utilized by the TGF-β, activin, and BMP receptors are different than those for receptors with intrinsic tyrosine kinase activity or that associate with intracellular tyrosine kinases
- **Protein Kinase C**: PKCs are involved in the signal transduction pathways initiated by certain hormones, growth factors, and neurotransmitters
    - The phosphorylation of various proteins, by PKC, can lead to either increased or decreased activity
    - Of particular importance is the phosphorylation of the EGF receptor by PKC, which down-regulates the tyrosine kinase activity of the receptor
- **MAP Kinases**: MAP kinases were identified by virtue of their activation in response to growth factor stimulation of cells in culture, hence the name mitogen activated protein kinases
    - MAP kinases are also called ERKs for extracellular-signal regulated kinases

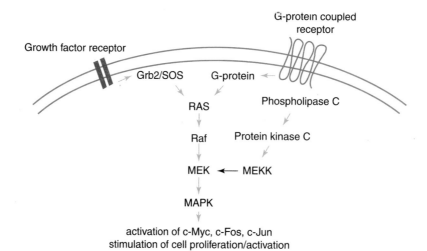

- **PI-3K**: PI-3K associates with and is activated by the PDGF, EGF, insulin, IGF-1, HGF, and NGF receptors
  - PI-3K phosphorylates various phosphatidylinositols at the 3 position of the inositol ring
  - This activity generates additional substrates for PLC-g allowing a cascade of DAG and IP3 to be generated by a single activated RTK or other protein tyrosine kinases

---

A 74-year-old female patient without a history of CAD or myocardial infarction has a marked lack of wall motion in the septal and inferior walls of her heart on an echocardiography imaging study. What is the most likely reason for this heart finding?

Chronic myocardial hypoxia induces apoptosis of cardiac myocytes and their ultimate replacement by fibroblasts and scar tissue.

Apoptosis

- Apoptosis is a tightly regulated form of programmed cell death
  - Morphologically, it is characterized by chromatin condensation and cell shrinkage in the early stage followed by fragmentation of the nucleus and cytoplasm, forming membrane-bound apoptotic bodies that can be engulfed by phagocytes
  - By contrast, cell necrosis is a different form of cell death in which cells swell and rupture
    - The released intracellular contents can damage surrounding cells and often cause inflammation
    - Potassium and lactic acid from ruptured cells can cause hyperkalemia and lactic acidosis
- During apoptosis, the cell is killed by a class of proteases called caspases
  - More than 10 caspases have been identified
    - Some (e.g., caspase 8 and 10) are involved in the initiation of apoptosis
    - Others (caspase 3, 6, and 7) execute the death order by destroying essential proteins in the cell
  - The apoptotic process can be summarized as follows:
    - Activation of initiating caspases by specific signals
    - Activation of executing caspases by the initiating caspases which can cleave inactive caspases at specific sites
    - Degradation of essential cellular proteins by the executing caspases with their protease activity

Targeted Therapies

Melanoma
Vemurafinib (Braf)
Ipilimumab (anti-CTLA4)

GIST
Imatinib (c-Kit)

HCC
Sorafinib (TKI)

Colon
Bevacizumab
(anti-VEGF)
Cetuximab
(anti-EGFR)

IBD
Infliximab (anti-TNF)
Adalimumab (anti-TNF)

Lung
Bevacizumab (non-
squamous)
Erlotinib (EGFR)
Crizotinib (ALK)

Breast
Trastuzumab (anti-Her2)

Pancreas
Erlotinib (EGFR)

**Rheumatoid
Arthritis**
Etanercept (TNF)
Adalimumab (anti TNF)
Tocilizumab (anti-IL6R)

- Apoptosis can be induced by death ligands (FasL/CD95L, TRAIL, APO-3L, and TNF)
  - Ligands bind to death receptors: Fas/CD95, DR4/DR5, DR3, and TNFR (tumor necrosis factor receptor)
  - Adaptors bind death ligands: FADD (Fas-associated death domain protein) and TRADD (TNFR-associated death domain protein)
  - Activation: Binding induces trimerization of their receptors, which then recruit adaptors and activate caspases
- Apoptosis can be induced by various stimuli, including growth factor withdrawal, UV light or irradiation, cytotoxic drugs, and death-receptor ligands.
- Two major signaling routes lead to apoptosis, the extrinsic pathway and the intrinsic pathway
  - The *extrinsic pathway* is initiated by binding ligands to specific death receptors on the cell surface
  - The *intrinsic pathway* is initiated at the mitochondria by various stimuli, such as cytotoxic drugs

A 6-year-old boy has a fever of 39.2°C during an episode of acute appendicitis. Which cytokine is directly responsible for causing his fever?

Cytokines are a large group of soluble proteins that mediate autocrine, paracrine, and endocrine signals between cells and tissues. IL-1 is the main cytokine responsible for altering the thermoregulatory set-point in the hypothalamus.

Cytokines and Innate Immunity

- Proinflammatory stimuli, including inflammation, infection, tissue injury and burns, generate a local, innate immune response by the involved cells that includes the release of the cytokines TNF-α, IL-1, and IL-6
- **TNF-α** (17kDa)
  - Made by mononuclear phagocytes, T cells and other cells
  - Activates inflammation in neutrophils and endothelial cells, targets the hypothalamus to produce fever, targets the liver to produce *acute phase reactants*, and targets muscle and fat to enter a catabolic state
  - Engages the NFkB signaling pathway in its target cells, which is primarily responsible for generating the inflammatory response
  - Alternatively, TNF-α can also induce apoptosis, which has a role in the resolution of local inflammation
  - Induces the production of IL-10, which suppresses TNF-α release and thus provides a negative feedback loop
- **IL-1** (17kDa)
  - Made by mononuclear phagocytes and others
  - Activates inflammation and coagulation pathways in endothelial cells
  - Targets the hypothalamus to produce fever, stimulates production of acute phase reactants in the liver, and induces costimulation in the thymus (thymocytes)
  - Is the primary mediator of pyrexia (fever) through its stimulation of prostaglandin E production in the hypothalamic-pituitary system
  - Is also involved in systemic prostaglandin release and elaboration of nitric oxide and other small molecules which interact with the vascular endothelium and induce hypotension as well a hypercoagulable state
- **IL-6** (26kDa)
  - Made by mononuclear phagocytes, endothelial cells, and T cells
  - Stimulates growth of mature B cells, production of acute phase reactants in liver, and co-stimulation of thymocytes

IL-6 is primary mediator of the hepatic response to inflammation through the elaboration of acute phase reactants.

- **Acute phase reactants**
  - Include proteins such as C-reactive protein, serum amyloid A, fibrinogen, ceruloplasmin, transferrin, and complement C3
  - These proteins play a role in homeostasis in response to injury and infection
- **Type I interferons (IFN-α and IFN-β)** are made by mononuclear phagocytes and fibroblasts.
  - They activate *natural killer* cells and increase MHC class I expression
  - These interferons are primarily responsible for inducing an antiviral state
- **Chemokines** are chemotactic cytokines that have the ability to direct leukocyte movement (**chemotaxis**) and induce motility (**chemokinesis**)
  - Structurally, these proteins contain two internal disulfide loops
    - The cysteine residues involved may be adjacent or separated by an amino acid, and this forms the basis for the division of chemokines into **CC** and **CXC** families
    - **CC** chemokines include monocyte chemotactic proteins 1,2, and 3; RANTES, monocyte inflammatory proteins 1a and 1b; and eotaxin
    - **CXC** chemokines include IL-8, platelet factor 4, stromal cell-derived factor 1, among others
    - Lymphotactin is a chemokine with a single disulfide loop
  - As can be surmised, most of these proteins have pro-inflammatory effects on their specific target cells

Specific Immunity

- Specific immunity refers to the immune system's response to specific antigens
- This process leads to the production of antigen-specific antibodies and antigen-specific T-cell responses, as well as immunologic memory
- **IL-2** (14-17 kDa)
  - Made by T-cells
  - Induces growth and cytokine production in T-cells, growth and activation in NK cells, and growth and antibody synthesis in B cells
  - Binding of IL-2 to its receptor induces signaling through Jak/STAT pathways
- **IL-4** (20 kDa)
  - Made by CD4$^+$ T-cells and mast cells
  - Induces isotype switching to IgE in B cells, induces growth and differentiation of T-cells into TH2 type cells, and activates endothelial cells
- **Transforming growth factor-β** (14 kDa),
  - Made by T-cells, mononuclear phagocytes and others
  - Is inhibitory to the activation and growth of many cell types and limits immune response
- **Interferon γ** (21-24 kDa)
  - Made by T-cells and NK cells
  - Activates mononuclear phagocytes and endothelial cells, increases expression of MHC class I and II molecules, and promotes T-cell differentiation to the TH1 subset and maturation of cytotoxic T lymphocytes (CTLs)
  - It also induces isotype switching in B-cells so that phagocyte-mediated elimination of microbes is maximized
- Lymphotoxins (21 to 24 kDa) are related to TNF and are made by activated T-cells.
  - They activate neutrophils and endothelial cells
  - They appear to be critical for the development of lymphoid organs such as lymph nodes, Peyer patches (small bowel), and splenic white pulp
- **IL-5** (20 kDa)
  - Made by TH2 subset of CD4$^+$ T-cells and mast cells
  - Stimulates the growth and differentiation of eosinophils and induces anti-helminthic activity

---

A patient with renal failure is chronically anemic despite iron supplementation. Which medications can be given to improve this situation?

Epoetin and darbepoetin are colony-stimulating factors for blood cell precursors. Endogenous erythropoietin is produced by the kidneys in response to hypoxia and anemia. Erythropoietin stimulates red cell precursors in the bone marrow to proliferate and mature. Other colony stimulating factors available for clinical use include G-CSF and GM-CSF. These agents are useful in treating myelosuppression associated with chemotherapy and granulocytopenia due to cancer, HIV, and other neutropenic conditions.

Hematopoiesis and Lymphopoiesis

- Colony stimulating factors (CSFs) stimulate expansion and differentiation of bone marrow progenitor cells
- **C-kit ligand**
  - Made by bone marrow stromal cells
  - Activates pluripotent stem cells to make them sensitive to the effects of other CSFs, sustains thymic T-cell viability and proliferation, and supports peripheral mast cells

- **IL-7**
  - Made by fibroblasts and bone marrow stromal cells
  - Stimulates immature progenitor cells to grow and differentiate into lymphocytes
- **IL-3**
  - Made by $CD4^+$ T-cells
  - Acts on immature progenitor cells and stimulates expansion and differentiation into all known mature cell types
- **Granulocyte-monocyte CSF (GM-CSF)**
  - Made by T-cells, mononuclear phagocytes, endothelial cells and fibroblasts
  - Stimulates immature progenitor cells to grow and differentiate into all cell types, stimulates committed progenitor cells to differentiate into granulocytes and mononuclear phagocytes, activates mononuclear phagocytes, and promotes the differentiation of Langerhans cells into dendritic cells

---

Bevacizumab (Avastin), used in combination with 5-fluorouracil-based chemotherapy, is indicated for first-line treatment of patients with metastatic carcinoma of the colon or rectum. How does it work?

Bevacizumab is a recombinant humanized antibody to vascular endothelial growth factor (VEGF) that binds to and inhibits VEGF, which, in theory, leads to the inhibition of angiogenesis. Current evidence suggests that the action of bevacizumab is considerably more complex in that it may "normalize" tumor vascular supply rather than inhibit it.

Angiogenesis

- Wound healing, tumor growth, revascularization following ischemia, and chronic inflammation all promote angiogenesis
- The first step in angiogenesis is stimulation of vascular endothelial cell proliferation
- Growth factors that stimulate endothelial cells include VEGF, FGF, macrophage-derived endothelial growth factor, TGF-β, and TGF-α
  - A stimulated endothelial cell must first break through the basement membrane and into the perivascular space
  - This process requires a protease enzyme
  - The endothelial cell subsequently migrates and divides
  - Vacuoles form in adjacent cells, which fuse to form capillary lumens
- Hypoxia stimulates angiogenesis, whereas increasing the oxygen concentration in the tissues may inhibit it

Targeted Chemotherapy Agents

- Monoclonal antibody-based agents
  - Are typically fully human or chimeric proteins generated to bind targets specifically, typically to inhibit function
  - The names of these agents end with "-mab"
  - Examples include trastuzumab (Herceptin), bevacizumab (Avastin), and cetuximab (Erbitux)
- Molecular inhibitors that are not antibodies
  - Include tyrosine kinase inhibitors (TKIs) that are typically small organic molecules designed to inhibit kinase function
  - TKIs may exhibit a high degree of specificity for specific targets, but most display considerable non-specific inhibition of other kinases
  - The names of these agents end with "-nib"
  - Examples include sorafenib (Nexavar), imatinib (Gleevec), and erlotinib (Tarceva)

42 Immunology

Srinevas K. Reddy and Sandhya Lagoo-Deenadayalan

A 43-year-old AIDS patient with a CD4 count of 50 develops an acute abdomen with pain and rebound tenderness localized to the right lower quadrant. On surgical exploration, the appendix is normal but a distal ileal perforation is noted. What is the most common etiology?

Immunocompromised patients are at high risk for Cytomegalovirus (CMV) enteritis.

Cytomegalovirus Infection

- Most cases are due to diagnoses related to an immunocompromised state
- Infective colitis
  - Infection results in vasculitis with thrombosis of submucosal blood vessels
  - Can lead to bowel perforation and toxic megacolon
  - Multiple sites of infection can occur simultaneously
  - Subtotal colectomy is the preferred operation
  - Anastomosis in the setting of peritonitis and severe immunocompromise should be avoided

Other Common GI Problems in the Immunocompromised Patient

- **Appendicitis** is most often associated with normal bacterial flora in the HIV/AIDS patient.
- **Non-Hodgkin Lymphoma**
  - The GI tract is the most common extra-nodal site of non-Hodgkin lymphoma
  - Most common site is the stomach, followed by rectum
  - Treatment of choice is chemotherapy
  - Reserve laparotomy for emergencies such as bleeding, perforation, or obstruction
- *Mycobacterium avium intracellulare* (MAI) and *Mycobacterium tuberculosis* infections
  - Can result in perforation of the intestinal tract
  - Even with optimal treatment, mortality is high
- **Histoplasmosis** of the colon
  - Acquired via inhalation of spores from soil contaminated with bat or bird droppings
  - Requires a histological diagnosis
  - Is treated with immediate and long-term administration of **itraconazole**

- Mild nausea and abdominal discomfort can also be attributed to HIV medications, antibiotics, or chemotherapy in the immunocompromised patient

Abdominal pain in the immunocompromised patient can be difficult to diagnose given the host of infections added to the differential diagnosis. Many of these infections are treated non-operatively.

A 25-year-old man arrives to the ER 12 hours after suffering a 6-cm long laceration on his leg after falling off of his tractor. The wound has several areas of devitalized tissue and he is unsure of his tetanus status. What tetanus prophylaxis should he be offered?

He should receive tetanus toxoid and human tetanus immune globulin.

Tetanus

- Tetanus is a severe progressive syndrome caused by a neurotoxin released by *Clostridium tetani*
- Even with ideal therapeutic intervention, mortality exceeds 30%
- *Tetanus prone wounds* have the following characteristics:
    - >6 hours old
    - Stellate wounds or avulsions
    - >1 cm in depth
    - Caused by missiles, crush, burns, or frostbite (not sharp injuries)
    - Have gross signs of infection, devitalized/denervated/ischemic tissue
    - Contamination with dirt, soil, or rust
- Removal of devitalized tissue and foreign bodies is key to preventing tetanus
- *Passive immunization* is provided by administering 250 units of human tetanus immunoglobulin
- *Active immunization* is provided by administering tetanus toxoid

Immunization status	Non-tetanus-prone wounds	Tetanus-prone wounds
Fully immunized	Give tetanus toxoid unless >3 doses of toxoid have already been given or last dose was given less than 10 years ago	Give tetanus toxoid unless >3 doses of toxoid have already been given or last dose was given less than 5 years ago
Partial or unknown status	Give tetanus toxoid	Give tetanus toxoid and human tetanus immune globulin

---

What are the major steps involved in migration of leukocytes from the vasculature into the extravascular space?

Leukocyte migration involves rolling of leukocytes along the endothelial surface, firm adhesion to the endothelial surface, release of endothelial damaging agents, and migration of leukocytes into the extravascular space by diapedeses.

Step 1
Attachment and rolling

Step 2
Activation

Step 3
Arrest and strengthening

Step 4
Transendothelial migration

Molecular signals

Leukocyte	Mucin-like molecules	Selectin	Seven membrane spanner receptor, G-protein linked	Integrin
	PSGL-1	L-selectin		LFA-1(CD11a/CD18)
				Mac-1(CD11b/CD18)
				p150, 95(CD11c/CD18)
				VLA-4(CD29/CD49d)
				LPAM-1(β7/CD/49d)

Endothelium	Selectin	Mucin-like molecules	Chemoattractant	Immunoglobulin family member
	E-selectin	GlyCAM-1	N-formyl peptides	ICAM-1,-2,-3
		CD34	C5a	Fibrinogen
		MadCAM-1	LTB$_4$	VCAM-1
			PAF	Fibronectin
			C-X-C chemokines (e.g. IL-8)	
			C-C chemokines (e.g. RANTES)	

Leukocyte migration. (With permission from Mulholland MW, Lillemoe KD, Doherty GM, Maier RV, Upchurch GR, eds. *Greenfield's Surgery.* 4th ed. Philadelphia, PA: Lippincott Williams & Wilkins; 2005.)

Leukocyte Migration

- Leukocyte adhesion and transmigration are regulated by
  - Binding of complementary adhesion molecules on leukocyte and endothelial surfaces
  - Chemical mediators (chemoattractants)
  - Cytokines modulating the surface expression or avidity of adhesion molecules
- Cells involved in the emigrating leukocyte response varies over time
  - Neutrophils predominate in the first 6 to 24 hours
  - Monocytes predominate in the next 24 to 48 hours
  - Lymphocytes may be the first cells in a viral infection
  - Eosinophilic granulocytes are the first to arrive in hypersensitivity reactions
- The initial rolling of leukocytes along endothelial surfaces is mediated by a family of proteins located on endothelial and leukocyte surfaces called selectins
  - Endothelial selectins
    - Cytokines including TNF, IL-1, and lipopolysaccharides induce expression of E-selectin and P-selectin
    - P-selectin is mobilized from intracellular storage granules as well as de novo synthesis with cytokine stimulation
    - E-selectin is made by de novo synthesis with cytokine stimulation
  - L-selectin is constitutively expressed on leukocytes
- This slowing of leukocytes allows for activation of β2 integrins, constitutively expressed on the leukocyte surface, by various chemokines

- Activated endothelial cells express ICAM-1 and ICAM-2, which bind to the β2 integrins, resulting in firm adhesion of leukocytes to the endothelial cells
- Release of proteases and oxidants by adhered leukocytes damages the endothelial cells and increases microvascular permeability, allowing the leukocytes to enter the extra-vascular space via diapedeses

A 62-year-old female ICU patient is febrile, breathing 32 times a minute, and has a white count of 16,500 cells/mm³. She is not on any pressors or inotropic support and has no positive cultures from any source. What is her inflammatory state?

She has systemic inflammatory response syndrome (SIRS).

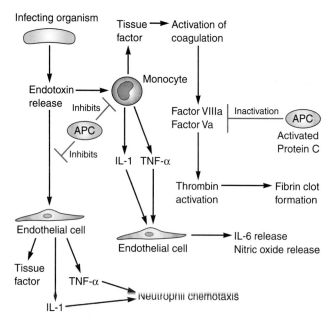

Cells and inflammatory mediators involved in SIRS. (With permission from Mulholland MW, Lillemoe KD, Doherty GM, Maier RV, Upchurch GR, eds. *Greenfield's Surgery.* 4th ed. Philadelphia, PA: Lippincott Williams & Wilkins; 2005.)

The Acute Phase Response in SIRS
- Fever due to exogenous pyrogens (bacterial products like lipopolysaccharide) that stimulate leukocytes to produce endogenous pyrogens (IL-1 and TNF-α), which together stimulate prostaglandin synthesis
  - This causes an increase in neurotransmitters like cyclic AMP that reset the temperature set point at a higher level
- IL-6, IL-1, and TNF-α increase the acute phase proteins synthesized by the liver and magnify the response to inflammation
- WBC increases, especially in the presence of a bacterial infection
  - The leukocytosis is initially because of an accelerated release of cells from the bone marrow's post-mitotic reserve pool and is associated with a rise in the number of more immature neutrophils in the blood (left shift)

A patient presenting with jaundice and right upper quadrant pain is suspected to have acute HBV infection. What will likely be detected in serum hepatitis studies?

HBV DNA, HBsAg, HBeAg, anti-HBsAb, and IgM anti-HBcAb

Hepatitis Antibodies

- Hepatitis B virus (HBV) is a double stranded virus with three major antigens (Ag):
    - HBsAg (envelope surface antigen)
    - HBcAg (core antigen)
    - HBeAg (a glycoprotein antigen associated with the core)
- The incubation time of HBV is 8 weeks
- The first serum indicator is HBsAg, which can precede symptoms
- Acute HBV infection is associated with serum HBV DNA and serum HbeAg
- IgM anti-HBc Antibody (Ab) occurs during clinical hepatitis at 4 to 12 weeks after infection
    - Presence of serum IgM anti-HBcAb is used to distinguish acute from chronic HBV infection
    - In most cases where chronic infection is not present, IgM anti-HbcAb does not persist beyond 6 months after infection
    - IgM anti-HBcAb is not protective against the disease
- Anti-HBeAb appears 4 months after infection, clears the HBeAg, but does not protect against the disease
- Anti-HBsAb starts to appear during recovery from acute hepatitis (as soon as 2 weeks after infection) and is associated with elimination of infection
- Hep B vaccine consists of recombinant HBsAg. Injection results in production of anti-HBsAb and is protective against reinfection.

Which cytokines are most important in stimulating hepatic acute phase proteins?

IL-6 and IL-1.

Hepatic Acute Phase Proteins

- The acute phase response to cell injury/trauma occurs 6 hours after the event
- Acute phase proteins change in concentration by at least 25% during this inflammation period
- Type I proteins: C-reactive protein (CRP), serum amyloid A (SAA), and C3
    - Stimulated by IL-1 and TNF
- Type II proteins: Fibrinogen, haptoglobin, ceruloplasmin, α_1-antitrypsin, α_1-antichymotrypsin
    - Stimulated by IL-6
- CRP
    - Activates complement
    - Recognizes foreign pathogens and binds to phagocytic cells
    - Activates tissue factor to initiate the coagulation cascade
    - Peaks 48 hours after the event and returns to baseline after 8 days
- Albumin and transferrin concentrations decrease in the acute phase response

---

A patient with diabetes mellitus is about to undergo a routine elective right hemicolectomy. Besides appropriate timing and choice of prophylactic antibiotic administration, what is the most important variable in preventing a surgical site infection?

Beyond intraoperative contamination, normoglycemia, both during and following a surgical procedure, is important in preventing a surgical site infection.

Postoperative Blood Glucose Control

- Immunologic deficiencies occur when blood glucose is poorly controlled
  - Impaired neutrophil chemotaxis and phagocytosis
  - Reduced CD4 cell counts
    - Both are reversible with the correction of hyperglycemia
  - Glucose toxicity injures the mitochondrial compartment and innate immunity

In diabetic surgical patients, both hyperglycemia and poor tissue perfusion due to microvascular and large vessel disease contribute to infection.

A patient is treated with prednisone for rheumatoid arthritis. What are the possible side effects of high-dose, prolonged steroid therapy?

Adrenal atrophy, impaired glucose control, immunosuppression, impaired wound healing, osteoporosis, glaucoma, cataracts, hypertension, and peptic ulcer disease.

Steroids

- Inhibit prostaglandin synthesis by repression of cyclooxygenase-2 transcription
- Induce MAPK phosphatase, preventing the transcription of genes encoding inflammatory proteins via the c-Jun transcription factor pathway
- Block NF-kB activity by direct binding to the glucocorticoid receptor in the nucleus
  - NF-kB stimulates transcription of cytokines, chemokines, complement factors, cell-adhesion molecules, and cyclooxygenase-2
- Side effects of high dose/prolonged steroid therapy
  - Adrenal atrophy
  - Testicular atrophy in men
  - Hypertension
    - Renal sodium retention and increase in blood volume
    - Potentiation of the effects of angiotensin II and catecholamines
  - Difficulty sleeping and "rage" behavior
  - GI bleeding, pancreatitis, and peptic ulcer disease
  - Immunosuppression
  - Delayed wound healing
    - Inhibition of collagen and matrix metalloproteinase synthesis
    - Decreased rate of epithelialization and fibroblast proliferation
    - Slowed capillary budding
    - All of the above impairments in wound healing (except wound contraction) can be reversed by supplemental **Vitamin A**
  - Acne, telangiectasia, purple striae, perioral dermatitis, and petechiae
  - Osteoporosis, retardation of longitudinal bone growth, and muscle atrophy
  - Glaucoma and cataracts
  - Delayed puberty, fetal growth retardation, and hypogonadism
  - Impaired glucose control by promotion of gluconeogenesis in the liver and degradation of muscle amino acids
  - Abrupt steroid withdrawal can cause severe depression and adrenal insufficiency

A patient has an anaphylactic reaction to a bee sting. What antibody mediates this response?

IgE is involved in a type I hypersensitivity reaction.

Hypersensitivity Reactions

- Type I reactions
  - IgE-mediated
  - Cross-linking of IgE on mast cells → activation and degranulation
  - Examples: Anaphylaxis, atopy
- Type II reactions
  - Antibody mediated
  - IgG or IgM binds to antigen on a cell surface → activates compliment cascade
  - Examples: ABO incompatibility, Grave disease, ITP
- Type III reactions
  - Immune complex mediated
  - IgG and IgM form circulating immune complexes
    - Complexes deposit in tissue or vascular epithelium
  - Examples: Serum sickness, rheumatoid arthritis, SLE
- Type IV reactions
  - Cell-mediated
  - Activated T cells will accumulate in an antigen-rich environment
    - Patients have to have had previous exposure to antigen
    - Occurs 24 to 48 hours post exposure
  - Examples: Contact dermatitis, TB skin test

A newborn baby is being breast-fed. What antibody is passed from the mother to her baby in her breast milk?

The most common antibody in breast milk is IgA.

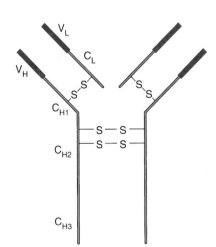

Antibody structure. (With permission from Mulholland MW, Lillemoe KD, Doherty GM, Maier RV, Upchurch GR, eds. *Greenfield's Surgery.* 4th ed. Philadelphia, PA: Lippincott Williams & Wilkins; 2005.)

Common Antibodies

- IgM exists as a pentamer and is the first antibody produced after antigen exposure
  - Associated with opsonin and complement fixation
- IgG is the primary antibody responsible for the secondary immune response
  - Crosses the placenta
  - Associated with opsonin and complement fixation
- IgA is found in secretions.
  - Binds antigen and prevents microbial adherence
  - Found in breast milk, tears, saliva, and bronchial fluid
  - Also found in Peyer patches of the small bowel
- IgD is a membrane-bound receptor on B cells
- IgE mediates type I hypersensitivity reactions
  - Helps defend against parasitic infections

An ICU patient has gram-negative rod sepsis. What is the key component of these organisms that causes SIRS?

Lipid A is a component of endotoxin common to many cases of gram-negative rod sepsis.

Endotoxins in Sepsis

- *E. coli* and *Pseudomonas aeruginosa* are the most common bacteria in gram-negative rod sepsis
- Lipopolysaccharide is released and triggers TNF
  - Lipid A is responsible for almost all the toxicity of endotoxin
  - LPS binds to lipopolysaccharide binding protein, which interacts with monocytes via the CD14 cell surface receptor, resulting in synthesis and release of cytokines
- The major sources of TNF are macrophages and the Kupffer cells of the liver
- The liver releases the largest quantities of TNF
  - Induces secretion and synthesis of cytokines, prostaglandins, leukotrienes, platelet activating factor, complement proteins, and activates components of the clotting pathway
  - Upregulates MHC class I and class II molecules
  - Results in fever (or hypothermia), tachycardia, increased cardiac output, and decreased systemic vascular resistance in sepsis

---

What are common supplements found in immune-enhancing enteral diets?

Enteral diets that are immune-enhancing are supplemented with glutamine, arginine, omega-3-polyunsaturated fatty acids, and/or nucleotides.

Dietary Supplements

- *Glutamine* is essential during stress and sepsis and is the primary fuel for cells lining the GI tract as well as immunological cells
- *Arginine* promotes proliferation of T cells after cytokine stimulation
- *Omega-3-polyunsaturated fatty acids* are metabolized into prostaglandins, thromboxanes, and leukotrienes
  - Reduce bacterial translocation and mortality
  - Increase resistance to infection by strengthening cell-mediated immunity

---

- *Nucleotides* are necessary for DNA/RNA synthesis
  - Deprivation of nucleotides suppresses T-cell function and IL-2 production

Glutamine is the primary energy source for cells lining the GI tract as well as immunological cells.

A patient being treated with whole-body radiation develops gram-negative rod sepsis. How does radiotherapy cause neutropenia?

The ionization damage to DNA triggers lymphocyte apoptosis.

Radiation Injury

- Radiotherapy targets sensitive tissues by ionization damage to DNA
- Acute effects of ionizing radiation:
  - High doses (>10Gy) cause overt necrosis
  - Intermediate doses (1 to 2Gy) kill proliferating cells (cancer, lymphocyte, hair)
  - Low doses (<0.5Gy) cause subcellular damage
- Acute radiation syndromes include 4 clinical categories: Subclinical, hematopoietic syndrome, gastrointestinal syndrome, and central nervous syndrome
- DNA damage in lymphoid and myeloid cell lineages triggers apoptosis with subsequent neutropenia and immunocompromise
- Neutropenia causes an increased propensity for infections

A patient with AIDS develops *Candida albicans* sepsis. Which type of immunity is primarily depressed in this patient?

Opportunistic infections move in when cell-mediated immunity is impaired.

Cell-Mediated Immunity

- Mediated by T lymphocytes
- $CD4^+$ and $CD8^+$ T lymphocytes perform distinct but somewhat overlapping functions
  - $CD4^+$ helper cells recognize and respond to an antigen only in the context of class II MHC molecules and produce IL-2 and IFN-γ upon activation
  - These cytokines stimulate $CD8^+$ cytotoxic T cells, which recognize cell bound antigens only in association with class I MHC molecules
  - A large number of antigen-specific lymphocytes are generated
    - Effector cells that eliminate the antigen that started the response
    - Memory cells that are long-lived and poised to respond rapidly to repeat encounters with the antigen
- Deficiencies in cell-mediated immunity impair defenses against
  - Intracellular bacterial infections: *Campylobacter jejuni, Mycobacterium avium intracellulare, Salmonella, Shigella*
  - Viral agents: Cytomegalovirus, Herpes Simplex Virus
  - Fungal infections: *Candida albicans, Histoplasma capsulatum*
  - Protozoal infections: *Blastocystis hominis, Cryptosporidium, Entamoeba histolytica, Giardia*

A woman in septic shock is hospitalized in the ICU. How does nitric oxide contribute to her hypotension?

Nitric oxide is a potent vasodilator and depresses the constrictive response to angiotensin II and catecholamines.

Nitric Oxide

- Nitric oxide (NO) levels are increased in sepsis
  - Nitric oxide is synthesized by iNOS, one of three isoforms of nitric oxide synthase
  - iNOS is highly expressed in endothelial cells in sepsis after stimulation by proinflammatory cytokines (IL-1, TNF, IFN-γ) and lipopolysaccharide
  - L-arginine is the substrate for NO production
- Effects of nitric oxide
  - Potent vasodilator and impairs vascular smooth muscle constriction in response to angiotensin II and catecholamines
  - Has negative inotropic effects and can result in liver and gut damage by disruption of microcirculatory regulation
  - Can lead to DNA and cell membrane damage through the formation of free radicals
- Treatment of patients in shock with nitric oxide synthase inhibitors has not been successful

A child with a known late complement component deficiency is hospitalized with sepsis. What is the most likely infecting agent?

Streptococcus pneumoniae is normally attacked by the body's complement pathway and is the most likely infection to occur when a complement component deficiency is present.

Opsonization

- Most inherited complement deficiencies are associated with a susceptibility to invasive bacterial infections caused by encapsulated bacteria
  - *Neisseria meningitidis, Neisseria gonorrhoeae, Haemophilus influenzae type b*, and *Streptococcus pneumoniae*
  - *S. pneumoniae* is the most common infecting agent
  - Susceptibility is due to a deficiency in the C5b-9 serum attack complex
- C2 deficiency is associated with atherosclerosis, lupus, and other rheumatic diseases
- The classic pathway is stimulated by antigen–antibody complexes.
  - C1, C2, and C4 are only found in the classic pathway
- The alternate pathway is stimulated by endotoxin and bacteria
  - Factor B, D, and P (properdin) are only found in the alternate pathway
- C3 is the convergence point of the classic and alternate pathways
- C3a, C4a, and C5a are anaphylatoxins that increase vascular permeability and activate mast cells and basophils
- C3b mediates opsonization

What is the main cytokine released by CD4$^+$ cells that stimulates the cellular immune response?

IL-2 is the main cytokine released by CD4$^+$ cells.

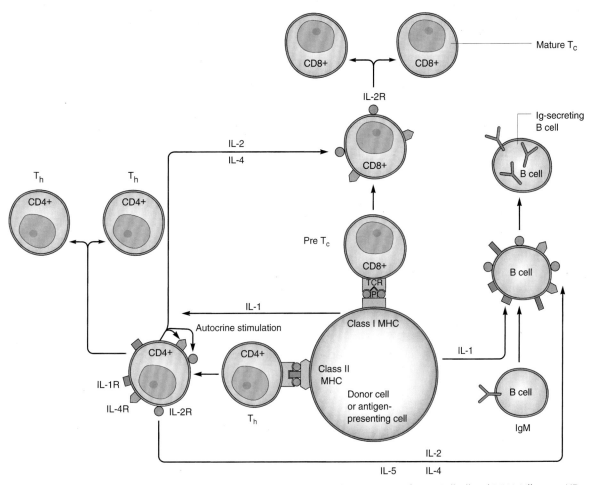

Interactions between CD4, CD8, and antigen presenting cells. (With permission from Mulholland MW, Lillemoe KD, Doherty GM, Maier RV, Upchurch GR, eds. *Greenfield's Surgery*. 4th ed. Philadelphia, PA: Lippincott Williams & Wilkins; 2005.)

T Cell Activation

- Signal 1
    - T Cell Receptor (TCR) is engaged by an MHC-bound antigen
    - Co-receptor (CD4 or CD8) binds to the MHC molecule
- Signal 2
    - CD28 molecule on T cells interacts with co-stimulatory molecules CD80 (B7-1) and CD86 (B7-2) expressed on antigen presenting cells

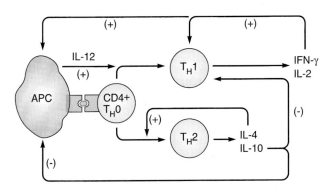

T cell activation. (With permission from Mulholland MW, Lillemoe KD, Doherty GM, Maier RV, Upchurch GR, eds. *Greenfield's Surgery*. 4th ed. Philadelphia, PA: Lippincott Williams & Wilkins; 2005.)

- Antigen presenting cells (APC) produce IL-1, which results in further stimulation of CD4$^+$ T cells (autocrine stimulation)
- CD4$^+$ T cells then release:
    - IL-2 to stimulate CD8$^+$ cells
    - IL-4 and IL-5 to stimulate B cells

Helper T cells (CD4$^+$)

- **Th1 Helper T cells**
    - Release pro-inflammatory cytokines (IL-2, IFN-γ)
    - Stimulate cellular immunity
    - Cytokine release results in maturation of cytotoxic T cells
    - Mediate delayed-type hypersensitivity
- **Th2 Helper T cells**
    - Release anti-inflammatory cytokines (IL-4, IL-5, and IL-10), which suppress T cell responses and inhibit macrophage production
    - Stimulate B cell proliferation, maturation, and immunoglobulin production

---

Which cells are the key effectors of the adaptive anti-tumor immune response?

CD8$^+$ T cells

Tumor Immune Response

- CD4$^+$/CD25$^+$ regulatory T cells
    - Found in high concentrations in the tumor microenvironment
    - Prevent the induction of tumor-associated antigen immunity by:
        - Directly killing CD8$^+$ T cells
        - Binding to and sequestering the proliferating agent IL-2
        - Inducing molecules on antigen presenting cells that upon binding to effector T cells result in T cell cycle arrest
        - Decreasing expression of MHC molecules on antigen presenting cells via IL-10
- Strategies for boosting host tumor immune response
    - Targeting regulatory cells by selectively blocking function, depleting cell number, or blocking differentiation
    - Stimulating tumor immune response by enhancing general immune response via administration of high dose cytokines, such as IL-2
    - Injection of dendritic antigen-presenting cells and/or tumor peptides

Cytokines in Transplantation

- The ability to transplant organs successfully depends on the response of the host to the allograft, known as the allograft response
    - CD4$^+$ T cells direct the allograft response by producing cytokines that coordinate the activities of macrophages, antigen-presenting dendritic cells, CD8$^+$ T cells, NK cells, and B cells
- IL-4, GM-CSF, and type I interferons have critical roles in the maturation of dendritic cells and their migration to the regional lymph nodes post-transplant.
    - Dendritic cells become the main antigen-presenting cells in the allograft response
    - Depending on their expression of co-stimulatory molecules (IL-10 and TGF-b), they can also be agents of tolerance

- Cytokines modulate T cell response to transplantation, having roles in both anergy and rejection
  - IL-2, IL-4, IL-7, IL-15 and IL-21 are all implicated in expansion of T cell populations
  - IL-2 is especially implicated in T cell rejection
  - IL-2 signaling through the calcineurin/NFAT pathway is specifically inhibited by such anti-rejection drugs as FK506 and mycophenolate mofetil

---

For which cancer has the most success been shown with IL-2 therapy?

IL-2 therapy is now a standard treatment in advanced stage melanoma.

Melanoma Immunology
- IL-2 is secreted by activated helper T cells
- In vitro or in vivo exposure of lymphoid cells to high concentrations of IL-2 generates lymphokine-activated killer (LAK) cells
  - LAK cells kill tumor cells nonspecifically
  - Response rate of melanoma to LAK cells + IL-2 is 20% to 25%
- IL-2 administration alone results in a 15% to 20% tumor response rate
  - The response is dose-dependent
  - Anti-tumor effects are due to the induction of LAKs, tumor-sensitized T cells, and the indirect secretion of other cytokines
  - High doses of IL-2 result in sepsis due to capillary leak syndrome caused by the induction of inflammatory mediators

While slicing a bagel for breakfast, a 27-year-old man accidentally lacerates his 4th finger requiring sutures to be placed. What sequence of events results in hemostasis in this healthy individual?

- *Vasoconstriction*
- *Platelet stimulation, adhesion, and aggregation (primary hemostasis)*
- *Activation and binding of coagulation factors forming thrombin (secondary hemostasis)*
- *Fibrin deposition to strengthen the platelet plug*

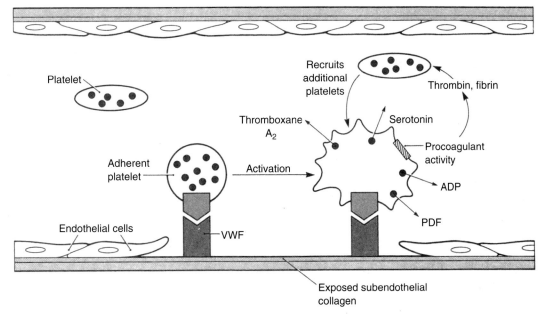

Sequence of events in normal hemostasis. (With permission from O'Leary JP, Tabuenca A, eds. *Physiologic Basis of Surgery*. 4th ed. Philadelphia, PA: Wolters Kluwer Health/Lippincott Williams & Wilkins; 2007.)

Normal Hemostasis

- Injury to vessel endothelium exposes collagen, which stimulates platelets
- Thrombin generation is also a major catalyst for platelet activation

- Vasoconstriction is endothelium-initiated
- Platelet adhesion is mediated by binding of platelet surface receptor GPIb to von Willebrand factor (vWF) within exposed collagen
- Platelet aggregation occurs when fibrinogen acts as a bridge between activated platelets via GPIIb/IIIa receptors
- Platelets then release granules containing ADP, serotonin, and arachidonic acid which is converted to thromboxane A2 by cyclooxygenase (COX)
    - Thromboxane A2 stimulates further vasoconstriction and platelet aggregation

Platelet adhesion: GPIb-vWF

↓

Platelet aggregation: GPIIb/IIIa-fibrinogen

↓ (ADP, ATP, Epi, TXA2, collagen, thrombin)

Activation of coagulation cascade

- Factor VIII-vWF is the only factor not made in the liver (made by endothelium)

Aspirin irreversibly inhibits the cyclooxygenase enzyme, which inhibits platelet aggregation (effect lasts up to 10 days).

The endothelium is an important factor in maintaining blood fluidity and preventing thrombosis in the face of vascular insults. What is the most potent endothelial factor responsible for preventing intravascular thrombosis?

Nitric oxide. Other factors include prostacyclin, thrombomodulin, heparin sulfate proteoglycan, and tissue plasminogen activator.

The Endothelium

- To prevent platelet aggregation, endothelium generates both nitric oxide (NO) and prostacyclin (PGI2)
- Natural heparin sulfate proteoglycan serves as a cofactor for antithrombin III, preventing thrombin formation
- Factors that disrupt the normal endothelial function (endotoxin, tumor necrosis factor alpha, interleukin-1, and hypoxemia) can lead to prothrombotic states

---

A 43-year-old man was diagnosed to have von Willebrand disease after prolonged bleeding following a tooth extraction. He now presents for an elective laparoscopic cholecystectomy. What measures should be performed to help prevent abnormal bleeding?

Desmopressin (1-deamine-8D arginine vasopressin, DDAVP) should be given prior to surgery to boost levels of vWF and Factor VIII. If unresponsive to DDAVP, factor VIII-vWF concentrates are available.

von Willebrand Disease

- Most common congenital bleeding disorder (1% prevalence)
- Characterized by a deficiency or dysfunction of von Willebrand factor (vWF)
    - Stored in endothelial cells and megakaryocytes
    - Assists in platelet adhesion
        - Carrier protein for factor VIII
        - Links GPIB receptors on platelets to collagen to cause platelet adhesion at the bleeding site
    - Type I: Quantitative decrease in vWF

- Type II: Qualitative decrease in vWF
  - Type IIa—abnormally small vWF (large multimers needed for platelet binding)
  - Type IIb—rapid clearance of large vWF multimers
  - Type III: Near absence of vWF
- PT is normal, aPTT normal/abnormal, bleeding time prolonged, ristocetin test is positive
- Presents with mucosal bleeding, petechiae, epistaxis, and menorrhagia
- Acquired forms of vWD (secondary to vWF directed antibodies) occur in lymphoproliferative disorders, malignancy, drugs, hypothyroidism, and autoimmune diseases
- Treatment
  - Desmopressin (DDAVP) causes release of endogenous stores of vWF from Weibel-Palade bodies in endothelium
    - Raises levels of factor VIII
    - Can induce flushing, tachycardia, and headaches due to vasoactive effects
    - Is not effective for all patients
  - Factor VIII-vWF concentrates
  - Cryoprecipitate may also be used if Factor VIII-vWF concentrates are not available
  - Aminocaproic acid and tranexamic acid can be administered as a mouthwash for dental procedures

---

A 25-year-old man is traveling through South America and becomes severely ill with malaria. He is given quinine and improves from his malarial infection. However, a few days later, he develops thrombocytopenia, anemia, altered mental status, and renal failure. What does he have and how can it be treated?

He has thrombotic thrombocytopenic purpura (TTP), which is most often idiopathic, but can be caused by quinines, some cancers, and immunosuppression.

Thrombotic Thrombocytopenic Purpura
- Caused by an inability to degrade large vWF multimers due to deficiency in protease ADAMTS13
- Signs: thrombocytopenia, hemolytic anemia, altered mental status, renal failure, and fever
  - Death is most commonly secondary to intracerebral hemorrhage or acute renal failure
- Treatment
  - Large volume plasmapheresis
  - Splenectomy is rarely indicated

Idiopathic Thrombocytopenic Purpura
- Caused by autoantibiodies (IgG) to platelets → platelet sequestration in the spleen and destruction
- Signs: Petechiae and bleeding gums
- Causes: Idiopathic, HIV, HCV, SLE
- Treatment: Steroids, IVIG, splenectomy
  - Splenectomy removes the source of IgG production and phagocytosis

Uremic Bleeding
- Platelet dysfunction due to decreased adhesion and aggregation mostly from altered GPIIb/IIIa
  - Also have abnormal expression of GPIb receptors, vWF and altered release of ADP, serotonin, and thromboxane A2
- Treatment: Dialysis, DDAVP

Glanzmann Thrombasthenia

- Defective glycoprotein IIb-IIIa receptors
  - Prevents platelet aggregation with fibrinogen
- Autosomal recessive
- Signs: Petechiae, bleeding gums, prolonged bleeding time
- Treatment: Platelet transfusion

Bernard-Soulier Syndrome

- Abnormality in the glycoprotein Ib (vWF receptor)-Factor V-Factor IX complex
  - Results in abnormal platelet adhesion
- Autosomal recessive
- Signs: Petechiae, bleeding gums, prolonged bleeding time
- Treatment: Platelet transfusion

A 5 year-old boy with a history of significant bleeding after small cuts is playing outside and comes in complaining of severe right knee pain. He states that he was just playing and did not fall on or injure the knee. On further workup, he is found to have hemorrhage into his right knee joint. What further hematologic workup should he have?

His story is consistent with hemophilia A or B and he should have mixing studies, which will normalize the factor deficiency if this is the diagnosis.

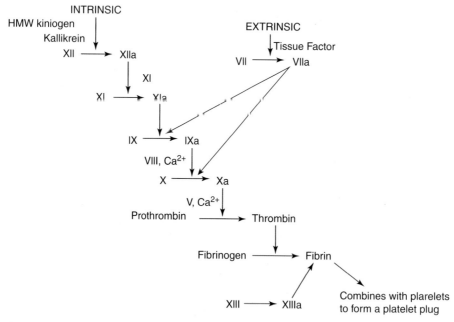

Coagulation cascade.

Hemophilia A (Inherited Factor VIII Deficiency)

- X-linked recessive (primarily affects men)
- Symptoms: Excessive bleeding, spontaneous hemarthroses
- Prolonged aPTT, normal PT, normal bleeding time
- Confirm with mixing studies, which should normalize the factor deficiency

- Factor VIII crosses the placenta and therefore newborns do not bleed at circumcision
- May use DDAVP to raise levels of factor VIII for simple surgical procedures
- Treat with recombinant factor VIII or FFP for severe cases
  - Do not aspirate a hemophiliac joint → use ice, keep joints mobile with physical therapy, and give factor VIII and cryoprecipitate
- Goal factor levels of 20% to 30% for minor surgery, 50% to 80% for major surgery

Hemophilia B (Inherited Factor IX Deficiency) "Christmas Disease"
- X-linked recessive
- Clinically indistinguishable from type A
- Laboratory findings similar to type A
- DDAVP not effective
- Treat with recombinant factor IX, FFP, or prothrombin complex concentrate

Inhibitors of the Coagulation Cascade
- Thrombomodulin
  - Binds and changes the shape of thrombin
  - Becomes a potent activator of protein C and S (anticoagulant)
  - Activates thrombin-activated fibrinolysis inhibitor (TAFI), which inhibits fibrinolysis
- Protein C and S
  - Potent inhibitors of factor VIII & V
- Antithrombin III
  - Does not require activation
  - Binds to thrombin
  - Inhibits factors VIIa, IXa, Xa, XIa, and plasmin
- Plasmin
  - Converted from plasminogen by tissue plasminogen activator (released from endothelium)
  - Cleaves fibrin, degrades factors V and VIII and fibrinogen
  - Levels also increased by Factor XII, prekallikrein, and HMWK
  - Inhibited by TAFI
  - Prostate surgery can result in release of urokinase → plasminogen activation to plasmin → thrombolysis
    - Treat with aminocaproic acid

A 38-year-old woman presents with a large pulmonary embolus with hemodynamic instability and cardiogenic shock. Catheter-directed thrombolysis is not available. What is the next step in management?

When catheter-based thrombolysis is ineffective or unavailable, a significant pulmonary embolus with hemodynamic instability is the rare indication for surgical pulmonary embolectomy (the Trendelenburg procedure).

Pulmonary Embolus
- Presents with shortness of breath, tachycardia, hypoxemia, and a normal or decreased $PaCO_2$
- Most deep vein thrombosis (DVT) originate above the knees
- Pulmonary embolectomy is rarely indicated
- Most patients will require lifetime anticoagulation therapy

A 35-year-old man is hospitalized after receiving multiple gunshot wounds resulting in a pelvic and right femur fracture. He develops a deep vein thrombosis on hospital day #4. What are the risk factors for deep vein thrombosis?

The risk factors are based on Virchow triad: damage to the endothelial lining, stasis and hypercoagulability.

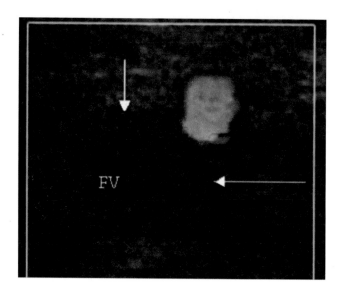

DVT on US. (With permission from Mulholland MW, Lillemoe KD, Doherty GM, Maier RV, Upchurch GR, eds. *Greenfield's Surgery.* 4th ed. Philadelphia, PA: Lippincott Williams & Wilkins; 2005.)

Deep Vein Thrombosis

- Most common site of a DVT in postoperative setting is the popliteal vein
- D-dimer test can be useful in the diagnosis of DVT and pulmonary embolus
  - Negative value helps exclude a DVT (high negative predictive value)
  - Positive value post-operatively is usually not helpful since it is commonly elevated following surgery (low positive predictive value)

Hypercoagulable States

- Acquired causes include surgery, trauma, immobilization, pregnancy, malignancy, and exogenous estrogen
- Genetic causes include Factor V Leiden, Protein C and S deficiency, antithrombin III deficiency, Prothrombin GP20210 mutation, antiphospholipid syndrome, and hyperhomocysteinemia

A 42-year-old woman presents with dyspnea and chest pain. Spiral CT scan shows a medium-sized pulmonary embolism in the right lower lung. Further questioning reveals that she had a DVT in the past, as well as two spontaneous abortions. What is the most likely diagnosis?

Factor V Leiden mutation is the most common genetic cause of hypercoagulability and is present in 50% of familial thrombophilia.

Factor V Leiden

- Factor V is resistant to inactivation by protein C
  - Due to a point mutation (substitution of arginine by glutamine)

- Autosomal dominant mutation with variable penetrance
- Most common inherited coagulation disorder (5%)
- Accounts for 20% to 30% of all spontaneous thromboses
    - Have spontaneous arterial and venous thrombosis
- Present with DVT, pulmonary embolism, pregnancy loss, or superficial thrombophlebitis

Prothrombin Gene GP20210 Mutation
- Second most common cause of genetic hypercoagulability
- Results in elevated levels of prothrombin

Protein C and S deficiency
- Autosomal dominant mutation
- Homozygotes die at birth
- Diagnosis: Protein activity assays, which use snake venom to inactivate protein C and S
- Usually requires lifelong anticoagulation after first DVT

Antithrombin III deficiency
- Autosomal dominant mutation
- Homozygotes die at birth
- Suspected in patients who cannot achieve adequate anticoagulation with heparin
- Anticoagulation with heparin may require FFP supplementation, which contains AT III
- Treated with lifelong (warfarin) anticoagulation

Antiphospholipid Antibody
- IgG and IgM antibodies against phospholipids: Anticardiolipin and beta-2 glycoprotein
- Diagnosed with positive Russell viper venom time: Prolonged aPTT in vitro, not corrected in mixing studies (Lupus anticoagulant)
- Diagnosis requires one clinical event and one laboratory study

Hyperhomocysteinemia
- Causes arterial and venous thrombosis
- Treat with folate and vitamin B_{12} supplementation

Hypercoagulable Testing While on Anticoagulation
- Accurate: Factor V Leiden mixing study, Prothrombin GP20210 gene mutation, anticardiolipin antibody, beta-2 glycoprotein, and plasma homocysteine levels
- Distorted by warfarin: Protein C and S levels
- Distorted by heparin: AT III
- Distorted by LMWH: Lupus anticoagulant

A 78-year-old woman is taking low-molecular weight heparin (LMWH) for a mechanical heart valve. What is the most common long-term complication?

Osteoporosis is a long-term complication of heparin associated with both LMWH as well as "unfractionated" forms of heparin (IV).

Action of Unfractionated Heparin

- $t_{1/2}$ of 1 hour
- Binds and potentiates the action of antithrombin III
- Inhibits all serine proteases (primarily Xa and thrombin)
- Directly inhibited by the administration of protamine
- Protamine may be associated with anaphylactic reactions, hypotension, and pulmonary hypertension

Low Molecular Weight Heparin

- Binds and catalyzes antithrombin III
- Inhibits factor Xa (but not thrombin)
- Advantages over unfractionated heparin include:
  - Increased bioavailability leading to a greater anti-Xa effect
  - Less platelet interference
  - Longer half life
  - Predictable dose-dependent plasma levels not requiring laboratory monitoring

Warfarin

- Depletes functional vitamin K reserves thereby reducing formation of vitamin K-dependent factors II, VII, IX, X, and Protein C and S
- Warfarin is teratogenic: Use heparin or LMWH during pregnancy
- Correction of supratherapeutic INR can be achieved with administration of vitamin K (takes 6 hours, IV infusion has higher risk of anaphylaxis) or FFP (immediate effect)

Administration of warfarin prior to heparin administration can lead to a transient pro-thrombotic state (and a complication known as warfarin-induced skin necrosis) since Protein C has a shorter half-life than factors II, IX, and X.

A 72-year-old woman is admitted to the surgical intensive care unit with severe intra-abdominal sepsis from a perforated colonic diverticula. After 3 hours of supportive care, she begins to bleed briskly from her nose, rectum, and IV sites. What is the next step in management?

Disseminated intravascular coagulation (DIC) is treated supportively; the main goal in therapy is to treat the underlying cause.

Disseminated Intravascular Coagulation

- DIC is a systemic process resulting in consumption of platelets and coagulation factors that ultimately produces both bleeding and thrombosis
- Common causes include sepsis (usually gram negative rods), malignancy, hemorrhage/trauma, and liver failure
  - Other causes include severe pancreatitis, snake bites, drugs, and obstetrical complications
- Pathogenesis is mostly related to over production of thrombin and activation of cytokines TNF, IL-1, and IL-6
  - Leads to widespread activation of the coagulation cascade
  - Results in extensive thrombosis, widespread deposition of fibrin, and finally massive secondary fibrinolysis

- Death is most commonly related to organ failure from thrombi in small and large arteries leading to tissue ischemia
- Laboratory abnormalities
  - Thrombocytopenia, prolonged PT
  - aPTT can be normal in some cases
  - Elevated fibrin degradation products and D-dimer
  - Decreased fibrinogen
- Treatment is largely supportive; however, high risk or actively bleeding patients can receive platelets, FFP, and/or cryoprecipitate

DIC is associated with decreased fibrinogen and increased fibrin split products. Management is geared towards addressing the underlying cause.

A 55-year-old woman with longstanding Crohn's disease is hospitalized for management of an enterocutaneous fistula. While in the hospital, she has a central venous catheter placed for total parenteral nutrition. Placement of the catheter was uncomplicated with the exception of prolonged bleeding, which required a transfusion. What is the etiology for the patient's coagulation abnormality?

Vitamin K deficiency is common in patients with malnutrition.

Vitamin K Deficiency

- Vitamin K is a fat-soluble vitamin found in leafy vegetables
- Antibiotics decrease intestinal *vitamin K–producing bacteria* in the normal flora
- For bleeding emergencies, FFP can be given
- Hepatic disease can cause bleeding because the liver synthesizes most of the coagulation factors and proteins
- Hepatic disease first manifests as a prolonged PT because factor VII has the shortest half-life of any of the coagulation factors
- Renal failure inhibits platelet function for unknown reasons
- In addition, uremia appears to adversely affect the function of von Willebrand factor and results in poor platelet aggregation

Coagulopathy associated with renal failure is best treated with dialysis or DDAVP.

One hour after an "on-pump" coronary artery bypass surgery, a 75-year-old man in the surgical intensive care unit continues to bleed from his mediastinal tube. His coagulation studies and platelet counts are normal and his previous dose of heparin has been fully reversed with protamine. Besides blood, what other product may help decrease his acute blood loss?

Coronary artery bypass causes a functional defect in platelet activity. Thus, even a normal platelet level may be deceiving. A platelet transfusion could help prevent further blood loss.

Additional Blood Component Therapy

- Platelets
  - Indicated for bleeding from thrombocytopenia or dysfunctional platelets
  - 1 unit raises platelet count by 30,000 to 60,000μL in 70 kg patient

- Higher risk of infection than other blood products because they are stored at room temperature
- Shelf life = 5 days
- Fresh frozen plasma (FFP)
  - A product of centrifugation of whole blood
  - Contains all components of plasma including coagulation factors and other proteins
    - High levels of factor V, factor VIII, Protein C and S, AT III
    - Does not contain thrombin
  - Has an immediate effect
  - Indicated for rapid reversal of coagulation defects
  - Can only be stored for up to 24 hours if thawed (1 year if frozen)
  - Carries the same risk of infection transmission as other blood products
- Cryoprecipitate
  - Obtained when FFP is thawed at 4°C
  - Concentrated source of factor VIII, vWF, and fibrinogen
  - Can be used in diseases such as hemophilia A and vWD
  - Also used as a source of fibrinogen in consumptive coagulopathies
  - Cryoprecipitate should not be used routinely for Hemophilia or von Willebrand disease because of the availability of DDAVP and recombinant products, which are safer
  - Shelf life = 1 year if frozen
- Recombinant factor VIII or IX
  - Use for hemophilia A or B
  - Needs to be reconstituted for use
- Factor VII
  - Use for refractory bleeding
  - High risk of arterial and venous clots
  - Needs to be reconstituted for use

During a national blood shortage, a 53-year-old woman with coronary artery disease and renal failure undergoes coronary artery bypass surgery and requires multiple transfusions with red blood cells that have been shelved for approximately 35 days. What is the patient's greatest risk in receiving a transfusion of blood with such a prolonged storage period?

As red cells are stored, potassium leaks from the cells and can approach 25 meq/L. This should be a special consideration in renal failure patients, where hyperkalemia can be a significant problem.

Packed Red Blood Cell Storage
- One unit of PRBCs has a volume of 250 mL, a hematocrit of 70% to 80%, and a storage life of 35 days
- Additives like citrate can increase the storage life to 42 days
- As cells are stored for long periods of time, the following changes occur:
  - Increased potassium levels due to leakage from stored cells
  - Decreased pH to as low as 6.7
  - Decreased 2,3-DPG level which increases hemoglobin oxygen binding and decreases the oxygen delivering capacity of red blood cells

- Increased concentration of inflammatory cytokines such as TNF, IL-1, and IL-6 which can cause fevers
- Leukocyte reduction can reduce the incidence of transfusion reactions and CMV transmission
- Each unit of blood can be expected to raise the hemoglobin by approximately 1 g/dL

Febrile, nonhemolytic reactions are the most common transfusion reactions and occur in approximately 1% of transfusions.

Six hours after transfusion of two units of PRBCs, a 60-year-old man develops severe hypoxemia and respiratory distress requiring endotracheal intubation. A chest X-ray reveals severe pulmonary edema. What is the most likely diagnosis?

Transfusion-related acute lung injury (TRALI) represents one of the many risks of a blood transfusion.

Acute Transfusion Reaction
- Symptoms include fever, chills, and lightheadedness
- Signs include hyperbilirubinemia, decreased haptoglobin, anemia, and low blood pressure
- Hemolytic reactions
  - Immune mediated
    - Due to complement-fixing antibodies attacking transfused RBCs
    - Acute hemolysis is the most common cause of a transfusion-related death
      - Caused by *human error* resulting in ABO incompatibility
      - Treat with fluid, histamine blockers, and pressors (if necessary)
    - Delayed hemolysis
      - Due to antibodies against minor antigens
      - Observe if stable; otherwise treatment as for acute hemolysis
  - Non-immune mediated
    - From infusing blood too quickly
    - Treatment: Fluid resuscitation
- Febrile non-hemolytic transfusion reaction
  - Most common transfusion reaction
  - Due to recipient antibodies against donor WBCs
  - Treatment: Stop transfusion and use WBC filter for subsequent transfusions
- Anaphylaxis is a rare reaction due to IgG or IgA antibodies attacking components of the donor plasma
  - Signs include hypotension, shock, dyspnea, bronchospasm, dizziness, and flushing
- Microbial contamination is an outcome that is more commonly seen with transfusion of platelets than RBCs because platelets are stored at room temperature
- When bacterial contamination is present, mortality can exceed 75%

The first intra-operative sign of a mismatched blood transfusion may be generalized bleeding.

TRALI (Transfusion-Related Acute Lung Injury)
- Life-threatening respiratory compromise manifested by non-cardiogenic pulmonary edema and hypoxemia
- Occurs in <0.1% of transfusions

- Believed to be due to reaction between donor anti-HLA or anti-leukocyte antibodies with antigen on recipient leukocytes leading to inflammatory response within pulmonary microvasculature
- Treatment is immediate cessation of transfusion and respiratory support
- Mechanical ventilation may be necessary and should follow the same principles as ARDS
- Not an absolute contraindication for future transfusion

Delayed Complications of Blood Transfusion

- The risk of contracting an infection is as follows:

Hepatitis C	1 in 1.2 million
Hepatitis B	1 in 150,000
HIV	1 in 1.4 million
Bacterial contamination	1 in 38,000

- A delayed hemolytic reaction can occur up to 2 weeks after a transfusion and is characterized by a late antibody response to the transfused blood

Infection with Parvovirus B19 is a common infection due to blood transfusion.

A 45-year-old man with a history significant for end stage renal failure due to polycystic kidney disease undergoes a cadaveric renal transplant. One month postoperatively, he develops headache and malaise. His hematocrit at that time is measured to be 62%. What is the most likely diagnosis?

Post-transplant erythrocytosis presents with a markedly elevated hematocrit following renal transplantation.

Post-transplant Erythrocytosis (PTE)

- PTE is defined as an elevated hematocrit greater than 51% after renal transplant
- 10% to 15% of renal transplant patients develop the condition
- Most patients present with malaise, headache, and lethargy
- 10% to 30% of patients may develop thromboembolic events
- PTE has a 1% to 2% mortality
- Treatment is supportive and consists of optimization of volume status and administration of an ace inhibitor

The greatest risk of death associated with receiving a blood transfusion is ABO incompatibility due to human error—a risk which supersedes the risk of an anaphylactic reaction.

44 | Statistics

Dora Syin and Peter J. Pronovost

A research study examining surgical approaches to hernia repair and length of stay found an outcome difference between open and laparoscopic surgery. Subsequent level I data with a much improved study design and larger sample size showed no difference in length of stay. What type of statistical error was made in the initial study?

The conclusion of the initial study was a Type I error. A Type I error refers to an incorrect rejection of the null hypothesis, when it is in fact true (i.e., the difference between observed values is declared statistically significant, when it really is not).

Type I Error

- Incorrect rejection of the null hypothesis when it is actually true
- "Convicting an innocent person"
- Probability denoted by the alpha statistic (α)
- Most common error in research (remember it as the #1 error that researchers make, i.e., to claim something is better when it really is not)
- The risk for Type 1 error is greater in observational studies than in randomized trials

A study comparing several antibiotic prophylaxis regimens for postoperative wound infections found no significant difference between treatment groups. The study's results were in contradiction with those of several larger studies. What type of statistical error was made in the initial study?

The conclusion of the initial study was a Type II error. A Type II error refers to a failure to reject the null hypothesis, when it is in fact false (i.e., no significant difference is declared, when there really is one).

Type II Error

- Failure to reject the null hypothesis when it is actually false
- "Letting a guilty person go free"
- Probability denoted by beta (β)

671

Ways to Prevent Type I and Type II Errors

- Raise the level of alpha
- Reduce population variability
- Make the difference between the conditions greater
- Increase the sample size

> A researcher compared hospital mortality or complications from 10 percutaneous tracheostomy procedures to 10 open tracheostomy procedures. What is the most likely principal design flaw of the study?

The sample size is small and lacks statistical power. Power is defined as the probability of correctly rejecting the null hypothesis when it is false (i.e., the probability of correctly declaring a significant difference between observed values, when one exists).

Power (1-β)

- Probability of correctly rejecting the null hypothesis when it is false
- Largely determined by:
  - Sample size (number of outcomes)
  - The difference the researcher wants to detect (the larger the difference detected, the greater the power)
  - The baseline variation (the greater the variation, the less the power)
  - The significance level (α) sought
- One of the most common problems in clinical research is when an underpowered study is negative
  - Readers are unable to determine whether the conclusion of no difference represents reality or low power
  - Studies with inadequate power are far too common and not informative
- Ideally, studies should have power levels of 0.80 or higher
  - This means that it will have an 80% chance or greater of finding an effect if one is really there

The greater the power of a test, the better able it is to correctly reject the null hypothesis and declare differences between values to be significant.

> A study is published on the surgical resection of liver metastases for gastric cancer. The 5-year survival rate of patients with a single metastasis was 61%, while no patients with multiple metastases survived for more than 3 years after surgery. The authors reported a significant survival difference in resected patients with single versus multiple metastases ($p = 0.011$). What is the meaning of the given *p*-value?

A p-value of 0.011 means that there is a 1.1% probability that the observed difference in patient survival is due to chance.

P-value

- Reflects the likelihood that a conclusion is due to chance rather than a real difference between the groups being compared
- Dependent on both the null hypothesis and the alternative hypothesis
  - Tests with a one-sided alternative hypothesis will generally have a lower *p*-value than tests with a two-sided alternative hypothesis, and thus are more likely to be significant

- One-sided tests require more stringent assumptions than two-sided tests and should only be used when applicable
- Importantly, a *p*-value does not tell you about the strength of the association between intervention and outcome
    - A *p*-value simply indicates how likely the results are due to chance
        - For example, a *p*-value of 0.0001 simply says the results are highly unlikely (only 0.01% likely) to occur due to chance
    - Measures such as relative risk or odds ratio provide information about the magnitude of the association

A *p*-value does not indicate how strongly the intervention is correlated to the outcome.

Following an experimental surgical procedure in six patients, the following data were collected for survival time (in months): 5, 10, 11, 4, 13, and 11.
What is the mean survival time? What is the median survival time? What is the mode survival time?

The mean survival time in the above data set is 9 months, the median survival time is 10.5 months, and the mode survival time is 11 months. A group of data can be described by their central distribution and degree of variation (scale statistics). Measures of central distribution include mean, median, and mode. Scale statistics describe the variability or spread of the sample data (i.e., how scattered or clustered the data are about the center of the distribution) and include variance, standard deviation, standard error of the mean, coefficient of variation, range, and interquartile range.

Mean

- Arithmetic average
- Appropriate for data that is normally distributed
- Equal to the sum of all the sample values divided by the sample size
- Strengths:
    - Calculated from all the sample values so makes maximum use of all available data
- Weaknesses:
    - Can be influenced by any extreme value (outlier)
    - Possible solutions include weighting or trimming the data set

Median

- Midpoint of a series of ordered values
- Appropriate for non-normally distributed data
- Determination involves arranging the numbers in sequence from smallest to largest, then finding the midpoint or calculating the average of two midpoints
- Most common way to report survival data
- Strengths:
    - Insensitive to outliers; may be preferred to the mean when dealing with skewed (non-normal, asymmetric) data
- Weaknesses:
    - Does not account for all data values; a mean generally is the preferred estimation of central tendency for symmetric distributions
- Relationship to mean
    - Symmetric distributions: mean = median
    - Left-skewed data: mean < median
    - Right-skewed data: mean > median

Mode

- Most frequently occurring value within the data set
- There may be more than one mode, or none at all
- Strength:
  - Less sensitive to skewed data than either the sample mean or median
- Weaknesses:
  - More subject to sample variation than either the sample mean or median
  - Limited applicability (samples may not have any repeated data values)

If the distribution is unimodal and symmetric, then the sample mean, median, and mode are all estimates of the same value, the population mean.

Standard Deviation

- Measure of spread, scatter, or dispersion of a sample
- When data are distributed normally, 1, 2, and 3 standard deviations from the mean encompass 68%, 95%, and 99% of the population respectively

Standard Error of the Mean

- Measure of the precision with which the mean is known
- Calculated by dividing the standard deviation by the square root of the sample size; it is always smaller than the standard deviation
- The choice between using standard deviation vs. standard error of the mean is controversial

Confidence Interval (CI)

- A range within which 95% (or other computed value, 1-α) of the population values being estimated would be expected to fall
- Reflects the strength (precision) of the evidence:
  - Wide confidence intervals indicate less precise estimates
  - Narrow confidence intervals indicate more precise estimates
- The larger the sample size, the narrower the confidence interval, and the greater the confidence that the true value is close to the stated value
- In a positive finding, the lower boundary of the confidence interval should remain important or clinically significant if the results are to be accepted
- In a negative finding, the upper boundary of the confidence interval is not clinically important for acceptance of the result

Validity

- Validity is the extent to which you measured what you intended to measure (accuracy)
- Internal validity is the integrity of a study's experimental design
- External validity refers to the ability to generalize the study's results to non-study patients or populations

Reliability

- Reliability is the reproducibility of your results (precision)
  - Different assessors making the same conclusions with the same data
  - One assessor making the same conclusions with the same data, on different occasions

> A recently published paper describes the circumstances, characteristics, and outcomes of one trauma group's clinical management of 15 cases of penetrating neck injury. What type of study is this?

A case series is a descriptive, observational study of a series of cases, which typically portrays the manifestations, clinical course, and prognosis of a condition or single intervention without a control group.

Study Designs

- Listed in the order of least to most robust study design
    - Case report (no control group)
    - Case series (no control group)
    - Cross-sectional study
    - Case–control study (select outcomes first and then look for exposures)
    - Cohort (select exposure first and then look for outcomes; can be retrospective or prospective)
    - Randomized controlled trial (lowest likelihood of bias)
    - Meta-analysis (pooled data)

Case Report

- Description of a single case, typically describing the manifestations, clinical course, and prognosis of that novel disease or intervention
- Strengths:
    - Disseminates new information quickly
    - Good for rare conditions
- Weaknesses:
    - Anecdotal evidence
    - Provides little empirical evidence to the clinician

Case Series

- Most common type of study in the surgical literature
- Represents a series of case reports
- Strengths:
    - Useful as a source of hypotheses for investigation by other study designs
- Weaknesses:
    - Provides weak empirical evidence because of the lack of comparability

> A study evaluated the long-term health status and quality of life of heart transplant recipients. 293 patients were asked to come in five years after their transplant, whereupon a full clinical examination and written survey were conducted. What type of study is this?

A cross-sectional study is a descriptive study of the relationship between diseases and other factors, within a defined population, at a specified point in time.

Cross-Sectional Study

- Also referred to as a prevalence study
- A prospective comparison of subjects with similar exposure at a certain point in time

- Strengths:
  - Good estimate of prevalence
  - Good generalizability
  - Good feasibility
- Weaknesses:
  - Cannot estimate incidence or temporal sequence
  - Cannot provide information on causality

A study seeking to quantify the association between diabetes mellitus and amputations examined 1000 individuals who had undergone non-traumatic lower limb amputations at 22 hospitals nationwide. These were compared to 1800 patients in the same hospitals over the same time period who underwent operations not likely to be associated with diabetes. Diabetes status was recorded for each participant. What type of study is this?

A case-control study is a retrospective, observational comparison of exposures of persons with disease (cases) to those of persons without disease (controls).

Case-Control Study

- A common association measure for a case-control study is the odds ratio
- Strengths:
  - Often used for initial and inexpensive evaluation of risk factors
  - Useful for rare conditions or for risk factors with long induction periods
  - Good generalizability
  - Good feasibility
  - Confounding/bias can be reduced with matching or nesting.
- Weaknesses:
  - Based on secondary data
  - Potential for many forms of bias (provides relatively weak empirical evidence even when properly executed)
  - Cannot estimate prevalence or incidence
  - Cases and/or control samples may not be representative of real diseased or non-diseased populations

To determine the risk of bone fracture before and after surgery for primary hyperparathyroidism, patients with the condition are tracked over the course of 20 years. Data on incident fractures are collected regularly, along with information on disease status, drug regimens, and surgery. What type of study is this?

This is a cohort study, which is a prospective comparison of subjects with the same disease and similar exposure.

Cohort Study

- Also referred to as incidence or longitudinal studies
- Follow-up of exposed and non-exposed defined groups comparing disease rates over the course of the studied time period
- Strengths:

- Prospective and observational, using primary data
- Can determine an association between an exposure and outcome
- Can collect incidence data or establish a temporal sequence
- More generalizable than RCT results (especially when inclusion criteria are broader)
- Enables analysis of a range of possible risk factors
- Weaknesses:
  - Sensitive to differential loss of follow-up (dropouts, deaths, migration, etc.), lack of controlled variables, and zero-time bias
  - Provides weaker empirical evidence than experimental studies
  - Cannot estimate prevalence
  - Cannot prove causality
  - Potential difficulty in differentiating/recruiting individuals "at risk"
  - Multiple comparisons may increase confounding and susceptibility to Type I error

---

A total of 180 patients with osteoarthritis of the knee were randomly assigned to receive arthroscopic debridement, arthroscopic lavage, or placebo surgery. Patients in the placebo group received skin incisions and underwent a simulated debridement without insertion of the arthroscope. Patients and assessors of outcome were blinded to the treatment-group assignment. What type of study is this?

This study was a prospective randomized controlled trial (RCT).

Prospective Study

- Study design where one or more clearly defined groups (cohorts) of individuals at risk are followed through time
- Data regarding exposures is collected prior to data on outcomes
- Strengths:
  - Primary data
  - Incorporates time and allows for evaluation of temporal relationships
  - May provide data on incidence
  - Enables use of more consistent patient inclusion criteria
  - Avoids potential biases of retrospective recall
- Weaknesses:
  - Limited to conditions that occur with relative frequency in the population
  - Ideal for conditions with short follow-up times so that a sufficient sample can be enrolled and followed within a reasonable period
  - Often expensive and requires long follow up

Retrospective Study

- Study design where all events of interest have already occurred and data are generated from historical records
- Strengths:
  - Relatively inexpensive
  - More efficient for studying rare conditions because affected individuals can be found in patient records rather than following a large number of individuals to find a few cases

- Weaknesses:
  - Secondary data
  - Cannot randomize subjects
  - No control of independent variables because they have already occurred
  - Higher possibility of incorrect interpretation
  - Subject to recall bias

Randomized Controlled Trial

- Assignments into different intervention groups are random
- Strict criteria are employed to ensure randomization is truly random
- If the sample size is large, the design minimizes bias and confounding by assuring that both known and unknown factors contributing to outcome are equally distributed between groups
- Strengths:
  - Prospective, experimental study using primary data
  - Represents the strongest empirical evidence of efficacy of preventive and therapeutic interventions when properly executed
  - Provides quantifiable data on any difference between experimental and control groups
  - Can collect causality and incidence data
  - Low risk for selection bias because enrollment is done by randomization and not the research team
- Weaknesses:
  - Does not provide information on prevalence
  - Less feasible to execute than other study designs
  - Limited generalizability
  - Not always compatible with surgery, because of several factors:
    - Patients often strongly prefer one type of operation (e.g. laparoscopic over open), which can lead to selection bias
    - Heterogeneity of preferences, procedural training or skill among surgeons participating in a trial can lead to confounding
    - Surgeons and often patients cannot be easily blinded to the procedure performed
    - Sham operations are unethical and previous studies have indicated that there is a placebo effect to any surgical procedure

Researchers wish to assess the effectiveness of a particular chemotherapy regimen plus surgery in reducing mortality for patients with resectable gastric cancer, compared to surgery alone. Data are compiled from 18 different studies and an aggregate median survival time for each treatment is determined. What type of study is this?

A meta-analysis study is an observational, analytical study based on aggregated secondary data.

Meta-Analysis Study

- Compiles data from several groups in different studies to make an aggregate conclusion
- Strengths:
  - High feasibility
- Weaknesses:
  - Provides weak empirical evidence since aggregated studies are often designed differently
  - Relationships at the individual level cannot be empirically determined, and instead are inferred from the group level

Researchers observe that a large proportion of patients with cervical cancer have a history of oral contraceptive use. They conclude that oral contraceptives are a risk factor for cervical cancer, when the real factors of interest are unprotected sex and HPV infection. What type of bias is present in their conclusion?

This is an example of confounding bias.

Bias

- Any systematic error in the design, conduct, or analysis of a study that results in a mistaken estimate of an exposure's effect on outcome or the risk of disease
- Can be reduced by proper study design and execution, but not by increasing sample size (increasing sample size only increases precision by reducing the opportunity for random chance deviation from a true value)
- Almost all studies have some bias
- Observational study designs are inherently more susceptible to bias than experimental study designs
- Types of bias include confounding, sampling, zero-time, measurement, and reader bias

Confounding Bias

- Occurs when a separate variable influencing outcome (confounding variable) is unequally distributed between study groups, distorting the relationship between the study variable and the outcome
- Can be accounted for if the confounding variables are measured and included in the statistical models of the cause–effect relationships
- Methods of compensation include restriction, matching, and adjustment during analysis

A study concludes that there is a significantly higher risk for morbidity after CABG than for angioplasty. However, the patients selected for the CABG procedure had, on average, a much greater number of negative predictors of outcome than the angioplasty group (more advanced disease, previous history of stroke, etc.). What type of bias is this?

This is an example of selection bias, a type of bias very common in the surgical literature.

Selection Bias

- Errors in sampling, selection, or allocation
- Occurs when there are differences in the baseline characteristics of the study groups, limiting their comparability
- Results in conclusions about interventions when the real difference may be attributable to other factors

Patients are recruited with an initial survey for a prospective cohort study assessing the progression of kidney disease. The questionnaire is not thorough and fails to exclude end-stage patients as well as those with significant comorbidities. The resulting cohort is heterogeneous and yields unusually variable data. What type of bias is this?

This is an example of zero-time bias.

Zero-Time Bias

- Occurs at patient enrollment when there are unintended differences between groups at the beginning of a prospective study
- Cohort studies are susceptible if the cohort is not assembled properly

Two percent of women who were positive for BRCA1 or BRCA2 oncogene and underwent double prophylactic mastectomy developed breast cancer within a 6-year follow-up period. In comparison, 49% of women with the same genetic mutation who did not undergo double prophylactic mastectomy developed breast cancer within the same time period. What is the relative risk reduction associated with the surgery?

The relative risk reduction (RRR) is the extent to which a treatment reduces a risk, in comparison to patients not receiving the treatment. In this case, it is 96%.

Relative Risk

- Relative risk = risk of disease in an exposed or treated group/risk of disease in an unexposed or untreated group
- RRR = (events/subjects in control group—events/subjects in experimental group)/(events/subjects in control group)
- Absolute risk reduction = events/subjects in control group—events/subjects in experimental group
- Number needed to treat = 1/Absolute risk reduction
- Referenced to a specified period of time
- Used in randomized trials and cohort studies

Odds Ratio

- Odds = probability of occurrence of an event/(1—probability of event occurrence)
- Odds ratio = odds in an exposed group/odds in an unexposed group
- An odds ratio greater than 1 indicates that the condition or event is more likely in the exposed group
- When is the odds ratio a good estimate of the relative risk?
  - When the case and control groups are representative of the populations from which the samples were drawn with regard to exposure history
  - When the disease being studied is relatively infrequent

Correlation

- Describes the linear association between two random variables (X and Y)
- Measured by a correlation coefficient such as Pearson's r, with a value ranging from -1 to 1:
  - If $r = 0$, X and Y are said to be non-correlated and have no linear association
  - If $r > 0$, a positive (direct) association exists: as X increases, the value of Y tends to increase linearly
  - If $r < 0$, a negative (inverse) association exists: as X increases, the value of Y tends to decrease linearly
- A correlation between X and Y suggests a link between the two factors, but not necessarily a causal relationship

A large university hospital serves a city population of 700,000 people. Out of 704 general surgical patients at this hospital during the last year, 68 presented with appendicitis. What was the incidence of appendicitis within the city population in the given time period?

In the last year there were 68 new cases of appendicitis among a city population of 700,000 people, making the incidence 0.000097, or about 9.7 cases per 100,000 people per year.

Incidence

- Number of *new* cases of illness occurring within a given population during a specified time period
- Can alternatively be presented as a proportion:

$$\text{Incidence} = \frac{\textbf{New cases within a given time period}}{\textbf{Total people at risk during that time period}}$$

In the same hospital as in the example above, the general surgery department decides to institute universal testing of patients for antibodies against Hepatitis C virus. Of 704 general surgical patients, 176 are found to test positive for anti-HCV. What is the prevalence of Hepatitis C among this hospital's general surgical population?

There are 176 positive patients among 704 surgical patients, making the prevalence 25%.

Prevalence

- Number of *existing* cases of illness within a given population at a specified time point
- Is greater than incidence in chronic diseases
- Can alternatively be presented as a proportion:

$$\text{Prevalence} = \frac{\textbf{Existing cases within a population at a specified time}}{\textbf{Total people in the population at that time}}$$

Case-Fatality Rate

- Percentage of persons with disease who die of that illness within a given time period
- Can alternatively be presented as a proportion:

$$\text{Case-fatality rate} = \frac{\textbf{Deaths from a disease with a given time period}}{\textbf{Total people with that disease in the same time period}}$$

A new diagnostic test is being evaluated against coronary angiography for early detection of coronary artery disease. Calculate sensitivity, specificity, positive predictive value (PPV), and negative predictive value (NPV) from the following data: true positives = 200; false positives = 80; false negatives = 240; true negatives = 560.

Sensitivity: 45.5%
Specificity: 87.5%
PPV: 71.4%
NPV: 70.0%

	Disease Present	Disease Not Present	
Test Positive	A (true positive)	B (false positive)	PPV = A/(A+B)
Test Negative	C (false negative	D (true negative)	NPV = D/(C+D)

Sensitivity = A/(A+C)   Specificity = D/(D+B)

Sensitivity

- Ability of a test to detect a disease when it is truly present (i.e., the proportion of people with disease, who test positive)
- Sensitivity = true positives/(true positives + false negatives)

Specificity

- Ability of a test to exclude the presence of a disease when it is truly absent (i.e., the proportion of people without disease, who test negative)
- Specificity = true negatives/(true negatives + false positives)

Positive Predictive Value (PPV)

- Probability that a person with a positive test is a true positive (i.e. the proportion of positive test results that are correct)
- Determined by the specificity of the test, and the prevalence of the condition for which the test is used
- Positive predictive value = true positives/(true positives + false positives)

Negative Predictive Value (NPV)

- Probability that a person with a negative test is a true negative (i.e. the proportion of negative test results that are correct)
- Negative predictive value = true negatives/(true negatives + false negatives)

45 | Patient Safety

Tinsay A. Woreta and Martin A. Makary

A patient develops a wound infection following a femoral-popliteal bypass with a prosthetic graft. Root-cause analysis identifies that the surgeon forgot to order perioperative antibiotics. How could this problem have been prevented?

Redesigning hospital systems to include standardized checks and prompts, such as prewritten orders, is increasingly being recognized as a way to maintain high standards of surgical care.

Systems Approach to Patient Safety

- An approach to increasing the quality of medical care by improving hospital systems
- Emphasizes teamwork, communication, and standardized checks
- Views medical errors as the consequence of faults in various systems

Innovative hospital systems, including preoperative briefings and checklists to streamline delivery of care, are associated with improved surgical outcomes.

A hospital claims that their surgical site infection rate is lower than the national average. What process of quality measurement provides standard benchmarks for participating departments of surgery?

The National Surgical Quality Improvement Program (NSQIP) is a standardized system for measuring adverse events using a risk adjustment method.

National Surgical Quality Improvement Program

- Patient data is entered into a national database for benchmarking
- Data is reported back as an observed-to-expected ratio for complications
- Participating hospitals see their outcomes relative to the national average
- Uses standardized definitions of preoperative morbidity and surgical complications

After a routine carotid endarterectomy for carotid artery stenosis, the patient suffers a cerebrovascular accident. This complication would be classified as what type of event?

This event is an "adverse event" because the patient experienced an injury as a result of medical management.

Adverse Event

- Injury caused by medical management rather than the underlying condition of the patient
- Prolongs hospitalization, produces a disability at discharge, or both
- Classified as preventable or unpreventable

A 60-year-old woman undergoes a Whipple procedure for pancreatic cancer. The patient does well postoperatively and is ready for discharge on POD#8. On the day of discharge, the patient complains to the staff of left calf pain but is discharged without evaluation. She presents to the emergency room that evening in cardiogenic shock and is found to have a massive pulmonary embolus. How is this event classified?

This event is a preventable adverse event due to negligence.

Negligence

- Care that falls below a recognized standard of care
- Standard of care is considered to be care a reasonable physician of similar knowledge, training, and experience would provide in similar circumstances

A 45-year-old woman with Type 2 diabetes is transferred from one hospital floor to another following an incision and drainage procedure for an infected toe. Following her transfer, her blood glucose levels are poorly controlled, and her insulin regimen is changed to achieve better control. Inadvertently, her previous regimen is not discontinued, and the patient is given two high doses of long-acting insulin. Despite the increased dose, the patient's blood glucose levels remain in the normal range. What type of event has occurred?

This event is classified as a "near miss" since the patient experienced no harm as a result of the error.

Near Miss

- An error that does not result in patient harm
- Analysis of near misses provides the opportunity to identify and remedy system failures before the occurrence of harm
- Sometimes referred to as a "Good Catch"

An 18-year-old boy has an ACL tear in his right knee. He came in for repair and after being put to sleep, the surgery resident prepped the left leg in error. No pre-op checklist was performed and the attending surgeon and resident proceeded to perform the operation on the wrong leg. What type of event is this?

This is a surgical never event.

Never Events

- These include wrong site/wrong patient surgery, an unintentional retained foreign body, and unexpected intra-operative death in an ASA class I patient
- Never events have become the most universally recognized quality indicator in surgery
- Surgical briefings and counts have decreased the incidence of these events

A 50-year-old man with Type 2 diabetes is undergoing a kidney transplant. Within minutes after reperfusion, the kidney becomes swollen and cyanotic. Subsequent review of the organ and recipient demonstrates a positive cross match that was missed preoperatively. What type of complication is this?

This is a sentinel event, a preventable adverse event involving serious patient injury.

Sentinel Event

- An unexpected occurrence involving death or serious physical or psychological injury
- The injury involves loss of limb or function
- This type of event requires immediate investigation and response
- Other examples
  - Hemolytic transfusion reaction involving administration of blood or blood products having major blood group incompatibilities
  - Never events are types of sentinal events
  - A medication error or other treatment-related error resulting in death

Communication failures are the most common cause of sentinel events when performing a root-cause analysis.

A 40-year-old woman is undergoing an abdominoplasty. In the process, the plastic surgeon performing the surgery inadvertently injures a segment of large bowel. A general surgeon is consulted and performs a limited resection of the injured bowel with a primary anastomosis. After the surgery, the surgeon does not inform the patient of the complication encountered and the additional procedure performed. What duty has the surgeon breached?

The surgeon has breached their duty to disclose the medical error to her patient.

Disclosure of Medical Error

- Failure to disclose errors to patients undermines public confidence in medicine and can create legal liability related to fraud
- Physicians' fear of litigation represents a major barrier to error disclosure
- Studies show that immediate disclosure of errors may actually lead to improved patient rapport, satisfaction, and fewer malpractice claims

Physicians have an ethical and professional responsibility to immediately disclose significant medical errors to patients.

A 66-year-old woman is scheduled to undergo a colectomy for colon cancer. During the surgery, she is found to have an 11 cm complex ovarian mass. What is the most appropriate course of action for the surgeon to take?

The surgeon should perform the colectomy and not remove the ovarian mass, as it does not represent a life-threatening condition.

Informed Consent

- Process in which a patient agrees to a procedure after being given sufficient information regarding the indications, potential risks and benefits, and alternatives to a procedure
- If a surgeon performs a procedure that the patient did not consent for, he or she may be accused of battery or criminal trespass; the exception is for potentially emergent life or limb-threatening conditions discovered at surgery
- Shared decision making is a program that seeks to better inform patients about the risks and potential benefits of a medical intervention

46 Medical Ethics and Palliative Care for the Surgeon

Steven J. Schwartz

As the surgical resident covering the emergency department, you are called to see a 78-year-old nursing home resident with severe dementia, labored breathing, a cold leg, and a blood pressure of 70/40. As you prepare to talk to the family about palliative care, his saturation drops to 60%. His family including eight children tell you that they want "everything done" because they know that their grandfather wants to live. What is the next step in management?

The patient should be intubated. This action is not medical futility because the ventilator provides oxygen and ventilation so the patient can breathe. It is not unnecessary pain and suffering because there are medications to relieve pain and suffering. It is not poor quality of life because quality of life is unknown and the desaturation could be very transient. It is not related to cost effectiveness because in the United States cost is not a factor in providing care to a patient in the emergency department.

Ethical Principles for Medical Decision Making

- Autonomy
- Nonmaleficence
- Beneficence
- Utility
- Distributive justice

Autonomy

- Self-determination
- A rational person is uniquely qualified to decide what is best for them
- A person should be allowed to do what they want even if it involves doing something others might view as foolish
- Respect for autonomy led to the development and requirement of informed consent procedures
- A competent individual has the right to refuse any treatment

Nonmaleficence

- The duty of a physician to not provide a treatment known to be ineffective
- A form of refraining from inflicting harm
- This is a daily issue when offering therapies, surgical procedures, and basic medications
- Most surgical procedures are fraught with risk and yet little is known about the benefits of some

Beneficence

- Requires positive actions to prevent evil or harm
- Physicians are trusted experts that are to act in the patient's best interest
- Providers are expected to make reasonable sacrifices for their patients

Utility

- Promotes the greatest benefit to the greatest number of individuals
- Fairness to individuals is compromised when focusing exclusively on a majority
- When trying to provide the most possible good to the community, some individual needs will not be met

Distributive Justice

- The concept of fairness among individuals
- Cases ought to be treated in a similar fashion
- Benefits and burdens should be equally shared within a society
- Goods should be distributed according to need
- Individuals should be rewarded for contributions made

An 81-year-old man with widely metastatic duodenal cancer underwent an exploratory laparotomy with intestinal bypass for obstruction. Days later, he develops shortness of breath on the floor and is transferred to the ICU. He is in minor distress and is unable to give consent. His advance directive states that he does not want any heroic measures or to be in a persistent vegetative state. His family is not present or immediately available. Would you intubate this patient?

There are two reasonable options in this situation which meet the goals of ethical care

- *Intubate the patient for a trial of 5 to 7 days to see if he improves on mechanical ventilation, during which time his wishes can be clarified with him and/or his family.*
- *Refrain from intubation if you believe this is what the patient wishes, based on your relationship with him.*
  - *Requires several physicians to document that mechanical ventilation will not benefit the patient*
  - *Continue to provide comfort therapy*

"For a patient with metastatic cancer and liver failure, respiratory support on a ventilator does not even have to be offered because it will only prolong a death rather than provide treatment of the disease." –Hening, 2001

The Advance Directive

- Completed in case a person becomes incapacitated and unable to participate in treatment decision making
- Three objectives
  - To maintain patient autonomy through "anticipatory decision making"
  - To help guide therapy in end-of-life circumstances by assigning a decision maker, thus avoiding the need for judicial involvement
  - To grant medical providers immunity from civil and criminal liability

The Living Will

- One form of an advance directive in which a competent adult can address his or her wishes for future specific medical therapies, should he or she become incompetent
- Specifies the life-prolonging measures an individual wants and does not want taken on his or her behalf in the event of a terminal illness

The Healthcare Proxy

- Sometimes referred to as a *durable power of attorney* for healthcare matters
- An individual designates an individual, usually a relative, or a close personal friend, to make health care decisions for someone when that person loses the capacity to make his or her own medical treatment decisions
- Can apply to any situation (not just terminal illnesses) in which an individual is incapable of making decisions

Statutes governing advanced directives, living wills, and healthcare proxies are determined by individual states. It is important to know the statutes in the state in which you practice. A hospital ethics, legal, or risk management office can help clarify state laws and hospital policies.

An 85-year-old male who sustained a motor vehicle crash arrives to the emergency department with extensive pelvic and facial fractures. He "codes" in the CT scanner, and CPR is performed for 20 minutes. He is transported to the ICU where he is on two vasopressors with a systolic blood pressure in the 70s after appropriate volume resuscitation. His family states that they "want everything done." What is the next step in management?

While continuing current management, hold a family meeting during which the family is presented with the patient's prognosis. In an open discussion, clarify what the family means by wanting "everything done."

Principles of Family Care

- Most families want reassurances that their loved one did not have a survivable incident and that all appropriate medical therapy was offered and performed
- Research shows that family members are highly concerned about their loved one being in pain in their final days and hours before death
- Ensure that the patient is receiving adequate pain control and reassure the family accordingly
- When feasible, the family should be present during a resuscitation event

---

A 93-year-old man with multiple rib fractures from a pedestrian-vehicle crash is ventilator-dependent for 6 months. His wife continues to "want everything done" so you continue all measures despite the fact that you think he will not recover. He develops renal failure. Should you begin weaning the ventilator?

Physicians are not obligated to provide care if it is believed to be of no medical benefit.

Medical Futility

- Ineffective medical therapy in the setting of terminal and irreversible disease
- Describes the preservation of permanent unconsciousness

"Physicians are not obligated to provide care they consider physiologically futile, even if a patient or family insists. If treatment cannot achieve its intended purpose, then to withhold it does not cause harm. Nor is failure to provide it a failure of standard of care." –Luce, 2001

"Physicians are not ethically obligated to deliver care that, in their best professional judgment, will not have a reasonable chance of benefiting their patients. Patients should not be given treatments simply because they demand them. Denial of treatment should be justified by reliance on openly stated ethical principles and acceptable standards of care, not on the concept of 'futility,' which cannot be meaningfully defined." –The American Medical Association

CPR

- Has a very low survival in hospitalized patients (15%)
- Not intended for irreversible illness for which death is imminent
- Unique among medical interventions as it requires a written order to preclude its use

"A physician's decision supported by consultants to withhold CPR is a medical decision and cannot be overridden. Patient autonomy and consumerism does not extend to medically futile care." –Weil, 2000

Levels of De-escalation of Support

- *Withholding* support is refraining from initiating a therapy to avoid a disproportionate burden while achieving reasonable or modest clinical goals
- *Withdrawing* treatment is distinguishable from purposely hastening death (intent)
- The distinction between failing to initiate therapy and stopping therapy can be artificial
- There is no obligation that once a treatment is begun, it must be continued
- *Euthanasia* is the explicit and intentional taking of a person's life in the setting of a terminal or unbearable illness
- Euthanasia is illegal in most countries
- *Assisted suicide* is the intentional taking of the life of a competent patient at his or her request

The consensual withdraw of therapy in a patient for whom no benefit is perceived is an accepted and long-standing medical practice.

A 14-year-old boy was hit by a car while riding his bicycle across the street. The patient arrives to the emergency department already intubated with a GCS of 6, and is now found to have a hemoglobin of 6.0. As you prepare to transfuse the patient, his parents tell you that they are Jehovah's Witnesses and refuse the blood transfusion. You tell them that without the transfusion, the patient is unlikely to survive. They respond that they are prepared for that possibility. What is the next step in management?

This patient should be transfused. Children do not have the life experiences to make decisions and are generally treated by a standard of care according to the broader cultural context, as opposed to their families' religious beliefs. This situation may require determination by the court.

Jehovah's Witnesses

- Disavow the use of allogenic blood or blood product transfusion
- Some accept alternatives to allogenic blood transfusion, such as auto-transfusion, erythropoietin, and iron
- Adolescents have a limited amount of autonomy corresponding with their advancing age (in cases concerning birth control, for example), but they are not considered competent to make independent medical decisions such as accepting a blood transfusion

> An 83-year-old former industrial worker has been hospitalized because of severe pain. He has pancreatic cancer with metastases to the liver and lung. He is experiencing severe abdominal pain. What is the best method of pain control?

Pain management should factor in a patient's life expectancy and the potential for narcotic complications. Aggressive pain control should be administered given this patient's imminent death.

Palliative Pain Management for Cancer

* When offering a therapy, it is the *intent* in offering a treatment that dictates whether the treatment is considered ethical medical practice
* Many physicians inappropriately assess the risk of an adverse event from narcotics
* Morphine-related toxicity will be evident in the sequential development of drowsiness, confusion, and loss of consciousness before a patient's respiratory drive is significantly compromised

If the intent in offering a treatment is desirable (to help the patient) and the potential outcome is positive (such as the relief of pain), administering the treatment is considered ethical, even in the face of an undesired adverse secondary event or potential negative outcome (such as death).

> The same 83-year-old lives in a state where the medical orders for life sustaining treatment are in effect. He has a completed MOLST form on his person that says he refuses all surgical interventions with the exception of pain control. He has the capacity to make decisions and refuses interventions. He has classified himself as a no CPR, no intubation and only treat for comfort. As his surgical consultant do you wait for him to become obtunded and convince his family to let you take him to the operating room for exploration?

A competent patient may refuse any procedure he or she wishes even if you as the surgeon believe it may benefit them. An obtunded patient with a MOLST form who is transported from the nursing home has the same rights to refuse as an awake patient.

Medical Orders for Life-Sustaining Treatment (MOLST)

* MOLST is a portable and enduring medical order form signed by a physician or nurse practitioner
* It contains orders about cardiopulmonary resuscitation and other life-sustaining treatments
* It must be completed for all individuals admitted to nursing homes, assisted living programs, hospices, home health agencies, dialysis centers, and all hospital inpatients being discharged to another hospital or any of the program types listed above
* Any individual who has the capacity to make decisions may ask their physician or nurse practitioner to complete the MOLST form
* MOLST helps to ensure that a patient's wishes to receive or decline care are honored throughout the health care system
* In every section of the order form, there are options to accept all medically indicated treatments or to limit intervention
* If a health care facility or program receives a MOLST order form signed by a practitioner who is not on their medical staff, the MOLST orders are still valid

The Surgeon and Palliative Care

* Palliative care consultative services are becoming commonplace in academic and community hospitals
* Patients and families often, although not always, have negative perceptions of palliative care and hospice—viewing such a discussion as signaling that the surgeon is "giving up on the patient" and that the reality of impending death must be faced

- For the attending surgeon, the decision to convey to a patient and family that a consultation is needed can provoke anxiety and they may fear such a discussion will provoke anxiety, anger, or a sense of hopelessness
- Steps in ordering a palliative care consult
  - First, decide why you want assistance from the palliative care team—typically, surgeons seek assistance in four domains
    - Pain and non-pain symptom assessment and management
    - Assistance in making difficult decisions, usually about continued use or withdrawal of potentially life-prolonging treatments such as feeding tubes, antibiotics, dialysis, or ventilators
    - Assistance in planning for the most appropriate care setting to meet patient/family goals for end-of-life care
    - Providing psychological support to patients, families and the health care team
  - Second, contact the palliative care team
    - Describe both what your goals are for the consultation, as well as what the family's/patient's goals may be
    - This is a good time to discuss any concerns you have about using the term palliative care with the patient or family
  - Third. engage the patient/family in a discussion of the current medical condition and goals of care
    - Introduce the topic of a consultation by saying something like: "to best meet some of the goals we've been discussing (fill in with the goals mentioned by the family/patient), I'd like to have some consultants from the palliative care team visit with you"
    - This can be followed by saying: "they are experts in treating the symptoms you are experiencing (fill in symptom)" and/or "they are also good at helping your family deal with all the changes brought on by your illness; they can answer your questions about (fill in previously discussed patient questions)"
  - You should not say that the reason you are asking palliative care to be involved is "that there is nothing more to do" or because "I have nothing more to offer"
  - Discuss the positive goals palliative care can help you and the patient achieve
  - Finally, offer your continued involvement and discuss the recommendations of the palliative care experts with the patients and ensure all of their questions are answered
- If a patient or family reacts negatively to the suggestion for a consultation, explore their concerns
  - It may be important to discuss that palliative care is compatible with aggressively treating the underlying disease
  - Emphasize the positive aspects of palliative care, rather than focusing on how the palliative care team will help them accept death and dying

---

A 45-year-old non-English speaking female from Sudan with a history of stage 4 ovarian cancer presents with a small bowel obstruction and sepsis. What is important in addressing the next steps in her care?

It is important to understand the patients beliefs about their care as well as the cultural context of these beliefs. For non-English speaking patients, it is imperative to have a translator.

Asking about Cultural Beliefs in Palliative Care

- C—Communication
  - Identify the patient's preferences regarding how and to whom medical information is shared
  - Some people want to know everything about their medical condition, and others do not

- For those who request that the physician discuss their condition with family members as if they would like you to speak with them alone, or if the patient would like to be present
  - Identify the main contacts to give information to about the patient's condition
  - Carefully explore with families requests to hide information from a patient
- U—Unique cultural values
  - Use respectful, curious, and open-ended questions about a patient's cultural heritage to identify their values
  - Ask if there anything that would be helpful for you to know about how their or their family's view of serious illness
  - Ask about cultural beliefs, practices, or preferences that affect the patient during times of significant illness
  - If the patient is open to discussing death, ask what concerns they have and what is important to the patient and their family
- L—Locus of decision making
  - For some patients, medical decision making is communally driven rather than individualistic
  - Multiple family members or a community elder or leader may need to be involved, often without prior official documentation because it is assumed or understood from the patient's perspective
- T—Translators
  - Language barriers are extremely challenging, especially during times of severe illness
  - Utilize medical interpreters frequently and effectively
- U—Understanding the patient and learning as a provider
  - Reassess what is being heard, understood, and agreed upon frequently, from both the patient's and clinician's standpoint
  - Specifically confirm the patient's understanding or agreement (beyond nodding or "yes" responses)
  - Ask the patient to tell you in their own words what they have heard from you and what's most important to them
- R—Ritualized practices and restrictions
  - Determine if there are specific customs the patient desires to be followed
  - These must be communicated to other health care providers, especially in the hospital setting
  - It may be necessary to advocate for the patient and negotiate with healthcare facility administrators to find an agreeable way to honor a patient's wishes
- E—Environment at home
  - Given that the majority of hospice care happens in the patient's home environment, respectfully explore whether there are any needs that can be met by the health care system, and how open the patient, family, or community is to receiving care at home
  - Recognize that patients may be hesitant to voice needs, or resistant to accepting help from outside the community
  - Even if a trusting, collaborative relationship has developed between a patient/family and clinicians in the hospital, this may not immediately translate into the home setting
  - With the patient's permission, expectations about cultural-specific aspects of a patient's care should be explicitly communicated to care providers outside the hospital

cleidocranial dysostosis, 97
Clostridium difficile, 139, 385–386
central nervous system infections, 26
coarctation of the aorta, 52
codons, 626
cohort study, 676–677, 679
collagen, 95, 108–110, 132, 411, 598–601, 650, 659–660
Colle fracture, 90
colon perforation, 377
colonic atresia, 155–156
colony stimulating factors, 643
colorectal cancer, 399–400
colorectal polyps, 397, 398–399
community-acquired pneumonia, 607, 616
condyloma acuminatum (anal condyloma, anal warts), 412–413
confidence interval (CI), 674
confounding bias, 676, 679
congenital
 cystic pulmonary adenomatoid malformation (CCAM), 176
 diaphragmatic hernia, 168–169
 lobar emphysema, 175
 lobar overinflation, 174, 175
 nevi, 442
 pyrophosphate disorder, 85
conjugated hyperbilirubinemia, 269
 differential diagnosis, 271–272
Conn syndrome (hyperaldosteronism), 346
connexons, 630
contents of platelet granules, 602
contralateral breast cancer, 469–470
coronary artery disease, 43, 44
correlation, 578, 680
Cowden syndrome, 396
COX-2 gene, 440
CPR, 534–535, 690
cricothyroidotomy, 525, 537
critical limb ischemia, 125–126
Crohn's disease, 200, 269–271, 284, 352, 360, 362, 363, 364–365, 367, 403, 411–412, 417, 418–419, 590, 609, 612, 667
Cronkhite-Canada syndrome, 396
cross match, 133
cross-sectional study, 675–676
cryptorchidism, 171
cerebrospinal fluid fistula, 5–6
cultural beliefs in palliative care, 692–693
Cushing syndrome (hypercortisolism), 347
 adrenalectomy in, 348
 screening test for, 344, 347
CXC, 642
cystosarcoma phyllodes tumor, 474
cytokine receptors, 639

cytokines
 and innate immunity, 642
 in transplantation, 656–657
 in wound healing, 601
cytomegalovirus (CMV) infection, 26, 139, 386, 645
cytoskeleton, 620, 628, 631

D

DCC (deleted in colorectal cancer) gene, 439
deamination, 293, 634–635
deep perforator (DIEP) flap, 485–486
deep vein thrombosis, 88, 663, 664
delta bilirubin, 277
depressed skull fracture, 6–7
dermatofibrosarcoma protuberans, 454–455
desmoid tumor, 394
desmosomes, 630
detoxification, 293
dexamethasone suppression test, 347
diabetes insipidus, central or neurogenic, 8
diagnostic peritoneal lavage (DPL), 538, 546
diaphragmatic injuries, 547
dietary supplements, 652–653
diffuse axonal injury, 5
diffuse esophageal spasm, 232–233
digoxin toxicity, 621–622
disability, 527, 684
disclosure of medical error, 685
disseminated intravascular coagulation, 298, 501, 528, 666–667
distinguishing adenoma vs. hyperplasia, 346
distributive justice, 687, 688
disulfide bonds, 627–628
diverticular
 disease, 379, 387, 390, 392
 fistulas, 392
diverticulitis, 164, 200, 294, 377, 379, 387, 391, 506, 520, 616
DNA replication, 624, 625
donor exclusion criteria, 136
ductal carcinoma in situ, 471
dumping syndrome, 240–241, 257
duodenal
 adenomas, 368–369
 atresia, 153–154, 155
 trauma, 549
 ulcer, 312, 371, 372
Dupuytren contracture, 95

E

E. coli, 199, 257, 293, 387, 578, 606, 609, 611, 652
Eaton-Lambert syndrome, 77

echinococcal cyst, 296–297
ectopic pregnancy, 197, 199–200, 377, 379
efferent loop syndrome, 256–257
Eisenmenger syndrome, 52
electrical burns, 573
electron transport chain, 633
elongation factors, 627
emphysematous gallbladder disease, 274
empyema, 58
enchondroma, 100
endocarditis, 50–51
endocrine pancreas, 310
endoleak, 116
endometrial cancer, 201, 207, 440, 471
endometrioma/endometriosis, 204
endoplasmic reticulum, 624–625, 627
endotoxins in sepsis, 652
end-tidal carbon dioxide, decreased, 502
energy yields of nutrients, 593
enteral feeding, 594
enterocutaneous fistula, 374, 581, 590, 594, 667
eotaxin, 642
epidural
 anesthesia, 498
 hematoma (EDH), 3
epiglottitis, 149
epistaxis, 32–33, 531, 661
erbitux (cetuximab), 436
escharotomy, 570, 572
esophageal
 cancer, 230–231, 234, 589
 caustic injury, 234–235
 diverticula, 227
 metaplasia and dysplasia, 229
 perforation (Boerhaave syndrome), 233–234
 rupture, 78, 233
 scleroderma, 229
etomidate, 492, 494
euthanasia, 690
Ewing tumor, 101
exocrine pancreas, 310
exons, 625
exploratory laparotomy/laparoscopy, 534
extended latissimus dorsi myocutaneous (ELD) flap, 487
extracellular matrix, 629–631
extremity
 compartment syndrome, 80, 573
 or trunk soft tissue sarcoma, 435
 trauma, 551
extrinsic pathway, 641
extubation, 507–508

low molecular weight heparin, 88, 128, 665–666
lower GI bleeding, 115–116, 164, 386–387
Ludwig angina, 31
lumbar disc herniation, physical exam findings, 21–22
lung cancer
  paraneoplastic syndromes, 76–77
  presentation of, 71–72
lymphangioma, 30
lymphotactin, 642
lymphotoxins, 643
lysine, 599, 625, 634–635

M
macrolides, 604, 608
major gastrointestinal hormones, 584
malate-aspartate shuttle, 632
male
  breast cancer, 478
  gynecomastia, 477–478
malignant
  hyperthermia, 501–502
  mesothelioma, 65
  mixed tumors, 36
  potential of islet cell tumors, 327
  small bowel tumors, 366–368
  thyroid nodule, 210
mallet deformity, 92–93
Mallory-Weiss syndrome, 242
malrotation, 152, 153, 154
mammography, 465–466, 478–479
MAP kinases, 639
marginal ulcers, 261
Marjolin ulcer, 453
massive hemoptysis, 56
massive transfusion protocol, 529
mastitis, 461, 468, 474
mastodynia, 462
matrix, 100, 600, 619, 624, 631
Mattox maneuver, 539
mean, 2, 78, 109, 124, 144, 204, 206, 673, 674
Meckel diverticulum, 164, 370, 379, 386
meconium ileus, 156–157
median nerve innervation, 91
mediastinal mass, 68, 176
mediastinal tumors by compartment, 68–69
medical futility, 687, 689
medical orders for life-sustaining treatment (MOLST), 691
medullary thyroid cancer, 216–217, 351–352, 438
melanoma, 445, 446
  Breslow system, 444
  Clark classification, 444

evaluation and categories, 444
immunology, 657
of the fingers and toes, 447
of the head and neck, 447
risk factors, 441
staging, 443
TNM classification, 442–443
MELD score formula, 306
MEN
  I, 351
  IIA, 220, 351
  IIB, 217, 352
meningioma, 23
Merkel cell carcinoma, 454
mesenteric ischemia, 372, 373
meta-analysis study, 678
metaphase, 623
metastasis (M), 417, 443
metastatic tumors
  liver, 302
  lung, 72
metronidazole, 296, 385, 419, 616–617
MHC Class II (DR, DP, DQ), 132
MIBG I131, 350
micronutrient deficiencies after obesity surgery, 261
microsatellite instability, 395, 623
microtubules, 629
microvilli, 629
minimum alveolar concentration (MAC), 493–494
Mirizzi syndrome, 278
mitosis, 623
mitotic spindle, 629
mitral regurgitation, 49
mitral stenosis, 49
mode, 673, 674
Mondor disease, 462
monocyte
  chemotactic proteins 1, 2, and 3, 642
  inflammatory proteins 1a, and 1b, 642
monomorphic adenoma, 34
monteggia fracture, 90
motilin, 359, 581–582, 584
MRI characteristics, 299
mRNA, 605, 609–611, 625–627
mucinous cystic neoplasm (MCN), 323
mucocele, 382
mucoepidermoid carcinoma, 35
mycophenolate mofetil, 137, 657
mycotic aneurysm, 18
myosin heads, 628–629

N
N-linked, 627–628
N-terminal, 627

Na$^+$/K$^+$ ATPase, 620
NADH, 632–633
nasal fracture, 33
National Institute of Health Criteria for Obesity Surgery, 249–250
National Surgical Quality Improvement Program (NSQIP), 683
natural killer, 642
NCAM, 631
near miss, 684–685
neck
  dissection, 34, 37–40, 107, 217, 234, 447–448, 453
  trauma, 532–533
  zones, 32
necrotizing
  enterocolitis (NEC), 161
  pancreatitis, 314–315
negative
  feedback loop, 642
  predictive value (NPV), 682
negligence, 684
neoadjuvant therapy, 75, 99, 230, 474, 477
nerve injury following hernia repair, 428
neuraxial (spinal/epidural) anesthesia, 497
neuroblastoma, 169–170
neurogenic
  diabetes insipidus, 8
  shock, 10
neurovascular injuries
  with orthopedic injuries, 79
nipple discharge, 462–463, 478
nitric oxide, 642, 648, 651, 660
nitrogen
  balance, 590–592
  metabolism, 634
node (N), 443
nodular melanoma, 445
nodule size
  doubling time of, 61
non-depolarizing neuromuscular blockers (NMB)
  monitoring effects of, 493–495
  reversal of, 495
non-Hodgkin lymphoma, 245, 336, 367, 645
non-receptor protein tyrosine kinase, 639
non-small cell lung cancer, 75
  TNM staging, 73
non-thyroid neck mass, 36
nonmaleficence, 687
normal hemostasis, 659–660
nuclear envelope, 623–624
nucleic acid metabolism, 636
nucleolus, 624

nucleotides, 595, 622, 626, 636, 652–653
nucleus, 622
nursemaid's elbow, 82
nutrient
    absorption, 356–358
    storage, 293
nutritional status, 589–590

O

O-linked, 627–628
obesity surgery complications, 256–257
obturator hernia, 429
odds ratio, 680
odontoid fracture, 12
Ogilvie syndrome, 388
Okazaki, 625
omega-3-polyunsaturated fatty acids, 652
omphalocele, 167–168
open fractures, 81
open pneumothorax, 561
open reading frame, 626
opsonization, 654
oral cavity and pharyngeal cancer, 40
organ donation, 136
ornithine, 635
orotic acid, 636
Osgood-Schlatter disease, 87
osteoarthritis (OA), 85–86
osteochondroma, 70
osteoid osteoma, 99
osteosarcoma, 99, 100
ovarian
    cancer, 202–203
    torsion, 197
    tumors, 201–202
overwhelming post-splenectomy infection, 340
oxaliplatin, 436
oxidative deamination, 634–635
oxygen
    delivery, 517–518
    extraction, 518–519

P

p-value, 672–673
p53 mutation, 399, 438, 450
packed red blood cell storage, 668–669
Paget disease, 468, 474, 475, 479
palliative pain management for cancer, 691
pancoast tumor, 74
pancreas
    blood supply, 309
    divisum, 311, 312

transplant technique, 134, 135
trauma, 549–550
pancreatic
    cancer, 285, 313, 317, 320, 321, 322, 437–441, 684, 691
    fistula, 315
    pseudocyst, 315–316
    tumors, 327
panel reactive antibody, 133
papillary thyroid cancer, 214–215, 218
parathyroid cancer, 224–225
parenteral nutrition, 594
paronychia, 93
parotid tumors, 34–36
parotidectomy, complications of, 34–35
passive immunization, 646
pectoralis major, 459–461, 472–473, 480–481, 488, 489
pectus excavatum, 137, 172
pediatric congenital hand disorders, 97
pelvic
    fractures, 191, 538, 544, 546, 551
    inflammatory disease (PID), 199–200
    surgery, 194
penicillins, 386, 605–606
peptide translocation complex, 627
percutaneous
    drainage, 142, 295, 314, 316, 378, 379–380, 391
    needle biopsy, 345
periampullary cancers, 317
perianal Crohn's disease, 418
periappendiceal abscess, 378, 379, 383
periduodenal hematomas, 547
perineal hernia, 432
perineural invasion, 36
peripheral
    nerve injuries, 82–83
    vascular trauma, 126
peritonsillar abscess, 41
pernicious anemia, 238
Peutz-Jeghers syndrome, 368, 394, 395–396, 439, 484
pharmacokinetics, 613–614
phenol burn injury, 93–94
phenylalanine, 625, 634
pheochromocytoma, 344–345, 349–351
phosphatidylinositols, 640
phospholipid bilayer, 619–620
phosphorylation, 631–633, 637, 639
phlegmon of the appendix, 379
phrenic nerve invasion, 70, 71
PI-3K, 640

pilonidal sinus, 420
pituitary adenoma, 25, 250, 323, 347
placenta previa, 198
placental abruption, 199
plasma membrane
    composition, 619
    proteins, 620
platelet
    degranulation, 602
    factor, 128, 602, 642
    transfusion guidelines, 528
pleomorphic adenoma, 33–34, 36
Poland syndrome, 461
polyadenylation, 625
polymastia, 460
polymerase, 625
polymixins, 605, 612
polysomes, 609, 627
polythelia, 460
popliteal artery aneurysm, 120–121
porcelain gallbladder, 278–279
porins, 620
porta hepatis
    anatomy, 264
portal hypertension, 307
    esophageal varices, 143
    extrahepatic causes, 308
    hepatic venous causes, 308
    intrahepatic causes, 308
positive end-expiratory pressure, 78
positive predictive value (PPV), 682
positron emission tomography (PET), 437
post-gastrectomy problems, 240–242
post-intubation stenosis, 61
post-splenectomy changes, 332
post-translational modification, 627
post-transplant erythrocytosis (PTE), 670
post-transplant patients, 140
post-TURP syndrome, 184
postoperative blood glucose control, 650
postoperative intensive care unit patient, 505–506
posttranscriptional, 624–625
potassium channel, 162, 620
power (1-β), 672
prealbumin, 589
pregnancy
    breast cancer and, 469
    breast changes in, 461
    chemotherapy and, 469
    trauma in, 197, 199
preperitoneal space danger zones, 429
prevalence, 32, 35, 122, 272, 344, 438, 614, 660, 675–678, 681–682

portions of, 356
transplant rejection, 118
transplantation, 363
tumors, 366
small cell lung cancer, 75, 58, 60
soft tissue sarcoma, 433
solitary pulmonary nodule (SPN), 56–57
somatostatin, 238, 310, 326, 327, 355, 581, 584–586
somatostatinoma, 326–327
specific immunity, 643
specificity, 122, 273, 644, 681, 682
spigelian hernia, 430
spinal
anesthesia, 497–499
cord trauma, 83
shock, 10, 527
tuberculosis, 85
spirometric parameters, 76
splenic
abscess, 339
arterial supply, 330
artery aneurysm, 121
cyst, 339
infarction, 332
microanatomy, 329–330
post-splenectomy changes, 332
products removed, 331
salvage techniques, 529
vein thrombosis, 332
spontaneous bacterial peritonitis, 143, 305
squamous cell carcinoma, 37, 38, 413, 451–452
standard deviation, 674
standard error of the mean, 674
stenosing tenosynovitis ("trigger finger"), 91
steroids
side effects, 650
in spinal cord injury, 11
wound healing in dependent patients, 601–602
Stewart-Treves syndrome, 470
stop codons, 626–627
strand, 137, 377, 620, 625, 627, 649
stress gastritis, 238, 511
stromal cell-derived factor 1, 642
study designs, 675, 678, 679
subarachnoid hemorrhage (SAH), 16
subdural hematoma (SDH), 4
succinylcholine, 491, 494–495, 501
sulfamylon (mafenide acetate), 574
sulfonamides, 570, 604, 610
sulindac, 394
superficial
spreading melanoma, 445
vs. deep classification, 566

super-obese patient, 253, 255
superior sulcus tumor, 74–75
superior vena cava syndrome, 63
supraceliac aortic control, 539
surgeon and palliative care, 691–692
Swan-Ganz catheter, 510–511, 521–523
symporters, 620
syndrome of inappropriate antidiuretic hormone (SIADH), 7, 77
systemic inflammatory response syndrome (SIRS), 513–515, 520, 648

T

tamoxifen, 217, 394, 440, 471–472, 478, 483
T cell activation, 655
TCA cycle, 632, 634–635
TCR, 639, 655
telophase, 623
tensile strength, 599
Tetralogy of Fallot, 52, 53
terminal ileum resection, 270–271, 363
tertiary
hyperaldosteronism, 347
hyperparathyroidism, 220
testicular
atrophy after hernia repair, 427
cancer, 191–192
torsion, 192
trauma, 192
tetanus prone wounds, 646
tetracyclines, 604, 609
TGF-b, 637, 639, 644, 656
Th1 helper T cells, 656
Th2 helper T cells, 656
thalassemia
major, 335
minor, 336
thiopental, 492, 494
third trimester bleeding, 198
thoracic
aortic dissection, 118–119
outlet syndrome, 64–65, 88
thoracoabdominal aortic aneurysm (TAAA), 117, 118
thoracodorsal artery perforator flap, 487
thoracolumbar spine fractures, 543–545
thoracotomy, 556–558
threonine, 625, 627, 634, 637, 639
thrombocytopenia, 33, 115, 128, 139, 145, 305, 331, 333, 456, 575, 595, 610, 661, 667
thrombosed hemorrhoid, 408

thrombotic thrombocytopenic purpura (TTP), 333–334
thymoma, 67–68
thyroglobulin, 210–211, 215, 218
thyroglossal duct cyst, 28–29, 31
thyroid
function tests, 211
nodule evaluation, 210
storm, 212
tight junctions, 629–630
tissue expanders and implants, 489
TNF-α (17kDa), 642
tobacco use, 34, 61, 70, 183
total body surface area (TBSA) burn determination, 567, 575
toxic epidermal necrolysis syndrome, 567
tracheoesophageal fistula, 149–151
tracheoinnominate artery fistula, 61, 62, 63
TRALI (transfusion related acute lung injury), 669
transamination, 293, 634–635
transcatheter arterial chemoembolization, 301
transcription, 624–625, 639, 650
transfer RNAs, 626
transferrin, 6, 296, 589, 642, 649
translation, 610, 624–626
transmembrane, 243, 619–620, 630–631, 639
spanning domains, 639
transporters, 620
transposition of the great arteries, 53
transverse rectus abdominis myocutaneous (TRAM) flap, 486–487
traumatic aneurysm, 18
traumatic pneumothorax/ hemothorax, 555–556
triacylglycerols, 636
trimethoprim, 476, 481
truncus arteriosus, 54
tryptophan, 367, 625, 634–635
tubular, 369, 377, 396, 398
tubulovillous, 368–369, 397, 398
tumor
ablation, 301
immune response, 642
suppressor genes, 438–439
(T), 417, 442
type I error, 671
type II error, 671
typhilitis, 404
typical carcinoid tumor, 65–66
tyrosine
kinases, 436, 637, 639, 640, 644
phosphatases, 637